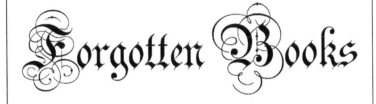

ISBN 978-0-266-99300-1
PIBN 11033823

1 MONTH OF
FREE
READING

at
www.ForgottenBooks.com

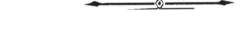

By purchasing this book you are eligible for one month membership to ForgottenBooks.com, giving you unlimited access to our entire collection of over 1,000,000 titles via our web site and mobile apps.

To claim your free month visit:
www.forgottenbooks.com/free1033823

English
Français
Deutsche
Italiano
Español
Português

www.forgottenbooks.com

Mythology Photography **Fiction**
Fishing Christianity **Art** Cooking
Essays Buddhism Freemasonry
Medicine **Biology** Music **Ancient
Egypt** Evolution Carpentry Physics
Dance Geology **Mathematics** Fitness
Shakespeare **Folklore** Yoga Marketing
Confidence Immortality Biographies
Poetry **Psychology** Witchcraft
Electronics Chemistry History **Law**
Accounting **Philosophy** Anthropology
Alchemy Drama Quantum Mechanics
Atheism Sexual Health **Ancient History**
Entrepreneurship Languages Sport
Paleontology Needlework Islam
Metaphysics Investment Archaeology
Parenting Statistics Criminology
Motivational

THE

AMERICAN

MEDICAL GAZETTE.

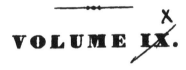

VOLUME IX.

D. MEREDITH REESE, M.D., LL.D.,

LATE ONE OF THE VICE PRESIDENTS OF THE AMERICAN MEDICAL ASSOCIATION,
FELLOW OF THE N. Y. ACADEMY OF MEDICINE, ETC.,

EDITOR AND PROPRIETOR,

No. 10 UNION SQUARE, NEW YORK.

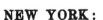

NEW YORK:

HALL, CLAYTON & CO., PRINTERS,

46 PINE STREET.

1858.

AMERICAN
MEDICAL GAZETTE.

Vol. X.   **JANUARY, 1859.**   **No. 1.**

ORIGINAL DEPARTMENT.

[From the XI volume of the "Transactions of the American Medical Association," held at the Smithsonian Institution, Washington, D. C., May, 1858.]

REPORT ON MORAL INSANITY

IN ITS RELATIONS TO MEDICAL JURISPRUDENCE.

By D. MEREDITH REESE, M.D., LL.D., &c., of New York.

There is no single topic in the whole range of medical inquiry which has so strong claims upon the earnest attention and pains-taking investigation of our profession, as the subject of *Insanity* in the various phases it assumes, all of which are included under this generic name. Happily for us and for the interests of humanity, many of the mightiest minds which have ever been enrolled among physicians, in our own and other countries, and in each succeeding generation, have consecrated their genius and intellect to this exclusive field of research. And hence, confessedly obscure as are the morbid phenomena of mind, in their etiology and causation, when latent, or even overt disease has begun its ravages upon the brain, yet there is no department of organic or functional malady to which our race is liable, upon which greater light has been thrown or greater improvements made, than in the prophylaxis, diagnosis, therapeutics and moral management of insanity. The present century especially, has been signalized by an entire revolution in the theory and practice in this department, honorable to our profession, and challenging the admiration of the world for the philanthropic results which have followed.

It is not our province or purpose, however, to discuss this general

1

subject of Medical Psychology, which, in its varied and multiform aspects, would be a task indeed for any but an acknowledged expert, who has made the selection of this department for special study and exclusive practice; and even he would require longer time and an ampler space than has been awarded to the author of the present paper, which must of necessity be brief.

"MORAL INSANITY" is the theme which has been assigned to us, and to this our inquiries and observations will be directed. And with the view to greater perspicuity, we propose to consider and discuss the following questions, viz:

I. What is "moral insanity," as defined by those who have introduced the term into our medical nomenclature, and who seek to connect it with our jurisprudence, and obtain its recognition by our tribunals of morals and law?

II. Wherein does "moral insanity" differ from "moral depravity," in any case in which "intellectual insanity" does not co-exist?

III. If insanity, whether intellectual or moral, be the result of physical disease in the brain, either functional or structural, are not the distinctions into partial or monomaniacal insanity—into mental and moral—wholly fabulous and visionary?

IV. In deciding all questions of responsibility and punishability, ought not the only distinction to be between *sane* and *insane*? The responsibility and "punishability" of the insane is prohibited by every code of law and morals, whether divine or human. The *sane*, and none else, are responsible and amenable to punishment, while the contrary may be infallibly predicated of the *insane*, whether the insanity be physical, intellectual or moral, or by Prichard's definition—"A disorder of the moral affections and propensities, without any symptoms of illusion or error impressed on the understanding."

I. "MORAL INSANITY" is distinctly defined by the phrase of Pinel to be "mania sine delirio;" or by that of Esquirol, "mania instinctive;" and as expressed in their works, "*A perversion of the natural feelings, affections, inclinations, temper, habits, moral dispositions or impulses; without any illusion or hallucination; the intellectual faculties being more or less weakened or impaired.*" Prichard and the disciples of Gall, Spurzheim and Combe, employ this term "Moral Insanity," as do also, among our own countrymen, Drs Ray, Brigham, &c., all of them deriving their views from the peculiar teachings of Phrenology, and all concurring in recognizing a distinct species of insanity, without delirium, without illusion or hallucination, and without any perceptible defect in the understanding or intellect, but manifesting itself only by a depraved perversion of the instincts and moral powers, whereby the power of self-control is alleged to be lost, and the individual hence ceases to be responsible. Dr. Spurzheim uses the term "*irresistibility*," as characterizing this form of insanity, signifying that the insane or depraved impulses are absolutely beyond successful resistance, and hence infers exemption from the obligations of law, and equal exemption from the penalties of its violation. All this is claimed in the absence of any perceptible aberration of the intellect, or alienation of the mental faculties, which are regarded as wholly distinct from the moral powers.

This phrenological distinction in the philosophy of mind, which recognizes the instincts, moral propensities and intellectual faculties as dependent upon certain separate portions of the brain, of which these several powers are the functions; and claiming that either of these functions of mind may be morbidly affected without the others being disturbed; has led to the whole theory of "moral insanity" as now propounded in some of our books, and taught in some of our schools. For if the mind itself be regarded as an individuality, and the brain its organ or instrument, a unit, through which all the various phenomena of mind are manifested, the idea of separating the intellect from the moral or instinctive faculties, and supposing one to be sound and the other unsound, both being the developments of the same mind, would never have been entertained. It is only on the theory that the brain is a congeries of organs, each of which has its appropriate function, and severally developing instinctive, moral or intellectual results; and on the still bolder hypothesis, that the organs of each separate function may be arbitrarily mapped out or designated by the "science," that this conception of moral insanity could ever have been engendered. Indeed, to render its existence plausible, even on this basis, it would seem to be necessary to wander into still wilder speculations, and either question the existence of mind as a distinctive and immaterial being; and hold, as many of this school teach, that all the attributes, mental and moral, are mere functions of the cerebrum and cerebellum, the cortical cineritious or medullary portions of the brain; or else to adopt the doctrine of the duality of the mind, and run into materialism outright in this direction.

There would seem to be a tendency in these investigations, looking to metaphysics and psychology, to lead to mysticism, if not essential heresy. All who employ the terms " Diseases of the mind," conceding that insanity in any form is thus accurately defined, most obviously deny the immateriality of the mind, and its immortality as well; for if liable to disease, the mind is *ex necessitate' rei*, liable to death.

But there is no occasion for dwelling upon these fine-spun subtleties, on a subject which, however difficult, is only rendered more obscure by this "philosophy, falsely so called." The *brain* is now recognized as the organ or instrument of the mind in every enlightened creed, either among jurists, theologians or physicians. The mind sits enthroned in its immaterial majesty, employing the brain and its continuous elongation in the nerves, not only in directing all the intellectual, moral and instinctive faculties, but in the perception by the several senses, and in the mobility of the voluntary muscles in obedience to the will; and in a subordinate way, by innervation, it may be regarded as enabling every organ and tissue in the human body to perform its destined function, in conformity to the vital laws.

"Insanity," says Dr. Brigham, "cannot be a disease of the immaterial mind itself, but of the brain." "The immortal and immaterial mind is in itself surely incapable of disease, decay or derangement;" for "if the mind could be deranged, independent of bodily disease, such a possibility would destroy the hope of immortality, which we gain from reason (and revelation), for that which is capable of disease and decay may die." Hence, "in all attempts to benefit and cure this unfortunate class of beings, they have been assigned to the physician and treated for a corporeal disease." "The phrase, derangement of mind, conveys an erroneous idea; for such derangement is only a symptom of disease of the head, and is not the primary affection. When moral or mental causes produce insanity, they first occasion functional or organic disease of the brain."

Dr. Haslam says, "Insanity is always connected with organic alterations of the brain."

Dr. Spurzheim "always found changes of structure in the heads of insane people," thus confirming the experience of Georget, Greding, Davidson, Esquirol, Combe and other scientific observers, who might be cited, if called for, almost without number. "Hence," says Dr. Parry, "that the brain is the material organ of all the mental faculties, scarcely at this period of science requires to be proved." These authorities will suffice, though they might be multiplied indefinitely.

If, then, this organ of the mind, the *brain*, in both its hemispheres, becomes from any cause diseased in its structure, or impaired in its functions, the intellectual and moral phenomena of mind must of necessity be hindered or perverted to a proportionate degree, and insanity to greater or less extent will be present. Nor is it at all rational to infer that the mind is itself diseased, because of either moral or intellectual perversions, if the instrument or organ through which it acts be the seat of morbid action. As well might we expect to have a harmonious concord of sweet melodious music from a broken or shattered piano, because a skillful musician was presiding at its keys; as to look for sound intellectual or moral action from the mind, when the instrument or organ upon and through which it acts, is suffering from some serious malady. The mind sees through the eye, but this organ must retain its transparent cornea and sensitive retina, else vision is precluded; the mind losing its power of vision, when the organs of vision are impaired, though itself still retains it, and when the eyes are restored to their function the mind again perceives as before.

Precisely thus, when disease of the brain results in insanity, the mind is no longer able to act in a normal way upon its shattered organ, though itself has undergone no change. But when, as is often the case, the diseased brain is restored to health, by nature or art, all the mental and moral and instinctive powers are again developed as before, the mind at once resuming the use of its organ, the capacity of which has been recovered.

But all history, all experience, and all observation have established the fact that partial mania, or monomania in any of its varieties, is only the indication and the precursor of general insanity; and this whether the morbid manifestations are intellectual or moral, and hence the attempted discrimination of "moral insanity" as a distinct species of mania is purely hypothetical; for as the mind is the source of both intellectual and moral developments, any serious disease in its organ or instrument, the brain, must by a physical necessity pervert both the intellectual and moral functions, whether the one or the other be the more prominently manifested. In either case the subject is insane, irresponsible and unpunishable, because of *insanity;* and hence the *moral depravity* in such case is the *fruit and the proof of diseased brain.* Insanity is none the less insanity, therefore, because its manifestations are chiefly or wholly exhibited by a perversion of the moral faculties only, if the other pathognomonic signs of diseased brain are present. If these latter are absent, then we may safely infer that either the insanity is *feigned,* or the moral perversion is the result of depravity, and there is *no insanity* in the case.

The term *Moral* insanity does not mean, as its use suggests, that

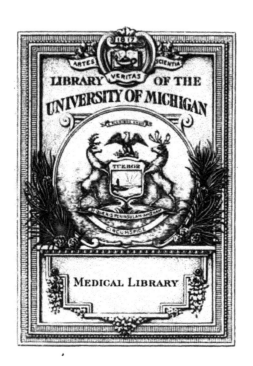

32

610.5
A 5
M 5
G 3

THE

AMERICAN

MEDICAL GAZETTE.

VOLUME I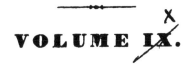.

D. MEREDITH REESE, M.D., LL.D.,

LATE ONE OF THE VICE PRESIDENTS OF THE AMERICAN MEDICAL ASSOCIATION,
FELLOW OF THE N. Y. ACADEMY OF MEDICINE, ETC.,

EDITOR AND PROPRIETOR,

No. 10 UNION SQUARE, NEW YORK.

NEW YORK:

HALL, CLAYTON & CO., PRINTERS,
46 PINE STREET.
1858.

and medical witnesses, each to define and discriminate at their own several option; and this even in works professedly written on the medical jurisprudence of the subject. And though it may be the fashion of the times to decry the decisions of the bench and bar, and denounce the verdicts of jurors and the judgment of the courts in our own country and in England; yet physicians should be better enlightened among themselves, and be able to present an intelligible and unexceptionable definition of what insanity is, before they so flippantly become the censors of the jurisprudence of insanity, of which they themselves know so little.

The bench and the bar have everywhere deferred to medical testimony, in all questions of forensic medicine, and especially in the jurisprudence of insanity. No man, in any civilized country, can be confined in an asylum, abridged of his liberty, deprived of the control of his property, or released from his responsibilities to civil and criminal law, without the judgment or testimony of medical men, as to the fact of his being "*non compos mentis*," or of "unsound mind," in the language of the law. The courts and juries everywhere rely upon physicians for their guidance in all such questions; and we owe it to this deference, everywhere extended to our profession in these important cases, to see to it that the administration of justice is not embarrassed by the incompetency of our representatives, for lack of adequate instruction being included in the training provided in our medical colleges and schools.

But how have we responded to the just demand of the legal profession in this regard? Dr. Pliny Earle justly complains that this "subject of insanity does not enter into the programme of lectures in any of our leading medical schools. It is safe, perhaps, to assert, that not one in ten of the graduates of those schools has ever read a treatise upon mental disorders." Indeed, the department of medical jurisprudence itself is either wholly ignored in the curriculum of our universities and colleges; or merely appended to some other chair or chairs, by way of formal recognition, and this for the most part *stat nominis umbra*.

In Germany, this subject attracts greater attention than in any other country. As early as 1811, the University of Leipsic founded the first professorship of Psychiatrie, which was long filled by the late Dr. Heinroth. Soon after, the establishment of clinical teaching in the asylums was sanctioned by government, and at the instance of the several faculties, attempts have been made to include such clinics among the requisites for graduation, on the rational ground that if physicians are to be intrusted with the treatment of insanity, they should be obliged to study the disease under capable and experienced teachers. It need scarcely be added that, with such opportunities in the German asylums, a multitude of students are found improving them, so that in most of the institutions for the insane in that country, those physicians who have been thus clinically trained are employed as Superintendents. It is full time that this subject should receive greater attention in the United States, as it doubtless will do under the enlightened guidance of the American Association of Superintendents, and the American Journal of Insanity. The demands of our civil and criminal courts all over the land, for competent and intelligent medical testimony, must be met by raising up an army of experts in every department of medical jurisprudence, and especially on this important topic of mental alienation; else the ignorance of too many physicians, displayed before the courts and juries, may lead to the undervaluation, if not the rejection, of medical evidence in all such cases.

In the Cyclopædia of Practical Medicine, the justly distinguished American editor strongly corroborates these views.

" In regard to the nature of the testimony relied upon in cases of insanity, and the mode of judging of the same, there is much room for animadversion. Too great weight appears to be given to medical testimony in such cases. It has always been the expressed conviction of the writer, that medical men are no better judges of the existence of mental alienation, than well-informed and discriminating individuals not of the profession. The only advantage at least which they can be presumed to have, is from the constant habits of observation and discrimination which the practical exercise of their profession requires. Yet for no other reason than that they belong to the medical profession, inferior men, whose judgments on any other subjects would be contemned, are often called upon to establish the existence or non-existence of a mental condition, which demands the most rigid and careful scrutiny." A modern able writer, in the Brit. and For. Medical Review, thinks it " essential for justice to abolish medical testimony as it is at present given on trials for crime, where insanity is the plea; and that questions of this important nature should be referred to a board of 12 or more competent men; the state of mind of a person accused of crime should not be left to be decided by those members of the profession whom the prisoner or his friends may select for their known support of his case. As to the questions of his responsibility and punishment, these should be intrusted to the authorities of the law. The whole subject is surrounded with difficulties, and hence much room is left for the ingenuity of counsel to act upon a jury, generally composed of men who are eminently unqualified for forming any correct judgment on the intricate subject submitted to their decision."

It is alleged that our legislative and judicial maxims on this obscure subject of Insanity are ancient, and indeed antiquated, in view of the increase of scientific light and knowledge which medical men have attained in this department, since those venerable maxims were adopted in jurisprudence. But how is it that, with all our boasted improvement, we still refuse to *define*, or submit any *test*, in which we are willing that courts and juries may confide? We object most strangely to the rule laid down by the law, and yet we propose no new rule, and even deny that there is any rule which can apply in all cases. But every physician, because he is such, speaks *ex-cathedra*, because he thinks himself an oracle, in announcing his medical opinion that a man is *sane* or *insane*, which many do with a confidence proportioned to their ignorance. And when called upon by the ministers of the law for the grounds or reasons upon which their opinion is based, they are " wiser than 20 men who can give a reason," while they reply, " no definition is possible, no test is reliable, but your ' right and wrong ' theory is arrant ' nonsense.' We doctors are the judges, and ' wisdom will die with us.' " Verily we assume that another Daniel has come to judgment.

That our brethren of the bench and bar should smile at our ludicrous assumption of infallibility, and that a common-sense jury should ignore such incoherent testimony, and even impute " moral insanity " to such doctors, is not at all marvellous.

But the profession of law, in view of our reciprocal relations and mutual responsibilities, are entitled to an intelligible explanation, if not a specific definition; as well as some reliable test on which they and we can rely, as characterizing those forms and degrees of insanity which are to be recognized as exempting from responsibility to the laws of the land, especially in criminal cases. It is only in the absence of any medical definition or test—our profession having failed to furnish either—that the bench has been appealed to by the bar for such definition or test. Hence the recorded decisions of the courts in every country have, with singular uniformity, concurred in the " knowledge of right and wrong," or the " knowledge that the act was contrary to the laws of God and nature" at the time of its commission, as the definition and test of *sanity*, for the guidance of juries. But many in our profession have been ever remonstrating against these legal decisions as defective and erroneous; and alleging that such " knowledge" is often possessed by the insane, who are unquestionably such. Still, however, we declare ourselves wholly unprepared to lay down any other or better rule of judgment; nor is there any other definition or test upon which the medical profession have ever agreed. Our highest authorities seem to content themselves with denying that any definition is practicable, or any test conclusive, although every medical sciolist and tyro expects his *ipse dixit* to be infallible, and the bench, the bar, and the jury are all profoundly to cower before a medical certificate of insanity; and the dictum of a professional man, that the solemn judgment of the fifteen judges of Great Britain and the House of Lords as to irresponsible insanity, is " absurd and nonsensical," must become the law of the land.

As an humble contribution towards a better state of understanding between our profession and that of the law, which may be regarded as hypothetical merely, we propose in this paper an attempt at a definition and test of insanity, which may be taken for what it may be worth.

Insanity, then, may be thus defined, viz: " A *disease of the brain*, by reason of which the functions of the mind are disturbed, perverted, or alienated, without the consciousness of the intellectual and moral change which has occurred."

This definition includes any and every disease of the brain, acute or chronic, primary or secondary, functional or organic, in which disturbance, perversion, or alienation of the moral or intellectual faculties occur without the consciousness of the change. In all such cases the subject is of unsound mind, *non compos mentis*, Insane.

The condition precedent is, any disease of the brain adequate to the suspension or overthrow of the functions of the mind. Of the signs of such disease there are at all times rational symptoms cognizable in some portion of the nervous tissue, which, in whatever part of the body, is but an elongation or distribution of the brain.

Hence the existence of corporeal disease located in the brain and nervous system, is a *test, and the only true test* of insanity, the presence or absence of which is proved or disproved by the morbid or healthy condition of the brain. If the brain and nervous system are in health, the mind can and does perform its functions; and *vice versa*, if the brain

and nervous system are diseased, the mind is hindered in its functions
in a degree proportioned to the nature and extent of such disease.
Sanity and insanity are thus *defined* by a practicable and reliable *text*.

Thus far, however, it must be obvious we have only defined insanity
to be "the disturbance, perversion, or alienation of the moral and intellectual faculties of the mind, because of a disease of the brain,
which renders the subject unconscious of the change."

The question as to the nature or extent of the insanity, in any
given case, is one which forms a subsequent inquiry, wholly distinct
from the former. It may amount only to singularity, eccentricity, or
waywardness, and may or may not develop itself as a serious malady.
It may, however, go beyond this, and yet be only melancholy, monomania, or partial insanity. And again, it may exhibit itself in the.
moral faculties being perverted, chiefly or exclusively; and in other
cases only the *intellect* may be disturbed, while in still others *both* the
moral and intellectual powers may be thus morbidly affected. In
some instances the *physical* functions may give equal evidence of abnormal derangement with the *mental;* while again the general *corporeal*
system may not exhibit any considerable departure from physical
health, while the functions of the *mind*, moral and intellectual, may be
overwhelmed with morbid action in the brain. So mysterious and
obscure are the mutual relations and dependence of the corporeal and
spiritual nature of man, that the effect of disease of the body upon
the mind, and the influence produced upon the body reciprocally when
the functions of the mind are deranged or impaired, is a problem
which, in the present state of our knowledge, remains unsolved. But
happily a solution of this problem is not essential to our inquiry; it
is the *fact*, and not the *manner* of the fact, which concerns us here.

Still, however, we have not reached the important topic of legal
and moral responsibility, except by indirection and implication. True,
we have defined Insanity, by showing in what it consists, and we have
seen a few of the phases it assumes, and indicated a number of these
varieties. But the question recurs, of what practical use are these
didactic averments in the jurisprudence of insanity? Let us see.

In the State of New York, as elsewhere, the Revised Statutes provide that

" *No insane person can be tried, sentenced to any punishment, or punished
for any crime or offence while he continues in that state.*" And again;

" *No act done by a person in a state of insanity can be punished as an
offence.*"

This last clause has, however, been authoritatively interpreted, by inserting after the word "insanity" the words "*in respect to such act;*" thus providing that it must be an "*insane act,*" and not merely the "*act of an insane person,*" which is exempt from punishment.

The language of this statute is sufficiently explicit, and would seem to be liberal enough in its terms to secure all the insane from "punishability," and protect our commonwealth from "judicial murder," so flippantly alleged by pseudo-philanthropy, as represented both in the legal and medical profession, when capital punishment has been inflicted—not upon the insane, for that were impossible under our law, which exempts all such even from trial, for any offence. But these clamors are put forth because the plea of insanity has not been sustained by proof. Either the evidence of insanity was not presented, or its character and amount were insufficient to convince the jury. Indeed it is scarcely possible under our law that any insane person can be tried, much less convicted or punished, for any offence whatever, so express and specific is the statute. The danger of escape from punishment under the feigned pretext of insanity, or by corrupt evidence, as through bribery or perjury, is infinitely greater. And it is so by design, for it were better that a hundred guilty men should escape than that one insane criminal should be punished.

It is plain, then, that the law in our own and other civilized countries provides and intends that no *insane* person shall be punished for any crime. The rule of the judiciary everywhere is, that the fact of insanity must be proved by competent testimony, and the medical evidence is very generally conclusive, where the witnesses are intelligent and honest. It is true that antiquated opinions of jurists and ancient decisions of courts often embarrass such inquiries, by introducing the dogmas of "*delusion, illusion, hallucination, irresistibility, impassivity, brutality,* &c., all of which, by the way, are terms for which our profession is responsible, by substituting theories for facts, and multiplying instead of simplifying definitions and tests, thus rendering "confusion worse confounded." Nor can we look for the correction of any errors on this or any other medical subject in the administration of the law by our tribunals of public justice, unless our profession shall furnish some standard authority for both definition and test, upon which we are willing to rest, and to which our judiciary, bar, and jury may appeal in weighing our evidence, as it is their right and duty to do.

That such standard definition and test is practicable we have only to prove, and both legislative and judicial action will soon substitute

these for the rules of law and the precedents found in the books. And
we submit that proposed here, only in the absence of a better, and until such a one shall be offered by wiser heads.

Let us now for illustration suppose that we testify, professionally,
that a man is *insane*, and this plea is urged in bar of trial, because of
our opinion and testimony under oath.

We are next interrogated as to the evidence on which our opinion
is founded. Our reply is, we find the man presenting the symptoms of a
diseased brain, which we describe to the court. These symptoms are
physical, intellectual, and *moral,* and though the first might raise the
presumption of insanity, yet, when accompanied by either or both of
the latter, they become unmistakable and conclusive.

If inquired of as to our theory on the subject, we reply:

1st. That the brain is the organ or instrument of the mind, of
which fact we cite the proofs.

2d. That the intellectual and moral faculties belong to the constitution of the mind, and that they are exercised through or by the
brain, and invariably correspond to the state of that organ, whether
healthy or morbid; and are temporary and partial, or permanent and
entire, as the nature and extent of the disease in the brain is greater
or less, functional or organic.

Is it next inquired what kind of insanity exists in this case? we
reply:

1st. An insanity which is the opposite of sanity, for the two states
cannot co-exist.

2d. It may or may not be entire, for this depends on the extent of
the disease to both hemispheres of the brain, which we may not be able
to affirm. It may or may not be partial—on one subject, or on many
subjects. It may be exhibited in the physical, intellectual, or moral
functions, either singly or in combination, and with more or less prominence in one or the other, but in either case the man is insane, and
this whether he have or have not lucid intervals, and whether longer
or shorter.

But it may be asked by the court, whether the man was insane when
he committed the crime? Of this the jury must be the judge by other
than the medical evidence, our opinion being founded on the existence
of physical disease at the time of our inquiries being made. The
known pathology of the brain may, however, be cited, that all maladies
of this organ are slow in their inception, and still slower in convalescence. If, therefore, insanity is proved to have existed shortly prior to

the act, and is found still to exist since, we may legitimately infer and testify in the affirmative.

Still, however, a much more difficult question may be propounded, if *moral* insanity only is alleged; and it may be inquired whether a perversion of the moral emotions, feelings, and propensities being proved to exist anterior and subsequent to the criminal act, while the intellectual powers were unaffected, be insanity at all—or such insanity as to give impunity to the offender?

To this we might safely reply, that this depends upon the evidence that such perversion depended on disease in the brain, and that no consciousness was betrayed of any change in the moral sense or status, for this is our definition and test. Such insanity arises from physical disease in the brain, the organ by which both moral and intellectual functions are performed, and the perversion of either or both, *if from this cause, is insanity.*

But in the absence of the pathognomonic signs of disease in the brain, if a criminal perversion of the *moral* powers be urged as a plea for irresponsibility to the obligations of law or its penalties, then it becomes the highest duty of our profession to rally to the rescue of morals and law, by protecting the administration of justice for the public security. For in the language of Forbes Winslow, Esq., the able British commentator on this subject:

"What are the peculiar or characteristic symptoms by which we are enabled to distinguish this form of insanity, in which the individual is not responsible for his conduct, from actions which are essentially vicious, and which'justly render the persons amenable to punishment? Can we safely draw the line of demarcation between vice and moral disease? Where does one commence, and the other terminate? If it be said that the impulse to commit murder is the result of a disease of the moral propensities, you will afford a ready and convenient palliation and excuse for the most atrocious offences. Society will no longer be safe. The prospect of punishment will not deter men from crime. The person disposed to murder may reason himself into the act, under the belief that he will be pronounced a moral maniac, and thus escape the consequences. I am not surprised that doubt should exist in the public mind as to the existence of the form of insanity termed homicidal, when we consider the natural tendency of the arguments advanced by those who have attempted to sustain this novel doctrine. Because a person may be proved to be strange and wayward in his character, to fancy himself a beggar when he may have the wealth of a Crœsus, or to be ill when he is in health—to believe that such a person ought of necessity to be exonerated from all responsibility, is a doctrine as unphilosophical and untenable as it is opposed to the safety and well-being of society."

In concluding this paper, and before presenting the practical inferences we have aimed to reach on the topic committed to us by the Association, we cannot refrain from alluding to the technical liability to prosecution to which physicians are often subjected by the performance of the duty they owe to society, and to the insane themselves, by certifying professionally to the insanity of parties, and thus procuring their arrest and confinement in an asylum or hospital. Even when there is just ground and imperative necessity to prevent homicide and suicide, after both have been attempted, by insane persons, the medical man, whose affidavit is indispensable to their confinement for their own safety and that of others, is liable under the existing laws to be sued for assault and battery or false imprisonment, and subjected to exorbitant bail bonds, and often years of expensive litigation, when the party is recovered, or, as he often is, discharged by habeas corpus during a lucid interval. Some of our profession have suffered such annoyance for public duty, even when performed gratuitously, that they decline officiating in such capacity without an indemnity bond for self-protection; and thus homicides, suicide, and other crimes of the insane are often the result of the reluctance of physicians to interfere, when the law affords them no protection in the discharge of this duty. A paroxysm of insanity is often known to the physician before the family or friends believe or suspect it, and his warnings of the danger of suicide are often disregarded until too late; and so when the impulse to homicide and other crimes is apparent, the wish to conceal the fact of insanity prompts the refusal to the restraint which is demanded for the safety of all concerned, unless the physician volunteers to take the responsibility of preventing crime by causing the arrest and transfer to the asylum of such insane patients. In these and similar cases ought not the laws to protect the doctor from the pains and penalties of a civil prosecution for discharging his duty to the community?

May we not confide in the legal profession for an effort to secure legislative enactments against such prosecutions, as obviously unjust as impolitic? Or, as in a similar liability to vexatious suits for malpractice, must we protect ourselves by requiring ample security from the wealthy friends of the insane before certifying to the facts, and this when these patients cannot be lawfully admitted into any asylum, or even be restrained of their liberty at home without such certificate ? And what is to be done with the insane paupers, whose families cannot give us indemnity ? Are they, when thirsting for blood, and even making insane attempts at self-destruction, to be suffered to go at large and let loose upon society, by our concerted refusal to incur the risks of such hazardous service ?

Unless we can with safety to ourselves interpose professionally in such cases, when humanity and the public security call for our action, it is our interest, and will become our duty, to decline interference. Very many heinous crimes are perpetrated and multiplied all over our country, and hundreds of suicides are reported, both the one and the other being the fruit of insanity. If these wretched victims of disease were humanely sheltered from harm on the first indications of the impulse to their bloody crimes, which physicians can generally discover before they have ripened into these deeds of blood, the moral sense of the community would not be shocked as now by the appalling repetition of self-murder. The reports daily and nightly recurring of persons found drowned, or poisoned, or butchered, might, to a very great extent, be prevented. But medical men, through whom alone this waste of human life can be prevented, by the early commitment of such parties to an asylum, are entitled to protection by the law and its ministers from such ungrateful return for their thankless services.

The practical conclusions to which we arrive are these, viz:

1st. Insanity is a *mental* phenomenon, symptomatic of a *physical* disease, having its seat in the *brain;* and hence can neither be *intellectual* nor *moral,* exclusively; but necessarily involves both *thought* and *feeling,* for the reason that the *mind* is the *source,* and the *brain* is the organ, of both.

2nd. No alleged Insanity, which is not preceded or accompanied by *positive disease in the brain,* of which the physical signs are cognizable and demonstrable, should be regarded, by our courts of civil or criminal jurisdiction, as justifying the judgment either of *incapacity* or *irresponsibility.*

3rd. When any disease of the brain is proved to exist, and a perversion or alienation of the moral or intellectual functions of the mind is present, while the subject is unconscious of any change in his mental or moral status; in all such cases insanity exists to an extent demanding impunity from the penalty of any law; and the protection of society, as well as the safety of the insane subject, requires that he be committed to the custody and remedial influences of an asylum or hospital ;

until his restoration to health and a sound mind is satisfactorily established by competent and adequate proof.

4th. All alleged "Moral Insanity," if unaccompanied by the preceding and simultaneous proofs of disease of the brain by characteristic symptoms, should be regarded as *moral depravity*, for which, as well as for its consequences, the party should be held accountable to the law.

5th. No metaphysical or psychological theory of "irresistibility," or the loss of "moral freedom," should receive the countenance of our profession in the absence of unequivocal evidence of physical disease involving the brain.

6th. Neither "delusion," "illusion," "hallucination," "systematic design," "knowledge of good from evil, or right from wrong, or that the act was lawful or unlawful, or contrary to the laws of God and nature," nor "impassivity or hereditary taint," can be safely relied on in deciding upon responsibility or irresponsibility; the presence or absence of disease in the *brain* being the only true criterion of sanity or insanity.

7th. In all cases of acquittal from crime on proof of insanity, perpetual restraint upon liberty during life by committal to an asylum, or until full proof of entire recovery, should be secured by statute law. The confinement of insane convicts should be in a separate and distinct institution, nor should they ever be admitted to the asylums or hospitals for other insane patients.

8th. Medical psychology, especially in its relations to juridical inquiries on the subject of insanity, should be made an integral part of medical education; and clinical teaching should be introduced into every asylum for the insane, as a measure of public policy, the duty to devolve upon the superintendent of each.

9th. Until a general provision is secured for the education of all students in medical psychology, no physician, who has not special qualifications, both by study and practice in this department, should consent to give testimony in cases of alleged insanity, unless after consultation and concurrence with an acknowledged expert. The reputation of the profession will else be jeoparded, if not compromised and destroyed, by indiscreet opinions, which the courts are obliged to overrule, or which are often notoriously disproved.

Meanwhile, let all the arbitrary distinctions into kinds and degrees of insanity, whether phrenological, metaphysical or psychological, be ignored when medical men are testifying in civil or criminal courts, and let their evidence be restricted to the relevant and single inquiry, whether the party is sane or insane. As to *insanity* on one subject only, with *sanity* on every other, it is a *myth*, as all practical men now admit, and hence the term monomania must soon become obsolete. So also *moral* insanity, co-existing with intellectual *sanity*, is a fable, unless *moral depravity* and intellectual purity can govern in the same mind at the same time, which is a mental and moral absurdity.

As a man *thinketh*, so is he. The appointed office of the *intellect* in man is to govern and control the moral feelings and conduct. If the intellect is sound, to prate of moral or legal irresponsibility is a farce; while, practically, it is to "throw the loosened rein upon the neck of headlong appetite," to abolish all distinction between vice and virtue, and overthrow all the standards of both morals and law.

Let physicians, then, keep within their province—the presence or absence of physical disease—and they will then be invulnerable to the cross-questioning of legal counsel. Leave the phrenology, psychology and metaphysics of insanity to the gentlemen of the long robe, but claim familiarity with the signs of diseased brain—a physical entity; and having hence pronounced our professional judgment on the sanity or insanity of the party, let us leave the law and its ministers to deal with abstractions, such as responsibility and punishability, which are questions foreign from our vocation, after we have acquitted ourselves of our own responsibilities in the premises. Our law will punish nobody who is proved to be *insane*. It is our province and duty to testify authoritatively, and when we shall have agreed what insanity is, our evidence will never be set aside, either by an intelligent jury or an honest judge, when we deal with facts and not with metaphysical distinctions.

On the Therapeutical Value of the Waters of Mineral Springs.

By John Bell, M.D.

Gifts freely dispensed are seldom appreciated at their just value, or received in a thankful spirit. Those so bountifully supplied by the Creator himself constitute no exception to this remark. The air which we breathe, and by which we live, would seem to be regarded by civilized man as something intrusive, if not positively noxious, which must be carefully shut out from his habitation, and from all the edifices in which he meets his fellow men for the purposes of religious worship, of commerce, of amusement, of law and legislation. The

water, which in a state of vapor fills and makes up so much of the
atmosphere, and which in its fluid state is both food and the vehicle
of all that is nutrimental in organized beings, and the imbibition of
which by them is a necessary condition for their growth, maturity and
fruition, is too often looked at askance, by the same civilized man
who takes all possible pains to alter the properties, while impairing
the purity of this universal fluid and menstruum by mixing it with
the distillations of art, and the products of the vat and the wine
press, not to speak of the so-called liquors and cordials compounded
of all these, and as if devilish ingenuity was still unsatisfied, drugged
with recognized poisons of every kind.   On the same line of gifts
beneficently bestowed on man, but either held at a cheap rate, or
neglected by him, are Mineral Waters, which jet out from nearly all
parts of the earth's surface; compounds, often of the most varied chemical elements, prepared in Nature's Laboratory and Nature's Pharmacy,
ready for use, and adapted to the cure of multifarious diseases, as
simple water is to the preservation of health.   What a contrast between, on the one hand, the alcoholic and narcotic adulterations of
water, to gratify a perverted appetite, and to excite and so generally
derange the functions of the organism; and, on the other hand, the addition of earthy and mineral salts which the water receives in its percola-
tion through different strata, and thus when it gushes up as a spring, it
is found to be endowed with sanitary and therapeutic virtues so great
and so diversified that it has sometimes been said, a region of mineral
springs is a region of miracles.   Equally striking is the difference between the destructive distillation of the nutritive cereals and fruits
into ardent spirits, and the conservative distillation of simple water,
when in its deep subterraneous course among primitive rocks it is subjected to central and volcanic fires, and converted into vapor, which,
ascending from this great natural alembic, is condensed in the upper
strata into thermal water, and a little later becomes in this state a
gushing thermal spring.   For the most part, the water, if of a temperature so elevated as to bring it under the category of a warm or
of a hot spring, is but slightly mineralized, and it is sometimes more
exempt from foreign substances than the water of common springs in
the same region of country.   It is with mineral waters as with most
of the articles of the Materia Medica.   Their remedial virtues were
known as matters of experience long before the basic elements and
proximate principles were discovered.   Chemical analysis, which has
revealed to us the intimate composition of these waters, is, if it be

viewed as a means of guiding us to an acquaintance with their therapeutical use, secondary in the order of time as it is in the scale of experimental observation. It may confirm, but does not originate our belief, and, at the best, it can only be regarded as suggestive in as far as it exhibits in the water of a recently discovered spring, a medicinal substance or medicinal substances identical with those in the water of a spring, the curative powers of which have been ascertained by long experience. A knowledge of the chemical constituents of a mineral water is also suggestive in another way, by leading the physician to more diversified clinical trials of the curative effects of the water than would otherwise have been attempted. Chemistry, in its suggestive relations to the therapeutics of mineral waters, enables us to improve our imperfect knowledge of those of our own country, by comparing them with those of Europe in a more precise and positive manner than could be done were we to rest the comparisons merely on their sensible properties. Thus, for example, from the long and fully recorded experience of the medicinal virtues of any one chemical division of the mineral waters of England, France, Germany, or Italy, we may obtain, if not rules, at least pregnant hints, to aid us in directing the use of waters of a similar chemical division in the United States. But even here we may be misled by apparent resemblances between two waters, which have an active principle—sulphur or iron, for instance, common to both, but which may differ materially in the number and proportion of their saline constituents. This circumstance must be continually borne in mind in the classification of mineral waters, which, like all classifications, is, at the best, but approximative, either as regards resemblances in the characteristics of the individual ones which, grouped together, constitute the class, or the differences which separate them from another group and another class. The chemical hypothesis of the operation of mineral waters offers an explanation of some of their effects as evinced in a change of the fluids of the organism. Lithic acid is neutralized by water holding in solution a large proportion of an alkali, and the predominance of this acid in the urine is destroyed, and the alkaline is substituted for the acid reaction, by the use of such a water as that of the Vichy Springs. Demonstrations of this kind do not, however, occur in such number and variety as to authorize a belief in a constant and intimate relation between the chemical constitution of a mineral water, and its chemical action on the organs, with the effect of restoring these latter to the healthy exercise of their functions.

In these cases it must be remembered that the removal of a symptom does not necessarily imply the removal of the disease, nor even always the cause of the symptom itself. There is something in the mode of combination of the several constituents of mineral waters, which gives them a therapeutic power not to be measured nor ascertained by an analysis and exhibition of each separate constituent or element. The active principle in a water resembles vitality in the organism, in its being only known by its effects. Looking at the subject in this light, Chaptal might well say that "chemists only analyze the cadaveric remains of mineral waters." Their life and their spirit disappear in the process of analysis. We must continue, notwithstanding, to look hopefully to chemistry, not indeed for a solution of the problem, but for an increase of the facts which give collateral aid to our causative researches into the subject.

From the latter part of the seventeenth century, when Boyle pointed out the right method of ascertaining the sensible and chemical properties, and the curative powers, of mineral waters, down to the present day, successive discoveries have been made of saline and other substances entering into their composition. About the middle of the last century the presence of muriate of magnesia was detected by Margraff, and the true nature of the sulphate of magnesia by Black. Venel discovered carbonic acid in mineral waters, and Bayen pointed out a few years later the means of detecting sulphur in those of the sulphureous class. Nearly about this time, Monet first, and afterwards Bergmann, discovered sulphureted hydrogen, then known under the name of hepatic air. In the present century, and within our own times, iodine, bromine and nitrogen gas, and quite recently arsenic, have been discovered in mineral waters. Their presence seems to explain the therapeutical activity of certain waters, which preceding and less skillfully conducted analyses had shown to be but slightly mineralized. I have now, beginning with the first observations of the kind which were made by M. Taupier on the waters of Hamam-mas-Koutin, in Algeria, and including those of a like purport on the waters of Wisbaden and Vichy, notes of between thirty and forty mineral springs, in the waters of which arsenic has been detected. The simple announcement of the fact of these waters containing active poisons might excite some alarm in the minds of those who had not at the same time been told of the very minute quantity, actual and proportionate, in which they are found in this form of combination. The fears of the most timid may be quieted by their learning that they could not, even if they would, produce toxical effects by the freest drinking of the iodureted or arseniated water of any known mineral spring. So wisely has it been ordered in this, as we ever find it to be in the other works of creation, that the quantity of iodine, or of arsenic, taken into the stomach, under these circumstances, would still fall short of an attenuated dose of these articles in extemporaneous prescription. We did not, however, need the aid of chemistry to give us assurance on this point. The long-continued use of the waters in question, previous to any analysis having been made, was experimental proof, not only of their innocuous character, but also of their therapeutical and even hygienic uses. It is a peculiar and very important feature in mineral waters that they constitute remedies which are always ready for immediate use, and which, unlike those furnished by vegetables and minerals, require no previous pharmaceutical preparation, and preserve for so many centuries their properties as unchanged as their flow from the earth is perennial. We may repeat now what was said at the beginning of these remarks, that, as regards the assistance which chemistry gives us towards our acquiring a knowledge of the operation and beneficial effects of mineral waters on the animal organism, it is but secondary, and in this relation explanatory and suggestive, but never initiative or truly guiding in the way of therapeutical discovery. Were therapeutical to follow chemical analysis, and the remedial value of each of the several substances held in solution in mineral waters to be carefully investigated and satisfactorily ascertained, we should still be far from a knowledge of the curative powers of all of them united in an apparently homogeneous fluid. Pharmacology has shown that we cannot predicate of the combination of different articles of the Materia Medica, even where no chemical change takes place—as, for instance, in compound pills and powders—a therapeutical result precisely corresponding with the known operation of each of these articles when given separately. How much more difficult to deduce a general result from particulars in the case of mineral waters, the ingredients of which are united by a complex play of affinties beyond, we might almost believe, those of pure chemistry—certainly with resulting compounds which, as yet, chemistry is unable fully to imitate. Some persons may be inclined to lay stress on the preference which has been commonly given to a chemical over a therapeutical classification of mineral waters; but this is based entirely on their chemical properties, and, as already intimated, is only useful as suggestive of the predominant ingredients, but not of the remedial value of waters of the several classes into which they are divided. It is like all classifications, an aid-memory and nothing more. Putting chemistry aside, as an unreliable guide for our reaching a knowledge of the therapeutical value of mineral waters, we can see no other way than that which was followed before any attempt was made to determine their composition and the nature of their ingredients by analysis.

The history of all medicinal springs is, in this respect, nearly the same. Tradition tells of some fortunate chance by which an individual obtained great relief, or even a cure of the disease under which he was suffering at the time, by his drinking the water or using it as a bath. His neighbors, hearing of the fact, made trials of this new medicament for their infirmities, and some of them with equally beneficial results. After a time, people at a distance were attracted to the spot, by the spreading fame of this healing fountain. The first visitors to the spring had very plain, if not primitive lodgings; convenience and accommodation were not applicable words; houses there were none, and tents or covered wagons were the indifferent substitutes. The cookery was in keeping with the lodging; and no person could talk, even by a figure of speech, of the pleasures of the table, when there was really no table on which to set the coarse viands, which, with the exception of now and then some game, shot in the adjoining forests, constituted the fare of the invalids. This "roughing it" was followed by the construction of cabins, and then an elementary hotel, in which something like regular lodging was procurable, although the fare was still sufficiently plain, and as little subject to the arts of a French cuisine as the most patriotic could desire. Notwithstanding all these impediments to a regulated use of the water therapeutically, each season was marked by an increase of visitors and of cures among those who were the subjects of disease. To traditional accounts of success in this way succeeded more formal, and in many cases even authenticated narratives, some of which were placed on record; and thus there was a beginning made towards a therapeutical history of the spring. So far belief was the growth of simple experience, without the bias of fashion or of imagination, neither of which could have enabled the hobbling martyr to gout or the limping victim to rheumatism to throw away his cane and crutch, and move and walk and disport himself in a way he had not done for a long time before. The cures at first were as real as the diseases, and so have they been since, although they are nearly overcrowded by the number of imaginary and nervous diseases, resulting from idleness and luxury, and which might be remedied anywhere by occupation, out-door exercise, and change of scene.

The benefits derived from the drinking of mineral water are not confined to the human species. Animals have sometimes, if we are to credit traditional story, led the way to a discovery of the healing virtues of the spring. Certain it is, in our own day, at some of the thermal establishments in France, provision is made for subjecting the sick cavalry horses of the army to a balneatory and also internal use of the waters of the spring, and with marked success. Great as may be the belief in the sagacity of the horse, no one will suppose that this animal is cured in these places by the powers of imagination. It has been said very justly in reference to the contested virtues of mineral waters and the influences of surrounding circumstances, that the sight of a new land-scape has never yet cured porigo or necrosis; and one has yet to hear of a paralysis which has disappeared at the sight of a cascade, how-ever picturesque it may be. Our belief, founded on accumulated evidence of the therapeutic powers of mineral waters, must not, how-ever, be allowed to run into a blind credulity which would invest them with the character of a panacea, a certain remedy for all dis-eases and for every stage of disease. The knowledge of their efficacy under circumstances favorable to their administration, implies, also, an admission of their injurious effects when given at random, and without a suitable selection of cases to which they would be applicable.

Mineral waters are, for the most part, exciting; and hence they are contra-indicated in acute diseases, and in those marked by much irri-tation or excessive excitability. They are illy adapted to those of a sanguine temperament or a plethoric habit, and, to those liable to cerebral congestion, hemoptysis. How often does it not happen that judicious resident physicians at the springs are obliged to send away patients suffering from hypertrophy of the heart, or aneurism of this organ and of the great vessels, or who have reached the last stage of phthisis. Physicians do not always seem to consider that chronic dis-ease, which has been intractable to a great variety of treatment, and is regarded as incurable, is therefore a fit subject for all kinds of ex-periments. That which is bad must not become worse under our hands—as when a chronic is converted into an acute inflammatory disease, and that which might have dragged its slow length along for years, is suddenly stopped short by death. The plea of giving the patient an additional chance of cure by sending him to watering places, either for the purpose of drinking mineral waters or of bathing, without a due appreciation both of the primary operation and subsequent effects, therapeutically considered, of the means thus employed, as well as of the precise character of the disease, is not a valid one. More than this is due by the physician to his patient. To recommend or assent to the use of a new remedy or a new plan of treatment, without making oneself master of what was previously known on the subject, or, at any rate, of the general results that may be expected, is worse than empiricism; for this does plead some analogous antecedents in its favor. We dare not say how many physicians, who send their patients to a mineral spring merely because it has acquired vogue, or has become a place of fashionable resort, come under this censure. The reputation of a mineral water ought to rest on something more positive than traditional or oral evidence; and yet, in many instances, it is sustained by little else than this. One season at the springs is but the echo of another, and of the crowd who resort to them from mingled motives of health and pleasure, how few come away with a clear perception of the influence which the use of the waters exerted on them, either for good or for evil. Many, perhaps we might say the majority of the invalids who visit these places, do so often in ignorance of their real malady, and with very vague notions of the efficacy of the water; which, notwithstanding, they set about drinking as if for a wager or in fulfilment of a vow. Nor can we attach much importance to the opinion of a medical man, whose experience is limited to·that gained by the stay of a week or two at the spring, and whose attention had not previously been directed to the entire subject of the therapeutical effects of the different kinds of mineral waters. Time is not given him to study their operation on himself, if he be the invalid, and still less on others, of whose antecedent history he is ignorant, and with whose treatment by the use of the waters he has not had an opportunity of superintending and becoming minutely and methodically acquainted through the means of a third party.

Of the little preliminary knowledge of this subject with which a physician is imbued before he visits the spring, we find an example in the published account of a visit to the Red Sulphur Spring of Virginia by one of the brethren, an intelligent and estimable man. He was laboring under hectic fever and other symptoms of phthisis. He arrived on the evening of the third day after leaving Washington

City, at the Warm Springs, Bath County, and immediately plunged into the delightful bath of that place—an imprudence against which he earnestly cautions invalids who arrive after a long journey, with the whole system exhausted by fatigue. If the writer had been aware of Count Rumford's personal experience of the effects of a warm bath taken in the evening, as contrasted with that of the morning, an account of which is given in more than one volume on baths, he would not have been thus imprudent: he would have learned that the state of fatigue does not contra-indicate the use of the warm bath, but rather the feverish condition or febricula, which is almost invariably induced by travel in an invalid, especially in one suffering from a pulmonary disease.

The next imprudence committed by this gentleman, was in drinking freely of the water of the White Sulphur Spring, Greenbriar County, during the two days which he spent there on his way to the Red Sulphur Spring. Had his attention been directed to the subject, he would have learned that most of the sulphureous waters, especially one which possesses the stimulating character of the White Sulphur Spring, are injurious, and that their use is prohibited in the state of confirmed hectic of pulmonary consumption; or if used at all by the predisposed to hemoptysis, it should be in small doses, and then diluted with milk, as recommended by some of the French writers on medical hydrology. The soothing effects of the water of another spring, the Red Sulphur, of the same class as the White Sulphur, of the former of which the gentleman just alluded to had such agreeable experience in his own person, show the necessity of studying each mineral water separately; for we may be sure that each has its own peculiar action on the organism.

Analyses and statistical and other returns may furnish general indications, but they fail to distinguish the characteristic shades of difference among springs of even the same class. The best, and, indeed, the only satisfactory means of obtaining an accurate acquaintance with the therapeutical effects of mineral waters, is carefully-made clinical records of cases treated by administering them on the spot. Opportunities for this purpose were furnished in France two centuries and a half ago, by edicts of Henry IV., whose early life was passed in the region of the Springs of the Pyrenees. He appointed officers who were charged with the supervision of the baths and mineral springs of the kingdom. His edicts on this subject were confirmed by Lewis XV. and Lewis XVI. In all directions the properties of these

waters were studied; by some, under the promptings of a scientific
zeal and in a spirit of philanthropy; by others, with the hope of finding a remedy for certain diseases of royal personages. Fagon, physician to Lewis XIV., examined with care the waters of Bonnes and
Bareges, in order to ascertain whether they would be adapted to the
cure of the fistula, with which that monarch was afflicted. Chirac directed his attention to the waters of Balaruc, and sought in them a
remedy for the wound of the Regent, the Duke of Orleans. A still
more formal and methodical plan of investigation was set on foot by
the appointment of resident medical superintendents, on whom it was
enjoined to keep a regular record of the cases of those invalid visitors
at the springs who came under their charge. By a royal decree, issued in 1823, the medical inspectors of the several springs were required to send, each year, to the Minister of Agriculture and Commerce
a report of the diseases which they had observed and treated, or seen
treated, during the season for the use of the waters. In order, however, to be able to discharge their duty in this respect, the concurrence or preliminary aid of the medical advisers of the invalids, in their
respective homes, is necessary, so that they should be informed of the
antecedent history, both of the character and progress of the disease,
and of its therapeutical treatment. Often the malady persists during
the period of the use of the waters, or the season, as it is called, of
three or at most four weeks' duration, and it may, on the return home
of the patient, become aggravated, or be amended or cused; circumstances these, which place it out of the power of the Medical Inspect-
or, or other resident physician, to complete his history of the cases of
those who resort to the spring for the purpose of either drinking its
water, or using it as a bath, or often employing it in both ways.
Then, again, many follow the directions, in these respects, of their own
professional advisers; others, after having consulted one or more physicians, follow ultimately their own notions. Of 4,500 persons who
took the baths at Rennes in the years 1847, 1848 and 1849, we are
told by M. Cazaintre, the Medical Inspector, that he had occasion to
see out of this number only 611. It is a lamentable thing, writes
M. C., in his report, to see numbers of persons take the baths and
drink the mineral waters to excess, without considering the nature
or stage of their malady, or the susceptibility of their organism.
Hence, in this irregular condition of things, some take the baths
who ought only to drink the waters, and others drink the waters who
ought only to bathe; a third party, in fine, have recourse to both

baths and drinking the water, in place of abstaining rigorously from all. How often, continues M. C., has it not happened to me to send away patients who labored under hypertrophy of the heart, or who had reached the last stage of pulmonary consumption, or who would have inevitably perished in the bath from a stroke of apoplexy, if chance or an aggravation of their sufferings had not in time enabled me to forbid all thermal treatment. In view of these abuses and evils, the Commission on mineral waters, appointed by the French government, in its report for the years 1849 and 1850, recommends strongly such stringent regulations as would prevent any person from making use of mineral waters without the authorization of the superintendent of mineral springs, or the prescription of some other physician.

The preceding picture falls short of representing the state of things at our own watering places, all of which are without medical superintendents, and not a few are destitute of resident physicians; and at which, more than in France, the visitors acting after certain notions of their rights, or perhaps often without a definite notion of any kind, commit all kinds of extravagances in bathing in and drinking the waters of mineral springs.

The most voluminous, and as yet the most detailed clinical records, illustrating the therapeutical action of mineral waters, are those kept by the Bordeu family—Antoine, the father, and Francis and Theophilus, the sons—who edited a journal, (*Journal de Bareges,*) in which were given accounts of two thousand cases. From this rich repertory the eminent Theophilus Bordeu drew largely for his work on " Chronic Diseases,"* in which the remedial nature of the thermo-mineral springs of the Pyrennees is exhibited with a clearness and method, not only unequaled, but after the lapse of the greater part of a century, down to the present time, scarcely imitated. The Journal of Bareges was the first, and, we believe, the last journal of medical hydrology ever published. Though we must not hope for such a periodical at the present time, we have, at least, the right to expect that resident physicians at our mineral springs, and medical men who pass an entire season at any one of them, shall keep a careful record of their clinical experience with the sick who are under their care, and making use of the water. From these records the writers can select for publication in

---

* Recherches sur les Maladies Chroniques, leur Rapports avec les Maladies Aigues, leur Periodes, leur Nature, et sur la Manière dont on les traite aux Eaux Minerales de Bareges et des autres Sources de l'Aquetaine, Paris, 1775.

medical journals the cases of most interest, not only on the score of
gravity and duration of the disease, but also of the regular and methodical administration of the water, and the minute details of its operation and immediate effects. Vague generalities will not serve any
useful purpose, and the parties, whose situation places it in their
power to impart the desired knowledge, must forego indulgence in unmeaning eulogy of their favorite waters, and, ceasing to view them as
panaceas, tell frankly their distinctive therapeutical character, and
the precise circumstances in the condition of the patient, to which, on
the one hand, they are adapted, and in which they have been found
serviceable; and, on the other, in which they are contra-indicated
and would prove detrimental.* An approach, at least, to accuracy
having been made on these points, the physician at home might venture with some confidence to give his patient directions for his guidance at the spring selected for him, and also to furnish him with a
chart of the different springs, which he would visit in succession, so as
by this means to carry out the indications presented in the successive
stages of his progress towards recovered health. Thus, for example,
the treatment of a case of visceral congestion might be begun by
drinking the water of a spring of the saline aperient class, and continued by that of a sulphureous, and then a chalybeate, with occasionally the judicious interposition of a gaseous one. A course of this
kind would be in harmony with that pursued in the treatment of most
diseases by ordinary therapeutic agents. It would secure, moreover, a
distribution of invalids among the different springs, and procure additional variety and change of scene, with fresh inspiring hopes in the
travel from one spring to another. There are some favored regions,
and even districts, so abounding in springs that the desired changes
may be made in succession or alternation in quite a small circle.

Much good might be, and often is done, in the treatment of various
chronic diseases, by the methodical administration of the waters of
mineral springs to patients at their own homes, both in town and country. It is true that some of the gaseous elements escape, and partial
precipitation of some of the bases may take place; but these drawbacks
are in a good measure balanced by the dietetic aids, and the more
tranquil sleep and regularity of life than are generally obtainable at

* We may look hopefully for instructive additions to our existing knowledge
on these points to Dr. Moorman, the experienced resident physician at the
celebrated White Sulphur Springs of Upper Virginia, in a new edition of his
work on the subject, which he is now preparing.

watering places. The physician, in such cases, is able to note for himself the immediate as well as the secondary or remote therapeutical effects of the water, and at the same time he acquires data for advising his patient as to the course to pursue in the selection of a spring, and the quantity of water to be drunk when the season for visiting such a place of resort has arrived. That our home clinics, both private and hospital, do not evince more of this kind of medication may be attributed, first, to the difficulty of procuring the water, and its apparent dearness; secondly, to the impatience on the part of the invalid, and hardly less on the part of the physician, to obtain speedy results, or 'at least to make a decided impression, such as both parties are accustomed to see when powerful drugs are administered. When the water is prescribed it is more with a view of obviating an annoying symptom or sensation than of bringing about a removal of the disease and entire restoration. Rarely is reliance placed in the curative power of the water alone, and hence its peculiar effects are intercepted, if not in a great degree prevented, by the use, at the same time, of drugs of the active mineral class, or of narcotics; in fine, of substances whose mode of action on the nervous and assimilating functions is often the very reverse of the secretory and depurative movements set up by a mineral water. On this point, when we reflect on the persistence of so many chronic maladies, notwithstanding the assaults to which they are subjected by the use of favorite articles of the materia medica, and frequently the sufferings of the poor stomach and bowels during this intestine war, we might wait with some degree of patience, and of hope too, for the more slow and remote effects of the use of mineral waters. Even under the disadvantages just stated, some of us, in this city, have had occasion to be pleased with the beneficial changes wrought on chronic cases by our patients drinking, as the case might be, Bedford or Saratoga water, including in the latter the two prominent varieties from the Congress and Empire Springs of the place, also the water of the Blue Lick, or salt sulphur, in Kentucky, all of which are sent on and procurable here. Reference was made to the reputed dearness of the water of mineral springs brought from a distance; but if we compare the cost of a given quantity used during a definite period, with that of medicines prescribed during the same time, the patient will have very little cause of complaint on this score.

Secondary only in importance to the selection of a mineral spring for an invalid is the quantity to be taken at any one time, and the hours for its use. Some writers, at the head of whom is Hoffmann, while they admit the curative powers of mineral springs, are disposed to attribute the chief efficacy to the water itself, rather than to the ingredients of which it is the menstruum. That a person who drinks twenty or thirty half-pint tumblersfull of simple water will experience, in consequence, a purgative effect, or at the least a great increase in his renal secretion, there can be no doubt. It is equally clear that if the skin be kept warm by clothing or external heat during this time, a copious flow of sweat will ensue, and take the place, in a great degree, of the discharges from the bowels and kidneys. But these results are not obtained, except in cases of intense thirst from fever, or the long privation of drink, without a feeling of discomfort and oppression, and sometimes nausea; in fact, sensations and effects differing very considerably from those which would ensue after the freest drinking of a mineral, and especially a saline mineral water. Absorption goes on more rapidly and extensively in the latter case, and the fluid entering into the current of the circulation stimulates the various secretory organs —kidneys, skin and liver, and the mucous surfaces of the gastro-intestinal, genito-urinary and laryngo-bronchial cavities. The sensible changes produced in the blood and the secreted fluids by the ingestion of mineral waters, and even by bathing in them, attest their physiological action, and at the same time the play of new chemical affinities and combinations, which cannot be without effect in modifying vital actions, and bringing about marked changes in the organism. As a diluent, and to a certain extent an alterant, simple water possesses decided therapeutic properties; but it fails to produce the varied and prolonged effects on the functions which are known to follow the use of a mineral water. The different results ensuing on introduction into the stomach of small quantities of each, places the matter in a clearer light. The toleration by the alimentary canal of large quantities of mineral water should not be received as an indication of its remedial value in any given case. We may read of De Thon drinking twenty-five glasses of the water of *Les Eaux Chaudes* every day, " more from choice than necessity," and of the exploits of a young German in his suite, who drank fifty glasses in an hour; but without our being induced in consequence to authorize any patient or friend to imitate such practices.   .

It will be prudent for the invalid to begin with a draught of a few ounces at one time of the water, and gradually to increase the quantity, but still to keep below the ordinary average for the first few days, and until the perturbating excitement, which almost always follows the drinking of the water during this period, has subsided. Some medical hydrologists assert that this excitement, bordering on the febrile, must replace the chronic languor and sluggish circulation, as a necessary condition for our obtaining the full therapeutical effects of the water. A discontinuance of the excitement is, however, soon expected to manifest itself in a crisis, as the Germans call it, consisting in copious purging, or diuresis, or sweating, or eruptions on the skin. When this state is induced by bathing, especially in water of an elevated temperature, it is called "bad sturm," a bath storm. After the first period of what might be termed seasoning the use of the water, which in some cases was suspended, is now resumed and given even in increased quantity. Reduced diet, diluent and demulcent drinks, and a moderately warm bath of 92° F., will commonly suffice for abating the excitement; and these means are to be preferred to actively reducing measures of a pharmaceutical character. During the first period in the drinking of a mineral water the general rule for an invalid will be to restrict himself to a simple diet, and to shun excess of every kind, even in his daily exercise. Throughout the entire treatment, indeed, they should adhere to the recognized laws of hygiene, if they wish not only to derive any permanent or substantial benefits, but also to prevent unpleasant effects from the use of the water. With this view all alcoholic stimulants, and even tea and coffee, should be dispensed with.

Mineral waters do not come under the head of heroic remedies, nor must we look to them for speedy results. On the contrary, by attempting a course of this kind we mar the cure of our patient, and diminish the chances, while retarding the period of his recovery. A hundred pints of the water, drank in three or four days, may drive the patient to his bed; the same quantity distributed over a period of three weeks may enable him to return home, so changed as to be in the direct road to recovery.

The most appropriate time for drinking mineral water is at an early hour in the morning, when the stomach is empty and the organism most susceptible to impressions of every kind. Absorption is also then more active, and the fluid drank finds a ready entrance into the circulation, and reaches the different organs, so as to produce its special effects on them with less disturbance than could be effected during the process of the first digestion. Next to early morning is an hour or two before dinner, when the stomach is in a great degree empty, and the im-

pressibility of the organs still active.   When the water is drunk after
dinner and at the decline of day, or in the evening, the system is subjected to two kinds of excitement—that of digestion, and that following the
imbibition of the water—each interfering with the regular course of
the other.   Most invalids suffer from a slight exacerbation of fever in
the evening, which of itself ought to be cause sufficient for refraining
from any disturbing influence.   If there be any concession made on
this point, it would be in favor of an alkaline or gaseous water, taken
in moderate quantity three or four hours after a solid meal, or of a
simple thermal water at bed time.

  The entire period of the invalid's stay at the spring will of course depend
on certain conditions, the adaptation of the water to his malady, and
the extent of relief obtained.   On the continent of Europe long usage
has fixed a certain period called a season, which on an average extends
from three to four weeks.   During this time opportunity is allowed to
test the curative powers of the water, so far as to allow of a judgment
being formed of its controlling or modifying influence on the disease,
and of the condition of things having been reached when it is desirable
to suspend the further use of the water for a week or two, and then
go through a second season, or to desist entirely from its use until
another year.   On one point, viz., the progress made in the cure of
the disease on the spot by the use of the water, the experience of the
greater number of medical hydrologists goes decidedly to show that
a cure under the circumstances just stated is the exception, and that
this desired result some time after the invalid's reaching home is the
rule.   Weeks, and even months, elapse after a season at the mineral
spring before returning health gives promise of the entire recovery
which ultimately takes place.

  The next division of our subject, if time and space were allowed,
would be an inquiry into the leading pathological conditions of the body
in which mineral waters can be used to advantage, and a specification of
the class of waters adapted to certain classes of disease.   I might
plead as excuse for not prosecuting this inquiry beyond the present
limits, by a reference to my recent labors in this line;* but much
yet remains to be said: on a theme of perpetually recurring, if not of
continued interest.

  ------

  * On the Mineral and Thermal Springs of the United States and Canada.
Parry & McMellan, Philadelphia.

The Anatomy and Physiology of the Placenta.

By JOHN O'REILLY, M.D.,

Licentiate and Fellow of the Royal College of Surgeons in Ireland, Resident Fellow of the New York Academy of Medicine.

The anatomy of the placenta, as well as its physiology, appears not to be thoroughly understood.

In *limine* it may be premised, that the uterus receives its supply of blood from the uterine and ovarian arteries, which it returns by the corresponding veins, and that it is furnished with nerves from the hypogastric, sacral and spermatic nerves.

It is quite certain that the placenta is continually receiving a supply of blood from the maternal circulation, by the uterine arteries, and reciprocally transmitting to the parent source the same quantity of venous blood, by the uterine veins.

It cannot be asserted that the branches of the uterine arteries anastomose with the branches of the umbilical veins, inasmuch as the latter cannot be injected from the former.

It is an ascertained fact, that injection thrown into the hypogastric arteries does not pass into the uterine veins.

The experiments of William and John Hunter are conclusive on these points.

It is an anatomical characteristic of arterial trunks to terminate in capillaries, as well as venous trunks to take their origin from corresponding vessels.

It therefore follows, as a consequence, that the uterine arteries, on passing through the placenta, must follow the prescribed law, and end in capillaries; and that on the same principle the maternal veins or sinuses must also owe their origin to capillary commencements.

The same rule holds good with respect to the hypogastric arteries and umbilical vein, as regards the capillary circulation of these vessels.

It must be readily understood that, unless there was a perfect arrangement of the blood vessels thus instituted, there would be a complete, or rather unavoidable commingling, of the maternal and fœtal blood; that, in truth, the arterial blood from the mother would mix with the venous blood of the fœtus.

It would not be *philosophical* to presuppose any such *complication*.

It is universally acknowledged that the placenta acts a prominent part in the arterialization of the blood for the fœtus.

The best anatomists of the present time consider the placenta is a double organ. They suppose this assumption is proved by the injections made of the maternal vessels, on the one side, and the fœtal on the other.

Assuming the correctness of *this theory*, it must be acknowledged that there must be a *vascular communication* between the respective organs.

Where is such *connection* demonstrated to exist? No person has pointed out the line of *demarcation* between the two bodies.

The idea, that the fœtal blood receives oxygen by the process of endosmosis, and exosmosis from maternal arterial blood, *presupposes* that the latter is in a condition to afford the requisite quantity of the vivifying agent, and that the uterine arteries, instead of terminating in *capillaries*, and thus containing necessarily blood of a venous character, present themselves in the shape of small *fountains* all over the *structure* of the *placenta*, separated by membranous partitions from the depots of fœtal blood in the *fœtal tufts;* in plain language, the reservoirs of the umbilical vein.

Taking for granted this ingenious *mechanical arrangement* is the *correct* one, it may be *asked* What *becomes* of the *carbon* displaced by the oxygen? The maternal blood *cannot* be *giving* oxygen and *receiving* carbon at the same time. In other words, the *oxygen* from the maternal blood would *unite* with the carbon from the fœtal. *Carbonic acid* would be formed. The *question* now *suggests* itself, What *becomes* of the carbonic acid, as there is no *channel* by which it can make its *escape?* There is no *organization resembling* the *bronchial tubes* or trachea to carry it off.

Another *argument* may be supplied against those who maintain that the fœtal blood becomes oxygenated by being *bathed* in the maternal blood, (here I would say, with due difference, that this is a *very soft* mode of *expression*,) that these authorities cannot *point* out the distinction between the fœtal and maternal blood in the placenta.

Now, what is the appearance of the *placenta?* Its name implies its form. Does it not *closely resemble* a *conglomerate* gland in conformation? Is it not *composed* of an *intricate* net-work, of blood vessels, connected together? Is it not divided into compartments by *membranous septa?* Does not a section of the placenta present a *lobular* or *granular* aspect? Is not the cut surface found *covered* with dots of blood? Are there any large caverns or sinuses to be found in its structure? I believe the answer must be in the negative. Can any *particular* set of *vessels* be *traced* to their ultimate distribution? Such has not been *yet done*. I now submit that the placenta is *composed* of lóbules, which William and John Hunter describe as cells or interstices; that *these lobules* are placed there for a *specific* purpose; that each *lobule* is *composed* of an uterine artery, uterine vein, hypogastric artery, and umbilical vein; that the *change* in the blood takes place in these *lobules;* that the uterine and hypogastric arteries inosculate in the lobule; that the carbonaceous matter is removed from the blood, and finds its way into the uterine veins, whilst the umbilical capillaries convey the *pure* blood to the fœtus.

The analogy of the anatomy and physiology of the liver and placenta, in my opinion, is very *evident.*

Does not the *liver contain* four sets of vessels? namely, the hepatic arteries, hepatic veins, venæ portæ and biliary ducts. Do not these vessels meet in the *lobule?*

Each lobule, according to Mr. Kernan, is *composed* of a *plexus* of *biliary ducts,* of a *venous plexus,* formed by branches of the portal vein, of a branch (intra-lobular), of an hepatic vein, and of minute arteries.

The vena porta and hepatic arteries represent the hypogastric and uterine arteries, whilst the hepatic vein represents the umbilical vein. The semblance still holds good with respect to the biliary ducts and uterine veins. The former contains the *excrementitious matter* derived from the portal circulation; whilst the latter *contains* the *impurities* of the maternal and fœtal blood, and in this respect may be said to be, to a certain extent, identical with the biliary ducts.

The doctrine I have now advanced may be deemed hypothetical. But do not certain facts go far to *substantiate* its *truth?* Is not the fœtus *developed* in *proportion* to the size of the placenta? If the placenta is diseased, does not the *fœtus* become *blighted?* Is not every *organ enlarged* in proportion to the work it has to *perform* in *the animal* economy? Would not a simple inosculation between the mouths of the uterine arteries and umbilical veins be sufficient, if the placenta was not destined to *discharge* a given *function* in regulating the quality of the blood for the fœtus?

If the fœtal blood is oxygenized by the process of endosmosis and exosmosis, how does it happen that a *fœtus, contaminated* by a *syphilitic* taint from the *father,* propagates the *virus* to the *mother.*

Is it not a fair deduction to arrive at the conclusion, that the impurities of the fœtal blood must not only be discharged from the fœtus itself, but likewise from the mother? Is there any provision made for the reception of any such effete matter in the placenta? If such cannot be found to exist, then how is the deleterious material disposed of? The answer appears to be, by the uterine veins. The supporters of the theory, that the fœtal blood is purified by the process of endosmosis and exosmosis, declare that a thin membranous septa, separates the maternal arterial blood from the fœtal blood in the fœtal tufts, and that the oxygen passes from the maternal to the fœtal blood. Again I ask, what becomes of the impurities of the fœtal blood?

Is there another membranous septum separating the fœtal arterial blood from the maternal venous blood?

Does the fœtal blood, by the process of endosmosis and exosmosis, give off the carbon and extraneous matter it contains to the venous blood?

I submit there are no direct proofs of any such construction of vessels and membranes.

Great importance is attached to the fact of demonstrating that the uterine arteries pass through the entire substance of the placenta. This truth can be no longer questioned. Prof. Dalton has established its correctness. But is there anything so extraordinary in the course pursued by these arteries? Do they not form a vascular net-work in the internal surface of the placenta? Is not the disposition of the uterine arteries in strict accordance with certain defined principles—as, for instance, the venal arteries? Do not the branches of the latter arteries proceed as far as the basis of the tubular bodies, before they commence their minute ramification. Is not the cortical substance of the kidneys almost entirely composed of terminations of capillaries?

Is it not true that the placenta is composed almost exclusively of blood vessels? Is not cellulary tissue required to connect the component parts together, as is the case in other organs?

Is not the pia mater a thin lamella of cellular tissue, permeated by innumerable arteries? Does it not dip in between the sulci of the cerebrum?

Is not the chorion composed of a structure closely allied in structure to cellular tissue? Is it not highly vascular? Does it not send prolongations into the substance of the placenta?

Is there not a strong resemblance between it and the pia mater? It may be objected that the brain is a non-secerning organ?

Is not phosphorus secreted from the brain? When a man overworks his brain is not phosphorus found in the urine? In corroboration of my views, I will quote a passage which bears on the subject, from the distinguished Mr. Kernan:

"But, Glisson's Capsule," observes Mr. Kernan, "is not mere cellular tissue; it is to the liver what the pia mater is to the brain; it is a cellulo-vascular membrane, in which the vessels devide and sub-divide to an extreme degree of minuteness; which lines the portal canals, forming sheaths for the larger vessels contained in them; and a web, in which the smaller vessels ramify; which enters the inter-lobular fissures, and, with the vessels, forms the capsules of the lobules, and which finally enters the lobules, and, with the blood vessels, expands itself over the secreting biliary ducts. Hence arises a natural division of the capsule into three portions—a vaginal, an inter-lobular, and a lobular portion." Having now endeavored to show the similarity between the chorion, pia mater and capsule of Glisson, I will direct attention to another point. It may be said, if the uterine veins commence in capillaries, how are the uterine sinuses accounted for? This interrogatory must be answered by asking how the cerebral sinuses are formed. In the former case the sinuses are enclosed between the decidua and the walls of the uterus; in the latter, between the walls of the cranium and the dura mater.

When the placenta is removed from the uterus, there is no appearance of sinuses; the same observation is nearly true of the encephalon. In the one case the capillary veins pierce the decidua to reach the sinuses, in the other they penetrate the dura mater to reach the sinuses. When the decidua is torn from the walls of the uterus the sinuses are laid open. The same remark is applicable to the cranium when the dura mater is torn off from the bone.[1]

What causes the hæmorrhage when the placenta presents itself over the os uteri? The separation of the decidua from the walls of the uterus, and the consequent destruction of the uterine sinuses.

Professor Simpson, in cases of placental presentation, recommends the removal of the placenta.

How does this operation prevent the hæmorrhage? As soon as the placenta is extracted the capillary supply to the sinuses is cut off, the walls of the uterus firmly contract on the fœtus, the uterine veins are thus firmly compressed, and no hæmorrhage can take place from them. With respect to the arteries, they are necessarily lacerated, and do not pour out their contents on the same principle that arrests or prevents hæmorrhage when a limb is torn from the trunk.

It may be said the fallacy of this explanation in shown, inasmuch as hæmorrhage occurs when the entire contents of the ovum are expelled from the uterus. It is well known that if the uterus is firmly contracted there is no hæmorrhage, and that it must be a flaccid state to admit such a casualty to take place. Now, when this is the case, the uterine veins having no valves, the blood regurgitates and escapes into the cavity of the uterus. The compress in the shape of the fœtus being abstracted, must not an artificial plug in the shape of the hand be introduced into the uterus to supply the deficiency specified?

What other proof is there that the capillaries perforate the decidua to pour their contents into the sinuses? The *bruit de soufflet.* Is not this phenomenon caused by the passage of the blood through a constructed orifice to a wider place? Does not the blood, in flowing from the mouths of the capillaries into the sinuses, afford an example of what the bruit depends on? Does not the blood flow from the small mouths of the capillary veins into the large uterine sinuses? Is it not the received opinion, that the bruit occurs in the walls of the uterus?

I now propose to show that there is a continued nervous connection between the fœtus and mother. Dr. Copeland says that the organic or ganglial nerves are chiefly distributed to the very internal membrane of the blood vessels, for the purpose of transmitting their vital influence to the blood itself. The experiments of Wilson Philip demonstrated that the nervous power acts a prominent part in the capillary circulation.

I will cite the experiments. "Doctor Philip passed a ligature round all the vessels attached to the heart of a frog, and then cut out the heart; on bringing the toes of one of the hind legs before the microscope, the circulation was found to be vigorous, and continued so for many minutes, at length gradually becoming more languid.

"Doctor Philip's next experiment. The web of one of the hind legs of a frog was brought before the microscope, and whilst Doctor Hastings observed the circulation, which was vigorous, Doctor Philip crushed the brain with a hammer. The vessels of the web instantly lost their power, the circulation ceasing. In a short time the blood began to move, but with less force than natural. The experiment was repeated with the same result. If the brain be not completely crushed, the blow increases the rapidity of the circulation in the web."

These experiments, I think, are satisfactory as to the presence of nerves in the capillaries.

The question now suggests itself, How does it happen that if a woman advanced in pregnancy receives a great shock, that the fœtus dies in utero, or is born with an arrest of development, or an idiot? If there is no vascular or nervous connection between the mother and fœtus, the explanation must indeed be difficult. How can the problem be solved? The solution of the difficulty, in my judgment, consists in recollecting that the internal coats of the blood vessels are lined by the expansion of the organic nerves, which, with the fœtal vessels, inosculate, and become continuous in the placental lobule, and thus that the excitement produced in the nervous system of the mother is directly communicated to the fœtus. It may be objected that this *modus operandi* of the nervous system is not capable of being proved.

However, do not the salivary glands of the epicure actively discharge their functions at the sight of a favorite dish? Does not the heart throb, or cease to beat, on the announcement of good or bad news? Do not the kidneys secrete urine when a person is terrified? Do not these facts incontrovertibly prove the nervous power existing between the cerebrum and the ganglionic nervous system? Did not the child leap inthe womb of Elizabeth on the entrance of Mary?* Is not this divine truth fully born out by physiological research? Is it not evident, therefore, that the organic nervous system presides over the organs of secretion? and may it not, *a priori*, be fairly assumed that the organic nerves effect the depuration of the blood in the placental lobule.

I am indebted to the writings of Doctor Copeland as well as Doctor Paine for my ideas on the action of the nervous system. I cannot pass by the latter authority without saying he is an ornament to the medical profession in the United States, and that he must be acknowledged to be the exponent of the great truths connected with the nervous system, which others have promulgated as their own discoveries.

It may be objected, as a fatal objection to my theory of the anatomy and physiology of the placenta, that the marsupial animals have no placenta. In order to dispose of this difficulty, I will quote a passage from Professor Owen in reference to the matter. In speaking of the Kangaroo, he says: "The fœtus and its appendages were enveloped in a large chorion puckered up into numerous folds, some of which were insinuated between folds of the vascular lining membrane of the uterus; but the greater portion was collected into a wrinkled mass. The entire ovum was removed without any opposition from placental villous adhesion to the uterus; the chorion was extremely thin and lacerated, and upon carefully examining its whole outer surface, no trace of villi or vessels could be perceived; detached portions were then placed on the field of the microscope, but without the slightest evidence of vascularity being discernible. The next membrane, whose nature and limits will be presently described, was seen extending from the umbilicus to the inner surface of the chorion, and was highly vascular. The fœtus was immediately enveloped in a transparent amnion. On turning the chorion away from the fœtus, it was found to adhere to the vascular membrane above mentioned, and to which the umbilical stem suddenly expanded. With a slight effort, however, the two membranes could be separated from each other without laceration, for the extent of an inch, but at this distance from the umbilicus the chorion gave way on every attempt to detach it from the internal vascular membrane, which here was plainly seen to end in well-defined ridges formed by the trunk of a blood vessel.

"When the whole of the vascular membrane was spread out, its figure appeared to be that of a cone, of which the apex was the umbilical chord, and the base the terminal vessel above mentioned. These vessels could be distinguished diverging from the umbilical chord, and ramifying over it. Two of these trunks contained coagulated blood, and were the immediate continuations of the terminal or marginal vessels. The third was smaller, empty, and evidently the arterial trunk. Besides the extensively membranous ramifications dispensed over the membrane, it differed from the chorion in being of a yellowish tint. The amnion was reflected from the umbilical chord, and formed, as usual, the immediate investment of the fœtus."

I think I am justified in stating that Professor Owen's dissection strengthens rather than weakens my position. It proves in the first place that the fœtal vessels end in capillaries; it further demonstrates that a secretion takes place from the capillaries; otherwise how account for the yellowish tint? Exhalation takes place from the capillaries, which gives rise to the coloring matter alluded to. The vascular membrane represents the placenta; the intimate connection of the two membranes points out the connection which subsists between the chorion and placenta; and further shows that the chorion forms the structure in which the blood vessels form their net-work in the placenta.

But let me inquire, does not the human ovum, in passing through the fallopian tube into the cavity of the uterus, simply enveloped in the amnion and chorion, possess an independent existence, inasmuch as it is not attached in any way, for a certain period, to the uterus?

Does it not follow, therefore, that the ovum of any other class of the mammalia may enjoy the same privilege for a given time? But it may be said the human ovum cannot prolong existence only for a little time, and that the shaggy part of the chorion, at a certain point, imbeds itself into the decidua, and thus gives rise to the formation of the placenta, through which it receives sustenance from the parent.

Now, this is all true; but is not the ovum of the kangaroo placed in a similar predicament as the human ovum? The kangaroo fœtus, after leaving the uterus, becomes attached to the nipple of the ovum, in a way not known, I believe, to naturalists, and receives nutriment from this source until it is able to maintain an independent existence. Now, it is clear neither the human ovum nor the fœtus of the kangaroo can prolong life without attachment to the parent. Therefore the sequence is clear, that the same law governs the human ovum as that of the kangaroo.[3]

230 Fourth Street, Washington Square,
December, 1858.

NOTES.

1 This may be said to be only half true, as no lamella of the dura mater separates the sinus from the bone. Now, this is of no consequence, as it is merely intended to show how the blood gets into the sinus by the capillaries.

2 The following passage from the Old Testament bears closely on the subject under discussion, showing how Jacob caused the cattle to be marked by different colors:

"And it came to pass, whensoever the stronger cattle did conceive, that Jacob laid the rods before the eyes of the cattle in the gutters, that they might conceive among the rods." Genesis 30: 41.

3 I am indebted to the "Historical Sketch on the Construction of the Human Placenta," by Francis Adams, LL.D., M.D., since writing the above article, which enables me to give a short epitome of the opinion of ancient and modern authorities on the Anatomy and Physiology of the Placenta.

"Galen maintained there was a vascular connection between the mother and fœtus in utero."

"Fabricius affirms that in the bitch, in the cow, and in the ewe, the vascular connection between the uterus and fœtus can be readily recognized."

"Hoboken, De Graef, Malpighi, Harvey, come to the conclusion, that in all the inferior classes of mammals there is no vascular connection between the mother and fœtus; that the latter is nourished by an alimentary juice which penetrates through the lining membrane of the uterus, and is imbibed through the inverting membrane of the fœtus."

"Doctor Alexander Monro, primus, says: Were I allowed to illustrate the communication between the mother and her child in the womb by a gross comparison, I would say, that the uterine sinuses are to a fœtus what the intestines are to an adult—the uterine blood poured into the sinuses being analogous to the recent ingestion of food and drink. The liquors sent by the umbilical arteries to be mixed with the uterine blood, resemble the bile, pancreatic juice, and other liquors separated from the blood. The umbilical veins, and those on the surface of the chorion, take up the former part of this composed mass, as the lacteal and meseraic veins do from the contents of the guts; but the grosser parts of the blood in the sinuses are carried back by the veins of the womb, as the excrescence of the gut are discharged by the anus."

"Haller says: I stick not to the belief that the red blood, as such, is brought from the mother to the fœtus, and transmitted from the fœtus to the mother as it were in a circle."

"John Hunter describes arteries about the size of a crow quill, passing from the surface of the uterus into the placenta, and terminating there in a very fine spongy substance; and that the veins originating from this same spongy substance pass obliquely through the decidua, and communicate with the proper veins of the uterus."

"Fyfe Compendium Anatomy, 1812. In the placenta are to be observed, on the side next the child, vessels forming the principal part of its substance; on the side next the mother, the ramification of the umbilical branches of the uterine arteries, almost of the size of crow quills, passing in a transluted manner between the uterus and placenta, and terminating in the latter veins, corresponding with the latter arteries, but flat, and of a good size, running obliquely from the placenta to the uterus, and in the substance of the placenta an appearance which has been supposed by many authors to be common cellular tissue, and easily ruptured by ingestion, but which is considered by late authors as a regular, spongy substance, similar to that in the body of the penis. The placenta receives blood from the uterus, and, according to the opinion of modern anatomists, purifies the blood as the lungs do in the adult for the nourishment of the fœtus. The blood is sent by the arteries of the uterus to the substance of the placenta."

"Doctor Lee (Philosophical Transactions, 1832,) states his observation on the result of the examination of six gravid uteri, and many placenta expelled in natural labor, which seemed to demonstrate that a cellular structure does not exist in the placenta, and that there is no connection between this organ and the uterus by great arteries and veins. He declares, in detaching the placenta carefully from the uterus, there is no vestige of the passage of any great blood vessel, either artery or vein, through the intervening decidua from the uterus to the placenta; nor has the appearance of the orifice of a vessel being discovered, even with the help of a magnifier on the uterine surface of the placenta; and further, that no cells are discernible in its structure on the minutest examination. He argues against a vascular connection between the uterus and placenta, from the surface of the latter appearing uniformly smooth, and covered with the deciduous membrane, which could not be the case did any large vessels connect it with the uterus, and from the circumstance that in the majority of cases it separated with the least possible force, and without hæmorrhage."

"Doctor Lee changed his opinion in 1842, and fully agreed with the Hunterian doctrine." "Velpeau combats the facts put forward by the Hunters; 1st. In extra uterine pregnancies such an arrangement is impossible; 2d. The placenta at first does not exist, and even until the third month it consists of agglomerated filaments only, and consequently no sinuses can exist between its lobules; 3d. A regular formed placenta has been found in connection with a fibrous polypus and hardened portion of the womb; 4th. Velpeau has seen the uterine surface of a recently delivered female hard, leathery, and without orifices."

"Wagner's Physiology, by Dr. R. Willis. The whole placenta, and therefore every individual lobule, consists of two distinct parts—the one a contraction of the chorion and vessels of the embryo, and the other a contraction of the membrana decidua and vessels of the uterus."

Baer's description coincides with Wagner's.

Doctor Knox, (Medical Gazette, 1840,) declares there are no cells or cavities in the placenta. He speaks of the decidua being interposed between the placenta and uterus. He further speaks of placental vessels penetrating through this decidua until they reached the surface of the uterus, when they floated in one of the venous sinuses of the uterus.

"Professor Goodsir represents a tuft, or a single point of the placenta. where it comes into immediate contact with the uterus." As neither Doctors Carpenter nor Adams seem to understand Goodsir's description, I pass it over.

Professor Dalton, New York, 1858: "I feel confident, indeed, from the facts which I shall immediately mention, that the blood vessels of the uterus do really penetrate into the substance of the placenta, as supposed by the Hunters, Dr. Reed, and Professor Goodsir, and that they constitute, with the tufts of the foetal chorion, an equal part of its mass."

It will be perceived that the theory propounded by me is positively sustained by the opinions of Galen, Fabricius, and Haller; is corroborated by the experiments of the Hunters, Reed, Goodsir, and Professor Dalton, who have demonstrated beyond a doubt that the uterine vessels perforate the placenta; is fully borne out by the observation of Knox, with respect to the decidua being interposed between the placenta and uterus, as well as the decidua being pierced with vessels; is negatively proved by Doctor Lee, who could discern no vessels on the smooth surface of the intervening decidua between the uterus and placenta. Dr. Lee was led to his very extraordinary conclusions by not being able to detect the small mouths of the capillaries perforating the membrana decidua. His views, although they influenced him to arrive at false deductions, admirably support the explanation I have put forward. I cannot help remarking, that it is strange how a man of Dr. Lee's penetration and sagacity could for a moment suppose that a child, a dozen pounds weight, could be formed in the uterus if it received no sustenance from the mother. His statement that the placenta can be removed without hæmorrhage may be true with respect to the dead subject; but everybody knows, who has attended a case of placental presentation, that it is not well founded with respect to the living, when an abundance of venous blood is discharged on every contraction of the uterus by the laceration of the sinuses. Velpeau's objections being overthrown by Doctor Dalton's able experiments, I pass them over. Wagner entertains the same ideas that I do with respect to the placenta being composed of lobules. Doctor Adams observes that De Graef, Doctor Lee, and others, argue that if the placenta was connected to the uterus by blood vessels of a considerable size, it would be impossible that the separation of the placenta could ever take place without hæmorrhage. The last remark was still more striking in the case of the inversion of the womb. Now, when the uterus is inverted no hæmorrhage can take place. The vessels

4

being firmly constricted at the cervix uteri, what opposes the reduction when in this condition? The answer has just been given.

The blood discharged in placental presentations is decidedly venous, whilst that in the umbilical vein is truly arterial. Such is Professor Barker's opinion, and other competent authorities.

OUR PHILADELPHIA CORRESPONDENT.

No. 10.

Reputation—The Blockley Hospital—The Influenza.

> " The world's all title page: there's no contents:
> The world's all face: the man who shows his heart
> Is hooted for his nudities, and scorned."—YOUNG.

> " Who breathes must suffer; and who thinks must mourn;
> And he alone is bless'd who ne'er was born."—PRIOR.

DEAR GAZETTE—Our city is filled with the popularity of a book, by our distinguished friend Oliver Wendell Holmes, entitled "The Autocrat of the Breakfast Table." We remember being introduced for the first time to Prof. Holmes, at the meeting of the "American Medical Association" held at Baltimore. During the first two days of the session we were much interested in a petite personage, with a large head, who moved rapidly up and down the aisles, nodding familiarly, gesticulating spiritedly, and conversing wittily with some of the brilliant spirits of the Association; and were surprised to learn that it was no other than the renowned professor of anatomy, writer of brilliant essays, poet, and philosopher, Dr. H——. We are under the impression that the most enduring and substantial reputation is that of the literary man and poet. The merely professional man has a comparatively small circle of influence in his time, and seldom lives beyond the century in which he was born. The man, therefore, who combines the scholar, and especially the poet, with the professional man, ensures for himself an immortality far more durable than that of the best compiler, or most chaste composer of merely professional subjects. "Cullen's Practice," "Cheselden's Anatomy," "Duncan's Dispensatory," were well written, and popular works in their day; but the "Vicar of Wakefield" and the "Deserted Village" will bear the name of *old Goldy* through ages of fame, long after those merely professional, but no doubt well-written books, shall have ceased to be read, or even to exist, except in the dusty corner of some antiquary's library. Query? How would it sound to hear the name of Oliver Wendell Holmes coupled with a petty investigation on the question, Whether Dr. Smith ever compounded and sold a prescription of his own, called a *"nostrum,"* or whether Dr. Smith's friend ever said a good word for him, and thus helped him to provide for a large and dependent family, in an honorable and ethical way? We do not mean by this that there is no such thing as a permanent professional reputation, or that, in order to acquire one, the man must be a poet or a philosopher; but we do say that literature gives wings to a professional reputation, and surrounds it with a bright and lasting lustre, and that those members of the profession who are grovelling in cliques, more intent on sliming the character of a professional brother than on building an enduring reputation for themselves, might learn a useful lesson from the example of the Boston poet and physician. A strong effort is being made by some of the professors and students of our city, through the press, secular and medical, as well as by private influence, to induce the Guardians of the Poor to open Blockley Hospital to clinical teaching. As yet the attempt has not been successful, but it is hoped that ere long the teachers will succeed in securing the use of this great institution to the profession. It is greatly to be lamented that the disputes and bickerings of wranglers and busy-bodies should result in closing so important and magnificent a hospital to the crowds of ambitious pupils who annually flock to Philadelphia to enjoy just such advantages as might be enjoyed in the Blockley. It cannot be but that the just representations now being made to the Board, and the public, will result in opening the doors of this hospital. On dit, that the late and present incumbents are now good friends, and arranging matters for the occupancy of the chieftainship of the hospital, and an important political office next year; it being understood that the question as to which office each shall occupy is to be decided by circumstances—chiefly or entirely of a political complexion.

The students' prayer meetings we fear are attended by few of the *boys* this winter, there being considerable *levity* among them—sometimes demanding bail by their professors or friends, to keep them out of the hands of his honor the Mayor.

Dec. 15th. This day the far-famed Blockley Hospital was once more opened to clinical instruction. The opening was accomplished by the present chief, who dwelt at length on the causes which have contributed to keep it closed for some years past. He was followed by a Satellite of the University, who, it seems, does most of the operatic surgery both for the venerable college and for the Blockley. Lots of old ulcers and a few unreduced luxations helped to make up the material of the clinic. A small operation on the eyelids of a patient constituted, we believe, nearly all the cutting. The Professor of Practice of the Jefferson College was elected in the beginning of this movement, but he has resigned, and the faculty of that institution is not now represented there. This we wonder at, inasmuch as some of that faculty deplored the loss of the great Blockley clinic very much, under the late administration. The present opening of the Blockley to the profession is due chiefly to the active energy of a medical man, a member of the Board of Guardians; but already we hear of dissensions among the doctors, which threaten to break up the clinic, as they have done in former times.

The present chief holds the chair of psychological medicine—an appointment we think quite appropriate on the homœopathic principle.

You noticed, Friend Gazette, some time ago, an event which occurred in our State Society among the Philadelphia delegates. This originated in the desire of a number of the most respectable members of the County Society to cut themselves off from a noisy rabble of talkers in that society; with this object, and the desire to be represented in the State and National Societies, they have taken up the charter of the old "Philadelphia Medical Society," founded by Dr. Wistar, and are modifying the constitution of the State Society, so as to admit a representation from the Philadelphia Medical Society. Some of the members of the College of Physicians tried this when the State Society was first formed, but failed because they could not frame the constitution in a way to admit them without admitting others. We fear the same difficulty will occur in the present case, and the gentlemen had better, perhaps, leave the State Society alone, and be satisfied with a representation in the National Association. The classes of the schools stand at present probably as follows: University 450; Jefferson 550; Pennsylvania and Philadelphia 150 each.

THE INFLUENZA.

The prevailing epidemic in and around Philadelphia this fall and winter is the influenza or grippe. The sore-throat feature is almost universal. In some cases severe neuralgic pains in the scalp, head, face, jaws, neck, or shoulders, one or all, are experienced by the sick. Cupping to the temples and back of the neck, followed by blisters behind the ears, have been found very beneficial in some cases. The local application of chloroform has also been followed with relief of pain. Complications of bronchial, pulmonary, cardiac, hepatic, and even renal affections have not been uncommon. Severe pains in the muscles and joints have been general, and in some cases a general rheumatic fever has prostrated the whole of the energies of the patient. No age, sex, or condition of life has been, or is, exempt from the disease. A patient this morning complained to me of paralysis of the ulnar nerves, together with general nervous prostration. Dover's powder, with small doses of calomel, has had a most excellent effect in soothing the pains, relaxing the skin, and restoring or correcting the secretions. The treatment, however, must vary with each case; and no routine treatment will do. When will a few leading spirits from outside of our city club together, and form a great third school here on principles in accordance with the demand of the times?

Yours, &c.,   SENECA.

MISCELLANEOUS ITEMS FROM FOREIGN JOURNALS.

By LOUIS BAUER, M.D.

—Dr. Schuppert recommends in the highest terms the aqua amygdalarum amarum against pertussis. Large doses every three hours will bring relief within three or four days. (Preuss. Vereins-Zeitung.)

—Dr. Bonorden, (Med. Zeitung, 1858,) pronounces ox-gall to be one, if not the very best remedy for resolving indurations, hypertrophy, and glandular engorgements. He states that he has repeatedly succeeded in relieving the like difficulties, that had already been threatened with the scalpel. The mode of using it is a mixture with olive oil, to which he adds extr. conii maculati, if the affections are very painful, or caustic ammonia, if they are torpid.

—Herpes tonsurans and other species of this dermatic disease of cattle, have been successfully transmitted by Prof. von Bärensprung, of Berlin, upon himself and Mr. Gerlash, one of the professors of the Berlin Veterinarian School. Spores were microscopically ascertained as the cause.

—The Wiener Med. Wochenschrift, Feb. 13th, 1858, reports that some most valuable researches have been instituted at the Imperial Hospital of Wieden, with iodide of potassium in lead poisoning, from which the following conclusions can be drawn:

1. The chemical test easily detects traces of lead in the urine, with or without the use of iodide of potassium; hence it is of great diagnostic and therapeutic importance.

2. The administration of iodide of potassium favors the elimination of lead through the urine.

3. This remedy should be so long continued until the lead disappears in the urine.

4. The elimination of lead by the uropœtic organs is co-existent with a dimunition of the phosphates of urea, the uric acid, and the specific gravity of the urine; whilst traces of albumen and grape-sugar appear simultaneously with lead.

5. Lead poisoning is by no means cured when the metal disappears in the urine, but only on the reappearance of phosphoric salts, and the specific gravity.

6. The diet with phosphoric food (meat and siliquosa,) seems to be ineffective as long as lead eliminates by urination. The latter having disappeared, those nutriments favor in a most conspicuous manner the elimination of phosphates, and the increase of specific gravity.

7. The symptoms of lead poisoning disappear earlier than the lead in the urine.

—Brueck's experiments (Virchow's Archiv. xii. Heft 1, 2,) tend to upset the views heretofore held, as to the coagulability of blood by atmospheric air. Since the introduction of air into the circulation of turtles and frogs leaves their blood perfectly liquid, he feels justified in premising other causes for the coagulation within (thrombosis,) or without the vessels. The facts ascertained by his researches seem to demonstrate, that the liquidity of blood depends upon the influence of the lining membrane of heart and vessels; but he is, as yet, unable to qualify that influence. Fibrine is but an atomistically altered albumen. The addition of a certain quantity of acid to the blood entirely deprives it of its spontaneous coagulation, and fibrine cannot be obtained in any way.

The studies of Prof. Brueck are likely to revolutionize the established doctrines, and to throw new light upon the physiology and pathology of blood.

—Very interesting observations on the sympatheticus maximus have just been published in the Gaz. Lomb., by Drs. Phillipe, Lussciana and Carlo Ambrasoli, the results of which may be observed in the following:

1. The term sympatheticus maximus is but conventional, and not physiological.

2. Its anatomical composition comprises:

(a.) Motor fibres from the spinal cord.

(b.) Sensitive fibres from the same.

(c.) Gray fibres partly originating from the cellular structure of the cord, and partly from the ganglionic cells of the sympatheticus itself.

3. The motor fibres terminate in the spinal cord; and therefore execute reflex motions, without, however, being subservient to the will.

4. The sensitive fibres bear the same relation to the cord; they are the excitors of reflex motion, and the carriers of pain, but not of sensation.

5. By virtue of its gray fibres and its ganglionic globules, the sympatheticus represents an independent nervous centre; by its connection with the spinal cord it becomes an appendix of this organ. It has no direct communication with the brain.

6. The sympatheticus is a composition of two distinctly different nervous provinces; a spinal or excito-motoric with peripheric distribution, and a ganglionic tropic, both central peripheral.

7. The gray fibres and their ganglionic globules preponderate in the structure, and consequently its tropic function.

8. The gray fibres are everywhere, even in the cerebro-spinal system, the representative of organic vascular function; their ganglia are the mediators and regulators of innervation.

9. The sympatheticus is no nerve, but a combination of nerves and ganglia.

SELECTIONS.

A CLERGYMAN'S IDEA OF A MODEL PHYSICIAN.

[Under this title the Rev. Duncan Kennedy, D.D., delivered an address to the graduating class at the late commencement of Albany Medical College, which the Faculty have deemed worthy of publication. It is an excellent discourse throughout, and we only regret that our limits oblige us to content ourselves with the following extracts:]

It is, furthermore, regarded as essential to a model physician, that he possess a high moral character. Without this he cannot meet the demands of his profession, nor satisfy the just claims of those who commit health and life to his care. Sound moral principle ever refuses to be the slave of impulse, or passion, or expediency. It allows no personal advantage, no momentary gratification, no selfish indulgence to become the rule of conduct, or constitute the measure of right and wrong. Such a man acknowledges no laws that are in conflict with his convictions of honor and right. He is ever alive to the sacred authority of conscience, and seeks to bow implicitly to its dictates. He is, therefore, incited to respect the rights of others, faithfully to render the service implied in the sphere of action he has chosen to occupy, and to adorn the various relations of life by the example of beneficent actions and moral virtues.

Upon principle, and without the stimulus of material reward, he will visit the poor and minister to their necessities as zealously and faithfully as he attends upon the rich. And when he once assumes the charge of a family, he will strive to be true to his trust. This he regards as a most solemn duty. And so it is. For, in the language of Dr. Rush, "to undertake the charge of sick people, and to neglect them afterwards, is a vice of a malignant dye in a physician. Many lives have been lost by the want of regular and punctual attention to the varying symptoms of diseases; but still more have been sacrificed by the criminal preference which has been given by physicians to ease, convivial company, or public pursuits, to the care of their patients. The most important contract that can be made is that which takes place between the sick man and his doctor. The subject of it is human life. The breach of this contract by wilful negligence, when followed by death, is murder; and it is because our penal laws are imperfect, that the punishment of that crime is not inflicted upon physicians who are guilty of it."* Inflexible moral principle will secure the model physician against all temptation to empiricism. Indeed, I cannot conceive how a man, who voluntarily stoops to the tricks and deceptions of quackery, can be an *honest man*. He may be well versed in all the learning of the profession, but when, for the sake of gain, he consents to sacrifice the high claims of his sacred mission, to trample under foot all that has for ages been achieved by medical investigation founded upon the certain laws of philosophical induction, and resorts to

---

* Rush's Lectures, p. 127.

some elixir which performs its magic cures by the influence of some hidden potency or supernatural charm, he is, and he must be an ingrained knave! He may make great pretensions to honor and benevolence, but the assumption of what is not really possessed is only the homage which hypocrisy pays to virtue. He may earnestly warn the public against counterfeits and impostures, but it is only the cry of "thief" in order to escape detection. But whatever be his pretensions or achievements, as to true honesty, he is a moral bankrupt!

I deem this a fitting time and place to allude to a complaint not unfrequently made against my profession, of evincing a disposition to endorse, by certificates and otherwise, the claimed efficacy of quack medicines. I feel very sensitive on this point, I confess, and am disposed to do my best to vindicate my brethren. I do so, in the first place, with a weapon furnished by one of your own profession—the venerable Dr. Alexander H. Stevens, who, when seeking to repel the imputation of the prevalence of skepticism among physicians, says: "We must go among the smaller men of our profession to find skeptics or infidels." I believe it. And in the same spirit I say, you must go down among the smaller men of our profession to find abettors and supporters of quackery. I do not think you will find them anywhere else. I say again, you must not take it for granted that every man is really a clergyman, to whose name in a quack advertisement you find "Reverend" or "D. D." attached. The titles of both our professions are constantly and surreptitiously assumed to give character and currency to some vile nostrum. There are many "distinguished benefactors of the race" bearing your insignia, whose names appear in print—but nowhere else—"Old Doctors," "Good Samaritans," "Retired Physicians," "whose sands are nearly run out," who, from a long residence in "India," or Africa, or somewhere else, have made discoveries that are to banish from the earth all the "ills that flesh is heir to." There are also many self-styled "Reverends," who, having for a season been called—mysteriously, and to the profound regret of the church universal—to lay aside the active duties of their profession, have been constrained, from a deep sense of duty, to make the attempt, and have finally succeeded, to discover some potent specific, which, by the "wondrous blessing of Divine Providence," has become entitled to the distinction of a sovereign panacea—so palatable that "the children cry for it," and so successful that the whole medical world is trembling with a jealous rage concerning it! These are all venerable men, animated by a pure, disinterested benevolence—until you happen

to meet them—when you behold them suddenly transformed into
sturdy impostors, arrant swindlers and liars! And shall we charge
upon each other the sins of such traffickers in fraud and villainy—
who, were they to receive the consideration to which their conduct
entitles them, would be furnished, at the public expense, with quiet
retreats, in such *retired* places as Sing Sing, or Auburn, or Clinton,
and for a period long enough to allow their sands to run entirely out?
I would indeed be sorry to believe that there is one in a thousand, of
the respectable members of my profession, who has voluntarily given
his endorsement to a quack medicine.

For myself, I believe I would suffer long and painfully under the
care of an intelligent, well-educated physician, before I would consent
to receive a certain cure at the hands of an empiric; for admitting
that by accident he cured me, yet by giving him my influence he
might have the opportunity of killing others, and I would be partaker
of his sin!

But the last and crowning attribute which completes the clergyman's idea of a model physician, is sincere piety. Not indeed that
high distinction in everything that is elevated and noble in professional
attainment may not be reached without this; but may it not be added,
that it is a most happy consummation, when with professional skill, refined tastes, unsullied honor and unimpeachable integrity, is united
the spirit of the humble, devout Christian? Whether the facts of the
case, at any past time, justified the charge of prevailing skepticism
against your profession, I cannot tell. But sure I am, that time has
passed away. The disgraceful proverbs have no longer any foundation in truth, " *Ubi tres medici, tres athei.*" " *Optimus inter medicos
ad gehennam.*" A splendid galaxy of names might here be rehearsed,
who have furnished to the world the noblest examples of living piety.
I will mention only a few, as referred to by Dr. Rush, among whom
his own holds a distinguished place.

Hippocrates and Galen were religious, according to the light which
they had, for they vigorously opposed the atheism of Greece and Rome,
with arguments drawn from the curious structure of the human body.
Botallus advises the physician, before visiting a patient, to offer prayer for the success of his prescriptions. Cheselden always implored the
blessing of heaven whenever he performed a surgical operation.
Sydenham was eminently a religious man. Boerhaave spent an hour
every morning in private religious devotion. Hoffman and Stahl were
not ashamed of the gospel of Christ; and Haller wrote a serious of

letters in defense of Christianity. Dr. Lobb had the motto "Deo adjuvante" inscribed upon the panels of his chariot. Dr. Fothergill's long life resembled an altar, from which incense of adoration and praise ascended daily to the Supreme Being. Dr. Hartley, whose works will probable perish only with time itself, was a devout Christian. To this slightly condensed record the author adds the just remark, that "the weight of their names alone, in favor of revelation, is sufficient to turn the scale against all the infidelity that has ever dishonored the science of medicine."* This catalogue of medical worthies might be indefinitely enlarged, by the addition of names of more recent date, but the occasion will not allow.

Gentlemen, in no secular pursuit in life is there so decided a demand for the possession of Christian principle, and the exercise of the Christian virtues, as in yours. From the fact of the conceded dignity and importance of your profession, and the universal confidence reposed in you, not only as physicians, but also as thinking and learned men, your known opinions have a great and deserved weight in the community. And how important is it, in this day of reckless speculation, of unrestrained radicalism, of wild fanaticism, and of open infidelity, that your influence be found distinctly and decidedly on the side of sound, conservative, eternal truth.

Besides, your calling leads you into scenes where the most favorable opportunities occur for benefiting, not only the body, but the mind and the heart. Knowing how conducive physical sufferings are to salutary reform, you may be instrumental in bringing back to virtue, as well as to health, those who by their vices have caused their own miseries, and upon whose minds a few kind words from your lips will make a deeper impression than the most solemn appeals from any other source. You will be frequently present where you will witness the last agonies of dissolution, and where the deep wail of bereavement will break upon the ear; there your tender sympathy and consolatory counsel may point the eye of the dying to the cross, and the faith of the living to sources of imperishable consolation. In thus acting you need not fear any intrusion into the sphere of the sacred ministry. You will excite no jealousy in our hearts. Doubly blessed is he who can do the work of the physician and the minister in the chamber of sickness and death.

----

* Rush's Lectures, pp. 128, 129. Some of the sentences changed for the purpose of abbreviation.

I trust it will not be deemed irrelevant to make a brief reference, at this point, to a matter which has occasioned some irritation between your profession and ours. You have sometimes found fault with us for seeming interference at the couch of sickness; and we have sometimes found fault with you for a seeming disregard of our prerogatives at the same place.

In regard to this, as indeed to most other grievances in this world, my conviction is, that there have been indiscretions and faults on both sides. There doubtless are clergymen who seem to know nothing about the proprieties of time, place and circumstance connected with anything with which they have to do; who are constitutionally dictatorial, rash and severe; who suppose themselves to be practicing the virtue of faithfulness in their calling, when it is only rudeness and insolence. On the other hand, there are physicians who, from a disregard to the salutary influence of religious sympathy, a conceit of professional superiority, or a spirit of rude indifference to the amenities of social intercourse, treat the pastor with less respect than they accord to the most ignorant menial in attendance. Now, is it surprising that such spirits should always be in trouble themselves, and should often occasion trouble to others? These are emphatically the "smaller" men of our respective professions; and I am happy in the conviction that they are "*few and far between.*"

Still it is well that we should comprehend our mutual rights in the premises. These, I contend, are in every respect equal. The duties of your profession lead you to visit your patient; the duties of mine lead me to visit my parishioner. And when the patient and the parishioner are found to be one and the same person, I ask, have we not equal rights there? You are there by the obligations of a contract; so am I, and by the obligations of a contract as binding and solemn as yours can be. The mission of the one is to do good; the mission of the other is precisely the same. You, then, have no right to interfere with my prerogatives, nor I with yours. How, then, is the matter to be cordially and amicably adjusted? Simply by the ruling of common sense, common courtesy, and a common conscience. It is not for us to quarrel over a dying bed, and there is no reason why we should. No clergyman, worthy the name, would seek to approach a patient, when a judicious physician had told him it would be hazardous to health or life. And no physician, worthy the name, would unnecessarily interfere to prevent the sympathizing pastor from seeking to awaken in the weary spirit—perhaps on the confines of the eternal state—the supporting energies of an unwavering faith and the joyous anticipations of an undying hope. Let us remember that our respective professions have a bond of union in the life of the great Physician, who, while on earth, made the body of man the subject of his miracles, and the soul of man the recipient of his heavenly doctrines. In Him we become bound in the ties of a common brotherhood. "Let there, then, be no strife between us, for we are brethren."

CHANCELLOR LINDSLEY

Opened the present session of medical lectures at the University of Nashville by an elaborate Introductory, of which we are only able to give the following striking extract:

Many of my hearers doubtless have visions of emolument, fat offices, easy times, honorable positions brought up with the mention of a medical professorship. Very wide, however, are they of the mark. As a class, no men are more poorly paid for the work, mental and corporeal, actually performed. Of the three hundred and twenty-one medical professors in the United States, many receive only two or three hundred dollars for their four or five months' work; others receive nothing; others less than nothing, actually paying for the privilege of wearing the professorial title and discharging the attendant duties. Some few receive a reasonable compensation for their labors, and others, the favored few, what may be regarded as quite handsome pay. It may be matter of surprise to some that under these circumstances so many are not only willing but anxious to engage in medical teaching. This may be explained by the fact that in our large cities there are real or supposed incidental advantages connected with these positions, which reward their occupants for the gratuitous labor performed. Besides, as managed in our country, medical teaching is a business, having many blanks for those engaged in it, and also a few very handsome prizes. Now, it is human nature to imagine hopefully that fortune will bestow the prize and not a blank; hence scores of physicians become professors, hoping that their schools will attain popularity, have a great run, and enrich them; they try it awhile, grow weary of waiting, and quit the business, leaving their places to other sanguine novices, who go through the same unprofitable round of experience. Thus we see a number of schools kept up with classes that do not pay expenses, and with faculties changing more or less completely every year. This must continue to be the case as long as medical teaching is in some respects a speculative business or trade.

As medical schools are more poorly endowed by the public than any other class of institutions, we find, not unnaturally, that medical. are more heavily taxed for their instruction that any other class of students. The law student may obtain his professional training at little or no expense, by reading with a lawyer and following the courts; the student of theology has to pay neither for tuition or lodging; the college student pays from twenty to sixty dollars per annum for instruction, board and lodging being furnished by the college at moderate and reduced rates; the student of medicine pays in most of the schools for his two courses of lectures about two hundred and fifty dollars, and at the same time must meet all the cost of living in expensive cities, What a contrast! Why should young men, mostly in limited circumstances, seeking a species of knowledge which enables them to emulate the gods in giving health to men, and which rarely enables them by severest toil to gain more than a bare support, be so much more heavily burthened than students of other professions? Why should not medical knowledge be rendered as accessible as theological, or classical, or legal knowledge? Were the profession alive to its own claims, would it not be speedily so rendered?

Where theological students pay nothing, where law students pay some few thousands, medical students pay annually hardly less than half a million of dollars for instruction. This large sum is very unequally distributed. The New England schools charge moderate fees, and with small classes receive but slender incomes. South of New England the greatest inequality exists among the schools as to numbers. The large schools are very large, and the small ones very small, a few being intermediate or respectable in size. Some schools have only two or three times as many students as professors. There are hardly six among the whole number in which a professorship is worth having on account of pecuniary emolument. But few teachers are really well paid, notwithstanding this enormous outlay by the body of students for tickets. A large proportion of their money is of no avail in promoting medical learning. A very large amount goes to meet the current expenses of schools, which are necessarily heavy; a still larger proportion is swallowed up in paying rent for the buildings used as colleges. Thus a large part of this by the students' illy spared half a million is consumed by expenditures for which there is no necessity, as in the case of the very small schools, which are evidently not wanted by the profession; or else for which the public should, and do generally provide, as in the case of private schools occupying rented premises.

In each of our large states there should be at least one fully endowed medical school, and a full endowment for a medical school should not be estimated at less than two hundred and seventy thousand dollars. One hundred thousand of which would, in most cases, be required for procuring grounds eligibly located and buildings suitably designed. A fund of fifty thousand dollars should be set apart for the continual increase of the museum and library, and at least thirty thousand dollars should be invested for the support of each of the elementary chairs. The practical chairs—surgery, medicine, and obstetrics—could be supported by moderate fees from the students, and the professional labors of the incumbents, it being an advantage to them as teachers that they should be fully engaged as practitioners. The incumbents of the elementary chairs should give all their time to their duties as professors, teaching and advancing science, and, being mainly supported by the funds of the school, should demand but moderate fees from the students. Medical would still be more grivously burdened than students of other professions, but yet the relief would be so great as to enable them to remain in the schools long enough to reap fully the many benefits they extend. Schools thus endowed would be placed beyond contingency, as to permanence and means of living; a large proportion of the professors, being removed from the clashings and jealousies engendered by the practice of their art, would become recognized leaders in the great field of medical observation, cordially receiving aid from hundreds of active practitioners; while rich museums and copious libraries, freely accessible to all, would stimulate and encourage a spirit of investigation and research. Such schools would become true and fruitful medical centres, and do much towards persuading physicians to forget the rivalry of artists, by cultivating the spirit of brethren in the study of nature for the sake of humanity. The hope and expectation that a goodly number of such schools will be established in our country at no distant day will not be regarded as wild and utopian by those who are acquainted with the deep interest now taken in medical education by the whole profession, and the great liberality manifested by the American public in endowing all manner of institutions fairly brought to its attention.

Whilst we find this great diversity in the history and endowment of our medical colleges, on one point we find a great similarity, namely, in the curriculum of studies as it is technically called; the length and arrangement of the courses of instruction, and the requirements for admission to the Doctorate, being very nearly uniform in all our colleges.* This is one among many instances showing the homogeny and common origin of our people, notwithstanding their dispersion over so vast a territory. The Medical College of St. Louis is but a copy, it may be with additions and improvements, of the University of Pennsylvania, from which a student might be transferred to the University of Louisiana without perceiving any great change. When one is described in its programme of lectures and appointments for teaching, all are described. This uniformity results in great practical good to the students, as they can commence and finish their studies in different schools without losing time or labor. It also renders it an easy matter for the schools to make such improvements, in their modes and means of teaching, as the voice of the profession may demand; since by concert of action among a few leading institutions such changes can be uniformly made, and other schools, in self-defense, will be compelled to adopt them.

The course of instruction as actually pursued in our schools at the present time was planned nearly a century ago, and has not since been materially changed. It was at the time a philosophical theory and a practically successful mode of teaching, admirably adapted to the condition and wants of the country. The student was expected to spend at least three years in acquiring his profession, much the larger portion of this time being passed in the office of his preceptor, and only some eight months at the school. It is obvious that his chief reliance was his preceptor, and not the school. He passed eighteen months with his teacher, a physician in full and active practice, reading under his advice and instruction the elementary books on medical science, and gaining as much practical knowledge of the art as it was in his teacher's power to furnish. He then went to the school, where he received a connected review in well-digested courses of lectures of the ground he had carefully travelled over, these lectures being made especially valuable by demonstrations and illustrations which ordinarily it was quite out of the power of the private teacher to give. After this he returned to the office, renewed his course of thorough reading and practical observation for eight months; and thence again to the school, to

* The University of Virginia is the principal exception.

attend upon a repetition of the demonstrative and recapitulatory lectures, and so finished his course, having during three years seen much of practice with his instructor, and through reading and lectures become well imbued with medical lore. At that day, with a scanty population widely diffused, cities were few and far between, schools still fewer, hospitals almost none, so that the student had to make a veritable pilgrimage to the shrine of medical learning, and naturally wished to get all that he could while there, and to get what he could not at home. It is difficult to say how the plan could have been improved upon for that time, and it is certain that under it was trained up a generation of physicians nowhere surpassed for skill and intelligence.

But in the lapse of this long period of time very great changes have taken place in our country. Cities are both numerous and accessible, and schools and hospitals are to be found within convenient distance of everybody; students and preceptors have changed their habits, and the schools remaining the same, the system of medical teaching has gradually become unsuited to the accomplishment of its design, and its symmetry has become marred by a number of serious blemishes and defects. That this is the case we have abundant and overwhelming proof in the fact that, during some fifteen years past, the pages of our medical journals and the proceedings of our medical societies have had so much to say about reform in medical education, and raising the qualifications for entrance into the profession; and that the great National Association, which for eleven years has gone on from strength to strength, was originated to effect this very object. Reform is often uselessly demanded, and all changes are far from being improvements, but surely a whole profession thus loudly speaking through every channel of utterance can hardly be mistaken upon a point like this, which so vitally concerns its well-being and very existence.

EDITOR'S TABLE.

SPECIAL NOTICE!

To the Subscribers of the American Medical Gazette.

This *January* number begins our TENTH VOLUME, the arrangements for which are such, that we can promise an improvement on any of its predecessors, in size, in the number of its collaborators, and in the variety of its contents.

☞ We are obliged to remind all our subscribers, *new and old*, that they are now indebted to us TWO DOLLARS IN ADVANCE, for the year 1859! which small amount they will greatly oblige by remitting *by mail at our risk*, in cash or postage stamps.

Delinquents for *one, two, three, four*, and even *five years!* are still on our books, to an extent, if all were paid, which would astonish those who are themselves delinquents, by neglect or forgetfulness.

BILLS TO BE SENT.

Those who do not *now* remit their arrearages, will receive their accounts by mail, and, unless promptly paid, they cannot expect to receive the GAZETTE any longer on credit. If any errors occur in distributing bills, they will be promptly corrected.

Paying subscribers, who wish to discontinue, will greatly oblige by giving notice.

☞ New subscribers should begin with the volume.
Back numbers can still be supplied.

TO SUBSCRIBERS AND MEDICAL MEN.

Those who enclose the names and address of TWO *new subscribers*, with the cash in advance, will receive their own copy *free* for the year. Thus we intend to make the GAZETTE the cheapest Journal in the country, and clubs as well as agents may avail themselves of these terms. All such may receive 80 pages monthly, at $1.83 per annum, our object being not to make money, but to extend our circulation and usefulness. Who will respond?

There are more than a hundred towns, having from five to ten physicians, in which we only send to one or two subscribers. Our friends will oblige us, in remitting their subscriptions now due, if they will send us the name of *one* medical man in their neighborhood, to whom we may send a specimen number,

FREE OF POSTAGE.

THE AMERICAN MEDICAL GAZETTE will be sent, *free of postage*, to all subscribers who pay during the months of *December* and *January*, in advance for 1859. The prompt transmission of *TWO DOLLARS*, by every subscriber, will bring them within this rule.

THE NEW YEAR.

The editor of the *American Medical Gazette* presents this *first* number of his TENTH VOLUME to his readers as a specimen of the improvements already made, and an earnest of what he is enabled to promise in the future, as the fruits of the prosperity of the Journal, which, single-handed and alone, he ventured to originate in 1850, and the success of which has gone on uninterruptedly, with an annual increase of subscribers to the present time. This professional and public favor has been gained by the freedom, independence, and impartiality with which the GAZETTE has ever been conducted, never having been shackled by "entangling alliances" with any college, hospital, school or clique, but doing equal and exact justice to all, irrespective of their location, in whatever part of our common country. The interests of the profession as a unit, have ever been paramount with the editor and his correspondents, and hence we have given no quarters to quackery or false pretence, whether in or out of the fraternity. Nor have we ever shrunk from our duty in this regard, smiting "iniquity in high places" whenever called for, and placing on the shelf, or consigning to Coventry, those who have sought to aggrandize themselves at the expense of the honor of the profession.

THE ENLARGEMENT OF THE GAZETTE.

The increase in size of our present number has been forced upon us by the accumulation of original material on our files, awaiting publication; much of which, including choice selections too important to be longer withheld, will now find a place in the present and succeeding numbers.

The amount of original matter in this number is greater than we have ever before been able to give, and exceeds in extent that of most of our contemporaries in journalism; while the value of most of the papers will bear comparison in point of interest and utility. The article on Mineral Springs, by the veteran Dr. Bell, of Philadelphia, and that by Dr. O'Reilly, of New York, on the Physiology of the Placenta, possess great novelty and merit.

The number and practical value of the original communications for our February number will be still greater than in the present issue. Among them will be found the report of the first successful operation for the removal of that terrible deformity in a female, viz., Congenital Exstrophia of the Urinary Bladder, performed by Professor Daniel Ayres, of the Long Island College Hospital, illustrated with photographic drawings taken from life. As also, contributions to the Physiology of Digestion, by Professor Busche, of the University of Bonn, translated and collaborated by Professor Louis Bauer, of the L. I. College Hospital, from whom we have received other similar favors.

May we not look to our friends at home and abroad for an appreciation of our efforts to furnish them with a larger and better journal, *without any increase in the subscription price?* And while receiving the *cheapest* medical periodical in the country, is it too much to ask that the subscribers should promptly remit for 1859 Two DOLLARS, for which they will obtain, *free of postage*, over 80 pages monthly, making annually over 1000 pages 8vo? Without such prompt remittance they tax themselves for postage, and cannot expect much longer to remain on our books.

New Subscribers will oblige by reporting themselves to commence with the new year.

☞ As bills are now sent out to Subscribers, if mistakes occur, let each correct the error in the amount of arrearages, and remit for 1859, including whatever back dues they know to be unpaid. Our books will be corrected accordingly.

UNIVERSITY OF MICHIGAN.

When we wrote the comments to be found in the November number of this Journal, on the action of the Regents of this University, and the part taken by two of its medical professors in relation to the *preparatory education* of medical students, we made no allusion to the general course of instruction given in the Medical Department of the University of Michigan, and intended to cast no reproaches upon the Faculty of, that Department touching the manner in which they perform their duty as teachers of elementary and practical medicine, whose fidelity in that regard is amply vindicated in the communication of Professors Palmer and Sager, which we took pleasure in inserting in our issue for December. Neither did we intend, by that act of courtesy to these gentlemen, to inculpate ourselves by the admission of any wrong on our part designedly done to them, for we spoke from the record of the Board of Regents, a transcript from which lay before us, that had been furnished to the newspapers at Detroit by authorized reporters. The character of the resolution commented upon, and the attitude in which these professors stood in relation to it, are neither of them changed essentially by their defence. On the contrary, the whole force of our remarks on the subject of preparatory education remains unbroken, and a careful reading of the defence makes the case worse than we had supposed or had dared to intimate. From the defence we learn that no inquiries are made into the qualifications of candidates for *admission* to the Medical Department of the University, as "it has been judged unadvisable to apply" "the rule *adhered to*" "to the student of the first year." The enormity of this custom will be best understood by supposing a case, which may be found on the pages of the annual catalogue of this growing institution for several years past. Suppose there are one hundred and fifty students in attendance upon the course of lectures annually delivered at the Medical School in Ann Arbor, and that twenty-five of this number are candidates for the honors of the institution. Suppose further, that the Faculty have thought best, "under the circumstances which have existed, to require these evidences of general knowledge, after full notice, and during the last year." And again, let us suppose that twenty-five is the average number of graduates from the Medical Department of the University of Michigan; who, then, becomes accountable for the introduction of the other hundred into the outer court of the Æsculapian temple, to dishonor and defile it? Is it not our friends Palmer and Sager (for such we regard them), and their colleagues of the Medical Faculty? Such is our opinion. And we still think that their conduct in perpetuating this custom, and in resisting its abrogation by the constitutional authorities of the University, demands the exercise of that moral power, the force of which we wot of.

The lines of defence set up by these gentlemen do not touch the point we had under our eye when we wrote what, as a journalist, we had to say on the proposed action of the Regents of the University, and the opposition made to it by the professors. We considered only the effect that the action of the one and the opposition of the other would have upon preparatory education, and were not thinking of their admirable chemical laboratory, their course of clinical instruction; or of the relation which the University bears to the State Normal School, the Agricultural College, the Union School, or the schools for the ragged children which supply the moral, mental and physical wants of a class not yet matriculants of the Medical Department of the University.

The first we know to be endowed for the purpose of disciplining the faculties and developing the powers of *professional* men; the second for the preparation of common school teachers; the third, to meet the intellectual wants of the cultivators of the soil; but we do not comprehend why certain studies of an elevating tendency should be excluded from the Medical Department of the State University, because they do not enter into the curriculum of a class or classes of school subordinate in position and secondary in influence.

The summing up of the defence to which these remarks have reference, amounts to this: the professors who have been aggrieved by our former remarks, admit that candidates for *admission* to the Medical Department of the school to which they belong, undergo no examination whatever, and that four-sixths of them are conducted by them into the outer court of the temple, regardless of qualifications, and confess their opposition to the resolution presented by the committee, but place it on the ground that the examination proposed was to be made by the Faculty of another department of the University. Wherein, then, have we done wrong to our friends, unless it be a wrong to give conspicuity to facts which have been carefully concealed from public view by the adroitness with which the language is used in which they were recorded. For one, we should have remained in ignorance of its import if we had not been urged to the inquiry by the accident of this discussion. Thus much we felt bound to say in self-justification. Our aim has been to place ourselves in the right—not others in the wrong. In this strife we intended to say naught that would cause us the loss of a single friend.

HON. TRUMAN SMITH, vs. DR. JOHN WATSON & CO.

The late U. S. Senator from Connecticut has replied to Dr. John Watson's article in the Times, which was intended to make a case for MORTON, the patentee of sulphuric ether, by a catalogue of medical names, who are made to endorse the patentee, whose imposture Mr. Truman Smith feels bound to unmask.

As an *argumentum ad hominum*, he now publishes in the Journal of Commerce the original *affidavits* of Drs. *Mott! Parker!* and *Francis!* the trio whose names are of more weight with the public than a regiment of the signers in Dr. Watson's article, each of whom *swears* that Dr. Horace Wells was the original and only discoverer of anæsthesia in surgical operations. They severally took this *oath* in 1852, and for the purpose of defeating the false pretences of this same Morton before Congress; whose fictitious pretensions Dr. Watson & Co. have now ensnared them into the endorsement of, and this in direct contradiction of their own affidavits, which they must have forgotten. For placing these gentlemen in this position, Dr. Watson and others are to blame. But Senator Smith may vindicate his course in the language of the indignant satirist:

> Ask you, what provocation I have had?
> The strong antipathy of good to bad !
> When honest truth an affront endures,
> The offence is *mine*, and should be *yours ;*
> *Mine*, as the foe to every false pretence,
> *Yours*, as the friend of truth and common sense.

We are happy to say that Morton's begging mission here has come to a dead halt. The President of the Board of Almshouse Governors, Washington Smith, Esq., has refused to sign the check for that $1500 which Gunther & Co. had promised to Morton out of the pauper funds. He is sustained, and will be, by the Hon. Richard Busteed, Corporation Counsel, and by the Courts, when that mandamus threatened is tried, in resisting this projected robbery of the city to pay Morton's printer and author of that book, called "Trials of a Public Benefactor," by a certain Dr. Rice. As Senator Smith says, "we hate imposture;" and that is our only motive for alluding to so loathsome a subject as Morton & Co.

A NEW JOURNAL.

Another *weekly* has made its appearance, closely resembling, in appearance and contents, the "Reporter" of Drs. Butler and Atkinson, of Philadelphia. The new-comer hails from New York, and is edited by Drs. *Kiernan* and *O'Meagher*, two of the younger members of the fraternity. Its tone is respectable and pacific in the first number, and its contents consist chiefly of magniloquent reports of the "college cliniques," professedly written by students, and adapted, we suppose, to circulate among the pupils of the several colleges, each being what is called a "student's number;" for so meagre material as these bogus cliniques furnish, cannot interest anybody else; but for this the reporters are not to blame. We fear that this "New York Medical Press" is destined to be short-lived, although, while the lectures last, it may serve as an advertising dodge for certain windy professors, who are seeking notoriety and specialities in practice. Our young brethren, who have started it in good faith, deserve encouragement, though we fear that they will find it a Herculean task to make it pay. We wish them better luck, however, than either of their competitors.

The following specimens of these bogus "cliniques" appear in the second number of this New York Medical Press:

ELEGANT EXTRACTS.

From the *Obstetric* Clinique of Professor Gunning S. Bedford, M.D.

Case of Uterine Erosion.

"My good woman, you have heard what I have said; will you permit me to do what I think is proper in order to relieve you?" "Yes, sir, I will submit to anything you may think best." "Very well, madam, if you will lie down on this bed, I will very soon make an application to your womb." Here, gentlemen, you see this cylindrical speculum; I introduce it, having previously lubricated it with oil, into the vagina; I now have the *os uteri* within the focus of the instrument; I introduce the moistened sponge for the purpose of removing from the ulcerated surface the mucous secretion, and then, as you observe, apply the solid nitrate to the affected part. "There my good woman, I have not hurt you, have I?" "Oh! no sir, I thought it would have been very painful." "Come back here, madam, next Monday, and if you will be a sensible woman, and submit to our directions, you will soon be quite well." "Thank you, sir." "Allow me, before you go, to ask you what is the state of your bowels?" "They are rather confined, sir."

Case of Nervous Prostration from Grief.

"Well, my good woman, what is the matter with you?" "I don't know, sir; I came here to have you tell me." "That's right, we shall endeavor to tell you all about it. How long have you been indisposed?" "I have been very miserable, sir, for the last six weeks." "What was the state of your health before that time?" "It was always excellent, sir, and I wish I could get it back again." "How have you been affected during the six weeks just passed?" "Oh! sir, I have been miserable—so nervous, and so easily frightened, I can't sleep, sir, and I am all the time afraid I shall lose my mind." "Have you any pain in your head?" "Yes, sir, I have shooting pains, and I am all the time trembling." "Do you know what produced this change in you?" "No, sir, I never had anything of it until I lost my poor little baby." "When did you lose it, my good friend?" "Just six weeks ago, sir; it was sick nearly a month, and I watched it all the time, hoping that it would get better." You cannot, gentlemen, but see how material it was for me to institute this examination by way of question and answer.

From the *Medical* Clinique of Professor John T. Metcalfe, M.D.

Case of Hypochondriasis.

Diagnosis.—This is either a case of tape worm, which I do not at all think likely, or the man is a hypochondriac. No amount of argument or assurance would persuade this man that he had not a vermiform appendix, and that this was the cause of his troubles. He will be a very hard case for us to cure. The way to inspire him with confidence in your professional capacity is to acknowledge your belief in his delusion, and to give him medicines " good for worms."

I once cured an old lady, affected in this way, by placing a worm in her chamber vessel and causing her to have a croton oil evacuation over it. When she had finished, she was so delighted to see the expatriated colonist, that she fairly *cackled like a hen over a newly-laid egg.* You may try this treatment with Mr. Flock. Perhaps it may succeed; but it needs caution and address in carrying it out.

We have no room at present for other and even richer specimens, but these will suffice to exhibit these cliniques in their true light, and hence the query made by the editors on the twenty-fifth page, viz:

"Why should medical students go to *Europe* in search of *medical and surgical knowledge!* now supplied in *this metropolis* in EQUAL PERFECTION AND ABUNDANCE?" Quid rides?

MEDICAL STUDENTS.

The *Medical and Surgical Reporter*, of Philadelphia, while protesting against the justice of its description, inserts in its columns the following coarse and vulgar portraiture of the present classes of students in the medical colleges of Philadelphia, by the editor of one of the daily papers of that city.

We ardently hope that it is a caricature, for the honor of the fraternity. The editor says:

"Their education, it must be allowed, is (in the majority of instances) neither finished nor respectable. They will pardon us for so severe a statement, but we make it because it is true—we make it because it should not be true, and because we wish to do them some good. It is true. A visit to the lecture rooms of our colleges will prove it to be true. What description of young men are to be seen in these places? *The roughest we ever saw in our lives. Most of them have a Texan Ranger look. Nobody in the world would pronounce them to be refined, liberally endowed young gentlemen. Hair as long as that of a savage, moustaches as fierce as the whiskers of a tiger, a reckless expression of the eye, a long, shuffling, clumsy gait, sword canes, dirk knives, revolvers, attire very unfashionably made, hard swearing, hard drinking, coarse language, cigars, tobacco quids and pools of tobacco spittle, are too prominent barriers for the formation of so flattering a judgment. The picture is not overdrawn.* We might make it a great deal less flattering, and then we would be absolutely true."

The editor of the *Reporter* is very indignant at this onslaught upon the students, and insists that they are a " very worthy class of young men."

VESICO-VAGINAL FISTULA.

In the surgical treatment of this formerly intractable disease, Dr. J. Marion Sims, of this city, has secured for his name a "mortal immortality," by demonstrating, in a multitude of examples, that this *opprobrium medicorum*, as it was justly regarded only seven years ago, is speedily and infallibly curable. This now established result is due chiefly, if not solely, to the patience, perseverance, igenuity, skill, and indomitable energy of Dr. Sims. The profession in his own country not only, but in Europe, have awarded to him the honor of being the pioneer, singly and alone, in this difficult path of discovery, and whatever of success other surgeons at home or abroad have since achieved, has been the legitimate fruit of his labors in this department of surgery.

As we were among the first to herald his success when still in Alabama, and to urge his removal hither in view of his broken and failing health, as well as furnishing a wider field for his reputation and usefulness, we cannot be indifferent to the systematic and persistent attempts made in various quarters to detract from his merits, and transfer to other brows the yet green laurels he wears in our own "Woman's Hospital," which is now the theatre of his toils and unparalleled successes. Hence, without detracting in the least from the merit of any useful modification or improvement, either in the instruments or operation of Dr. Sims, we still claim for him the original and prior right to the discovery and demonstration that the resources of surgery are adequate to the cure of every case of vesico and recto-vaginal fis-

'tula, and by a method peculiarly his own. That he gave all to the profession and the world, by publishing his cases, his processes, his instrumentalities, his defeats, and his ultimate triumph over this formidable malady, should endear him to every lover of science and humanity—while it proves him to be a worthy member of a liberal and benevolent profession, whose glory it is to conceal nothing which can benefit the public health or prolong the span of human life.

We have been led to these reminiscences, and prompted to these reclamatory remarks, by the receipt of a pamphlet from London, by Dr. J. Baker Brown, in which he reports *eleven* cases of the successful treatment of this malady by an operation which he confesses was first "*suggested* by Dr. Marion Sims," and yet laying so much stress upon the "button introduced by Dr. Bozeman," that he dedicates his pamphlet to the *latter*, as a tribute to his having "brought the operation for vesico-vaginal fistula to the highest perfection!"

Still, however, this Dr. Brown says that he cured one case by the "plan of Dr. Hayward, of Boston," and ten by that of Dr. Bozeman; and he then adds, "I claim no merit beyond that of having been the *first* to adopt and successfully carry out *Sims's and Bozeman's* SUGGESTIONS!" Indeed! Dr. Sims then only suggested a suggestion, which Dr. Bozeman repeated as a suggestion from America, while this Dr. Brown claims, in the "British Association," that he was the "first to carry out successfully!"

Now, what are the facts? Dr. Sims "suggested" nothing, until he had successfully carried out his own operations so frequently, that he was able to report them to the profession, and the world in detail, which he did as early as the year 1852; while Dr. Brown's first attempt at the operation was in 1856! and this two years after Dr. Bozeman's pamphlet reporting similar successes, and his suggested modifications of Dr. Sims's method. He may have been the first to repeat in *England* the operation of Dr. Sims with Dr. Bozeman's suggestions, after both had established its success, and not merely "suggested" it for Dr. Brown.

But the latter gentleman is not content with ignoring the true merits of Dr. Sims in originating and perfecting the operation of which both Dr. Bozeman and himself have since availed themselves with so much success; but he denies to Dr. Sims the merit of introducing *silver* sutures, because a Mr. Gossett, of London, used *golden* sutures in the same operation some twenty-five years ago. Hence, he announces that "the merit of being the first to apply *metallic* sutures to these cases is undoubtedly due to Mr. Gossett, of London, and not to Professor Sims, of New York." His friend, Professor Simpson, "could have informed him better; for *metallic* sutures were used in this country long before the times of this "Mr. Gossett, of London," *lead* being chosen for the purpose; and before Dr. J. Baker Brown was born.

Dr. Bozeman, now on a tour to Europe, seems to have been present at some of these operations of Dr. Brown, in London, and aiding him by his suggestions. But we cannot believe that he could have been privy to the studied concealment of Dr. Sims's real merits, which characterizes the pamphlet; for, as his former pupil and friend, he could not connive at such injustice. We are sorry to learn that Dr. Bozeman has not been so successful as at home, in the few operations he has himself performed in Europe. His reception abroad has been highly honorable to himself and to his country, at which we rejoice, for we are not insensible to his surgical merits. We should, however, honor him still more if he based his claims to distinction on being the improver of Dr. Sims's operation, instead of urging his pretensions to a new method of his own. This Dr. Brown, however, aims to rob *American* surgery, including both Sims and Bozeman, of all but the "suggestion" of an operation, which he, in England, was the first to carry out successfully. Against this enormity Dr. Bozeman will unite with us in protesting, for the honor of our common country.

THE HEALTH OFFICE.

This politico-medical prize is again in the market, and the new Governor will soon nominate some one out of the score of applicants from city and country, who are already circulating their petitions.

From this city we have heard the names of numerous candidates, among whom are Drs. Woodward, Harris, Sanger, Wells, Sayre, Gunn, Sterling, &c., besides those from Staten Island. Dr. Jones, from Onondaga, is said to head the list of the country doctors who apply. We hope the Legislature will abolish the fees, and fix a stated salary, before any appointment is made.

CITY INSPECTOR.

Drs. McNulty, Griscom, and Harris are on the Mayor's slate for this office, if a medical man is to be chosen, which is not yet certain. We should not be surprised if the doctors should all be laid on the shelf, and the old wheel-horse of the Democracy should receive the nomination.

THE OLIVE BRANCH.

What is the matter with our friend, the senior editor of the Nashville Journal of Medicine and Surgery? He seems to have grown sour and cross of late, which is in strange contrast with the cheerful equanimity of temper which aforetime was characteristic. He pitches into our correspondent, Dr. Lee, as though he meant to annihilate him, as he lately did Dr. Gross. He pounces upon our old friend, Dr. Davis, of Chicago, "pugnibus, calcibus, et ungues," as if he owed him an old grudge. While in his irate frenzy, he raves at others of his brethren as "Big Flunkies, Little Flunkies, Barnacles," and even compares them to "lice among dogs!"

We are almost afraid to say what we think, and only repeat our inquiry, "Is this the style to do good with?" although we fear the retort "Happy is the man who condemneth not himself in the thing which he alloweth;" for of our own infirmities we are sadly conscious. We may, however, safely whisper in his ear the counsel of our grandfather, "Always use soft words—they cost nothing."

We hope he may recover his equanimity of corporeality and intellectuality before May, and be at Louisville "himself again;" for in his present mood it might he hazardous to encounter him.

NEW YORK ACADEMY OF MEDICINE.

The annual oration was delivered by Professor E. R. Peaslee, Nov. 25th, at the rooms of the Historical Society, and gave great satisfaction to the large audience assembled. It was a learned and able performance, vastly superior to those listened to on similar occasions for a number of years past, when the orator has seemed to have been oblivious of the duty he was called to perform. Dr. P's discourse, when published, will speak for itself.

At the last meeting of the Academy, the time was chiefly occupied by M. Groux, the stranger whose extraordinary physical structure of the anterior portion of the thorax, the sternum being nearly absent, or substituted by a fissure, rendering the heart's action palpable to the sight and touch. A paper on the placenta and its physiology, by Dr. O'Reilly, was read, and remarked upon by Dr. Dalton and others. The time was then occupied with Dr. Corson's twaddle about the position of the shoulders in auscultation—a matter more germain to the gymnast than the physician.

MISCELLANEOUS ITEMS.

Dr. John C. Draper has been appointed Professor of Analytical Chemistry in the University of New York. His father, Dr. John W. Draper, retains the Chair of General Chemistry as heretofore.

Drs. Mott, Parker, and Francis have published a card, explaining that, in their *affidavits* in favor of Dr. Wells, as the discoverer of anæsthesia, they were influenced by the solicitation of Senator Truman Smith. This will be regarded as a very inadequate reason for *swearing one way, and certifying another.* The veteran Senator is on their track, and hangs them on either horn of the dilemma. Far better would be their defence, if they could truly say, that Dr. Watson and this Morton persuaded them to certify that they had sworn falsely. We commend them to an old book, which says, "The good man sweareth to his own hurt, and changeth not." Tuckerman, the mail-robber, now in the State Prison for feloniously raising money in aid of this Morton swindle, might have escaped his sad fate, if he had known that the sworn testimony of these doctors would be contradicted by their own certificates. Their oaths defeated Morton, and ruined Tuckerman, but they are now aiding these men by recommending a national testimonial to pay the debts of both, incurred by their joint imposture.

Hints to Craniographers.—Dr. J. Aitken Meigs, of Philadelphia, who devotes himself to ethnological researches, has published, under this title, a loud call upon the profession for human skulls, for the collocation of which he has a passion. Catalogues of crania in public or private collections will be highly acceptable, and more so if with a description of the source and history of each. The museums of the several medical colleges in Philadelphia contain 450 skulls, and the Mortonian collection in the same city is the largest in the world, and belongs to the Academy of Sciences, contains 1,100 crania, and represents 170 different races and tribes of the human family.

An epidemic anginose affection has been singularly fatal in Albany of late, which, from the descriptions we have seen, resembles what was formerly known as putrid sore throat, and differing but little from scarlatina maligna. Nothing satisfactory on the subject has yet appeared in the journals. We hear that Dr. Brinsmade, of Troy, President of our State Medical Society, is investigating it.

The Albany Medical College will henceforth hold but *one session annually.* See announcement on another page.

Medical men seem to have a proclivity to public life. The Governors of New Jersey and Delaware are both physicians. Dr. Frank Tuthill is now a member of the New York State Legislature, and will again make himself useful at Albany.

Among the recent deaths of medical men in our country, which we have failed to chronicle, we have been reminded of the following, viz:

Dr. Bissell, of Buffalo, N. Y.,

Dr. Clanton, of Warsaw, Ala.,

Prof. Picton, of the N. O. School of Medicine,

Dr. J. S. Duval, of Houston, Texas,

all of whom were men of influence and reputation. It is a remarkable fact that, during the year now closing, we have lost 17 of our subscribers by death.

New Books.—The following are received from Blanchard & Lea, Philadelphia, viz:

Erichsen's Surgery—Condie on Diseases of Children—Ricord and Hunter on Venereal—West on the Diseases of Women, Part II.

Lindsay & Blakiston's Annual Diary and Memoranda for Physicians has also reached us.

We can only announce them in this number.

BOOK NOTICES.

CONTRIBUTIONS TO OPERATIVE SURGERY AND SURGICAL PATHOLOGY. By J. M. Carnochan, Professor of Surgery in the New York Medical College, Surgeon-in-Chief to the State Emigrants' Hospital, &c. With illustrations drawn from nature. Philadelphia: Lindsay & Blakiston. 1858.

The second part of this serial quarto has appeared, and will be found of still greater interest to the profession than the first, which we have had occasion to commend, in a former number of the Gazette. It contains a case of Exsection of the entire Ulna, an original and highly meritorious operation, the successful result of which might be regarded as a triumph by any living surgeon at home or abroad. The other papers in this number possess equal novelty and interest, both relating to Facial Neuralgia, with cases of the most persistent and formidable character, in which operations alike ingenious and difficult have been successfully performed, after the failure of all other remedies, and in one case after numerous attempts by other surgeons to afford relief by division, cauterization, and excision of nerves. Dr. Carnochan's new and original operation consists in the excision of the *trunk* of the second branch of the fifth pair of nerves, *beyond the ganglion of Meckel;* and this he has proven to be a radical cure of this terrific malady, in a number of desperate cases which are reported in detail in this number, with remarks on their pathology.

The illustrations, drawn from nature, are elegantly colored lithographs, while the paper and typography of this beautiful quarto are super-excellent.

Dr. Carnochan appears to be laying a deep and broad foundation for a surgical reputation, second to no man in the country, and the publication of this series cannot fail to elevate him to high rank abroad as well as at home.

PROCEEDINGS OF THE AMERICAN PHARMACEUTICAL ASSOCIATION, at the seventh annual meeting, held in Washington, D. C., 1858. Philadelphia: 1858.

This volume approaches in size, and closely resembles in appearance, the "Transactions of the American Medical Association," and emanates from a kindred body, closely allied to us, in our reciprocal relations to the public health.

It numbers among its members very many able and liberal-minded men, whom the medical profession ought to recognize as worthy co-workers in contributing to the growth, improvement, and usefulness of the healing art. Our mutual interests should prompt physicians everywhere to promote the objects of this American Pharmaceutical Association, by word and deed, for the education and training of Apothecaries, so that their important functions shall no longer be usurped by unqualified persons, is a desideratum with the profession and the public. This volume contains much valuable matter, and is highly creditable to the fraternity. We heartily wish them success, as we do to their Journals and Colleges of Pharmacy everywhere, all of which merit higher appreciation.

RECEIPTS to 1858, for Subscription to Gazette.

Drs. Greene, Bartlett, H. Lindsley, Whaley, Dodge, Hallet, Sanger, Byrne, Mitchell, Brown.

RECEIPTS for 1859.

Dr. H. N. Wells, Budd, E. H. Davis, March, Gindrat, Oliffe, Quackenbush, Rouse, W. Maney, Lenoir, Armsby, F. H. Hamilton, S. Jackson, G. B. Wood, La Roche, W. P. Reese, R. E. Rodgers, F. G. Smith, J. M. Warren, Brinsmade. D. Ayres, S. Avery, Messenger, G. Greene, F. S. Greene, Atlanta Medical College 5; Pennsylvania Medical College 10; N. Y. Medical College 10; Albany Medical College 15; New Orleans School of Medicine 15; Brown, T. Green, Blatchford, Marvin, Phillips.

CONTENTS.

AMERICAN
MEDICAL GAZETTE.

Vol. X.   FEBRUARY, 1859.   No. 2.

ORIGINAL DEPARTMENT.

Congenital Exstrophy of the Urinary Bladder, Complicated with Prolapsus Uteri following Pregnancy: Successfully Treated by a New Plastic Operation. (Illustrated.) By DANIEL AYRES, M.D., LL.D., Surgeon to
the Long Island College Hospital, &c., &c.

Exstrophy, or extroversion of the urinary bladder, is a congenital
malformation, which Prof. Gross, in his excellent work on the Urinary
Organs, says "amounts to a hideous monstrosity."

Such cases are, comparatively, seldom met with, except in large
cities, to which they resort for pecuniary assistance. Excluded as they
are from the avenues of honest industry by a condition at once disgusting and repulsive, they are (unless born in affluence) literally
outcasts from society, and may occasionally be found ekeing out a
precarious subsistence by exhibiting themselves as surgical curiosities
to the classes of our various medical schools.

Little is to be found on this subject in systematic works of surgery;
but excellent descriptive monographs have been contributed by different countries. Among them will be found that of Dr. Monro, contained in Vol. I. of the Edinburgh Medical and Surgical Journal. In
France, Thiebault has contributed some cases; and an article by Bres-
chat will be found in the Dic. des Med. Sciences, tome xiv.

Von Ammon has recorded instances in his "Congenital Diseases of
Man," vol. 1, p. 14; and Heyfelder has furnished a paper on the sub-
ject to the transactions of the Royal Leopoldinean Academy of Natural
Philosophers.

In the London Medical Gazette for 1845, Prof. Errichsen details
a series of highly interesting experiments on the elimination of differ-

ent substances by the kidneys, in a person under his inspection with this deformity.

Other cases have been noted in various professional journals from time to time. The general type to be observed in all the instances which have been described is much the same; shades of difference and peculiarities of sex constituting the chief points of variety.

The essential characteristic of these malformations consists in a deficiency or absence of the symphesis and bodies of the pubis. The osseous keystone of the pelvic arch in front, which is the natural point of insertion for the abdominal parietes being absent, the pelvic bones terminate abruptly on either side, leaving a hiatus varying from two to five inches in width. The recti, and other abdominal muscles necessarily inclining off, to be inserted at these abutments, removes all anterior support from the viscera situated in this region. The bladder is consequently pressed forward during the early period of foetal life to occupy the vacant space, and becomes fused with the integuments at that point where the placental vessels traverse the abdominal walls.

But it may be pertinently asked, What is the *initial* cause of this failure of ossific union at the pubis? It is scarcely an answer to such a question to call it " an arrest of nutrition," for we naturally seek to know the *cause* of such " an arrest."

It has been noticed that the umbilicus is uniformly absent in all these cases, proving that the mechanism of the maternal and foetal union is intimately connected with, if it does not determine this malformation.

An instance occurred in the practice of Dr. McPhail, of this city, in which the urachus was continued several inches into the umbilical cord, and was therefore included very naturally within the ligature applied at the usual point of deligation. A fatal peritonitis was the result, and a post-mortem examination revealed the fact. Now, may not such an occasional prolongation of the urachus into the cord be looked upon as an intermediate form of development, which, when aggravated, may determine the difficulty in question, acting in this position as a foreign body to prevent the osseous union and consolidation of the pubic arch? Such an explanation of the rationale of this species of deformity certainly requires no inordinate stretch of the imagination, and may be worthy of attention in the absence of any more plausible hypothesis.

The absence of a bony support is partially supplied by fibro-cellular tissue between the abutments, whilst above there is probably an expansion of the aponeurosis of the external oblique, conjoined tendons, fascia transversalis, and peritoneum, all of which are firmly attached around the base of the posterior wall of the bladder, which is here gathered into an oblong, oval body varying in size, from a filbert to a large fist. This tumor is found to become larger when the patient is standing, and smaller when the recumbent position is assumed. It exhibits a deep vermilion color; is exquisitely sensitive to the touch; bleeding upon very slight irritation, and surrounded by integument which near its base resembles mucous membrane. In elderly subjects it is said that the surface of this tumor is sometimes changed, becoming invested with a kind of cuticle, whilst its sensibility is greatly diminished. On close inspection, the mouths of the ureters will be detected emerging from the inferior portion of the tumor near its base, from which urine constantly dribbles, unless the parts are irritated or pressed upon, when it is discharged per saltum. This constant wetting of the parts is not productive of so much irritation or excoriation as might be anticipated, provided tolerable attention is paid to cleanliness, and the parts are not subjected to much friction; for it seems that the renal secretion exhibits less acrimony when immediately extruded from the kidneys, and is consequently indebted for much of this quality to its retention in the bladder, where probably some of its watery constituents are reabsorbed, and the remainder becomes subject to chemical changes.

It will be observed that the integuments which are here usually covered with hair, are, as it were, split, whilst on both sides the hair is found growing luxuriantly in lines curving outwards towards the iliac spines.

It has been remarked, that the greatest variations among these cases arise from the imperfect development, malposition, or entire absence of different portions of the genital organs; and the amount of venereal desire seems to be in proportion to their perfection. In the male, a rudimentary penis and urethra are generally discovered below the cystic tumor, and the testicles, if present, are in an equally undeveloped condition.

In the female, the genital organs are also occasionally very imperfectly formed. The clitoris is most frequently absent, or not to be detected, and, as we might expect, there is seldom any trace of a urethra. In other respects, the organs may be normal; the uterus, ovaries, and vagina being perfect, and the subject capable of procreation, as was shown in one of the cases related by Thiebault, and noted as a very interesting and remarkable fact. Similar capacities existed in the subject of the present memoir, and a hope of mitigating the deplorable results of parturition first prompted an extension of surgical art to the melioration of a hitherto intractable deformity.

The patient (whose name is omitted by special request) was admitted to the Long Island College Hospital November 1st, 1858, and a history of the case recorded by the House Surgeon, Dr. Ostrander.

She is 28 years of age, born of healthy parents, both of whom were free from deformity; her height is below the average of females, and she is unmarried. She declares her health to have always been good, appetite and digestion excellent, bowels regular, and the catamenia in all respects normal.

She states that, on the 5th of July preceding, she was delivered of a well-developed child, having carried it to maturity without extraordinary difficulty.

Labor commenced with free hæmorrhage, (footling presentation,) and lasted two hours, at the end of which time the child was born, having died in process of delivery. Perineum uninjured.

She reports having made a tolerable recovery, though for a long time weak, and her present appearance is somewhat anæmic.

Shortly after she began walking about, symptoms of prolapsus uteri came on, becoming gradually worse, until the organ projected external to the vulva, attended with dorsal, dragging pain, difficulty of locomotion, and gastric disturbance.

In quest of relief, she entered the Brooklyn City Hospital on the 1st of September following her confinement, and remained there one month. Here she states that a variety of pessaries were tried, none of which could be retained, and finally a surgical operation was performed, the nature and character of which is not very apparent.*

Finally, a species of stem-pessary was contrived, which was intended to support the uterus, whilst kept in position by strings passed around the thighs. This, however, proved very inefficient—the uterus

---

* Since the above was in press, a short article, descriptive of this case, has appeared in the *Virginia Medical Journal* for January, 1859, written by the House Surgeon of that Institution. The writer states, that an attempt was made to retain the prolapsed uterus " by removing an inch of mucous membrane from the bottom and sides of the vulva, and uniting them by two figure of 8 sutures, which were removed on the sixth day, when no adhesion was found to have taken place." The writer continues: " The patient was allowed to get up on the fourteenth day, when the prolapsus was found to exist nearly as much as before," &c.

It is obvious that no effort was made to relieve the congenital deformity, and that she was discharged in much the same condition as when she entered.

slipping by the instrument upon the slightest extra exertion. Moreover, the parts had now assumed an irritable condition, partly due to increased friction of the apparatus, and undue attention to cleanliness, added to the causes already noted; altogether her deplorable condition was scarcely susceptible of being made worse.

I may here remark, that the figures, both before and after the operation, have been photographed from accurate plaster casts, taken directly from the patient—a very difficult and delicate procedure, for which I am much indebted to the skill and kindness of my colleague, Dr. Bauer, and our valuable assistant, Mr. J. F. Esslinger.

Fig. 1, is an exact representation of the parts at the time of presentation to the clinical class of the Long Island College Hospital, for the purpose of critical examination. The prolapsus having been carefully and completely reduced, was found to retain its place so long as the patient maintained the recumbent position.

The distance between pubic abutments was estimated at about three inches.

The bladder (a) forming an oval, eliptical tumor, mammillated upon the surface, which in the recumbent position measured two inches in its long, and one and a quarter inches in its short diameter. This was soft, elastic, of bright vermilion color, and covered with a thick tenacious mucus; bleeding readily when rudely handled, and so exquisitely sensitive, that whilst under the full influence of chloroform, and insensible to the knife, a sponge passed over the exposed bladder excited reflex motions.

The integuments immediately surrounding the bladder were found red and puckered, but very soft, delicate, and free from hair between the bladder and point of sternum. The labia majora (o. o.), thick, fleshy, and luxuriantly covered with hair, were gathered into folds swelling away towards either thigh; these were carefully shaved previous to taking the cast and performing the operation.

The nymphæ occupied isolated positions on each side of the vulva, and are designated in all the figures by the letters b. b.

Between these and the vagina below no trace of clitoris or urethra could be distinguished, but the whole surface was covered with mucous membrane, continuous with the vaginal lining.

Here, then, we had to contend with two formidable difficulties, either of which was a problem in itself, viz., aggravated prolapsus from an entire absence of anterior support, added to the original congenital malformation.

To form an estimate of the value attached to surgical operations in these cases, we cannot do better than quote the opinion of Prof. Errichsen, of University College, London.   Having collected the experience of the profession on this topic, his eminent position at the centre of surgical science, added to his well known and extensively recognized erudition, renders him at once a reliable and compendious authority on the subject.

" This malformation," says he, " is incurable.   Operations have been planned, and performed with a view of closing in the exposed bladder by plastic procedures, but they have *never* proved successful, and have terminated in some instances in the patient's death; they do not, therefore, afford much encouragement for repetition."

So unsatisfactory have been the results of these operations, that the profession has not been favored with their general plan, their details, nor the causes of failure.   It must be evident, however, that operations based upon the principles of plastic surgery alone offer prospects of success.

The most probable source of failure, and one which challenged our early attention, was the disastrous result to be apprehended from urinary infiltration, which, by its irritating character, would necessarily destroy all prospect of union, if it did not induce extensive sloughing of the abdominal parietes: peritonitis and purulent phlebitis are likewise probable sources of danger, unless carefully guarded against. Indeed these may all become inevitable consequences of attempting to accomplish too much at one time; and it was therefore determined to arrange our proceedings with a special view, if possible, to avoid them.   The indications which it was proposed to follow were:

1st. To form an anterior wall for the exposed bladder.

2d. To restore the urinary canal.

3d. To establish the anterior fourchette of the vulva.

4th. To supply means to prevent the prolapsus, and to collect the renal secretions.

The delicate character of the integuments above the bladder, and its well-known transmutability into the conditions of a mucous membrane, peculiarly adapted it to supply the anterior cystic wall, and thus fulfil the primary indication.

With these objects in view, the operative proceedings were divided into two stages.

The first consisted in raising a flap from the anterior portion of the abdomen, including the superficial fascia, turning its cuticular surface

FIG. 3.

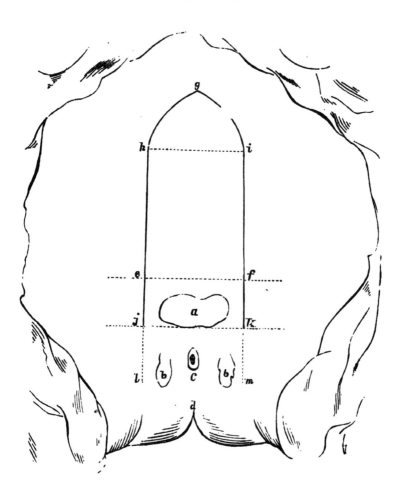

a, BLADDER.   b, b, NYMPHÆ.   c, VAGINA.   d, ANUS.

down over the exposed bladder as far as its inferior border, and securing the lateral union of the flap in that position, whilst a free exit below was maintained for the urinary discharge; an important result, still further assisted by the dependent situation of the outlet of the ureters already alluded to.

By these means it was proposed to accustom the highly sensitive bladder to a gradual and methodical compression, whilst the flap itself was insured ample space to undergo such swelling as might be anticipated from its new position, and the unusual stimulation of a new secretion. Time was likewise given for the necessary transmutation of tissues to make some progress.

The steps of this procedure will perhaps be better understood by a more detailed statement of the first operation in connection with the diagramatic plates, figs. 3 and 4.

It was performed on the 16th of November last, the patient being thoroughly under the influence of chloroform, and a sugar-loaf shaped flap having been previously marked out upon the abdominal integuments; its base e. f., three inches in width, was situated three-fourths of an inch above the cystic tumor, and extended five inches in length, with its apex towards the ensiform cartilage. The dark line e. h. g. i. f., (fig. 3,) indicates its form, position, and the line of incision.

This flap being left sufficiently large to meet the elevated form of the bladder, and allow for shrinkage, was quickly but carefully separated from its cellular attachments, down to the line e. f., whilst two lateral incisions e. j. and f. k. were continued directly downwards, and towards the nymphæ, to serve as beds for receiving the sides of the new flap.

The integuments covering the lateral and inferior portions of the abdomen, extending from g. to j. on one side, and from g. to k. on the other, were now sufficiently separated from their cellular attachments to the muscles beneath to insure their sliding freely, and meeting without tension at the mesial line g. N., (fig. 4.) When brought into this position they completely covered from view the raw surface of the flap already turned over, and investing the bladder, with the exception of a triangular space, j. N. k., (fig. 4,) formed by the coaptation of the lateral flaps; this was temporarily covered by reflecting back upon itself the corresponding triangular free end of the deep flap, j. c. k., (fig. 4,) and attaching it along the line j. N. k. Numerous points of interrupted suture were used to retain the parts in situ, assisted by long strips of adhesive plaster, compresses, and a retentive bandage around the body. It will be observed, that the lower portion of the cystic tumor was thus temporarily left free and partially exposed, whilst no portion of cut or denuded surface remained uncovered.

The patient received a large dose of opium, and was strictly maintained in the recumbent position upon a bed, properly protected; such additional measures being adopted as would secure cleanliness.

As the parts subjected to operation began to swell, she complained of irritation and pressure upon the bladder, which, however, was promptly met with morphine alone, and subsided in the course of a few days. Now was exhibited the great importance of leaving the tumor partially uncovered, whilst all the cut surfaces were in close contact, and thus freed from the action of irritating secretions; important facts, duly dwelt upon and recently enforced with great stress by the distinguished Prof. Syme, of Edinburgh, whose contributions to the surgical treatment of the urinary organs have alone placed both hemispheres under permanent obligation to him.

On the fourth day after the operation all sutures were removed, the wounds having all healed by first intention or primary adhesion, with the exception of a spot the size of a ten cent piece, situated just above the point of the triangle, and where the deep flap had been reflected over the bladder. At this point the lateral abdominal flaps were necessarily raised up from the tissues beneath, and could not be brought into contact even by the use of compresses. This, however, granulated kindly, and was nearly cicatrized on the 7th of December, when the second and last operation was performed, as follows:

The patient, being under the influence of chloroform, the lower triangular flap $j. N. k.$, (fig. 4,) was dissected from its recent and temporary attachments, both lateral and deep, and turned down over the vulva, as indicated by the dotted line $j. c. k.$

Two incisions $j. l.$ and $k. m.$ were now carried from the external angles of this triangle, perpendicularly towards and terminating just behind the nymphæ, $b. b.$

The lateral flaps bounded by the lines $N. j. l.$ and $N. k. m.$, and including the labia majora, were then freely dissected from over the abutments of the pubic bones, until they could be readily slid to meet each other at the central line $N. c.$, which, being a continuation of the line $g. N.$, reduced the whole to a single linear wound, occupying the "linea alba." See fig. 2.

During the operation several arterial branches bled freely, and were arrested by torsion and the free application of ice, after which the flaps were confined at the mesial line by points of interrupted

FIG. 4.

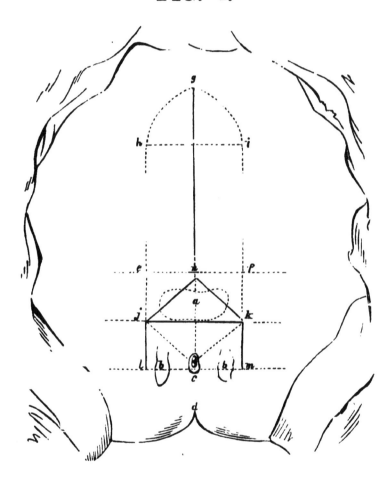

a, BLADDER COVERED BY DEEP FLAPS. b, b, NYMPHÆ. c, VAGINA.
d, ANUS.

suture; the most inferior one, viz., at *l.* and *m.*, being made to include the apex *c.* of the triangular flap.

Fearing to depend on sutures alone to secure the approximated flaps, and the use of adhesive plaster being excluded by the irregularity and position of the parts, the whole surface between the points of suture was hermetically encased by strips of patent lint, soaked in collodion, and accurately applied. In addition to this, pieces of muslin were by the same method firmly attached to the labia majora, at some distance from the mesial line, and to these suture silk was fastened in such a manner as to form a lacing across and over the wound. By means of this dressing all tension was removed from the sutures, urine was totally excluded, whilst rapid and perfect adhesion soon followed.

Thus a urinary canal was formed, which would admit the little finger to be passed up one and a half inches. The anterior fourchette of the vulva was firmly established, and the mons veneris assumed its prominent and natural appearance.

The last cast of the parts representing her present condition, (fig. 2,) was taken on the 4th of January, 1859, previous to which time, the parts being all firmly united, she was permitted freely to walk about, and left the hospital to spend the holidays with her friends. No artificial support whatever was applied in order to ascertain how far the operation would succeed in preventing the prolapsus.

After a severe test, the anterior fold of the vagina alone descended, and that for a short distance, forming a pale oedematous tumor, occupying the vulva, about the size of an English walnut. The anterior fourchette of the vulva remaining firm and resisting, a light oval pessary, made of vulcanized rubber, and perforated, was introduced into the vagina and readily retained in situ. After thorough trial, this was found to support the parts completely, and without the slightest uneasiness, even under active exertion and straining.

This was a better result than had been anticipated, inasmuch as it was intended to rely mainly upon a disc-shaped pessary, supported by a foot attached to a simple apparatus, which we had constructed, to act as a reservoir for the urine.

January 20th.—The patient was again examined at the hospital, in the presence of a number of medical gentlemen, she having walked a distance of two miles without experiencing any inconvenience. The parts were all found sound and firm, and her general health and spirits much improved.

156 MONTAGUE PLACE, BROOKLYN.

BOOK NOTICES.

TRANSACTIONS OF THE AMERICAN MEDICAL ASSOCIATION. Vol. XI. Philadelphia: 1858.

This formidable octavo, of 1,027 pages, has appeared, but our copy reaches us too late to allow of more than a brief statement of its contents, the variety and value of which will be found to be quite equal to any of its predecessors. It is printed in beautiful style, but has been delayed in its passage through the press by causes beyond the control of the publishing committee.

After the usual detail of the business at the late Annual Meeting in Washington, D.C., in May last, we have the following papers, viz:

1. President's Address. By Paul F. Eve, M.D.

2. Report on the Medical Topography and Epidemic Diseases of Kentucky. By W. L. Sutton, M.D.

3. Report on Epidemics of Ohio. By G. Mendenhall, M.D.

4. Report on the Topography and Epidemics of New Jersey. By Lyndon A. Smith, M.D.

5. Report on Medical Education. By J. R. Wood, M.D.

6. Report on Spontaneous Umbilical Hæmorrhage of the Newly Born. By J. F. Jenkins, M.D.

7. Report on Marriages of Consanguinity. By S. M. Bemiss, M.D.

8. Report on the Functions of the Cerebellum. By E. Andrews, M.D.

9. Report on the Treatment best adapted to each variety of Cataract. By Mark Stephenson, M.D.

10. Report on the Medical Jurisprudence of Insanity. By C. B. Coventry, M.D.

11. Report on the Law of Registration of Births, Marriages, and Deaths. By Edward Jarvis, M.D.

12. Report on the Nervous System in Febrile Diseases, and the Classification of Fevers, &c. By H. F. Campbell, M.D.

13. Report on Moral Insanity, in its Relations to Medical Jurisprudence. By D. Meredith Reese, M.D., LL.D., &c.

14. Report on Stomatitis Materna. By D. L. McGugin, M.D.

15. Report on the True Position and Value of Operative Surgery as a Therapeutic Agent. By J. B. Flint, M.D.

16. A Method of Preserving Membranous Pathological Specimens. By R. D. Arnold, M.D.

17. Letter of E. D. Fenner, M.D., to Paul F. Eve, M.D., President of the Association.

18. PRIZE ESSAYS, viz: The Clinical Study of the Heart-Sounds, in Health and Disease. By Austin Flint, M.D. And

Vision and some of its Anomalies, as revealed by the Ophthalmoscope. By M. A. Pallen, M.D.

The volume concludes with the plan of organization, Code of Ethics, and list of officers and permanent members.

A TREATISE ON HUMAN PHYSIOLOGY, designed for the use of Students and Practitioners of Medicine. By John C. Dalton, Jr., M.D., Professor of Physiology
and Microscopic Anatomy in the College of Physicians and Surgeons, of New
York, &c., &c. Philadelphia: Blanchard & Lea. 1859.

This is a new and original work, though on a trite subject, and one in relation to which it may be said "of making books there is no end." And yet Dr.
Dalton needed no apology for giving us another work on Physiology, especially
as by excluding from his plan much that is unsettled, and more that is purely
hypothetical in the science, he has made a book which is more readable and instructive to students as well as physicians, than any other we have seen.
The author is well known to be an enthusiast in physiological research, in the
experimental part of which he has already made his mark, though comparatively
a young man. As a writer he has few equals, and as a teacher no superior,
while the work before us is chiefly the result of his own ardent and deligent
study, his experimental facts being founded to a great extent upon personal
observation. Of this the illustrations in the volume, numbering 254, are in
evidence, nearly all of them being entirely new, and they are exquisitely done
in the finest style of finished art. We take pleasure in expressing our high
gratification at this new work emanating from New York, and trust that it is
only the harbinger of other evidences like it, of the industry and literary capacity
of many of our medical men. We shall be surprised and disappointed if Dr.
Dalton's work does not receive high commendation from our brethren whose
journals are capable of inserting critical reviews, for we are certain that it has
strong claims to both novelty and merit.

A TREATISE ON DISEASES OF THE AIR-PASSAGES, &c. By Horace Green. M.D.,
LL.D., &c. New York: Wiley & Halsted. 1859.

Under the title of "Green on Bronchitis" this work has been well known for
many years, and the author been extensively reviewed at home and abroad. A
fourth edition has now been issued, revised and enlarged, with an appendix containing an epitome of the foreign works on kindred topics, and what is doing
abroad by topical medication in laryngeal and tracheal disease. Whatever differences of opinion may exist among the profession, as to the extent to which
topical medication is adapted, and may be made available, in anginose, tracheal,
bronchial, and pulmonary affections, all now concur in the general views which
Dr. Green has been so persistent in promulgating, and which he has been practically carrying out to an extraordinary extent. In France the subject is at-
tracting great attention, and Dr. Green is there honored more than at home, for
he has encountered in his own country very great, and even unscrupulous hostility, such as is the fate of all who practise a specialty, or claim any novel or
exclusive pretensions in any department. His errors have been those incidental
to riding any hobby, prompting him to run into extremes; but we doubt whether
his experience has not corrected many of these, for we think this apparent in
the new edition of his book. That he has merit is undeniable, and all must
respect him for his perseverance in teaching what he believes, and in defending
himself against every assault, relying, as he seems to do, that ultimately the
profession will do him justice. The last edition of this book is the best, and
is gotten up by the publishers in handsome style.

THE SCIENCE AND ART OF SURGERY; being a Treatise on Surgical Injuries, Diseases, and Operations. By John Errichsen, Professor of Surgery, &c., in University College, London, &c. Philadelphia: Blanchard & Lea. 1859.

The present is an improved American edition, from the latest revision and enlargement by the author. The high character attained by the former issue of this book will be enhanced by the present issue, which is superior in every respect. Its typography is super-excellent, and the engravings, numbering more than 400, are admirably executed. It cannot be necessary to say more than that no surgical student should be without this new edition.

A PRACTICAL TREATISE ON THE DISEASES OF CHILDREN. By D. Francis Condie, M.D., &c. Philadelphia: Blanchard & Lea. 1858.

The success of this standard book, for such it is long destined to be, is a sufficient guarantee of its merits. A fifth edition has now been demanded, and the author has availed himself of the opportunity thus afforded to revise, enlarge, and improve it by extensive additions, which will be found pertinent and valuable, embodying everything recent in this department, whether at home or abroad. The publishers have done their part well in the issue of this beautiful volume.

FAVORITE PRESCRIPTIONS FROM AMERICAN PRACTITIONERS. By Horace Green, M.D., LL.D., President and Professor of the N. Y. Medical College, &c. New York: Wiley & Halsted. 1859.

This is one of a class of books of which we retain the opinion heretofore expressed, that they are neither meritorious nor useful. The apothecaries loudly complain of these prescriptions being numbered from 1 to 263, and so ordered; which they denounce as a ruse to make them buy the book, which could not have been intended by the author.

A TREATISE ON THE VENEREAL DISEASE. By John Hunter, F.R.S., with copious additions by Dr. Philip Ricord, of Paris. Translated and edited, with notes, by F. J. Bumstead, M.D., &c., of New York. Philadelphia: Blanchard & Lea. 1859.

This is the second edition, revised, of a work to which we have heretofore referred. Both Hunter and Ricord are recognized as authorities in this department, and the translator has aimed to do them both justice; and has included the recent lectures of Ricord on Chancres. We fancy that our syphilitic literature is now sufficiently extensive, and cannot subscribe to all that is now taught by recent writers, who are multiplying theories and trying experiments, the animus and the morale of which are at least questionable. This work, however, will be found to comprise everything really worth knowing on the subject, and as such we commend it to students.

LECTURES ON THE DISEASES OF WOMEN. By Charles West, M.D., &c. Part II. Diseases of the Ovaries, Vagina, Bladder and External Organs. Philadelphia: Blanchard & Lea. 1859.

Those who have read Part I. of these lectures will welcome the completion of the author's work by the issue of this volume. Nor will they be disappointed in the interesting and practical manner in which all the subjects are treated. We heartily recommend the book to both physicians and students, who cannot rise from its perusal without profit.

LINDSAY & BLAKISTON's DIARY AND MEMORANDA FOR 1859 reached us too late to repeat, at the beginning of the year, our high sense of its value to practitioners, founded on its constant use for many years. In none of the rival publications we have seen is there any claim to improvement. They are all but awkward imitations, and some of them encumbered with trash and quackery.

[We insert the following critique from the last number of the N. O. Medical News and Hospital Gazette, in proof that we are not alone in the views we have expressed in our last, of the books of Dr. Bigelow and Dr. Forbes. From other sources, including some of the ablest professional men in the country, we have received personal assurances of their approval of our criticisms.]

BRIEF EXPOSITIONS OF RATIONAL MEDICINE: to which is prefixed THE PARADISE OF DOCTORS—A Fable. By Jacob Bigelow, M.D., late President of the Massachusetts Medical Society, etc. Boston. 1858.

When we very recently noticed the receipt of Sir John Forbes' late book, entitled "Nature and Art in the Cure of Diseases," and, in the mildest terms we could, put our condemnation on it, we were in hopes that we should never again be called on to read a book, from a respectable source, so little calculated to do any good and so eminently calculated to do harm; so far from expecting to find a single respectable endorser of such a work, we have looked, with confidence, for nought but terms of condemnation from the pen of any and every respectable medical man who should deign to notice the book at all.

Who is Sir John Forbes? and what has he done? We will only detain the reader with answers almost as short as the questions themselves. Sir John Forbes is "Fellow of the Royal College of Physicians, London, and Physician of the Queen's household, etc., etc." Sir John Forbes has been a regular practitioner of medicine for fifty years, has amassed a princely fortune by practicing as other physicians do, and now issues a book to inform the world that art can effect nothing in the cure of disease—that nature does the whole work. Comment is scarcely necessary. To have maintained his position in the Queen's household he must have practiced medicine legitimately—he must have aided those who were really sick with the known useful appliances of our art: he must have given purgatives to overcome constipation, emetics to unload the stomach, quinine to prevent paroxysms of intermittent fever, etc., etc., etc., etc.; and he must have vaccinated to prevent small-pox. If he administered these and many other known useful remedies, without believing in their efficacy, then was he receiving princely pay for the grossest deception; if he administered bread pills in their stead, and clandestinely, then was he not only guilty of the same offence, but he should be despised for not having the moral courage to have come out long ago and proclaimed the views he now sets forth. We can only reconcile his conduct with his dotage; we are bound to presume that his proper position is beside the venerable Prof. Hare, who in his old age fell a victim to the miserable humbug, Spiritualism.

But in Dr. Jacob Bigelow, of Boston, we now find a champion of Sir John Forbes. He, too, writes a little book, (a very small one,) in which he endorses all that his oracle has said, and prefixes a fable, "The Paradise of Doctors." Shade of Æsop! come to the assistance of the modern fable writer. In the name of science and common sense, give him a theme, and then invigorate his pen.

To read these little books of Sir John Forbes and Dr. Bigelow, one would suppose that they were the only "rational" medical men in the civilized world. They tell us of "Artificial" doctors, "Expectant" doctors, "Homœopathic" doctors, "Exclusive" doctors, "Hydropathic" doctors, and, lastly, "Rational" doctors. All those who read their books must belong to one or another of the five first named; while *they* are, *par excellance*, the "rational" doctors. We look around us and find that the course pursued by respectable medical men is about as "rational" as the frailties of the human mind will admit—that no conscientious and well-informed man is solely the one or the other—that every such man sifts from each all that is good, and eschews all that he deems evil, and yet all are irrational practitioners, and the bright day of "rational medicine" is just dawning in Boston and London. Sir John Forbes and Dr. Bigelow had better, old as they are, study human nature a little farther; they will surely find that, although the tendency of man is to run into extremes, there is a conservative balance ever existing, and the march of science and art is onward—the march of medicine is onward. Thus far they have lived long lives to little purpose, outside the little circle of self; and now they are establishing the unenviable reputation, at least with their professional brethren, of having long practiced an art, the utility of which they only ignore when they are looking into their graves—or, when they no longer need the bread and meat and raiment which the practice brings.

The North American Medical Reporter. Edited by W. Elmer, M.D.

This is the title of a new journal published by W. A. Townsend & Co., New York, the publishers of Braithwaite's Retrospect. It is to be regretted that a journal which is evidently designed to be issued in a kind of connection with such a work as Braithwaite's should not take a more dignified position than the one before us. It is designed to present an index of the interesting articles which appear in the various periodicals to which it has access; so far it is good; but in addition, even the first number, which it would be policy to keep free from everything objectionable, we regret to say, contains many things which the regular profession cannot but condemn. We should not have mentioned this publication, had it appeared under the guise of an eclectic or homœopathic journal; but the position which it aspires to assume, the circulation which it hopes to obtain among the regular profession, and especially its apparent connection with the reprint of Braithwaite's Retrospect, make it necessary for us to speak of its claims on the profession. A journal which contains a favorable notice of "The American Family Physician or Domestic Guide to Health," by John King, M.D., Professor of Obstetrics and Diseases of Women and Children in the *Eclectic* College of Medicine, Cincinnati; and the "Pronouncing Medical Lexicon," by C. H. Cleaveland, M.D., Professor in the same institution, cannot demand our support or sanction. We say nothing of an editorial article which reads as though it had been copied from the advertising sheet of a daily paper, announcing a new hair invigorator, the formula "to be found in a subsequent part of this number, which constitutes one of the best if not the only *rational* preparation for restoring the hair to its original or healthful condition." These are undignified and unprofessional, and we cannot commend a publication which, like this, either panders to the interests of an eclectic, or the discoverer of a hair wash, or puts himself on a level with them, and endorses their opinions.—*Buffalo Med. Journ.*

[We adopt the following from our contemporary at Richmond, in lieu of the notice we had prepared, because better than anything we could write, and too good to be lost.—Ed. Gaz.]

CONCENTRATED ORGANIC MEDICINES. A Practical Exposition of their Therapeutic Properties and Clinical Employments, &c., &c. By GROVER COE, M.D. Published by B. Keith & Co. New York. 1858.

Imagine for a moment the feeling of hopeless depression with which the student, fresh from the tedious pages of "Pareira" or "the Dispensatory," will undertake the perusal of this work. After all his patient labors, he finds himself face to face with an entirely new set of remedies, "*the combined proximate medicinal extracts;*" and his flesh quails at the formidable catalogue before him. Nearly *one* hundred of these "organic medicines," all rejoicing in sonorous names, present themselves to his astonished view for the first time, and his brain is bewildered with the polysyllabic music of the hamamelin, caulophyllin, the cypripedin, or the menispermin, running up and down the alphabetic gamut, from amphelopsin to xanthoxylin.

Soon, however, will this sadness be turned to joy, as the investigation proceeds; and he who began with a sinking heart, will presently cry out, Eureka —no more difficulty now—no more misgivings about the method of treatment. Dr. Grover Coe has written a book, and B. Keith & Co. have published it.

And here let us perform that always pleasant duty, of bestowing praise when it is justly merited. On the authority of Dr. Grover Coe, we can state that, but for the liberality of the enterprising publishers, B. Keith & Co., this valuable production might never have seen the light! Nay, we can go farther. "To this enterprising firm we owe all of these inestimable organic medicines. They have invented them in their laboratory," 590 Houston Street. Mr. B. Keith has for six years been "testing in clinical practice these preparations, which his scientific skill had succeeded in bringing to a state as near perfection as possible;" and indeed "to this gentleman and his colaborers in the field of organic chemistry belong the credit (for which they now want the cash) of being the first to discover, describe, and introduce to the profession all but two of the concentrated preparations enumerated in this work"—p. 110.

Not only has Mr. B. Keith prepared and made ready these invincible specifics, thoroughly tested in practice by himself and his author, Dr. Grover Coe, but the latter individual has, in this book of four hundred pages, brought together a mass of evidence in favor of the organic extracts when used in the treatment of incurable diseases, which we may safely say is unparalleled.*

After so much to praise, we regret to find a serious and glaring cause of complaint. Our duty as critics compel us, however, to speak. There are two portraits in this book—one of "Yours respectfully, B. Keith;" the other, of "Very respectfully yours, &c., Grover Coe." Of the first we must say, that after the philanthropic labors in the laboratory, 590 Houston Street, for the good of humanity—after in *six years* doing more than all the rest of the world in twenty centuries, we *must* say that it is a disgrace to see this great and good man LIBELED in this atrocious manner. Why, reader, if you were to meet a passenger in an omnibus with such a face as this *falsely* called "Yours respectfully, B. Keith," you would instantly put your hand on your pocket book. We don't

*As an evidence of the wonderful nerve of the author, see the following "extract" from his preface: "Some few typographical errors have undoubtedly crept in, consequent upon family afflictions and professional cares, *by which our attention has been much diverted.*"

care who did it. A man in New York named Orr, says *he did it*, but we never, never will believe that this is anything like the great originator of the concentrated organic medicines.

Let us turn for a moment to " Very respectfully, &c., Grover Coe." It can't be like that gentleman. Where is the laughing face, " diverted with typographical errors and family afflictions." It is impossible to believe that one who has found out (in the laboratory of B. Keith & Co.) a certain cure for all diseases ever sported *such a beard*. Cross Tom. Hyer upon the Benicia boy, and the attempt would be a failure. But we can't speak of these *shameful caricatures* as they deserve.

In this book, then, reader, you will find *the remedy* for every disease! All that you have to do is to write to B. Keith & Co. (e), and you are ready for action. "The indomitable energy and skill of this firm" have surmounted all obstacles. Take the gelsemin, for instance—" fevers of almost every type may be controlled in from *six* to *eighteen* hours." But B. Keith & Co. (e) have a great many other extracts to sell you; and the more you mix them the better they are. So put with gelsemin, podephyllin and euphorbin, and rheumatism stands no chance. Add leptandin, pneumonia vanishes; but for a scarlet fever, don't forget asclepin. Female disorders, however, require to be added caulophyllin, viburin, corhein and cerasin.

. All that we have said, however, fades into insignificance, when we approach the invincible *veratrin*. Here our author, who truly says in his preface that he had " not sought to charm the sense by elegance of diction," surpasses himself. It cures every ill to which flesh is heir, and even is successfully employed in the removal of *pin worms from the rectum.*

" Its positive, yet kindly control of the heart and arterial system—by means of which we may say to the turbulent currents of the blood, 'peace, be still'— constitutes it a *sine qua non* in the treatment of febrile diseases." And lastly— oh! ignorant pretenders and deluded followers of the healing art—throw away your calomel vials, burn down the drug stores, and send an order to B. Keith & Co. (e) for the true elixer of life. Give it to your patient, " and you can truly pronounce him *well. when he is discharged*—no ptyalism; no loosening of the teeth; no sloughing of the soft parts; no lesions of the mucous membranes or other tissues; no morbid discharges from the eyes or ears, as is frequently the case in scarlatina and measles; no troublesome eczema to harass the weary sufferer; no barometric pains to announce approaching meteoric changes; no fœtid ulcers discharging their filthy ooze from fountains of corrupt and stagnated se- ᐧcretions within; but a system renovated and invigorated—the vital currents *leaping* in LIVING JOY through their unobstructed channels—the unfettered nerves *harmoniously* obedient to the mandates of the organic intelligence, and the *rose of health* blooming in grateful acknowledgment over the INTEGRITY of the SOUL'S CITADEL."†—*Va. Med. Journ.*

---

* "FIVE to TEN drops in THREE or FOUR ounces of water" have been used, but Dr. Grover Coe says that *he* would prefer it mixed with a "*thin mucilage of slippery elm* or a *solution of molasses and water;*" and we agree with him most decidedly.

† As another evidence of the power of these organics, see p. 246, where, by a combination of lobelia and podophyllin, Dr. Coe removed from the stomach of a child eight months old, *one and a half pint of solid casein*. When we recollect that for this proportion of casein, the stomach must have also taken in 1¼ pint of butter, 1½ pint of sugar of milk, and about *thirty pints of water*, besides various salts, can we hesitate to confess the value of the remedy? Our author, in this case, considered the "so-called congestion of brain to be nothing but acrid ingesta in the alimentary canal;" and we say he was *right*.

Synopsis of Contributions to the Physiology of Digestion.

By Prof. W. Busch, of Bonn.

Collaborated by Louis Bauer, M.D., M.R.C.S.,Eng.; Surg. to the L. I. College Hospital, Brooklyn, &c.

With the aid of experiment, the physiology of digestion has been elaborated beyond anticipation; yet doubts are still entertained whether experiments upon the higher mammalia permit conclusive inferences to be drawn upon the digestive functions in man. For this reason the contributions of the talented professor of surgery at the University of Bonn, as contained in the recent number of Virchow's Archives of Pathological Anatomy and Physiology, (Vol. xiv., No. 2,) will be received with great satisfaction, having had the rare opportunity of testing upon human digestion the various views on that process hitherto entertained.

A woman, thirty-one years of age, was introduced to the professor, who, from injuries received, presented fistulous openings, which completely separated the superior portion of the intestinal track (stomach, duodenum and a short fragment of the jejunum) from the lower one.

As not the least communication existed between the two portions, and as the alimentary contents of the stomach and duodenum, conjointly with the gastric, enteric and pancreati csuccus and bile, were discharged separately, from the contents and secretions of the lower portion, a series of experiments could thus be instituted that were well calculated to throw light upon some obscure points in the physiology of digestion, whilst it affirms others, thus converting hypothesis into established facts.

The woman in question was in her sixth month with her fourth child, when she was assailed by a bull. One horn lacerated her abdominal parieties, midway between the pubic symphysis and umbilicus, whilst the other caused but a trifling ecchymosis. The wound (in the parieties) was five inches in length, and transversely to the mesian line of the body. The prolapsed intestines seemed not to be injured. They were replaced, and the wound closed by sutures.

During the subsequent three days the patient passed one alvine evacuation, and felt comparatively comfortable; but then violent pains commenced, the wound reopened, stools became obstructed, and, with increased pain and suffering, food and fæces forced their way through the opening. A week after, the patient was prematurely confined with a still-born child.

7

Although the pains very soon after entirely subsided, and although a most ravenous appetite set in, yet the patient became so rapidly reduced in flesh and strength, that her relatives decided upon her removal to Bonn. It appears from collateral statement, that the intestinal track had not been injured at first, but had subsequently become inflamed and sloughed.

When Professor Busch first saw the patient, she had the appearance of a woman double her age, presenting a rare degree of emaciation, without the slightest trace of fat. The epiphyses of the bones were everywhere prominent, and the muscles attached flabby, relaxed, and seemingly atrophied. It hardly needs mentioning, that the patient was equally debilitated and prostrate; that she had scarcely strength enough to move her lips, and that her expression of countenance was that of profound indifference and indolence. Pulse rarely exceeded 50, and was of small, empty, thready calibre; respiration correspondingly rare (10 to 12 in a minute,) and superficial, with a weak, hoarse and toneless voice.

On examining the abdominal parieties, which were drawn towards the spine and excavated, an oval distension presented itself, about midway between the pubic symphysis and umbilicus, similar to abdominal hernia. On the lower half of said projection there was a cutaneous defect of about one and a half inches, with two openings, a left and superior and a right and inferior one. The finger, or a middle-sized elastic tube, could easily enter the former, from which a yellowish liquid issued, occasionally mixed with fragments of food. The latter was surrounded by a prolapsed ring of mucous membrane, which also admitted the finger, but only for a short distance, where a valve or stricture stayed its progress. Dilatation soon overcame the difficulty, so that no further interruption existed between that opening and the anus.

From this pathological condition, it follows that there was a perfect artificial anus of the intestine, which had no communication whatsoever with the lower portion of the track.

The seat of the superior fistula close to the umbilicus, the density of Kerkring's connivent valves, and the liquid state of chyme with unaltered fragments of food, rendered it highly probable that it connected not only with the smaller intestine, but that its connection could not be far from the diverticulo Vateri. This supposition was still more strengthened by the fact, that in the morning, and prior to breakfast, the bile discharged was green as grass, whilst that color was not met with in a lower portion of the bowels; and still more by the rapid waste of the patient, despite of rapacity for, and abundance of aliments consumed.

Unfortunately, the patient's weight was not ascertained when admitted to the University Hospital, but her emaciation may be imagined by comparison, for after considerable improvement of nutrition, she weighed, eight weeks after, no more than 68 lbs. 2 oz.; whereas, thirteen weeks after, she weighed 75 lbs.; and twenty-one weeks after, 85 lbs.

An operation, purposing to connect the two fragments of the intestinal tube, was, of course, out of the question at that juncture, and the whole attention was directed upon leading the contents of the upper portion into the lower by artificial means. But, failing repeatedly in that attempt with various appliances, another course of feeding the patient was determined on and followed up successfully. At first protein substances were injected into the lower opening, alternately with amylaceous, and subsequently eggs and meats were stuffed in by the finger. The result was most surprising, and admitted no comparison with the previously adopted feeding through the mouth. Although there was not commensurate increase of the volume of the patient, yet the muscles manifested more tone, the features lost their death-like expression, the eyes became bright, the voice returned, and the patient could sit up in the erect posture.

After the patient had acquired a certain degree of strength and weight, the food was taken through the mouth, which almost sufficed to maintain nutrition, needing but rare additional support through the lower portion of the intestine.

Professor Busch had thus ample time and scope for his digestive experiments and observation, which the following will illustrate:

1. *Consequences of Wear and Tear with Deficient Assimilation.*

When the patient entered the hospital, the immediate effects of the injuries received had passed off, and her morbid appearances were solely attributable to the immense loss of digestive fluids, amounting to several pounds a day, without adequate supply. Bidder and Schmidt observed the same effects in dogs, with artificial fistulæ of the small intestine. The disappearance of fat; the sequent loss of muscular strength; somnolence and decrease of temperature, are well-known facts. The latter is, however, but subjective, and not confirmed by the thermometer. With the progressive improvement of the patient, she became more comfortable and wakeful. When her prostration was greatest, her time was actually divided between eating and sleeping; but at a later period she required no more sleep than a healthy individual. Hoarseness and voicelessness had no other cause than inanition; for when, at a later period, the closure of the fistula was attempted, and the patient voluntarily abstained from taking any food for several days, in order not to disturb the healing process, both returned to a certain extent for the time being. Vox cholerica may be ascribed to an analogous cause.

Highly interesting were the statements of the patient as to sensation of hunger. She devoured incredible quantities of food, and for a length of time; while still eating, the food first taken would make its appearance in the superior fistula, and, on being questioned, she would state that, although feeling better, her strong desire for food was not satiated. In fact, though her stomach might be filled, she nevertheless felt an irresistible desire for aliments, being of course materially increased by abstinence.

The case was decidedly most favorable as to the physiological character of hunger, the two factors of which were clearly discernible, viz., that general sensation, originating with the extreme want of supply, and that appertaining to the emptiness of the first passages themselves. The latter could be temporarily satisfied; the former did not subside before the supply had somewhat restored the balance with the continuous waste and drainage. Another proof of the dualism of hunger was rendered by the observation that the stuffing of the lower section of the intestinal tube reduced the hungry feeling more effectually and permanently than the continuous reception of food by the stomach.

2. *Peristaltic Motion.*

The entire absence of adipose tissue, and the extreme attenuation of the skin in general, would have enabled the observer to watch and to follow the peristaltic movements of the bowels. But this case was still more favorable for such observations, by the co-existence of abdominal hernia and the direct exposure of a portion of the entrails.

Under ordinary circumstances the peristaltic motions were uniform in all parts of the bowels; but when, as it occasionally happened, a prolapsed invagination took place through the superior fistula, the invaginated portion would move vehemently until retracted, and sometimes tonic spasms would befall it so as to be hard and erect. This, however, only happened when the prolapse measured more than two inches.

According to Ludwig's and Schwarzenberg's observations, the peristaltic motions are periodical, alternating with perfect rest of the intestines, and this was found to be correct in the case of Prof. Busch. The latter saw, oftentimes, during 10–15 minutes, not the slightest alteration in the calibre of the bowels. Nor could he find that the difference of temperature, or a moderate mechanical stimulus (for instance, the introduction of a finger) made any difference. Nay, even food did not always disturb the quietude. The same would, however, suffice to increase or rather accelerate the peristaltic actions. Moreover, the latter could be observed early in the morning, before the patient had taken food, showing a certain independence of external influences. During night rest seemed to supervene, when also the discharge ceased from the superior section, commencing again at 4 or 5 o'clock, A.M. Light food, taken late, would entirely escape before night; heavier victuals would eliminate in part, and the rest in the morning. Sleep or waking made no difference at any time. The respective contents of the intestines are not propelled in a continuous column, but with interruption. Substantial food would be pressed out like part of a soft sausage; liquids would issue briskly forth, and then a pause would ensue, and so on. If not attributable to the adhesion of the bowels to the abdominal parieties, gotten up for the purpose of freeing itself, and consequently connected with the morbid condition of the patient, there is also a longitudinal locomotion of the intestinal track. For the peristaltic movement is not exclusively circular, but also longitudinal, and has been clearly observed so in the present instance. A finger being introduced in the intestinal tube, the latter would close around it, and cause a sensation as if the finger was drawn deeper in. The intestine would also glide over the finger, and then contract to expel the foreign body. In the expulsion of food and digestive liquids the same could be observed in the periodical protrusion and retraction of the mucous membrane through the superior fistulous opening.

The experiments of Ludwig and Schwarzenberg upon dogs, as to the direction of the peristaltic motion, tending to show that it is invariably towards the anus, could not be confirmed in Prof. Busch's case, the lower section of the intestinal tube being repeatedly observed to move anti-peristaltically, and disturb thereby the experiments in progress. Thus not only food, hours and days after being taken, was returned from the inferior opening, but also a gauze bag filled with articles of food, and deeply introduced. Soon after the dilatation of the lower fistula, mucus was ordinarily thrown out by regurgitation.

The various experiments instituted, with a view to ascertain the exact amount of the propelling powers of the peristaltic action, had to contend with considerable difficulties, the want of a proper apparatus, and its fastening within, or to the intestine, being the chief ones.

A glass tube was bent in appropriate angles and intimately connected with two small funnels, one to surround hermetically the superior fistula, and the other to be used as a recipient of water or any other fluid. This apparatus being applied and filled with cold water, produced at first contraction and firm closure of the opening; but after a while it relaxed, when the water descended, and disappeared within the fistula. The repeated contraction, and relaxations of the entrail, thus raised and lowered the column of water in the glass tube. Gradually more water was added, so as to form a column 24″ in height. ·The pressure of the intestine upon its contents was amply sufficient to counterbalance it, (that is, a vertical column of water 24″ high,) nay, raising it even beyond its original level, and conjointly forcing out some alimentary contents.

Much beyond a column of water of the stated height the intestine could not balance, and though it acted with great vehemence, yet it could not prevent the water escaping into the artificial anus.

This experiment, however inefficient, tends nevertheless to prove:

1st. That during the peristaltic action the walls of the intestines come in so close contact as to prevent the entrance of water.

2d. That the strength of the peristaltic action is amply proportioned to the pressure of a column of water 24 inches in height.

Again, a strong glass tube closed on one hand, and filled with 12 ounces of hydrargyrum vivum, was inserted in an acute angle to the horizon, and likewise propelled with great ease. Still other experiments were contemplated to measure the peristaltic force more accurately, but the patient objecting, they had to be abandoned.

3. *Succus Entericus.*

Its quantity is yet in dispute. Frerichs separated a portion of small intestine by ligature, and after a while it was filled with alkaline liquid. Bidder and Schmidt, however, state that the enteric juice just suffices to moisten the surface. The observations of Prof. Busch confirm the latter. By introducing a two-leafed speculum into the lower opening, a part of the mucous membrane became thus exposed. The surface, either pale or rose-colored, presented at no time an abundance of secretion; nay, there was mostly not sufficient to moisten a stripe of litmus paper, if not left for a great while. Again, cane sugar brought into the lower opening in a gauze bag was, after 15 minutes' exposure to the action of the enteric juice, not entirely dissolved. Hence it seems that this digestive fluid under physiological conditions is secreted, but in moderate quantity, and that its averted abundance is attributable either to bile, gastric and pancreatic juices admixed, or to a morbid state. Mechanical irritation of the mucous membrane repeatedly augmented and deteriorated the enteric juice, converting it into a thick viscid substance not unlike the nasal mucus. The fluctuating consistency of enteric juice justifies the supposition that there is a difference in the proportion of fixed and liquid constituents. Bidder and Schmidt estimate the former at $1\frac{1}{2}$ per cent. Busch has observed them to be as high as 7.04, and as low as 3.87, therefore an average of 5.47 solids.

Chemical reaction of enteric juice was throughout alkaline.

4. Digestive Properties of Succus Entericus.

On this head the views of physiologists are almost diametrically opposed to each other. Frerichs has acquainted us with the power of this fluid to convert amylum into grape sugar, but disputes its effects upon protein substances, as asserted by Bidder and Schmidt. None of them had as good a chance in deciding the pending question more conclusively than Prof. Busch, on account of having enteric juice unadulterated, for his observations.

As the first experiment may be admitted, the feeding of the patient through the lower opening, with a diversity of nutriment, (beef tea, beer, farina soups, hard-boiled eggs, and meat.) During six weeks prior to her entering the hospital the patient had had but one alvine evacuation of the size of a chestnut, consisting probably but of mucous and epithelial cells. Subsequently she had every 24 hours a copious one of ordinary consistence, though of a grayish white color, on account of the total absence of bile. Most conspicuous was their foetid odor. Digestion seemed otherwise to be perfect, and the faeces retained no traces of nutriments taken. These facts, with the steady improvement of the patient, would seem to demonstrate the dissolving properties of enteric juice upon protein bodies.

In order to test separately the action of succus entericus upon various articles of food, they were introduced singly by means of permeable bags, whilst their respective weights were ascertained by the method of Bidder and Schmidt—that is, they were dried by 100° C., and their liquid parts evaporated prior to their insertion. After having remained in the bowel for some time they were carefully washed with distilled water, again reduced to a dry state by evaporation, and the difference of weight noted. This method gives as near as possible an accurate result; inevitable accidental losses of food may be supposed compensated by retaining some of the mucous or enteric juice, notwithstanding the subjects of experiment being washed.

5. *Action of Enteric Juice upon Protein Substances.*

All experiments instituted for the purpose of ascertaining the solving faculties of enteric juice upon protein, resulted in a positive reduction and disintegration of the test substance. Although the loss of weight was but trifling, yet that is accounted for in the first place by the test substance being retained at a certain distance from the fistulous opening, where but a small quantity of the secreted juice could act upon it, and moreover that itself was freed from water, and hence in a very concentrated state.

When the test substances were removed from the bowel, they had lost their firmness, form and color. The cubical pieces of egg had lost their corners and appeared like cheese; they crumbled in small fragments. Meat had become quite pale, and parted in rags and fibres. At the same time all presented evidences of advanced decomposition; a fœtid odor and the contact with muriatic acid would cause the rise of ammonia vapors. That the latter originated in the putrescence of the nitrogenic articles, could not be doubted, for empty bags, or one filled with powdered charcoal, and for some time inserted into the bowel, would present no similar phenomena. Nor can it be said that the exposure of organic bodies to moisture and warm temperature would have produced those marks, as none of the experiments extended over 7 hours, but some were limited to $1\frac{1}{2}$.

1. Experiment with Albumen.—1901 grains of hard-boiled albumen in a clean gauze bag, being introduced $6\frac{1}{2}$ hours, then removed, washed and dried. It weighed 189 grains. 5589 grains of the same substance was also dried in the same manner, weighed 859 grains. According to that proportion 189 grs. dry represents 1229 grs. wet, leaving a balance of 672 grs. consumed by enteric digestion. Loss, 35.085 per ct.

2. Experiment with Albumen.—2298 grains hard-boiled albumen inserted for 5½ hours, afterward washed and dried, when it weighed 312 grs. For comparison, 4194 grs. of same egg being dried showed a remnant of 0,609 grs.; consequently 312 grs. dry are equal to 2148 grs. undried albumen, showing a loss of 105 grs. or 6.05 per ct. by digestion.

Similar differences are noticed by Bidder and Schmidt.

1st Experiment with Meat.—On the 15th of January. 1605 grs. of boiled beef, in cubic pieces, were brought into the lower fistula. After 7 hours' exposure to the enteric juice it was removed and dried, when it weighed 0,528 grs. 4895 grs. of the same meat are equal to 2297 grs. when exsiccated. In that proportion, 0,528 grs. dry are equal to 1125 grs. of undried meat, and the loss sustained by digestion is therefore 0,480 grs., or 29.090 per ct.

2nd Experiment with Meat.—3754 grs. boiled beef was subjected to the same process, and after 5 hours its weight was ascertained to be 1,479 grs. dry. In a balancing experiment, 5094 grs. of same meat dried and reduced by evaporation to 2,124 grs.; a proportion from 3547 grs. to 1479, being equal to a loss of 5.03 per ct. by digestion.

6. *Action of Enteric Juice upon Starch.*

The enteric secretion acts by far more powerfully upon amylaceous substances, for the lowest per centage of loss by enteric digestion considerably exceeds the loss of protein, although variations were equally observed. In order to secure as correct a result as possible, Prof. Busch inserted the dried paste.

1st Experiment.—1286 grs. dried pap in a gauze bag, inserted for 5½ hours. When removed and perfectly dried, it weighed 0,469 grs., leaving a loss of 0,817 grs. by digestion.

2nd Experiment.—1404 grs. dried paste, after 6 hours' exposure, leave 0,863 grs.; a loss of 0,541 grs. or 38.5 per ct.

3rd Experiment.—A glass with starch water was injected, and after 48 hours an injection was made of sulphate of magnesia, producing two stools; chemico-microscopical examinations of the latter show the perfect absence of amylum bodies. Whereas iodine solves them first red, gradually changing into pale violet. In all probability the fæces contained some dextrin, though no reduction of oxyde of copper could be effected.

The solution of starch in the intestine is attained by its being con-

verted into grape sugar, and experiments to that effect showed invariably positive results under Fehling's test.

7. *Action upon Cane Sugar.*

Enteric juice does not change cane sugar.

1st Experiment.—A bag with small pieces of cane sugar was
suspended in the lower opening; 17 minutes after they were not quite
dissolved. The test gives no evidence of grape sugar, but sulphuric
acid chemically verifies cane sugar.

2nd Experiment.—Cane sugar was suspended for some hours in
the bowel; the bag when removed contained no more pieces of sugar.
Test, no grape, but cane sugar.

3d Experiment.—The bowels were cleared by a solution of Epsom
salts. In proper time a solution of ʒii. of sugar is injected, and ʒiss.
is added in 10 hours. Shortly before the latter injection, patient had
a serous stool, and soon after a second; chemical inspection of both,
slightly sour, no grape, but so much cane sugar was found that after
the liquid had been reduced by evaporation, a drop running down the
wall of the vessel would have crystals along its course. The quantitative analysis yielded more than ʒi. of cane sugar.

4th Experiment.—A very weak solution of sugar ʒii. to 600 cm.
water was injected at 4 different times. Before, the stool was carefully examined and no sugar detected. After the second injection, a
stool, in which was found, by careful proceeding, 5 grs. of cane sugar,
but no grape sugar.

Prof. Busch is inclined to believe that the previous administration
of sulphate of magnesia may have had some prejudicial influence upon
the absorbents, yet his experiments clearly demonstrate that cane
sugar is not converted into grape sugar by means of enteric juice. It
should also be mentioned, that the chemico-microscopical analysis of
the urine gave no evidence of either kind of sugar.

8. *Action of Enteric Juice upon Fat.*

There being no bile or pancreatic juice in the lower section of the
intestinal track, it was a matter of great interest to ascertain what
changes, if any, fat would undergo by the mere contact with enteric
juice. For this special purpose Prof. Busch instituted the following
experiment:

During 10 days the patient received small quantities of melted butter, in all ʒiii. Unfortunately the anti-peristaltic motion ejected, at
different times, small, whitish-gray and sausage-formed substance, that

proved to be fat, mechanically mixed with mucus and epithelium, *without forming* an intimate emulsion. The quantity thus eliminated from the fistulous opening could not be fixed.

On the 10th day, the patient had the first spontaneous discharge from the rectum, being whitish, and of a highly offensive odor. When cold it seemed to be enveloped with a hard fatty substance like tallow. The rest presented itself under the microscope as consisting of amorphous and crystallized fat, freely mixed with epithelium; the entire mass reacted sour, and the smell manifested rancid acid. By repeatedly shaking the fæces with sulphuric ether and subsequent evaporation, about ℥ss. of fat could be collected.

In another experiment ℥iv. of oleum jecoris Aselli were injected at intermissions. A good deal was lost by anti-peristaltic motion. The small evacuation that ensued 14 days after, consisted of large fat drops with mucus and epithelium. About the fæces there was more than an ounce of liquid oil.

Observations upon the Superior Portion of the Alimentary Track.

It will be remembered that the left fistulous opening terminated the superior section of the intestinal track at about the beginning of the jejunum. Before breakfast, synchronistic with the peristaltic motion, a discharge of digestive fluids was observed that was rendered frothy by the atmospheric air in the intestine.

The statements of Beaumont and other observers, indicate, that food requires some considerable time before it leaves the stomach. Prof. Busch says, however, meat, eggs and vegetables appear at the opening from 15 to 30 minutes after being taken. From a large number of observations on this point, he relates, that

Boiled Eggs were discharged in . . . . . . 20, 26, 35 minutes.
" Cabbage " . . . . . .15 to 19 "
" Meat " . . . . . . .22 to 30 "
" Carrots " 12
" Potatoes " . . . . . . .15 "

A sumptuous meal required from 3 to 4 hours for its entire removal; but traces could be detected even beyond that time, and among nourishments subsequently consumed.

With evening meals it was different; but a part was discharged, and the rest next morning.

The chemical reaction of digestive fluids in the morning was always neutral; the enteric juice, however, alkaline. When mixed with food, the reaction differed so much as not to elicit any stationary rule. Although solids appeared to the eye unaltered, yet a mere touch indicated their disintegration and softening. As stated by others, the microscope revealed the muscular fibres being split lengthways and broken across; and in a greater measure, when the meat had previously been hashed so as to expose more surface.

Mixed food was always discharged with a large quantity of digestive fluids, so as to swim in it; uniform aliments and some vegetables, cabbage, turnips, carrots, and potatoes, diminished the latter considerably. Amylaceous substances were but in part converted into grape sugar; protein ones gave ordinarily no evidence of albumen, from which, however, two slight exceptions were noticed.

The digestive fluids were so intimately mixed as to render examination almost useless. But one point was decided, namely, the complete absence of saliva by the negative result upon rhodanpotassium, caused either by previous resorption or chemical appropriation. The considerable quantity of digestive fluids discharged in the morning justified the supposition, that the gastric juice supplied a large proportion, which did, however, not conform with the average amount of ashes by dry distillation, namely, 2.048 per cent., whilst gastric juice is said to furnish 3 per cent. solids.

The number of heterologous substances entering upon the composition of ordinary chyme would render any examination doubtful in result, hence the experiments had to be directed upon simple material.

1. *Cane Sugar.*

The action of gastric juice upon cane sugar is yet a question of dispute. Bouchardat contends that sugar is first to be converted into grape sugar before it is capable of being absorbed; this conversion he ascribes to the effects of gastric juice, whereas Frerichs believes that the simple solution of cane sugar is directly absorbed by the stomach.

In order to render the experiments conclusive, the patient was permitted to take no other food, on the previous day, than meat and eggs. The digestive fluids, despite the presence of bile, presented next morning *no evidence of grape sugar.* After this negative fact had been ascertained, 2 ounces of cane sugar were dissolved in 28 ounces of water, and gradually taken by the patient. Under the same precautions ʒiii. of cane sugar dissolved in a large quantity of water were at another time administered to the patient. In both instances but grape sugar was discharged from the fistulous opening, and no trace of cane sugar; proving conclusively the entire conversion of the latter into grape sugar.

2. *Fluid Albumen.*

With a view of testing the coagulability of albumen by gastric juice being still asserted by some physiologists, the patient received the albuminous portion of four eggs, diluted in water. During the following four hours a moderate quantity of an opaque sticky and alkaline fluid was discharged and collected, in which no fragment of coagulated albumen could be noticed. Part of that fluid, diluted with distilled water, was subjected to the following tests:

(*a.*) *Boiling* produces coagulation.

(*b.*) *Alcohol* precipitates numerous flakes.

(*c.*) *Nitric acid* in minimo: coagulation; being boiled, perfect solution; refrigerated, precipitates again; acid added and boiled, dissolves and remains so.

(*d.*) *Acetic acid* in minimo: no effect; boiled, coagulates; acid added, dissolves the precipitate· liquid cold, opalesces; becomes clear again on boiling.

The same results were attained by the same tests upon fresh albumen.

From the preceding it follows that albumen experiences no change by the stomach.

How much of it is absorbed by this organ could not be ascertained with any degree of certainty, on account of its being intimately mixed with mucus, bile, &c. However, some experiments were made to that effect.

In one instance the patient, having received on the evening previous *but* vegetable food, took 38 drachms raw albumen. In order to control the experiment, 349 grains of raw albumen were dried, the water free remnant amounting to 2,708 grains. The discharged fluid being collected, acidulated and boiled; the precipitate washed with water, alcohol, and ether, in order to free it as much as possible of choleviridine, bile, fat, and other foreign substance, finally dried, leaves 6,137 grains solids. In proportion with the former ℥xxii. had been absorbed, and the rest passed into the small intestine.

3. *Gummi.*

One morning the patient took ℥i. gum arabic with water. Unfortunately its entire elimination could not be waited for, because the patient was so much tortured by hunger as to demand satiation after two hours. During this time 142 cm. of a sticky, green and neutral substance had run out, in which there was *no sugar*.   15 cm. of it were diluted with water, by which it became almost transparent. With alcohol it forms a considerable white and thick precipitate. The latter being filtered and warmed with water, dissolves again, leaving but a few particles (mucus.)   The quantity of water being increased, all filtered, and in fine evaporated, the solids weigh 2,126 grains, according to which 142 cm. contain 20,126 grains of gum. It follows that within the short period of two hours about two-thirds of gum consumed had again been discharged.

In another experiment patient had taken along with soup in the morning and noon a considerable quantity of gum arabic. The same process was gone through as in the former experiment, and its result was materially confirmative.

4. *Gelatina.*

Before breakfast ʒv. of gelatina, with an addition of wine to render it palatable. Within 3½ hours a sticky neutral fluid issued from the aperture. It was carefully examined, and found that two-thirds had been absorbed.

5. *Milk.*

After taking milk a sour liquid was collected, in which small crumbs, and not large pieces of casein, as seen in children, were swimming. Being filtered, acetic acid caused some coagulation, soluble on adding acid.   In that solution Cyanoretum ferro-potassii effected opalescence, nitric, muriatic and sulphuric acids, bi-chloride of mercury, alum and alcohol produce precipitation, which precipitate would dissolve again by adding more test substance.

Examining upon sugar—positive result.

Evidently had not all casein coagulated, and in part remained solved in the fluid.

6. *Fat.*

In the morning cod-liver oil; discharge of a large quantity of fluid ensued, disproportionate with the amount of oil taken.

1st Experiment.—Ol. jecoris Aselli ʒxiv., within three hours almost ʒx. of dark gray fluid escaped.

2d Experiment.—Ol. jecoris Aselli ʒxv., in same time ʒxii. ʒvi. fluid run out.

Reaction different, mostly sour, yet occasionally alkaline; in the latter case the fat was so finely diffused as not to be noticed by the naked eye. Under the microscope, however, it appears as infinite small fat molcules. The liquid, when sour, represented as near as possible a perfect emulsion, yet some oil drops would swim on its surface. If the primarily alkaline liquid, by exposure to air and temperature, had subsequently turned sour, a part of the fat would separate and swim on the surface, as before mentioned.

7. Digestibility of Different Aliments.

To determine the digestibility of food is of so great and practical interest, that various means have been devised and employed. The case of Busch seemed to be particularly calculated of serving for such experiments.

With reference to sugar, it has already been stated that in one instance (ℨii.) the thirtieth, and in another (ℨiii.) the fifteenth part had entered the small intestines, whilst the rest had been appropriated on its way towards the fistulous aperture. As to fluid albumen, the proportions absorbed to those appearing in the jejunum are 5, 6 : 3, 2, and to gelatine about 2 : 1.

The plan adopted by Prof. Busch, of ascertaining as near as possible the relative digestibility of consumptibles was:

(a.) That in the morning a certain quantity of a certain aliment was given to the patient.

(b.) That the solids of that aliment were exactly made out by drying.

(c.) That the fluid discharged thereupon was collected until the fragments of that aliment disappeared, then weighed, filtered, and reduced to dry state by evaporation.

(d.) That its relative proportions were ascertained arithmetically.

As a matter of course, those calculations are not exact, because it is impossible to fix the amount of digestive fluid partaking in the formation of chyme, though it was duly taken in consideration that certain alimentary articles employed a larger proportion of digestive fluids than others.

1st Experiment.—Patient takes thirty-nine drams of soft-boiled eggs; 3,975 grs. contain 985 grs. solids, equal to 24.78 per cent.; the patient has consequently received 585 grs. of solids. During the experiment no drinks permitted. After four hours the evidences of albumen disappeared; the entire liquid collected within this time amounts to ℨxiii., 150 grs.; part of the fluid well stirred and dried, leave but 6.86 per cent.; another well filtered and dried, leave but 4.8 per cent.

2d Experiment.—ℨiv., ℨvss. of hashed roast veal eaten by the patient; 6,415 grs. when dried leave 2,466 grs. or 38.4 per cent. solids, equal to ℨj., ℨiv., grs. 40 of solids in the veal consumed. After three hours and forty minutes, ℨviij., ℨj. of fluid have been collected, when no further traces of meat could be noticed. Part of the liquid being filtered and dried, it shows 5.4 per cent. solids, the non-filtered leaves 7.78 per cent.

3d Experiment.—℥xvii., ℨvi. milk are drank; 26,105 grs. dried give 8.19 per cent.; in all there are 2,907 solids. In four and a half hours ℥xxii., ℨii. of a sour fluid have been collected, which being dried the filtered furnished 3.4 per cent., the non-filtered 4.08 per cent.

4th Experiment.—℥xxx., ℨvj. cabbage, cooked with fat, eaten; 15,596 grs. of it leave 1,586 grs. or 10.2 per cent., equal to ℥iij., ℨj. solids. The first pieces of cabbage discharged were almost unaltered, and but comparatively little fluid could be collected during the subsequent four hours. The latter, treated with distilled water, and well filtered, furnished 2.64 per cent. solids, the non-filtered 6.6 per cent.

5th Experiment.—℔ii., ℥ix, ℨiii. boiled carrots, eaten; 17,646 grs. contain 2,818 grs. or 1,597 solids. After four and a half hours, ℔iij., ℥ij., ℨvi. of a consistent pap is discharged; 17,985 grs. being filtered and dried, return 0,560 grs. or 3.1 per cent. solids in solution; the rest being subject to same process without filtration, return 6.4 per cent.

6th Experiment.—℔ij., ℥xii., ℨij. potato pap, prepared with broth and some fat. In 12,986 grs. of this food, 2,926 grs. or 22.5 per cent. are solids. After four and a half hours, but mere traces of potato can be observed. During that time ℔ij., ℨvi. of a thin saccharine pap has been collected; 24,029 grs. filtered and washed. In a soluble state 1,548 grs. or 6.4 per cent. of solids are found; 21,465 grs. are dried without filtration, and 10.6 per cent. are found.

The result of these and other experiments elicit:

	Proportionate weight between Aliment taken and Chyme discharged.	Proportionate weight of Solids taken, to the Solids in Chyme.	Proportionate weight of solved, to insolved Solids in Chyme.
Fat................	1·6,0	......	......
Gelatine............	1·3,675	1·0,94	......
Boiled Eggs........	1·2,73	1·0,76	1·2,3
Meat............	1·1,73	1·0,35	1·2,27
Milk...............	1·1,25	1·0,62	1·4,3
Carrots....	1·1,2	1·0,49	1·0,94
Cabbage	1·0,91	1·0,58	1·0,66
Potato	1·0,7	1·0,53	1.1,5

·. The first column of the preceding table demonstrates clearly the quantitative differences of digestive fluid required by different aliment- ary material.' Oleous and protein substances employ by far a larger quantity than vegetables.

The chyme being made poorer in solids than the aliments taken, is consequently· a higher dilution with water, the loss of which the patient had to replace by frequent drinks.

The solids introduced exceed considerably the solids discharged, despite the profuse admixture of digestive fluids; yet the comparison of the different figures in the several columns above could not be con- sidered positive, without calculating also the quantity of digestive fluids employed, (vide gelatine.) But the conclusion seems to war- rant, that meat is more digestible than eggs; carrots more than pota- toes; and the latter more than cabbage.

With a view to ascertain the difference in the appropriation of alimentary material of purely animal or mixed diet, the following ex- periments were instituted:

Consumed in twenty-four hours, were—

Beef tea, mixed with 3 eggs,	℔2	24⅝	loth.*
Two boiled eggs,	0	5⅝	"
Roast pork,	0	8½	"
Beef,	0	17⅝	"
Smoked tongue and cold roast veal,	0	18½	"
Water	℔2	2½	"
	℔6	12¹⁹	"
From the fistulous aperture discharge	5	9¼	"
Balance,	1	3¹¹	"
Urine,		28²⁷	"
Rest.		6½	"

On another occasion—

Coffee,	℔2·	1	loth.
Broth, mixed with eggs,	2	29½	"
Bread (rye bread),	0	16¼	"
Rusk, (wheat bread,)	0	8	
Meat,	0	11	
Carrots and potatoes,	1	5¾	

* 1 loth of German weight = ℥iv.

Soup (amylaceous),.........................℔1   2   loth.
Wine,..................................   0 15⅞   "
Water,.................................   1 17½   "
                                         ————————
                                         10 10⅞
From the fistula discharge,...............   7   3¾
                                         ————————
Balance   3   7⅛
Urine secreted in same period,............   14⁵₁₆
                                         ————————
Remains, ...   2 24¹¹₁₆ ..

From the first experiment may be inferred that, after deducting the urinary secretion and the discharge from the fistulous opening from the weight of food and drinks received, no balance remained sufficient to sustain the other expenditure of the body through lungs and skin; whilst the second experiment left a sufficient balance for the purposes of the organism.

Most conspicuous were the changes in the chyme of the first experiment, when compared with the beginning and termination. The discharged chyme was warm examined every three hours. At first but a liquid run out, in which crumbs of egg, meat, &c., swam; gradually the amount of digestive fluid decreased in the same ratio as the solids increased, so that, particularly in the morning, a consistent pap eliminated from the opening, looking and smelling like fresh meat, without being even colored by biliciridrose. In the latter experiment the chyme remained fluid throughout, with an exception at noon, when it became for a short while more consistent.

8. *The Solving Power of Digestive Fluid.*

On filtering the chymes in which fragments of egg or meat were suspended, it was noticed that their solution proceeded in the open air without putrescence, and that but a small quantity remained undissolved upon the filterer. This took place, whether the digestive liquids were neutral or alkaline. All those protein substances having for a time been exposed to the exclusive action of gastric juice, it became a point of interest to learn how much of fish, egg or meat might be dissolved by the conjoint action of all digestive fluids; and for this purpose the following experiments were undertaken:

1st Experiment.—After the taking of raw albumen, the alkaline reacting liquid was collected, and 910 grs. of boiled albumen suspended in a gauze bag, part of the latter having previously been dried, and its solids fixed upon, 15.3 per cent. After six hours' exposure, the cubic-shaped pieces had lost their contours, and showed a tendency of dissolving in small particles and flakes. They had in weight, collectively, lost 41 grs. (This artificial digestion had been effected in low temperature, to avoid fermentation.)

2d Experiment.—The patient having previously consumed some meat, the liquid portion of discharged chyme, being neutral, was mixed with 1,648 grs. of cold roast veal, cut in square pieces, and placed for twenty hours in a cold room. At the termination of the experiment, no putrescence; the surface of the meat is very soft and imbued by biline liquid. The examination elicited a loss of 555 grs. of meat.

It is obvious that the neutral, and even alkaline mixture of digestive fluids, retain their digestive powers upon protein substances without the body, although not in the same degree; and the exterior juice being also endowed with digestive properties, it seems to be conclusive, that the gastric digestion is the prominent one, and the other merely supplementary.

9. *Quantity of Digestive Fluids.*

The patient received for 12 hours but $2\frac{1}{4}$ lbs. of black rye bread and water at pleasure. The first chyme was neutral; the latter sour. A good quantity of tolerably consistent bread chyme was discharged before the clear, digestive fluid appeared. The entire liquid collected during 24 hours amounted to 5 lb. $21\frac{1}{8}$ loth. After deducting the weight of the bread it would leave a fluid balance of 3 lb. $5\frac{1}{8}$ loth. Yet this calculation is considerably altered by the fact that the bread contained $42\frac{88}{100}$ loth, (21 oz.,) whilst the entire discharge contains but about 1 lb. of solids, including the uncountable solids of the digestive fluids. Dr. Busch assumes that about 4 lbs. of digestive fluids have been expended in the experiment, which was the seventeenth part of the entire weight of the body, (68 lbs.)

Prof. Busch summons up the results of his experiments as follows.

1. Hunger is constituted by two sensations; the first is represented by the nervous system in general, and derived from the impoverished condition of the tissues; the second originates with the nerves of the digestive organs, indicating their emptiness. The former is removed only by the required assimilation of nutritive elements, and not by merely filling the first passages.

2. The peristaltic motion of the intestines takes place with the same

power within the abdominal cavity as when exposed to the atmospheric air.   Its propelling power equals a column of water 24 inches high.

3. The alimentary canal has its periods of rest and action.

4 The quantity of enteric juice secreted is invariably small, and of alkaline reaction.   Its percentage of solids averages 5.47.

5. Enteric juice is capable of digesting amylaceous and protein substances.

6. Enteric juice converts starch into grape sugar.

7. Enteric juice prepares protein substances for assimilation under the phenomena of putrescence.

8. Enteric juice leaves cane sugar unchanged.

9. Cane sugar, absorbed as such, is not discharged in the urine.

10. Fat, unless exposed to the action of bile or pancreatic juice, is absorbed either not at all or in insignificant quantity.

11. Food appears between 15 and 30 minutes after being taken in the superior third of the thin intestine.

12 Solution of cane sugar disappears in part before entering the small intestine; all that enters the latter is converted into grape sugar.

13. Raw albumen taken from hens' eggs is directly absorbed in the stomach and the adjoining portion of the small intestine.   All that descends to the lower portion of the latter is unchanged.

14. Gum is not converted into sugar, but remains unchanged.

15. Gelatine is dissolved, and loses thereby its coagulability.

16. Casein remains partly dissolved in the digestive fluids.

17. Fat is entirely emulgated by the digestive fluids when alkaline or neutral, but partially when acid.

18. The digestive liquids of the small intestines possess digestive powers over protein substances.

19. The minimum of all digestive fluids entering the small intestine in the course of 24 hours, amounts to more than the seventeenth part of the weight of the body.

SELECTIONS.

[From the Journal of Practical Medicine and Surgery, of Paris.]

On immediate Straightening and Cauterization under Starch Bandages in the Treatment of White Swellings.—Utility of Chloroform in discriminating between Muscular Contraction and Coxalgia.—Croup: Cutaneous Anæsthesia: Tubing of the Glottis substituted for Tracheotomy.

A communication made to the Academy of Sciences, by Dr. Bonnet of Lyons, on the treatment of white swellings by instantaneous straightening, has, in latter times, created a very lively sensation in the medical world.

In many diseases of the joints, says Dr. Bonnet, articular lesions coexist with deviations and incomplete luxations. Prudence sometimes points out the propriety of not interfering with these mal-formations, but it is often requisite to replace the limb in its proper direction. Now, when straightening is necessary, there are two modes of effecting it; immediate straightening by forcible extension, and slow and gradual straightening by machinery. Great experience in both, which he has compared, has proved to Mr. Bonnet the superiority of the former of these modes over the latter.

Dr. Bonnet already proclaimed, seven years since, its excellency in coxalgia attended with fibrous adhesions. This surgeon now shows that in all deformities without organic lesion, or coexistent with rheumatic, or scrofulous white swelling in progress of increase, or resolution, the mode of straightening to be preferred is that which requires but one operation, followed by protracted immobilization for several weeks.

The essential and general rule to be followed in such cases is, first to loosen the articulation during artificial anæsthesia, and to restore its mobility completely. This may be accomplished by an alternate series of gentle flexions and extensions, graduated and carried to the extreme limit of the natural movements. The adhesions being destroyed and mobility restored, the straightening of the deformity and the reduction of the displacement may be proceeded with. Proper tractions and pressure are then sufficient, and success is in proportion to the mobility obtained.

When the limb operated on has resumed the best possible direction, nothing further is required but to fix it in its new position with all due precaution, in order to prevent or attenuate the consequent pains. Grooves constructed with annealed iron wire, properly lined, may be employed for this purpose. But these grooves are not indispensable, and, in Dr. Bonnet's estimation, it is preferable to use a wadded and starched pasteboard bandage. Some days ago, Mr. Bonnet applied his apparatus, in the presence of a great number of persons, at the clinical lecture of Dr. Nélaton; and we remarked the minute care with which he arranged its various parts. The surgeon first rolled round the limb thick strips of wadding, which he fixed in their places by a few turns of a linen roller; pasteboard splints impregnated with liquid starch paste were placed over it, and were in their turn covered with starch bandages of considerable length; in order to give this apparatus immediate solidity, Mr. Bonnet applied over all annealed iron-wire splints, which he prefers to Mr. Seutin's dry pasteboard ones.

Thus constituted, the starch bandage must be left in its place for three weeks or a month. At the end of that time it is removed, the diseased parts are examined, and the surgeon, by applying either a new bandage of the same nature or some other apparatus, completes the straightening, and endeavors to obviate the return of the deformity, which long preserves a great tendency to recur.

But how brilliant soever the result of the straightening may be, when viewed with reference to form, to functional aptitude, or to the rapid improvement of the inflammatory state and the removal of pain, it does not, however, directly tend to cure the disease itself. To obtain this ultimate benefit, Mr. Bonnet practises cauterization under the starch bandage.

This cauterization can be performed with caustic potash, Vienna paste, or chloride of zinc. Mr. Bonnet usually employs potash lozenges wrapped up in wadding, so that the escharotic liquid may not extend beyond the point to be acted on.

Whatever caustic may be selected, it is important that the bandage applied after cauterization should extend far enough to procure absolute immobility and a complete protecting cover. Thus, for instance, after an operation on the knee, the bandage should extend from the extremity of the foot to the pelvis, and thus render motionless the foot and even the hip. In this manner the counter-irritants act exclusively on the skin and the cellular tissue, without the local inflammation which follows the application of caustic being communicated to the diseased synovial membranes, as would happen were the limbs abandoned to their natural movements.

. Dr. Bonnet began, in the spring of 1857, cauterizations in combination with immobility and occlusion, and since that period sixty cases, referring to white swellings of the foot, knee, elbow and hip, have testified in favor of this method. In the fifteen months which have just expired, Dr. Bonnet has cured, or improved to a degree bordering on cure, three white swellings of the foot, as many of the knee, and one of the elbow, all attended with numerous abscesses proceeding from the joints, and in conditions which, according to habitual surgical practice, would have justified amputation.

We should add that, during the period of cicatrization of the cauterized parts, the limbs remain supported in grooves which, while they insure immobility, expose to view the regions which require to be dressed. At the same time, a treatment calculated to modify the general state of the patient is instituted, and during the convalescence light supports are used, which can be placed and removed at pleasure— an indispensable prop to limbs weakened by too long protracted inaction. Such is the method expounded by Dr. Bonnet, not only before the Academy of Sciences, but before the greater part of the learned societies of Paris. Several members of the Society of Surgery expressed a desire that Mr. Bonnet should state with precision the circumstances in which immediate straightening may be practised in coxalgia. Mr. Bonnet replied that for four months past he had attempted straightening eight times in that articular disease, and that he had succeeded seven times. He attributed this enormous proportion of success to the fact of having operated on subjects under fifteen years of age. Before the twelfth year, straightening, applied to coxalgia, presents chances of success so numerous as almost to amount to certainty, unless the deformation is of several years' standing, and presents many closed sinuses. Above the age of fifteen, the difficulties of straightening are extreme, particularly if the injury is of more than six months' date. The effects of counter-irritant cauterizations are then but uncertain, and deep and direct cauterizations may be attended with danger. Relatively to the circumstances of the disease being acute or chronic, Mr. Bonnet has always found that, far from being counter-indicated by the acute state, straightening and immobilization are the best means of treatment which can be opposed to the inflammatory action. In the chronic period, straightening in children is still applicable, when any traces of mobility remain. Complete anchylosis at any age and in every case is a formal counter-indication to straightening. To confute the objections raised on the subject of the inflammatory accidents, which might be induced in a diseased articulation by his operation, the skillful surgeon of Lyons had but to invoke his own experience. By resorting to methodical movements alone, by keeping up a uniform temperature around the diseased limb, by means of the thick layer of wadding with which his apparatus is provided, by rendering the limb immovable after it has been straightened, Dr. Bonnet has never had to deplore any serious accident, even when, to attain his object, he has been compelled to perform the subcutaneous section of the contracted muscles.

— We shall certainly revert to a question which promises to afford for a length of time matter for discussion at the meetings of our learned societies; but we have deemed it a duty at once to call the attention of our readers to one important result obtained by the application of Dr. Bonnet's method. We allude to the facility with which artificial anæsthesia generally enables the practitioner to discriminate between mere muscular contraction and real coxalgia.

The *Gazette des Hôpitaux* has published on this subject several interesting cases, one of which was observed in Dr. Robert's wards, at the hospital of the Hôtel Dieu in Paris.

A young woman twenty-five years of age, occupying the bed No. 8 of Saint Paul's ward, presented the last four months all the symptoms of coxalgia, viz., pain in the hip, improper attitude of the limb which was bent upon the pelvis, placed in adduction and slightly rotated inwards with consecutive deviation of the pelvis, immobility, resistance to straightening, attempts to effect which occasioned much pain, etc. Dr. Verneuil, who at present supplies the place of Dr. Robert, desirous of applying Dr. Bonnet's method in this case, had her conveyed to the operating theatre, where, previously to any operation, she inhaled chloroform. Mr. Verneuil expected that he should have to use great strength, and he had secured the co-operation of numerous assistants, when, to his surprise, the limb reduced itself, as if spontaneously, at the first efforts of the operator. It was then easy to cause the thigh to perform without the least violence the most extensive physiological movements, without experiencing any resistance whatever, and without the hand or the ear detecting the smallest amount of friction. The limb, replaced in its proper position, was maintained by means of Mr. Bonnet's apparatus.

We read on the other hand, in the *Gazette Hebdomadaire*, that, in a girl of eighteen, who had been for three years thought to be laboring under coxalgia, anæsthesia, employed for the purpose of immediate straightening, enabled Mr. Robert to ascertain the complete integrity of the coxo-femoral articulation, and to discover a muscular contraction, which was most successfully treated by walking, electricity, and general tonics.

The same journal relates another fact, well worthy·of attention. Dr. Laugier had to treat, in his wards of the Hôtel Dieu, a boy who had been suffering for three years in the right hip. The pain felt by this patient was at times so intense that for a fortnight he remained seated on the edge of the bed, with his feet resting on a chair, his thigh bent and in outward rotation.

Mr. Laugier, unable by ordinary means to relieve this child, put him under the influence of chloroform, and performed instantaneous straightening without encountering any serious difficulties; a mechanical apparatus was then applied, to render the extension permanent. The pain ceased as it were by magic, and the patient was soon able to walk with crutches.

Facts, such as these, are so much the more deserving of remark, that the muscles, as Dr. Jules Guérin has observed, play an extremely important part in coxalgia. Sometimes they are in a state of contraction, i. e., of spasm, and susceptible of immediate return to their normal length and consistency; at other times they are in a state of retraction or of organic shortening, and do not resume their physiological dimensions unless by laceration or tenotomy. This surgeon even considers muscular contraction the essential symptom, one of the earliest in coxalgia, so that it may exist without disease of the bones, as it, at times, is superadded to a morbid condition of the bones, and is then merely an accessory phenomenon. The benefit which may be derived in these various cases, from an agent that alleviates pain, enlightens diagnosis, and becomes the first element of rational therapeutics, will be readily conceived.

— Within the last six weeks more than twenty children attacked with croup have been operated on at the Saint Eugenie Hospital. The attention of the physicians of this hospital has, therefore, been much engaged in the observation of this disease, and the clinical studies, to which Dr. Bouchut in particular has devoted himself, have produced results which we deem it our duty to lay before our readers.

We would first notice the existence of a new symptom of croup, which affords an indication for tracheotomy. Since Professor Trousseau has again brought this operation into favor, the question has often been asked at what time, except that of asphyxia with suffocation, the operation should be performed on children attacked with croup. We stated, some years since, in this journal, that Dr. Trousseau was of opinion that it should not take place before the last stage of the disease had fairly set in; more recently the eminent professor has pronounced in favor of an early operation. Increasing asphyxia is with the major part of practitioners the determining consideration; but it is known that certain children die with their faces pale, without cyanosis or apnœa; in short, without any apparent traces of asphyxia. With regard to the latter, therefore, the practitioner has no indication to guide him.

Now there is, in Mr. Bouchut's estimation, a more certain sign of asphyxia, viz., *cutaneous anæsthesia.*

Whether asphyxia be *latent* or *apparent*, when the obstacle to hæmatosis has lasted for some days, and the disease is approaching a fatal termination, the skin gradually becomes insensible, and it may be pricked or cut without occasioning any pain, or at least any movement indicative of suffering. If croup requires tracheotomy, it is not rare to see children undergo the operation without manifesting the least sensibility. Dr. Créquy, formerly Dr. Barthez's house surgeon, has just published in his inaugural thesis the case of a little girl of six years of age operated on for croup, who, having recovered from the operation, declared she had felt no pain. Dr. Demarquay has similarly ascertained the existence of anæsthesia in a woman on whom tracheotomy was performed for an accidental fit of suffocation. Anæsthesia is not, therefore, an effect of diphtheritis, but of the interruption of hæmatosis, and, as experiments on animals have proved, the result of the presence of too large a proportion of carbonic acid in the blood. Now, what is the clinical importance of this phenomenon? As we have said above, it affords one indication more for the performance of tracheotomy, and this indication will be particularly useful in the case of *latent asphyxia.*

Mr. Bouchut has thus contributed to increase perhaps the favorable chances of this operation. But his ambition did not stop here, and he has recently communicated to the Academy of Medicine an idea which, already carried out with two children attacked with croup, would tend to nothing less than the suppression of tracheotomy as an ultimate resource henceforth useless.

After all the attempts made to arrive at the cure of croup by the introduction of the catheter into the larynx, Mr. Bouchut has drawn from that practice the principal of a new method, which he designates by the name of *tubing of the glottis,* and which consists in introducing and leaving for a time in this orifice a metallic ring.

The instruments he has used twice on living subjects are: 1. curved male catheter of different sizes, open at both ends, and intended to penetrate into the larynx as guides to the ring which this organ is to receive; 2. straight cylindrical silver rings, of from $\frac{1}{2}$ to $\frac{3}{4}$ of an inch long, provided at their extremities with two ridges at the distance of a quarter of an inch, and pierced with a hole for the passage of a silk thread, the function of which is to preserve a hold upon the ring from without; 3. a ring to protect the fore-finger, or an instrument destined to keep the jaws open. When provided with these instruments, Mr. Bouchut employed them first on a dead subject, and he ascertained, to his own satisfaction and that of his colleagues, that after having been introduced into the larynx, the upper edge of the ring was engaged beneath the superior vocal chord in the ventricles of the larynx; that the movements of the epiglottis and the arytænoid cartilages were not obstructed; that the inferior vocal chord placed itself between the two ridges of the canula, and consequently that it was above the lower ridge corresponding with the internal face of the cricoïd cartilage.

This being accomplished, it became necessary to apply the method on the living. An opportunity soon presented itself, but it was during the dreadful epidemic, which in the month of August sent to the Saint Eugenie Hospital fifteen cases of croup, which terminated fatally. Diphtheritis was generalized; and in addition, as Mr. Bouchut acknowledges, had the two children, on whom the *tubing* was performed, recovered, nothing positive could be concluded from the circumstance. All that can be said, and Mr. Bouchut has kindly permitted us to witness the operation, is that the tubing of the larynx is not a difficult process; that the canula remaining in the glottis for thirty-six hours was perfectly harmless; that the two children could speak distinctly, and take liquids without swallowing them the wrong way, and that there was, in every respect, a temporary improvement analogous to that which follows tracheotomy.

MEDICAL COSSACKS.

The professors of the healing art, numbering in the United States alone not less than fifty thousand, may aptly be compared to a huge army, assembled to resist the invasion of an insidious and obstinate enemy. The war is long and desperate, for the king of terrors is a foe worse than tyrant or conqueror; and hence, as we find many elements entering into the composition of on army—some for good and some for evil—the same is also the case with those who profess to defend the people from the ravages of death and disease.

The great body of the profession are the rank and file of this gallant host, who bear the brunt of the battle. They are the regiments of the line, upon whose bravery and perseverance victory depends. These are the faithful and hard-working country doctors, the general practitioner, not known to fame perhaps, and probably not remarkable either for learning or originality, but true followers of the old fathers in medicine, under whose banners they wage the war as long as health and life lasts. All honor to the humble common soldier of medicine: Others may win the renown, but he it is who does the work and deserves the laurel crown.

Ever and anon we meet with the heavy artillery of medicine— the great guns, who make loud (and long) reports, and frequently do great execution. Their fame is heard over the whole land. The celebrated surgeon and popular lecturer belongs to this class. Occasionally we have even a Paixhan or a Lancaster, who makes a tremendous noise and much smoke, but is apt to explode unexpectedly, spreading terror and dismay among surrounding groups of friends and admirers.*

The flying artillery is also deserving of mention. This branch of the service is very showy and fashionable. They rush about with extreme celerity, fire a broadside, and off again in a twinkling. They wear out a chaise in a few months, drive a horse off his legs in less time, and produce a powerful effect upon the public at least.

We must hasten on to describe the various *irregular* troops which are clustering around the main body—the voltigeurs, the lancers, and the hussars of medicine. One regiment is armed with long silver canulas, and wear in their caps, in place of a pompon, the sponge probang. These are they who carry the " nitrate crayon" into the minute ramifications of the lungs, and route the enemy in his citadel. Others march by, bearing speculums of silver, ivory or glass—are very much admired by some of the other sex, especially old nurses, who are occasionally favored with a peep at the mysteries of the " ulcerated os."

Wandering off still further from the main column, are found the hot-water quacks, who, like the inimitable Jenny Dennison at the siege of Tillietudlum, are prepared to give the enemy a warm reception. The cold-water quacks fight on the opposite principle, and believe that disease, like an old witch, can only be cured by a ducking. The homeo-quacks should not be forgotten; for while they depend mainly upon small shot, yet, like the poisoners of old, much may be done with a globule (especially if it is made of strychnia or arsenic.)

Now we have reached the outskirts of the army, and we find ourselves among the predatory hordes which always follow the column,

* May not this sometimes happen from *over-charging ?—Printer's Devil.*

and spread rapine and murder through the surrounding country. These are the Pariahs of medicine, who watch about and pick up the despairing victims of cancers, tubercles, and other incurable diseases, who, getting no comfort from the honest and truthful, are ready to clutch at anything which promises relief. For such the artful and unscrupulous Cossack eagerly seeks, promises everything they desire, fans dexterously for a time the flame of hope, robs them of their last dollar, and deserts them, to follow up another whose purse promises a better reward, and whose credulity is not exhausted. These miscreants are like the ghouls, who fatten upon the substance of dying men, and beguile with lying words the poor sufferer who falls into their hands. They are the foul blots upon a noble profession, and yet they will never be exterminated. The drowning mariner will cry out for a sail, although the pirate crew will plunder his pockets and make him walk the plank. Poor human nature instinctively shrinks from the embrace of the last dread foe, and, when all else fails him, he will run anywhere for succor.

Let us at least draw a moral from our parallel, which may be useful and instructive. The brave soldier stands by his comrade shoulder to shoulder, strikes with him his last blow, and falls with him when the charge is sounded. He observes the strictest discipline, obeys explicitly the code of martial law, and drives with scorn and contempt from his presence the plunderers and camp followers who linger about his path. Let the true-hearted members of our army imitate this example. We too have a code of honor, which tends to promote good order in our ranks. Discarding petty jealousies and impatient longings after fame or fortune, let us stand, each one supporting the other; defending his brother, protecting his reputation, and advancing his interest. Above all, turn away with unhesitating contempt from any contact with these adventurers, who will bribe you to countenance them, but for whose sake you will assuredly sacrifice the good opinion of honest men. Such a well-ordered union in our ranks would greatly increase the dignity and efficiency of the calling, and would curtail largely the domain of the irregulars, who now thrive by our dissensions and profit by our confusion.— *Virginia Med. Journ.*

QUACKERY.

We were much pleased with an editorial which appeared in the last number of the Belmont Medical Journal, on Quackery. It is undoubtedly true that there is a vast amount of ignorance and charlatanism among many of those who have had the degree of Doctor of Medicine conferred on them by Medical Colleges, and it is not surprising that the public should feel quite as much disposed to place confidence in persons who claim to possess skill in the art of healing without having a diploma, as in the graduates of Medical Institutions. Success is the only test of qualification which they can apply to Medical practitioners, and only those who are successful in the long run can expect to be entrusted with the treatment of their diseases.

Were the power of granting diplomas taken from Medical Colleges, and conferred upon a Board of Examiners appointed by the State government, who, having no interest to graduate any except those who were qualified, should examine all candidates for medical degrees as rigidly as the candidates for medical appointments in the army and navy are, this evil would be obviated, and the profession would take the rank which it ought to hold, and the title of Doctor would mean something more than that its possessor had paid lecture and graduation fees at a medical school.

There are now forty-one medical colleges in our country, all anxious to have as many students as possible, and many, we fear, less desirous of sending out well-educated physicians, than of swelling the number of names on their catalogues, and pocketing their fees. The writer of the article before alluded to remarks:

"The verriest ignoramus that we have seen for many a day, was one carrying a diploma from the principal college in New York city. How he came by it God only knows, for it must have been evident that none of the professors belonging to the college could have given a satisfactory explanation, or have signed it as a guarantee of his scientific acquirements. But by such a diploma the young man was thrown upon the world in a false position—in a position that he had necessarily to act the charlatan, and disgrace the profession. Such things are, however, not confined to New York, or Philadelphia, or Baltimore. The celebrated institutions of Europe are equally culpable ; all proceeding on the principle of ' you tickle me, and I'll tickle you.' Our readers, if they wish a comprehensive view of the subject, will do well to peruse an article on medical education, in the July number of the Westminster Review. Here is a specimen of evidence on the state of the medical profession, given before a parliamentary committee.

"Mr. Guthrie, in his evidence, says: ' I know too well that from various parts, certificates, diplomas, and all other papers, come very improperly sometimes, and that they are very often deceptive. . . . .

I do not hesitate to say, that among those attending my surgical lectures, I have, at this moment, three or four who have paid me their
money whom I have never seen; and when, last season, I called their
names over, I found them absent. They had paid their money and
walked off to the country, and had relied upon my never discovering
the fact; and at the end of the season they would have come to me
and asked for a certificate, and probably they would have got it. I
was once (?) deceived in that way, and gave a false certificate.' The
College of Surgeons, in 1834, called upon teachers to be more discriminating in giving their certificates; 'but,' says Mr. Guthrie, 'I
do not believe they have given themselves any trouble about it, either
students or teachers; and, in fact, it is not their interest so to do, unless the rule is general.' Mr. Green affirms that students are likely to
abandon any school where regular attention on lecture is enforced.
That the certificate system must generate loose notions of moral obligation in both teachers and pupils, there can, we think, be little doubt.
We heard a young man ask for a certificate of having attended a
course of lectures, not one of which he had been present at. The lecturer began to fill up the certificate, but before completing his signature he said to the student, 'Have I ever seen your face before?'
After considerable equivocation, the student admitted that he had not
attended more than one lecture. The lecturer then said that on
evidence of attending one lecture, he would sign the certificate of his
having attended the course. The student finally admitted that he
had not attended one lecture, and that he did not even know in which
quarter of the year the course was given. But he pleaded illness as
an excuse for non-attention, and having paid his hospital fees, he persisted in trying to convince the physician that if he refused the certificate, he would not only be guilty of a great unkindness, but a great
injustice! He evidently considered that in paying his fees he had actually bought the certificate, and that the lectures were given into the
bargain, to be attended or refused at his option.

"In olden times diplomas were of some account. It is not so now.
Every man, with brain not in excess of the barnacle, may buy one
with his money or some deceptious art. And what makes the title
still more discreditable is the fact, that colleges of all doctrines have
spread over our country, spewing out Eclectic, Homœopathic, Hydri-
atic and Gyneocratic M.D's, until the whole land stinks. Seeing,
then, that the cognomen is no evidence of skill in the profession,
would it not be well for the true Æsculapian to drop the title and
leave it in the hands of the mountebanks? For all purposes, a name

expressive of a person's identity is sufficient; and for character, let the scriptural rule, ' By their fruits shall ye know them,' be applied. If we must have titles, let them be such that not only scientific men, but that the vulgar also, will feel assured of the merits of the possessor."—*Maine M. and S. Reporter.*

MENSTRUATION DURING PREGNANCY.

By Dr. Elsasser.

This contribution to a disputed topic is founded upon 50 cases, extracted from the journal of the Stuttgart Lying-in Hospital—cases which are said to rest upon the most certain information. The subjects were 15 primiparæ and 36 pluriparæ, who, with the exception of two women (aged 36 and 41), were between 20 and 30 years of age. Of the 51 children born, 34 were boys and 17 girls, 36 being mature and 15 immature. The menstruation during pregnancy occurred in 50 women in the following manner: Once in 8, twice in 10, three in 12, four in 5, five in 6, eight in 5, and nine in 2. In 13 cases the peculiarities of the rhythm of the discharge were inquired into, and the rhythm was found regular in 4, in 1 it occurred at the sixth week, in 3 there were pauses between the epochs, in 2 the menstruation first appeared after the second month, in 2 after the fourth, and in 1 after the fifth month. In one case the menstruation first appeared in the middle of gestation, and henceforth came on every four weeks, lasting three or four days. The child, perceived but feebly at first, was strongly felt during the last four or five weeks. Hæmorrhage occurred twice within a week before delivery, but a mature, living infant was born. Indications as to the amount of discharge were furnished in 26 cases, and in 18 of them it was less than in the non-pregnant condition. The weight of the 35 mature infants varied from 5 lbs. to 9 lbs.

Dr. Elsasser observes that, although he is unable to state the proportion of cases in which menstruation occurs during pregnancy, it is by no means so exceptional an occurrence as supposed by some authors. It occurs more frequently in pluriparæ than in primiparæ; and it takes place much more frequently during the first half of pregnancy, and especially in the earlier months of this, than during the latter half. The amount of discharge, too, is smaller than in the normal menstruation. The duration of the pregnancy was normal in more than two-thirds of these cases (36), while in nearly one-third

(14) of the cases it was interrupted—in 4 during its first, and in 10 during its latter half. As regards the development of the child, which by some authors has been supposed to be impeded by the occurrence of menstruation, this was found to be normal, or more than normal in three-fourths of the cases.—*American Journal of the Medical Sciences.*

AN EXAMPLE

[From the Baltimore Christian Advocate of Dr. Bond.]

Patent Medicines.—We have received several applications to publish advertisements of an empirical character, all of which we have declined. To prevent such applications in future, we will now state that it is our purpose to refuse all advertisements of the kind.

We have before us an advertisement from a manufacturer of lozenges in Boston, supported by a number of commendatory extracts from papers religious and secular, which we are instructed to insert, and "print just like the copy."

In this advertisement it is stated that these lozenges will "instantly relieve" Coughs, Bronchitis, Asthma, &c. This is utterly untrue. Anybody who knows the nature of these affections, knows that the pretension to cure them by lozenges is false. To sell these lozenges to people under this pretense, is to obtain their money without equivalent, and through false representations. More than this, it is cruelty to speculate upon the necessities of the sick; to pillage those who have the strongest claim to our sympathy by abusing their confidence; and still more, it is to trifle with health and life by inducing the afflicted to postpone the use of rational means of cure, until their diseases becomes more formidable, perhaps intractable. In this abominable business we will have no participation. No pecuniary advantage can tempt us to abuse the confidence of our readers by publishing advertisements of the above description.

We do not mean to say that the proprietors and advertisers of patent and secret medicines are all as culpable as we would be if we should publish them. They may not know as much about such things as we do.

ARTIFICIAL DILATATION OF THE LARYNX IN CROUP.

Much discussion has of late taken place at Paris respecting a bold measure in croup—viz., actual catheterism of the larynx and trachea, followed by caustic injections, proposed and successfully practised by M. Loiseau, of Montmartre, near Paris. This operation is to prevent

9

the necessity of tracheotomy, and has been warmly supported by M. Trousseau, in a report presented by this physician to the Academy of Medicine. Several successful cases have been quoted: one, however, proved fatal in August last.

The Academy has very recently heard another paper on the "Dilatation of the Larynx in Croup," to render tracheotomy unnecessary. The author is M. Bouchut, an eminent hospital physician of Paris. Trials were first made on the dead body, and a silver, truncated, hollow cone, a little smaller than a common thimble, was passed into the larynx, and was felt to dilate that passage perfectly. A series of instruments were contrived by M. Bouchut for the introduction of the cone, or canula, to which a silk thread is fixed, which hangs out of the mouth. Two children, affected with diphtherite, have been operated upon by the dilator, full details being given by M. Bouchut in a paper presented to the Academy of Medicine. Although the results have not been favorable in one case, it has been proved by these operations that a hollow, truncated cone can, in the paroxysms of suffocation of diphtherite, be introduced into the larynx, and there left for several hours, to the great relief of the child. Respiration, in both cases, became perfectly tranquil after the cone was introduced, the same being subsequently removed with the greatest ease. Further trials will prove whether this method of admitting air is preferable to tracheotomy.—*Lancet*, *October 2d*, 1858.

CLINICAL INSTRUCTION—JOCOSE "CLINICS!"

We have an exalted idea of the value of true clinical teaching; and have not failed, long since, to express our views in the JOURNAL upon this important subject. Whether the instruction be strictly clinical—that is, imparted at the bed-side—or such as the material afforded daily at our Dispensary Central Offices and Hospitals, to which out-patients now come in great numbers, offers abundant opportunities to descant upon, the chances of practical information to the medical student are large and increasing. This is a privilege which we, in our student days, did not enjoy; and these are the cases which will most frequently occur to the young and inexperienced practitioner; they should, therefore, be as familiar to him as "household words." The study of the *physiognomy of disease*, only to be acquired by this personal confrontation of the student with the examples of morbid affections, and by a reiteration of observations, patiently, day by day,

is one of the chief means efficient in forming an acute and useful practitioner. We are glad to observe that much attention is paid to this
department of medical study; the Faculty of our Medical College
evince their appreciation of its value by setting apart a portion of
time from the lecture routine, to be devoted to this object.

If it is desirable—nay, essential—that students have ample opportunities for the observation and appreciation of actual cases—it is
even more so, that the teaching to which they listen should be of that
character which will impress them with the importance and the true
dignity of their profession. In the management of what are now
termed "*clinics*," much tact is required. This is true in two different
senses: first, no little share of ingenuity is often demanded in order to
elicit, from the class of patients to be found in hospitals and in dispensary practice, the information absolutely needed, in order to prescribe judiciously for their ailments. Next, it is not an easy task to
communicate information upon medical and surgical topics, in such a
manner as will at once enlist the attention, and interest the minds of
students. Too dry and circumstantial details, often repeated, and never
varied, will weary—and an occasional departure from the stiff and
precise forms of mere scientific communication, is not only often justifiable, but exceedingly useful. There are many patients, too, who
can best be approached in a jocose way; and who are led to disclose
certain important facts by a species of bantering. Harmless jokes
may often pass between the patients and their medical attendant, or,
occasionally, be hazarded by the latter alone, with benefit This has
been, at times, our own experience. We differ, however, widely, from
those who think that the *publication* of these jokes, or of the ordinary
conversation, necessarily taking place, between the practitioner and
his patients, at the institutions to which we have referred, is desirable,
or proper. For our own part, we are pained to see a tendency to
adopt that *ad captandum* style, in reporting the preceedings of certain
cliniques, which, to our mind, is always in bad taste, and lowers the
dignity of the profession, in all eyes. We cannot understand how men,
deservedly distinguished in their calling, can allow themselves to be
thus shown up. Is it necessary, we would ask, to chronicle all the
chit-chat, both relevant and irrelevant, which occurs during the examination of clinical-lecture patients, or of such as present themselves as
out-patients at hospitals and dispensaries? Let the said chit-chat go
on, if you please—make the "clinic" as pleasant as possible, to both
patients and lookers-on—there is need enough of it, usually—but don't

have it all strung out in type—it really is not creditable, to say the least.

We do not wish to be invidious, or captious, in our remarks—but where else, we would ask, do we see this sort of thing except in our own country? And do not those journals, and those authors of books who adopt it, suffer, sooner or later, not only in the opinion of their medical brethren, but in that of "outsiders," who happen to get wind of the thing? We confess to a feeling of disappointment, when we take up a book of real value—such, for instance, as *Professor Gunning S. Bedford's* indisputably is—and have to wade through long and profitless *conversations*, before we reach the gist of the matter. It really strikes us as only an appeal to the public, and a poor one at that.

Of course the remarks offered by distinguished practitioners (at the New York *cliniques*, for example) could not be published, entire, without their sanction—and yet we are treated, in the pages of the *New York Medical Press*, to specimens like the following, from gentlemen for whose scientific reputation and private character we have the very highest respect—yet to whose course, in this matter, we cannot but take exception. For instance, would it not have been more in accordance, not only with scientific interests, but with propriety and good taste, to have stated the treatment of the cases, simply, and to the point, without giving the detailed conversations which we quote? "Now, Madam, be kind enough to take your position on the bed, and I will very soon do what is right for you." "Thank you, Sir." "You perceive, gentlemen, I introduce this cylindrical speculum; I now have the cervix within the focus of the instrument, and, as you see, freely cauterize it with the solid nitrate." "Return here, Madam, next Monday; I will repeat the same thing again." "I shall, Sir." "Madam" was certainly very cool and collected after her *expose*, and conversed with great nonchalance! We conclude that, shortly after "next Monday," we shall be favored with a little more small talk of the same sort.

In the same number of the journal we have cited, there occurs another conversation, of about a quarter of a column, wherein the patient (who is styled by the prescriber his "good friend," twice, within the compass of a few lines) affords some amusement to the bystanders—and is *supposed* to do so to the readers of the above journal—by having misunderstood the doctor's language. A uterine tumor had been discovered; the questioner asks, "What did I call the tumor, my good friend?" "A *porpus*, Sir." "Oh! no, you misunderstood me; I said a polypus." "Well, Sir, I know it sounded something like a *porpus!*" * * Now we submit that while it may be all very well to laugh at such a mistake, and air the joke, for a few minutes, at the time it is enunciated, the reproduction of it in a medical journal, as a part of the proceedings of a medical *clinique*, is worse than absurd—it is "flat, stale and unprofitable"—out of place and out of taste. The same kind of twaddle, upon the next page, is fully as objectionable: "Now, my good woman, if you will be kind enough to place yourself on this bed, I will remove the polypus." "Thank you, Sir."

But by far the most offensive specimens of so-termed clinical reports are to be found a few pages in advance of the latter extracts. In the midst of much instructive information, communicated by *Prof. Willard Parker*, the reporter thereof has seen fit to interlard the text with frequent informations of the occurrence of hilarity. The word "laughter" is parenthetically inserted no less than three times within a dozen lines. This reminds one of the similar interpolation of the words "applause," or "cheers," in political or other popular addresses. The only difference is, that in the latter case it is proper; in the former, anything but that. Still farther on, no less a person than *Professor Alonzo Clark* is reported as taking *his* turn at the same species of jocosity. "Will you tell us some features in your case?" "I don't remember any at present except that my heart feels large." (Laughter.) "That's no evidence, Madam, of its being so." "Let us look, gentlemen, into the objective symptoms." "Throw off your cape and furs, Madam, and arrange your dress in such a way that I may listen to your heart." "I have had dyspepsia for a long time, doctor." "We will consider that." Even the account of the "auscultatory signs," which follows, is given in a loose, affected style; and is terminated by a narration setting forth the action of tobacco on the heart of a medical brother, whose "beautiful wife" did not become a widow when he thought she would!

We cannot suppose for a moment that these gentlemen, so widely and creditably known, gave their clinical remarks, with their little interludes, (proper enough in *moderation* in the hospital ward or dispensary room,) in the expectation that they would be thus reported, in such very significant and *insignificant* detail; but the question will arise, why do they *allow* their publication, after once seeing them? And, in this connection, we cannot but remark the striking contrast of the report from Bellevue Hospital, by Charles Phelps, M.D., House

Surgeon. This is done in the style it should be; and conveys a clear idea of the circumstances of the case, in the terse terms which befit such communications. A weekly journal can hardly, we should think, devote much of its space, continuously, with advantage to its subscribers or credit to itself, to miscellaneous conversation, or to a jumble of that and scientific statements.

We have none but the best feelings and wishes to express toward any and every medical journal which seeks to enlighten the profession and to be its medium of communication; but we hold, that management of the sort to which we have referred, is, to say the very least, a *grave mistake.*

We confess to being somewhat amused by the closing sentences of the leading editorial of the New York journal mentioned; and we present them, as worthy of consideration: "We are well aware that other cities of our Union have made an advancement in medical matters, in ratio to their increase, commensurate with our own, and the knowledge of this fact gives us sincere pleasure, as it places our country, in that respect, not a whit behind the older nations, whose medical records filled many a heavy tome ere ours began; yet we maintain that Gotham is *The Metropolis.*" For a journal, which, at the time the above was printed (Dec. 25th, 1858), bore on its cover "Vol. I., No. 4," we contend that the sentiments—and particularly the last—are "pro——digious!"—*Boston Med. and Surg. Journ.*

EDITOR'S TABLE.

TO OUR SUBSCRIBERS.

All who have paid their subscriptions for 1859, (see "Receipts" in the present and last numbers,) will receive their numbers *free of postage.*

If any find themselves taxed with *postage,* they are thus reminded that they are *delinquent* on our books, and may relieve themselves by *promptly* remitting their dues.

Our paying subscribers have our thanks, and we need a few more such; although new subscribers come in fast enough to take the places of a few who are offended at the truth, and essay to punish us by stopping that $2, the price they pay to be let alone. *Certain brethren cannot bear the light, but it will shine none the less in the* GAZETTE.

☞ As *advance payment* is the rule, we have begun to curtail and prune our list, and shall stop the GAZETTE *after this month* to all delinquents, who have *received their bills and failed to pay.* Let none complain after this notice.

If any mistakes occur, they will be promptly corrected on hearing from the parties.

DEATH OF SAMUEL S. WHITNEY, ESQ.

Testimony of his physicians, DRS. J. C. BEALES, VALENTINE MOTT, and HORACE GREEN. Official report of the *post-mortem* by DR. ALEXANDER B. MOTT. *Cause of death,* as certified to the CITY INSPECTOR. Explanations and vindications, statements and counter-statements, criminations and recriminations, before the N. Y. Academy of Medicine on the part of the doctors. The latest *Parisian* fashion of attempting a *diagnosis* after the patient is *dead!* and blundering at that!

> " The doctors found, when she was dead,
> Her last disorder *mortal.*"
> MADAM BLAIZE.

The last excitement among the public and the profession of New York has arisen from the death of Mr. Whitney, a respectable and wealthy citizen, who, as will be seen, himself ascribed his last illness and death to the topical treatment of his throat with the sponge probang by Dr. Horace Green. So vehemently did he assert this opinion, that his family and friends not merely, but his physicians, as will appear, were so fully impressed with its truth, that even before his death the rumor became general through the city that the probang had perforated the trachea or larynx, and to this malpractice the accompanying emphysema of the neck, face and chest was attributed, which indeed was a very natural inference from the premises, had the latter been true. The newspapers at home and abroad took up the rumor, that our neighbor, Dr. Green, had killed his patient, and both he and his method of cauterizing the throat were suitably denounced. Our medical brethren who are very generally in the daily use of similar instruments in analogous cases, as well as their patients, were startled at these rumors, and this mode of practice seemed to be coming to a dead halt.

But the death of Mr. Whitney occurring after several days of suffering from obstructed deglutition and respiration—during which time his physicians, Drs. Beales and Mott, made every effort for his relief—

an opportunity was afforded for verifying the diagnosis of the patient, which was that also of the two doctors, for they had found it impossible even to look into his throat. The post-mortem was resolved upon; but unhappily Drs. Beales and Mott consented to make it, so far as Dr. Green was concerned, clandestinely—since Dr. Mott's son was employed for the purpose, but neither Dr. Green nor any of his friends were allowed to be present; and this, though all the gentlemen expected to find a perforated larynx or trachea, and a consequent implication of Dr. Green in his charge of having killed the patient, "not intentionally" to be sure, but by awkwardness or unskillfulness, which would have been fatal to his reputation. But even under such circumstances no notice was given to Dr. Green; a right which courtesy and ethical propriety alike demanded, and one which has never before been withheld in the annals of honorable medicine. But what must have been the surprise of this dissecting caucus, when on opening the larynx and trachea they found no perforation or other lesion in either, the mucous membrane of these organs being a perfect type of health? Their surprise, while it overthrew the diagnosis of the patient, in which they had fully acquiesced, only forced the conviction that the cause of death had yet to be discovered, for it was not where they expected to find it. Hence they proceeded posteriorly, when the scalpel detected pus anteriorly, laterally and posteriorly to the pharynx, where an acute abscess existed, as " large as a hen's egg," and which, though full, "*had a hole in it large enough to admit the finger!*" Now they learned, for the first time, why the patient could not swallow, and why his respiration was obstructed. Supposing that they had now reached the cause of death, a new theory was started, viz., that the sponge probang of Dr. Green had created this abscess, by lacerating the pharynx, and this, though the opening was in a part of the organ which the instrument could not by possibility reach. Still this was a happy thought, for it seemed to favor the discovery of the sapient committee of the Academy, that Dr. Green in his operations only enters the pharynx, when he claims to enter the trachea.

Unfortunately for the theory, however, they had to open the thorax, and here they seem to have found another cause of death in an anomalous abscess in the lung, and the mysterious emphysema was found to have arisen from ulcerated openings in the pleura! All this mischief in the chest seems to have been ascribed to Dr. Green, who had injected into the lung a drachm of the solution of the nitrate of silver, 15 grs. to the ounce, some ten days before death occurred. Unless, indeed, the *tube* only entered the pharynx, in which case the injection never reached the lung, and that apparent sloughing, spoken of in the post-mortem, would be nowhere. But now came up the question, what report shall be made to the City Inspector of the "cause of death," so many causes having been found. The theory of Dr. Beales, after the perforated trachea was not to be found, seems to have been that death was the result of the abscess behind the larynx and pharynx, and that this was caused by Dr. Green's probang. He did not so report, however, either to the City Inspector or to the Academy. To the former he says, "*Effusion into the lungs!*" and to the latter, "He died partly from *exhaustion* and partly from *asphyxia!*"

Dr. Mott, however, more wary than his colleague, ascribed very numerous causes of death, confessing himself at his wit's end to decide, even *after* the post-mortem, which of Mr. Whitney's complicated diseases killed him; and hence enumerated before the Academy, as "causes of death," each and every pathological lesion discovered, whether in the pharynx, or bronchia, or lung, or pleura; adding, "he died of all these, being blown up with emphysema!" All of which incongruity and prevarication might have been spared, had the simple fact been stated, that the "*direct*" cause of death was *suffocation*, and the "*indirect*" cause an *abscess* near the œsophagus, which mechanically prevented deglutition and respiration. But this plain statement would have exonerated Dr. Green, and implicated nobody, though it would have disappointed the scandal mongers, whether in the profession or out of it.

In this brief reference to the medical aspects of this case from a professional stand-point we only perform our duty as a public journalist. We disclaim any, the least prejudice or partiality for or against either of the medical men concerned, all of whom we regard as personal friends, worthy of all honor as men, and as physicians. But believing, as we do, that Dr. Green has been wrongfully blamed before the public, and that his treatment of Mr. Whitney had no agency in the fatal result, it is our opinion that the two medical gentlemen into whose hands the case fell should have insisted that Dr. Green, or some one to represent him, should be present at the post-mortem, and that they greatly erred in consenting to such an inquiry in the absence of a professional brother, their equal in every respect, who was expected to be implicated by the result. We regret their course for their own sake, rather than Dr. Green's, who has thus been placed in the vantage ground with that portion of the profession and the public who can appreciate right and justice.

We think, moreover, that they greatly erred in not silencing the public clamor against their professional brother and equal, by authoritatively exonerating him from the rumors they had countenanced, so soon as the post-mortem had proved that no lesion had been made in the larynx or trachea. The fiction that the patient was dying of an inaccessible abscess in the throat, in two hours after the last introduction of the probang, is too idle for belief. That this abscess had a sufficient volume to compress the œsophagus, with a hole in its wall large enough to admit the finger, while yet filled with pus, is the very error of the moon. While to ascribe the chronic abscess in the lung and ulcerated pleura to either of Dr. Green's operations, is the climax of absurdity. Neither Dr. Beales nor Dr. Mott should have indulged these and the like speculations, but admitted frankly the now obvious truth, that they failed to find out what was the matter during life, or what was the "cause of death" by the *post-mortem*. This would have been no reproach to their professional sagacity and reputation, but would have exalted both, for equally great men have been equally at fault in obscure cases, and gracefully recorded it for the instruction of posterity. Lastly, the certificate of death given to the City Inspector, viz., "Death from effusion into the lungs," was singularly unscientific, and worse, it did not conform to the fact by their own showing. We repeat that the man died of *suffocation*, of which "exhaustion, asphyxia," and even "pulmonary effusion," could only be the fruits or sequela. The emphysema was traceable to the pleuritic and pulmonic lesion, and to this alone. Had our brethren only stated the facts, injustice would have been done to nobody.

The attention of the reader is now invited to the documentary history upon which our opinions are based. They were spread before the N. Y. Academy of Medicine, and are, viz.:

Dr. Horace Green's Statement.—His Treatment of Mr. Whitney.

The doctor stated that this unfortunate case was first presented to his notice on the 25th of October last. Mr. Whitney came in with the rest of his patients, and made two calls at his office before he saw him. His assistant informed him that the gentleman had called, but would not wait for his turn, and wished to see him at once; to which he replied that his rule in such cases should be adhered to, and that, unless in the case of a lady, the patients should wait for their turn. Mr. Whitney then came in in his turn, and entered his name on the doctor's book, as all his patients did. He stated to him that he had been in ill health for two or three years, and that for the last two months he had quite a bad cough, and he also complained of his throat and chest He stated also that some physician had examined him before, and had told him his lungs were affected. He (Dr. Green) then made an examination of his chest by auscultation, in the presence of his assistant, Dr. Richards, who, as usual in all cases which he examines, made a note of it at the time. He found the chest thin, a little depression on the left thoracic wall; percussion gave a flat sound over all the upper portion of the left lung. On applying the ear to the chest a distinct mucous rale or click was heard below the left clavicle in both inspiration and expiration. These symptoms when accompanying the signs, were indicative, in his (Dr. Green's) experience, of the presence of tubercular softening. Mr. Whitney's throat appeared granulated and inflamed, and the left tonsil was slightly enlarged and ulcerated, the epiglottis was thickened, and its border whitened with a line of erosion. The doctor then gave an account of the several interviews which he had with Mr. Whitney from the 26th of October to the 14th of December, and his treatment on these occasions—the application of a solution of nitrate of silver to the fossæ, epiglottis, and into the glottis, and the use of the "probang." The visits of the patient occurred at such long intervals that he found that the parts were not prepared for the introduction of the tube; but as Mr. Whitney had several times expressed a desire to have it used, he (Dr. Green) resolved, on the 6th of December, to make the attempt. The tube was therefore introduced, and the nitrate of silver applied. Dr. Green then proceeded at length to detail the facts of the case, and stated that he had not seen Mr. Whitney from the 14th of December until he heard of his death. He was most willing that the matter should be discussed by the Academy, and he left the matter entirely in their hands. Dr. Green continued at some length.

Remarks by Dr. Foy, who saw the Application upon the Deceased.

The President then said Dr. Foy should next be heard.

DR. FOY rose and said: I was present on the occasion described by Dr. Horace Green, and saw the application made upon Mr. Whitney. Dr. Green has stated exactly the particulars of that occurrence. On introducing the probang into the throat of the decedent, he made a sudden motion of the head, and gave an expression of pain. The pain was not greater than I myself have felt upon having the uvula touched with nitrate of silver. The date of that visit is fixed upon my mind with certainty; so, also, is the size of the probang, for I remember noticing it very particularly, and telling Dr. Green that I

could not get even a small probang, nor one thus curved, at the druggist's. Mr. Whitney left the office before I did, and left it not suffering any particular inconvenience.

Statement of Dr. J. C. Beales.

I find myself in a very disagreeable situation. It is the first time
I was ever engaged in any controversy with any of my professional
friends; and you have never known me to enter into any professional dispute of any kind before. I always have avoided it. Upon
the present occasion I shall be forced to take a position antagonistic
to Dr. Green, for which I have abundance of evidence; and I assure
you it is not voluntarily assumed, but forced upon me.

In the statement of the case I am about to read to you I am sorry
to say that there are some expressions in the commencement which
are put in with very great reluctance, but owing to the different reports that have been circulated, I felt it necessary to insert them, that
you may have a just comprehension of the state and feeling of the
patient.

Condition and Feeling of Mr. Whitney between his Last Treatment by Dr. Green and his Death.

Dec. 14, 1858.—About one in the afternoon I was called to see
Samuel S. Whitney; I found him surrounded by several members of
his family, in a state of the most intense excitement, suffering and
terror; in answer to my inquiries as to what had happened, he answered, "Sit down, Beales, and I will tell you the truth; I was such a
fool as to go to Dr. Green to be operated upon, and the d—d villain
has killed me." His countenance was pale and haggard, and had all
the appearance of a man whose nervous system had received a severe
shock; his breathing was occasionally irregular, and almost spasmodic,
coughing almost incessantly, and speaking with great difficulty and pain,
in a hoarse and unnatural tone of voice; his skin was cold and clammy,
and covered with perspiration; the pulse was extremely frequent, feeble,
irregular and intermittent; he was excessively restless, not remaining
in the same place more than a few minutes at a time; complaining of
intense pain in the region of the larynx, shooting through to the cervical vertebræ, and down the course of the trachea to the chest; he
kept grasping the larynx, and reiterating every few minutes that he
was murdered; I endeavored to calm the excitement of the patient,
and tried to examine his fauces and throat, which appeared in a state
of great inflammation; I discovered no lesion, as, in fact, on account

of the pain and terror of the patient, the examination was necessarily very imperfect, as he would scarcely allow the spoon to touch his tongue, and I concluded, therefore, to defer the examination till he should become more quiet; I gradually ascertained, partly from the family and partly from himself, that he had been several times to see Dr. Green; on the first occasion his tonsils had been amputated; on a subsequent occasion, ten or twelve days previously, (the exact dates were not told to the relator,) "a hollow tube had been passed into his lungs, and about a teaspoonful of solution of nitrate of silver had been injected into them by touching a spring at the top of the tube." Whether this was done more than once the relator does not recollect to have been stated. On the 14th of December Mr. Whitney breakfasted with his family, appearing to be in his usual health; he afterwards went to Dr. Green's office; "the doctor passed an instrument into his throat, and finding some obstruction, he pushed the instrument with some force; he (Mr. W.) felt something give way, immediately experienced severe pain about the top of the windpipe, and told the doctor he had hurt him;" he returned home, informed the family of what had occurred, and I was called as before stated. 1 P. M., I saw him with the symptoms, and in the state previously described; it was evident that, under these circumstances, the only indications that could be followed were to rally the patient's strength, to produce some reaction and to moderate the local irritation in the fauces; to this effect I ordered him to be immediately put in bed, bottles of hot water to the feet, with sinapisms to the extremities and chest, and flaxseed poultices to the throat; a teaspoonful of chloric ether or volatile tincture of valerian in water occasionally, till reaction should be established, and a mixture composed as follows: br. ol. amygd. dulc. syrup papav. som. mucilag G. acac. liquor, potass., a dessert spoonful to be slowly swallowed occasionally. For nourishment he was allowed arrowroot and flaxseed tea.

Dec. 14, 7 P. M.—Is suffering severe pain, described to be in the larynx down the course of the trachea to the chest, and round to the cervical vertebræ; pulse 112, feeble and irregular; still excessively restless; other symptoms are about the same; insisted on my remaining with him all night. R. antimonial solu. S. morph. syrup gummi, ing aq. distill, a dessert spoonful every four hours; to inhale the vapor of infusion of flaxseed and poppy heads.

Dec. 15, 3 A. M.—They called me, as they observed the face to be swelling; I found extensive emphysema all round the neck, and partially in the face, rather more noticeable on the left side; he had continued exceedingly restless, scarcely dozing for a few minutes, breathing very irregular; pulse 106; urine scanty, very high colored, and turbid. Continued the same remedies and nourishment.

1 P. M.—Heat of surface more natural; scarcely any pain in the chest, emphysema very much increased round the throat and face, and extending down the chest; has not slept; has taken scarcely any nourishment on account of the pain in swallowing; could not continue the inhalations, although they rather relieved him temporarily. Anodyne liniment to be applied to the throat and chest.

8 P. M.—Dr. Valentine Mott saw him, in consultation with me. Is decidedly worse; emphysema very much increased; neck and face enormously swollen, it has extended all over the chest, but lower down on the right side; breathing somewhat labored; pulse very feeble, irregular, and 112; skin is again covered with clammy perspiration, and about the neck and chest of a purplish erysipelatous appearance; does not particularly complain of pain, except on talking or swallowing. Dr. Mott gave a very unfavorable prognosis. Continue anodyne, and take alternately a teaspoonful of ammoniated tincture of valerian.

Dec. 16, 6 A. M.—Upon the whole has passed a more comfortable night; symptoms are all a shade better; the emphysema rather less in the face, but the throat and the chest are enormous, the mammæ resembling those of a stout nursing woman. Continue wine whey.

1 P. M.—With Dr. Mott. The emphysema extends to Poupart's ligament, on the right side; but only as low as the umbilicus on the left; cough less frequent, except when he swallows; pulse 108, and rather firmer. Same remedies and nourishment.

9 P. M.—With Dr. Mott. Is not so well; emphysematous swelling increasing; cannot open his eyes till the air is carefully pressed out of the lids; chest and abdomen still more swollen; pulse more feeble, 122, although he had taken nourishment more freely. Same remedies.

Dec. 17, 6 A. M.—Has slept more during the night, sometimes for nearly an hour at a time; has taken more nourishment, but there begins to be considerable mucous secretion, which interrupts his respiration, and gives him great trouble to expectorate; pulse very irregular and feeble; the slightest movement increases its frequency; it averages about 108.

1 P. M.—With Dr. Mott. There is no observable change in the symptoms, although he says he feels more comfortable; several attempts have been made from time to time to examine the fauces and adjacent parts, but the excessive swelling rendered them useless.

9 P. M.—With Dr. Mott. There is again a slight lull in the symptoms, excepting the pulse, which is extremely irregular at 108; same remedies.

Dec. 18, 6 A. M.—Has passed the best night since the attack; there is a decided improvement in all his symptoms; emphysema slightly subsiding; pulse 90; is rather more hopeful.

1 P. M.—With Dr. Mott. We consider him decidedly improving; all the symptoms are milder; he is slightly flighty from the effects of the anodyne.

9 A. M.—Is not so well again, without any other apparent cause than he would get up during my absence and sit for about an hour in a chair; the pulse is more frequent and irregular; the difficulty of swallowing is also evidently increasing, the attempt to do so bringing on coughing, partial strangulation, and some regurgitation of the fluids.

Dec. 19, 6 A. M.—Passed a very bad night, principally owing to the great increase of the mucous secretion, that keeps him almost constantly coughing and expectorating, which he does with great difficulty and suffering; the pulse very frequent, feeble, and excessively irregular; take half the dose of the anodyne at a time:—(R. Ammon. carbonat, grs. iv.; emuls. amygd. dulc., dr. i., every four hours, in place of the tinc. valerian ammoniat); although it is certain that there is some serious lesion in the vicinity of the glottis, yet it is utterly impossible to ascertain the state of the parts; the emphysema has rather subsided about the upper part of the face, so that he can partially open his eyes.

1 P. M.—With Dr. Mott. Has slightly rallied, but the mucous secretion is increasing; the cough more frequent, and difficulty of swallowing greater; bowels have not acted for three days; continue remedies; injection; give as much nourishment as possible.

9 P. M.—All his symptoms much worse; pulse more feeble, 120; difficulty of swallowing, with the coughing and strangulation very much increased; consequently has not been able to take so much nourishment.

Dec. 20, 6 A. M. Has passed a very bad night; breathing labored, and all the difficulties of swallowing, &c., increasing; the emphysema rapidly disappearing from the face and throat; abdomen distended and tympanitic; injection did not operate; a tablespoon full of castor oil.

1 P. M.—With Dr. Mott. All the symptoms gradually becoming more serious.

10 P. M.—Is very much worse in every respect; respiration excessively labored; the slightest attempt to doze threatens suffocation from the accumulation of mucus; can with difficulty be induced to swallow; the oil operated twice, and he was excessively exhausted; pulse extremely feeble and irregular, 126; he is evidently sinking.

Dec. 21, 7 A. M.—During the night he became rapidly worse; did not swallow after 2 A. M., and died rather suddenly at 8 A. M., partly from exhaustion and partly by asphyxia.

Note.—A number of trifling circumstances, such as the varying appearance of the urine, the continual slight changes in the symptoms, &c., as not throwing additional light on the case, have been omitted, in order not to make the statement too tedious.

J. C. BEALES, M. D.

As far as relates to this case, from the time I was called in, it is a faithful narrative.

VALENTINE MOTT, M. D.

I certify that this is a faithful copy of the original.

J. C. BEALES, M. D.

NEW YORK, *Jan.* 18, 1859.

Post Mortem of Samuel S. Whitney.

NEW YORK, *Dec.* 22, 1858.

Thirty hours after death nothing peculiar in the appearance of the body. Rigor mortis quite moderate. On making an incision from under the chin, in the mesial line of the sternum, it was remarked that the anterior projection of the thyroid cartilage was more than ordinary. Directly as the knife divided the deep cervical fascia on the left side of the thyroid cartilage, pus issued out; a little further division opened into a cavity, containing pus, about the size of a large hen's egg, and extending a little in front of the pharynx, and downward behind and below the thyroid cartilage. At the upper and posterior part of this abscess there was an opening into the pharynx, large enough to admit the end of the forefinger. This abscess was lined by a large quantity of destroyed filamentous tissue, hanging from different parts of it like wetted tow. The entrance into the œsophagus immediately below this was perfectly sound, internally and externally. The larynx was now laid open from behind, and at the first glimpse, a red point about the size and shape of a grain of wheat on the left side, a little below the left chorda vocalis, and running longitudinally, led us to exclaim there is the point of laceration of the mucous membrane, by which the air has escaped into the cellular tissue to constitute the emphysema. On close inspection, and wiping the part with a sponge, no abrasion or aperture could be discovered. Every other part of the larynx and trachea, as far as removed, presented on its internal surface a perfectly normal appearance. Indeed, we all remarked, that we had never seen a larynx and trachea more natural and healthy. We next concluded to have a look at the bronchi and lungs. Perhaps about an inch above the division of the trachea, the most beautiful vermilion redness that we ever saw on a mucous surface commenced and extended into each bronchus, but greatest in the left, and extended down each lung. Over this peculiar redness there was a cloudy shade, which vanished after a short exposure to the air. On opening the pleura, the upper lobe of the left side, at first glance, seemed covered with white thick pus. But, on close examination, it proved to be soft, strumous-like fibrin, easily rubbed off. This, on the side and posterior part, connected that lobe in patches to the pleura costalis. These imperfect adhesions were easily broken down with the fingers. The whole of the upper part of this lobe was very red and solid—hepatized. Just at the root, or at the commencement of the bronchial ramifications, there was an open cavity, about the size of a small black walnut, of a reddish brown color, and irregular villous surface, as though a slough had separated. At the upper and anterior part of this cavity there was a small opening through both pleuras. This lobe was cut into in different directions, but no tubercles could be found. The lower lobe was perfectly healthy. The redness of the mucous membrane of the right bronchus extend to the lung of that side, but the three lobes were perfectly normal. There were no old adhesions on either side of the cavity of the chest. Some little appearance of the emphysema remained.

(Signed,)   VALENTINE MOTT, M.D.

J. C. BEALES, M.D.

ALEX'R B. MOTT, M.D.

Statement of Dr. Beales.

DR. BEALES said: During the number of years that I have attended Mr. Whitney's family, I have not known Mr. Samuel Whitney to be seriously ill, so as to be confined to his bed; but he has for a long time been subject to various derangements of the digestive organs, such as want of appetite, torpidity of the bowels, deficiency of the bilious secretions, and occasionally a bronchial cough. For these I have frequently prescribed for him; but during the whole or greater part of the last year (as I have been informed by the family) he placed himself under the care of a homœopathic physician, so that, with two or three trifling exceptions, I was not called on to prescribe for him until the present occurrence. Toward the end of October his sister informed me that her brother was very low-spirited and depressed, as some physician had informed him his lungs were very much affected. He wanted me, therefore, to examine him, but did not want me to know that he had consulted any other physician. I was not told who it was, nor do I know to this day, although I now presume it to have been Dr. Green. Sir, I wish to state that I appreciate the stethoscope as highly as most men; I believe it, as most others do, one of the greatest discoveries in our profession, but I frankly confess that I do not believe in its infallibility, even aided by percussion. I do not believe that any man can at all times discover one or two, nor even a few tubercles, scattered about the upper lobes of the lungs. I am sure that every man, if he would frankly tell the truth, would admit that he had occasionally been mistaken. For myself, I do not pretend to any extraordinary skill with this instrument, but, independent of my private practice, I have been for fifteen years examiner for various life insurance companies, and therefore I constantly make use of it, and ought to know something about it. Now, under these circumstances, well knowing the opinion of the other physician, I examined Mr. Whitney with all the care and accuracy of which I am capable; I declared to him that I could not discover any tubercles in his lungs, and that I did not believe that any existed. [No notes of the examination.] Now, Sir, on turning to the report of the postmortem examination, it will be seen that a "cavity" was found, but not a single tubercle. I will not, of course, assert that such a thing as a tuberculous cavity never exists without the presence of other tubercles, but I do say, that it is a most rare and exceptional circumstance; but I wish to make a few remarks on this "cavity." Was this a *tuberculous* cavity? It neither contained any kind of fluid, nor was it lined with lymph, nor the slightest appearance of false membrane, nor were there any remains of *tuberculous* deposit, and *I* at least have never seen a tuberculous cavity similar to it—in fact, although that word was used in the report as probably most readily occurring, it could scarcely be justly so called; it was rather a shallow depression or scooping out of the actual apex or superfices of the lung; its surface was not like that of a "cavity," but rough and irregular, and had that peculiar appearance, that all present remarked it looked as though a slough had separated. Communicating with it was a perforation in the pleura, sufficiently large to admit the little finger of the gentleman who had operated; all other appearances about the lung were of the most recent disease, the hepatization was in its earliest stage, and the adhesions spoken of were so recent that the folds of the pleura were, more properly speaking, glued together, than adhered. We did not discover the slightest sign of chronic disease in or about the lung, and so striking was this fact, that Dr. Mott told the family, after the post-mortem examination, that we had not seen any disease that might not have been produced within a week. But Dr. Mott is here to speak for himself. Dr. Green says that the epiglottis was thickened and its border whitened with a line of erosions. At the post-mortem, this part was very minutely and carefully examined, and found to be extraordinarily healthy and free from the slightest vestige of disease. Under all these circumstances, I am forced to believe that Dr. Green erred in his diagnosis, and that these various operations were unnecessary and uncalled for. I do not say that the operation of tubing caused the disease in the lung, because I confess myself ignorant of the effects of nitrate of silver on the substance of the lungs; but for the operation itself, I do not hesitate to express my conviction that it is at all times attended with extreme peril and risk of the patient's life. I have never heard of or seen a single case of phthisis where it has effected a cure, and therefore I believe it to be perfectly unjustifiable. I believe that a slough or eschar was formed at the apex of the lung, involving the pleura, and which, at the time of the unfortunate occurrence, became separated by the violent exertions and spasmodic coughing—the air percolated into the cellular substance, and produced the emphysema which formed so prominent a symptom. I will now leave this part of the case, and go on to that which was, after all, undoubtedly the immediate cause of the death of the patient. I mean the lesion of the pharynx. By referring once more to the post-mortem examination, it will be seen that there was a lacerated opening in the pharynx communicating with a large abscess. I have heard it rumored—and, indeed, it has been stated in the public papers, especially in an article in the *Tri-. bune*, which is evidently from a suspicious source—that this abscess was chronic. Insinuations were made against Dr. Mott and myself in regard to it. If, Sir, the friends of Dr. Green have given currency to this idea, or intend in any way to suggest it, then has the Doctor ample reason to say "Defend me from my friends." It appears by his own statement, that for two months previously to his death Mr. Whitney was under the professional care of Dr. Green; for my own part, I solemnly declare, I have never prescribed for nor heard him complain of his throat. Early in October, the Doctor cut out one of the tonsils. Did the chronic abscess then exist? If so, how was it that the Doctor did not discover it? He several times applied the sponge and probang—did the abscess then exist? On the 8th of December Dr. Green states that he passed the tube down the trachea. This, at all events, whatever we may think of the operation itself, requires a careful observation of the parts; did the abscess then exist, and the Doctor not discover it? But, Sir, on the very day of the last unfortunate operation, Dr. Green was showing to Dr. Foy how he applied the sponge to the larynx, and showed why it only entered the pharynx—of course the organs were closely observed—how was it that the Doctor did not diagnose this chronic abscess? Why, Sir, the reason that Dr. Green did not see this chronic abscess, was because it did not exist. Sir, I do not believe that among all those who are now listening to me there are two opinions. At all events, to my mind, the evidence is irresistible, that in the last unfortunate operation, on the 14th of December, the pharynx was accidentally lacerated by the probang; the first effects, as we have seen, were excessive irritation of the parts, and a severe shock, increased, no doubt, by the nervous temperament of the patient, and his conviction that the injury was fatal. Afterwards, doubtless, portions of the various foreign bodies he attempted to swallow, food and medicine, were forced into the wound. After three or four days, a sloughy abscess began to be formed, which, gradually increasing in size, formed a mechanical obstruction to swallowing; by pressure on the adjoining parts, prevented the epiglottis from properly closing, and produced the strangulation and regurgitation which we have noticed, till at length the unfortunate patient sank from exhaustion and asphyxia. I wish now, Sir, with your kind permission, to make a few remarks with respect to the post-mortem examination. I perceive by statements in the public papers, the source of which can easily be understood, that we are censured for not having Dr. Green present. I need not say that, as the case progressed, the excitement and feeling in the family did not diminish. I do not think that on this point I have the right to judge Dr. Green; he doubtless did what he thought right in the matter; but had he, by sending inquiries, shown any sympathy with the misfortune of the family, it would have afforded an occasion to Dr. Mott and myself to have introduced him; that he did not so act, was repeatedly remarked by many of the family. Now, under these circumstances, it was no pleasant thing to ask permission of the family, and I frankly allow we did not; but, for myself, I solemnly declare, that I went to that examination without the slightest idea of criminating Dr. Green, but with the earnest desire to ascertain the nature and extent of the injury. But let me ask, What do these insinuations mean? I will tell you how the post-mortem examination was arranged: I asked Dr. Mott who he would wish to perform it; he replied, his son, Dr. Alexander; and on the day of that operation I was introduced and spoke to that gentleman for the first time in my life. The insinuations to which I have alluded either mean that we were not competent for the examination, (if so, let the truth be told,) or that the examination or report was distorted to meet particular views. On this point I shall merely remark that Dr. Alexander Mott has never, till to-night, heard me say a word as to my views of the case. I do not know his. We have never interchanged a word on the subject. Both he and his father hold such positions in the profession and society, as ought to place them beyond such calumnies. As for myself, those who know me, Sir, will not, I am proud to believe, imagine me capable of misrepresenting solemn facts, for any purpose whatever; and this is all, Sir, I think it needful to say in answer to these unmerited and disgraceful inuendoes.

DR. VALENTINE MOTT followed, strongly substantiating the post-mortem examination, which, he said, was prepared by himself, and controverting Dr. Green's theory of the case.

DR. GREEN said: I do not rise, Mr. President, to make any speech. So far as I am concerned, I am willing to leave this whole subject to my professional brethren connected with the Academy, and to the profession throughout the whole world. In the first place, however, I may be allowed to say that there are some insinuations to which Dr. Beales has referred, which are improper and groundless. It has been inferred that I have sought to keep this *post-mortem* examination from the public. I should have been very glad at any time to have it published, as its publication would have saved a great many persons from having exposed themselves to heavy damages for libel, for it shows that there was no perforation, and no injury done to Mr. Whitney at the time; but that was not my reason for withholding it. I came before you, gentlemen, and stated the case candidly. It was at the urgent re-

quest of my friend Dr. Mott, (for I shall so consider him, notwithstanding all this,) that nothing should be brought before the public in
relation to this, except through the Academy, that I refused to give
this *post-mortem* over for publication. I have his written request here,
and I offer to read it if he will allow me. Since the last meeting of
the Academy I have been visited by, I presume, no less than ten editors, desiring me to surrender that *post-mortem;* and there are some
of the gentlemen here present to whom it was positively refused. I
declined also to give it, at the advice of my friends, and in conformity
with my own feelings, and these gentlemen of the Press can testify
whether I did not so refuse. If I am permitted, I will read from
Rokitansky's *Pathological Anatomy*—an authority on the subject
which no one here will question—a description of one variety of tuberculous cavity, which, I think, will hardly be found to concur with
the inferences of the gentlemen by whom this *post-mortem* examination
was made. At page 103 of the Sydenham Society's edition, he says:

"*Infiltrated tubercle*, unlike interstitial tubercle, is actually deposited in the cavities of the air-cells. It arises from a more or less extensive croupous pneumonia, whose products, under the influence of a
tuberculous infiltration, becomes variously discolored and converted
into yellow tubercle, instead of being absorbed or dissolving into pus.
Hence tuberculous infiltration presents the form of *hepatization,* induced by a tuberculous product."   *   *   *   *   *

And again, at page 112:

"The contents of tuberculous cavities present many differences.
Sometimes, and especially when the infiltrated tubercles begin to soft-
en, these caverns contain a yellow and somewhat thickish pus; more
frequently, however, they contain a thin, whey-like fluid, (tuberculous
ichor,) in which may be observed numerous grayish and yellowish,
friable, cheesy, purulent flocculi and particles, whose quantity, however, is not in itself sufficient to explain the profuse expectoration
which so often occurs in phthisis. This fluid is often of a grayish red,
or reddish brown—(mark the similarity of the phrases here and in
the gentleman's report)—or chocolate color, from the admixture of
blood; or of an ash or blackish gray color, from the pigment which it
takes up during the softening of the tissue. Moreover, the caverns
sometimes contain smaller or larger fragments of lung, resembling the
parenchyma contained in their walls, and chalky concretions are occasionally found in them."

In the next place, I would say that the inference is left to be made by the members of the Academy, that this sloughing was produced by an injection administered on the 6th of December, between which and the date of Mr. Whitney's death (on the 21st, I think,) an interval of fifteen days elapsed. Now, every gentleman of the Academy who understands what they are now doing in France, knows well that during its last five sessions the French Academy has been occupied in discussing this very subject of injection and cauterization in diseases of the air-passages, admitting unanimously that this operation is not only performed with safety, but that great beneficial results follow therefrom. And within the last few months large numbers of young and delicate children—1, 2, 3, 4 and 5 years of age—have been treated for croup by injection with nitrate of silver into the larynx, by such men as MM. Trousseau, Loiseau, Bouchut, and others. Professor Bennet, of Edinburg, in describing his use of the introduction of the tube and injection into the lungs, says:

"My period of attendance on the clinical wards having expired in January, it was not until last May that I had an opportunity of making a series of observations on this subject. I was then fortunately assisted by Prof. Barker, of New York, who showed me the kind of catheter he had seen Dr. Green employ, and demonstrated the manner in which the operation was performed. Without entering into minute particulars, I have only to say that I have confirmed the statements made by Dr. Horace Green. I have introduced the catheter publicly in the clinical wards of the Royal Infirmary in seven patients. Of these, five were affected with phthisis in various stages; one had chronic laryngitis, with bronchitis; and one chronic bronchitis, with severe paroxysms of asthma. In several other cases in which I attempted to pass the tube, it was found to be impossible—in some because the epiglottis could not be fairly exposed, and in others on account of the irritability of the fauces and too ready irritation of cough from pressure of the spatula.

"My experience of this treatment is as yet too limited to permit my saying anything of its permanent effects. In the case of bronchitis with asthma—a female, aged 24—I have now injected the lungs eleven times, at first throwing in two drachms of a solution of nitrate of silver, of the strength of half drachms of the crystalized salt to one ounce of distilled water, and latterly I have thrown in half ounce of a solution of the strength of two scruples to one ounce. She declares that no remedy has had such powerful effect in lessening the cough, diminishing the expectoration, or delaying the asthmatic paroxysms.

She breathes and blows through the tube, when inserted four inches below the larynx, and I have been surprised at the circumstance of the injections not being followed by the slightest irritation whatever, but rather by a pleasant feeling of warmth in the chest, (some have experienced a sensation of coolness,) followed by ease' to the cough, and a check for a time to all expectoration.

"I think it of importance that these facts should be known to the profession, as a homage justly due to the talents of a distinguished Trans-atlantic physician, and with the view of recommending a practice which, if judiciously employed, may form a new era in the treatment of pulmonary diseases." [Applause.]

I have only one word more. I never go, unless requested by some one, to see a patient. I did not desire Mr. Whitney to come and see me. He came of his own accord. I treated him legitimately, and, I believe, properly. When he left me and went under the care of another physician, should I lower myself by dogging him, and thus degrade the profession? [Applause, and cries of "Good!"] Never. Had they sent for me, (I having had several cases of retro-pharyngeal abscess, where I have saved the lives of the patients by opening those abscesses,) I would not have hesitated to go. I saved my 2 or 3 patients in this city by opening the abscess; they failed to do so. Why should they not come out as magnanimously as Carmichael did, when, having lost two patients from having overlooked a pharyngeal abscess which was not discovered until after death, he bravely acknowledged it? Dr. Beales has himself described the rage of the family toward me. And how did they meet it? Why was it not lulled at first, as I would have endeavored to do for you, Sir, or for any member of this Academy? [Applause.] Why was not this done by the physician in attendance on the family? I merely ask the question. He has declared that if I had ventured to come near the house I should, in all possibility, have suffered personal violence. This is one reason, perhaps, why, even if I had been called on, I should not have gone. But I would have gone, nevertheless. To these remarks, Mr. President, I wish to add one other. Having understood that a *post-mortem* examination was to be made, several of my medical friends called upon me and urged that either I, myself, or my representative should be present. At length, when the day arrived, Dr. Carnochan, my colleague, said it was injudicious to permit the examination to be made without one of us being there. I deputed him, therefore, to claim of Dr. Mott the privilege of being present. In accordance with this arrangement he drove down in his carriage, but was too late; the examination had already taken place. [Applause, which was immediately put down.]

A debate ensued, which was terminated by a motion to lay the whole subject on the table, when the Academy adjourned.

The reader has now before him the whole case, so that each may form his own conclusions, it being our purpose to do equal and exact justice to all parties. If either of them are dissatisfied, our columns will be open, and we shall take pleasure in correcting any errors or supplying any omissions.

ANÆSTHESIA AND DR. HORACE WELLS.

A large and spirited meeting of the citizens of Hartford, Conn., was lately held in that city, in which the physicians, dentists, and scientific men of Connecticut participated. The Hon. Truman Smith delivered an address, in which he reviewed the recent course of Dr. Willard Parker, Dr. Mott, and Dr. Francis, of this city, with great causticity, reading their affidavits in favor of Dr. Wells, and their late contradictory letters, certificates, &c., in aid of Morton's swindle. We observe that Judges Williams, Storrs, Ellsworth, Brockway, and other legal gentlemen were present. The following resolutions were then adopted:

Resolved, That this meeting return their thanks to the Hon. Truman Smith, for his generous and able vindication of the rights of the late Dr. Horace Wells, of this city, as the discoverer of the principle of anæsthesia as applied to medicine and surgery.

Resolved, That it is the sense of this meeting that the credit of having made the aforesaid discovery, and of successfully introducing it into practice, is due to Horace Wells, M.D., and we cherish for his memory a sentiment of profound respect for having conferred so great a boon on humanity.

Resolved, That whatever benefactions the generous and philanthropic may be disposed to accord to its author. will, in the judgment of this meeting, be misdirected and misapplied, unless the same be bestowed on the family of Dr. Wells, now resident in this city.

Resolved, That we believe this subject is pre-eminently worthy the attention of our citizens, that the claims of Dr. Wells, a public benefactor, may be asserted, and we advise that a subscription be taken up for the purpose of bringing the facts more fully before the world.

Resolved, That Doctors P. W. Ellsworth, G. W. Russell, G. B. Hawley, P. M. Hastings, and B. G. Whitman, Esq., be a committee to take such measures as they may deem expedient to realize the object above mentioned.

NEW YORK SANITARY ASSOCIATION.

This is among the new projects of the day, and after numerous caucuses a Constitution has been agreed upon, and organization will follow. Drs. Harris, Reid, Griscom and Watson seem to be the leaders in this movement for reform in the Health Department of the city, and they are nobly aided by public-spirited citizens, who concur that something should be done in this regard irrespective of politics, and agree with the claims of our profession, that medical offices should be filled by medical men, and not by party demagogues who know nothing of sanitary science, and care less, going in only for the spoils.

The Hon. Mayor of the city favors this view, as he has shown by nominating a medical man for the office of City Inspector, who, by the City Charter, is the Executive head of the Health Department, and whose office is nevertheless burdened with the business of cleaning streets, the care of the public markets, &c. The confirmation rests with the Board of Alderman, with whom the patronage of the office in appointing subordinates, &c., is so important, that their action is delayed, and our lucky neighbor who has the nomination is meanwhile suspended *in dubio.* The former City Inspector holds over until his successor is appointed—an event which, while the Aldermen linger over the new nomination, is uncertain. Political considerations, both at Albany and here, prompt to the anticipation of still farther delay, so that the result cannot be predicted at present. If the present nominee should be rejected, the Mayor will name another immediately according to law, but while they suffer the nomination to be delayed in the Committee to whom it is referred, no appointment is possible.

Central Ohio Lunatic Asylum, Columbus, Ohio.

The 20th Annual Report is before us, and authorizes the inference, that under the superintendency of Dr. R. Hills and his able assistants, the institution is prosperous and useful.

NEW YORK STATE INEBRIATE ASYLUM.

A full account of the ceremonies, addresses, &c., at the laying of the corner stone of this great and noble institution, in Binghamton, N. Y., has just appeared, with an appeal in its behalf, by J. Edward Turner, M.D., addressed to the present Governor.

The death of its first President, B. F. Butler, Esq., is a severe blow thus early in its history. We observe, however, that he remembered this charity in his will.

NEW JOURNALS AGAIN!

The Semi-monthly Medical News, Edited by Professors S. M. Bemiss and J. W. Benson, and published at Louisville, Ky., has just reached us. The first number is excellent, and we welcome it to our list of exchanges. Price $3 per annum, in advance. A novel feature is, that Jacob Smyser, Esq., sustains the enterprise, and receives its dedication. We should like to dedicate ours on the same terms.

Another! a "Medical Gazette" is announced at Louisville, also a semi-monthly, edited by a Dr. Frazee. We have not seen it, nor care to see it, unless the editor can find a *name* for it without stealing ours.

DR. McCORMAC, OF BELFAST,

Is out with another pamphlet, "Theory of Consumption," which he addresses to the French Imperial Academy of Medicine. He still stoutly maintains, that the great cause of pulmonary consumption is breathing vitiated air; and that prevention and cure are to be sought chiefly by the ventilation of sleeping chambers everywhere, but especially in the habitations of the poor. His zeal and industry are commendable.

EXSECTION OF THE OS CALCIS.

This operation was performed successfully at the Emigrants' Hospital, by Professor Carnochan, on his last clinical day; as also a single and double amputation, by the same surgeon. The opportunities for students to learn clinical surgery on Ward's Island are unsurpassed, so numerous are the patients, and so frequent are operations in that large hospital.

NOVEL SURGICAL PROCEEDING.

Professor Carnochan, last month, tied the common carotid for elephantiasis, involving the right side of the head and face. The tumor, which was immense, became considerably softer after the ligature was tied. The artery was unusually deep, on account of the extent of the morbid mass below the lower jaw.

JOCOSE CLINICS!

We advise all to turn to the article on this subject, from our Boston contemporary, which we reproduce in this number. It shows how the ludicrous twaddle of certain bogus clinical teaching in New York strikes others, and we hope that Bedford & Co. will "reform it altogether," or at least keep it out of the press; else we shall be tempted to republish Prof. Puffer's Lecture in the University of the Moon! The attempt made to revive the defunct American Medical Lancet, of Plattsburg, under another name, in New York, begins to be understood. We are sorry to see that several of our brethren have consented to ride in the tail-end of the cart, for the ventilation of the Professor of Gas. It is surely a "psychological phenomenon."

Chancellor Ferris, of the N. Y. University, delivered an able address on the founding of the Law Department. It is dignified, laudatory and hopeful. Judge Clerke has led off the Law Faculty in fine style. He is scholarly and eloquent in a high degree, and it is said that this Law Faculty is not excelled in the country. We wish them success.

RECEIPTS for 1859—Continued.

Drs. Meakim, Paine, Goldsmith, Chalmers, Roberts, Voss, Levings, Linsly, Passmore, Stillwell, Chilton. Eager, Pratt, Mott, Hartt, Heywood, Crane, Hoffman, J. Davis, Parmly, Fitch, Kennedy, Woodward, Sharrock, Barstow, Cullen, Doremus, Harris, Miner, Jr., Storer, Griswold, H. Green, Beales, Sayre, Belden, Frankel, Cairns, Osborne, Hyslop, Francis, Freeman, N. Y. Hospital, Miner, Sen., Brown, T. T. Green, Underhill, N. Allen, McCall, Thweatt, Coon, P. Van Buren, Sims, Jackson, J. Miller, Regensburger, J. M. Smith, Marcy, Emmet, Cammann, Post, Miller, Telkampf, J. R. Wood, Newby, McClelland, Rowe. Bergold, Belcher, Hannay, Pope, Darnell, Swift, Clark, Peaslee, Collins, Morton, Hoyt, Elder, Van Antwerp, H. G. Cox, Monkur, Platt, N. Palmer, A. Smith, Farlin.

CONTENTS.

AMERICAN
MEDICAL GAZETTE.

Vol. X.   MARCH, 1859.   No. 3.

ORIGINAL DEPARTMENT.

The Connection of the Nervous Centres of Animal and Organic Life.

By John O'Reilly, M.D., Licentiate and Fellow of the Royal College of Surgeons in Ireland, Resident Fellow of the N. Y. Academy of Medicine.

It is generally admitted that the secretions from all glandular bodies, as well as the skin and mucous membrane, depend on the presence as well as the agency of the organic nerves. Acknowledging this to be true, it must be confessed that it is just as difficult to trace nervous filaments in their structure as in the maternal or fœtal vessels in the placenta. The deduction to be arrived at from the observations just made, is, that if it were possible to remove every particle of the body with the exception of the substance of the organic nervous system, that the outline of the body would remain perfect, as well as a true delineation of all the viscera, as well as the blood vessels and muscles.

The retina is the termination or the expansion of the optic nerve. The optic nerve takes its origin from the corpus geniculatum externum and a white fasciculus sent from the nates. The pineal gland rests on the tubercula quadrigemina, and is attached to the inner margins of the optic thalami by two bands of white cerebral matter. In color and appearance it bears a strong resemblance to a ganglion belonging to the organic nervous system. The third nerve arises from the inner border of the crus cerebri. It is distributed to the lavator palpebræ and all the muscles attached to the eyeball with the exception of the

11

superior oblique and external rectus; it communicates by a small branch with the lenticular ganglion. The ganglion is an exceedingly small body. It sends several filaments to the iris, some of which are lost on the ciliary ligament. I am stating facts, without entering into minute particulars.

The movements of the iris show that the nerves which supply it must come from a source endowed with vital intelligence and instinct. Every person knows that the iris adjusts itself to meet circumstances, and that, it vigorously contracts when the retina is threatened with danger by too strong a light being thrown on it. If the lenticular ganglion possesses the faculties just stated, and that it is only connected to the brain by a small branch of the third nerve, I think it may be fairly asked why the pineal gland, (which I look on in the light of the chief ganglion of the organic nervous system,) which communicates with the brain itself, should not have similar characteristics. That the mind's eye must see objects pictured on the retina before the iris discharges its functions, is evident from what occurs in cases of amaurosis resulting from a disorganized condition of the brain, the pupil in such cases continuing dilated. It follows as a consequence, that the nerves proceeding from the lenticular ganglion must act in concert with a sound condition of the brain. As the conservatism of life rests with the ganglionic nervous centres, it is expedient to the well being of the body that the mind should have free communication with the centre of organic life, so as to be capable of imparting to it, as well as receiving from it, the rules for governing the other nervous centres of organic life.

Ocular demonstration declares that the mind and the ganglion operate consentaneously, as is witnessed in the case of the retina when exposed to light or darkness, and the movements of the iris under such contingencies. The division of the communicating branch of the third nerve demonstrates that the ganglion does not act without corresponding with the brain and central organic ganglion. The cornea, in persons who are obliged to look at very small objects, is rendered convex by the action of the muscles receiving branches from the third nerve, and the axis of vision is properly directed by the action of the muscles specified. How is this matter to be accounted for? The mind becomes conscious through the retina that the latter requires assistance; it is not able to afford the aid required; it communes with the central ganglion, (the pineal gland,) receives power, which it directs to the lenticular ganglion; reflex action takes place through the branch of communication of the third nerve; the muscles are thus enabled to co-operate in harmony with the mind. It follows as a sequence, that the ganglion must have knowledge of what is passing in the mind, and this is further proved by recollecting that the third nerve is a motor nerve, not guided by intelligence, and that neither the fourth nor sixth nerves, which are distributed to muscles whose action would be to distort the eyes from the proper focus, have any connection with the ganglion.

When a person is overwhelmed with grief tears are freely shed; the nose as well as the eyes become suffused; the mind, as in the former instance, communicates its troubles to the central ganglion, and by reflex action through it to the lenticular ganglion, through the nasal branch of the fifth nerve which is distributed to the pituitary membrane, the integuments at the extremity of the nose, the upper eyelid, the tensor tarsi muscle, the root of the nose, the lachrymal sac, and caruncala lachrymalis; hence the source of the tears is easily explained.

When a person is anxious to hear a sound at a distance, the tympanum is rendered tense by the action of the tensor tympani muscle. Before this can take place, the mind must be made acquainted by the portio mollis of the necessity of further assistance; it communicates with the central ganglion. What is the position of the parts concerned? The tensor tympani is supplied with motor branches from the facial nerve; the mind cannot effect anything through it, but the muscle receives branches from the otic ganglion, which is under the influence of the central ganglion, which inosculate with the branches of the facial nerve, and thus the muscle is capable of acting in unison with the mind. Can it be doubted but that the otic ganglion is co-equal in intelligence with the mind in regulating the action of the muscle to meet the requirements of the mind?

That such small bodies as the ganglions alluded to should possess so much instinct, is marvelous in the highest degree. It also follows a fortiori, that all the other ganglia are possessed of the same faculties in guiding the actions of the organs they are established to preside over.

A man that has made a speculation in railroad stock in which he is interested to a large extent, is told that the directors are a band of swindlers; that the concern is a mere bubble. The mind becomes deranged; it sympathizes with the central ganglion, with which it is united. Now, I should remark, the cerebrum is placed in the same position with respect to the ganglion that the motor nerve of the third or sensitive branch of the fifth nerves is connected with the lenticular ganglion; the announcement is forwarded by the par vagum to the pulmonic plexus; hurried respiration succeeds to the cardiac plexus, inducing violent palpitation to the solar plexus, causing the stomach to refuse food to the hepatic plexus, producing a secretion of bile; to the mesenteric plexus, causing diarrhœa; to the renal plexus, inducing a secretion of urine to the hypogastric and sacral plexus, throwing the sphincter vesicæ off its guard, followed by wetting of the pantaloons; and, in case of woman a short time pregnant, abortion produced by contraction of uterus. From this exposition, the fatal consequences attendant on the division of the par vagum must be manifest, as it actually severs the connecting thread of life. This is proved by recollecting, when a man gets a blow on the semi-lunar ganglion, that death instantaneously follows. The unity of action between the mind and the ganglia is rendered apparent when a man is about making a large leap; the mind surveys the distance; the will acts through the spinal chord, under the reflex influence of the central ganglion; the motor nerves are summoned to action; the intervertebral ganglia sends them filaments to accompany and instruct them how to exercise their power on the muscles, acting on the same principle that governs the lenticular ganglion and third nerve; and thus it is that the muscles act in strict harmony with the mind, propelling the body to the distance contemplated.

The inference from what has been stated is clear, that the spinal nerves are a triple compound, composed of sensitive motor and organic filaments, so that wherever one is found, the other two must be present. The nerves of organic life act consentaneously with the will wherever located, provided there is a nervous connection established between them. For instance, when a man is playing on a musical instrument, he has his mind fixed on the music book; his fingers move rapidly in harmony with his mind. Now, the nerves distributed to the fingers are branches of the brachial plexus; are capable of giving sensation and motion, as well as organic life, to the parts they are destined to supply in consequence of being connected with the organic ganglia at the roots of the nerves. The otic and lenticular ganglia again explain the phenomenon.

I presume it must be conceded that physiologists, in experimenting on the hind legs of frogs, have committed a most palpable mistake. They appear to have lost sight of the fact that the spinal nerves are a triple compound. I think the peculiarities of the afferent, efferent, and excito-motor nerves can be readily accounted for when the triple compound nature of the spinal nerves is duly studied. The action of these nerves is attributable to the organic nervous filament they contain.

When a person suffers from irritation in the bowels, caused by worms or indigestible food—here I must observe, that the intestines are exclusively supplied with nerves from the ganglionic system, and that the muscular fibres contract without the agency of motor nerves from the spinal chord. This fact proves that the iris does not require to have the ciliary nerves influenced by a reflected action of the tubercula quadrigemina through the communicating branch of the third. To revert to the patient—he is attacked with convulsions; the irritation is propagated to the brain; from thence to the central ganglion, and by reflex action from it to the brain and spinal chord; and next through the motor roots of the nerves to the intervertebral ganglia, the organic filament communicates with the muscles—the result is alternate relaxation and contraction of the muscles. Now, this is an action of the muscles independent of the will, and cannot be imitated by the most strenuous exertions of the will.

Again, a man gets a lacerated wound in the palm of the hand; the first thing he complains of, if he is about to get tetanus, is that he has caught cold, that his throat is sore, and·that he cannot swallow; in some time the muscles about the neck and face become rigidly contracted; next, the muscles of the upper part of the trunk, and finally the muscles of the lower part. This condition of the muscles could not be produced by the motor spinal nerves, inasmuch as the muscles would relax; no man can continue muscular exertion over a given period. What happens can be thus explained: the irritation is conveyed through the organic filament, to the cervical ganglia, and then the muscles of the neck, which are furnished with nerves from these ganglia, become contracted; here I need scarcely remark the superior cervical ganglion furnishes the pharynx with nerves. All the ganglia in due time become affected, those connected with the spinal nerves, and similar consequences are the result.

When an individual takes an over-dose of strychnine the muscles become rigidly contracted. Here the poison acts on the organic nerves, and through them on the muscles. It therefore follows, when the muscles are paralyzed, that strychnine excites spasms in the muscles—a fact which is too well known to need comment.

A man gets a dislocation of the shoulder; by throwing him off his guard it is easily reduced; but let him see what you are going to do, although he is most anxious to assist your efforts, the muscles will become forcible contracted, and baffle your attempts to accomplish your object.' Here, too, the mind and the muscles act together, through the influence of the ganglia placed at the roots of the brachial plexus.

When chloroform is administered it first acts on the organic nerves in the bronchial ramifications; secondarily, on the brain, known by the delirium that takes place; thirdly, on the central organic ganglion, and from it, by reflex action, on the brain and spinal chord; and through the nerves of the latter on the intervertebral ganglia, and ultimately the filaments which proceed from the latter to the muscles. That chloroform operates in the manner described is made painfully true, when the heart of man, under its influence, ceases to beat, when all human efforts will prove futile in some instances to restore its vital action—and thus demonstrating, by death, that chloroform is able to destroy an organ endowed with the greatest degree of muscular strength.

When a man gets drunk, the intoxicating liquor makes its first impression on the organic nerves in the coats of the stomach; the par vagum announces its presence to the brain, which becomes exhilarated, and after some time it shares its insidious sensation with the central organic ganglion, which reflects the intelligence through the brain and spinal chord to the intervertebral ganglia, and from the latter to the filaments destined to supply the muscles. This description is literally true; when witnessing the movements of a drunken man, his lower extremities will be observed not to obey his will, his legs cross one another, he stumbles from side to side, and, if he has imbibed too much, the muscles refuse to move, and he falls prostrate to the earth, perhaps to awaken in another world. Here it is evident that the faulty movements of the muscles, as well as their loss of power, is caused by the ganglia at the roots of the lumbar and sacral plexus, and that death is caused by the destruction of the ganglionic system; post-mortem examination fails to discover any lesion. My friend, Dr. Finnell, who has made such an immense number of examinations of the dead bodies of drunkards and others, can corroborate this statement.

I hope I have now given ample proof that the muscular fibres of the muscles are furnished with nerves from the organic nervous system; that the muscles owe their enormous power to their connection with the nerves in question. It may be said no nervous filament can be discovered in the muscular fibre; but the same observation is true of capillary arteries and veins, although no person doubts their presence.

When a drop of prussic acid is placed on the tongue of the subject, as Dr. Copeland remarks, he dies before the poison has time to get into the circulation; post-mortem examination discloses that the blood is fluid and dark colored in the blood vessels, caused by the death of the organic nerves in the internal coats of the vessels.

If a man is subjected to great violence, and sustains a compound dislocation, he will quickly fall into a state of collapse. The surface of the body will grow cold, the heart will almost cease to beat, the sphincters will be relaxed, and if a surgeon is so imprudent as to perform amputation under such circumstances, it is ten to one but the operation will be attended with fatal consequences, inasmuch as the patient's organic nervous system is unable to bear an additional shock.

Surgeons attribute this condition of the patient to sympathy; but it is more—it is direct and continued communication of the nerves in the part injured with the nerves in other parts. How is the cold on the surface of the body to be accounted for? By the vitality of the organic nerves in the skin being impaired in vitality, and by their being unable to eliminate the oxygen from the capillary arteries; (this is an hypothesis.)

When a person is seized with Asiatic cholera, on the hottest day in summer the body becomes colder than the surrounding atmosphere, the powers of life quickly give way, and the patient falls a victim to the poisonous influence exercised on the organic nervous system. The state of the patient in cholera goes to prove what I have just stated, that the production of animal heat is a vital action depending on the integral condition of the organic nerves.

As some persons may say that all I have said about the pineal gland being the great organic nervous centre of organic life is mere speculation, I must remark that if the wisest man in the world a century ago was shown a galvanic battery, and told that it was susceptible of generating an immaterial agent that could send a message by a small wire from one extremity of the globe to the other in a second, he would look on the individual giving him such assurance as a man laboring under mental alienation. I cannot help remarking there is an analogy between the pineal gland and the battery; the particles of gritty matter resemble the metallic plates, and the gelatinous matter the acid mixture. The Omnipotent Creator, who showed such infinite wisdom and unity of design in the construction of the organs of sense, did not place the pineal gland in such an important locality for a useless purpose. I strongly conjecture that the ganglion is so constructed as to regulate the *aura vitæ*.

It may be objected, that the gland or ganglion cannot receive and give impressions at the same time. The gland is connected with the brain itself; the nerves proceeding from the brain may be said to be continuations of it. The lenticular ganglion receives impressions from the brain through the branch of the third nerve, and sends communications to the muscles of the eyeball by the same nerve at the same instant. This matter, I think, is now fully elucidated; what is true of the one organ is equally true of the other. I now submit that life is centred in the organic nervous system; that the brain and its append-ages are attached for the purpose of affording a seat for the organs of sense, intellect, judgment, volition, sensation, and motion. That the ganglionic system is capable of influencing all the functions of the body, as relates to its preservation and harmonious action, as well as the preservation of the species; that the attributes of the cerebro-spinal system are instituted for man's guidance and connection with the world—that whereas man has the power to control his mind, he has no control over his life.

The will is seated in the brain; this is an admitted fact. The will has no influence over the organs of life. The lenticular ganglion is an organ of life, therefore the brain can have no power over it.

The lenticular ganglion is connected with the brain by a small nerve, and acts in concert with it.

It is the law of the organic ganglia to act in communion with one another.

Therefore, as the lenticular ganglion acts in consequence of being con-nected with the brain, it follows that there must be an organic ganglion located within the brain. And such is the fact; and placed, too, in the very centre of the brain, and in direct communication with it, called the pineal gland, but more worthy of the title of being styled the president of the organic nervous system.

That there is a close and intimate connection between the organs of animal and organic life, is a matter that cannot be disputed, and such close union is necessary for the well being of man. Life is the special gift of the Deity.

"And the Lord God formed man of the slime of the earth, and

breathed into his face the breath of life; and Man became a living soul." GENESIS, chap. v., 7.

Having traced the effects of the nervous system to their final cause, I will conclude. I could have entered more fully into details, but I deemed it would be superfluous to do so, having found the master-key to unlock the difficulties connected with the nervous system.

230 FOURTH STREET, WASHINGTON SQUARE,
   (formerly of White Street.)
January, 1859.

POSTSCRIPT.

Since writing the foregoing article, I have read Bernard's experiments on the nerves entering the sub-maxillary gland. His remarks, with respect to the blood becoming arterial, and the blood vessels becoming dilated when the tympano-facial nerve is acting, and consequently the secretion of saliva is susceptible of explanation precisely on the same principles as those governing the connection between the nasal branch of the fifth and its communication with the lenticular ganglion; in the one case, tears are secreted; in the other, saliva. With respect to the blood vessels contracting and the blood becoming venous, when the tympano-facial nerve is in a state of quiescence, being caused by the action of the organic nerves derived from the carotid plexus, it is clear these nerves preside over the circulation of the blood in the gland; the former condition of the nerves described is destined to make the mind act in concert with the vital action of the organic nerves, whilst the latter is instituted for the preservation of the gland itself.

Browne-Sequard has demonstrated that irritation of the skin at certain points causes epilepsy. Now, I submit that the phenomenon produced in the organic nervous filament, which communicates with a sensitive nerve, and thus, in some instances, conveyed directly to the brain; in others, to the spinal chord and thence to the brain. The irritation thus propagated being extended to the central ganglion, and, by reflex action, from the ganglia to the brain and spinal chord; thence to the ganglia at the roots of the nerves; and, finally, to the nervous filaments supplying the muscles. Here the brain is known to be implicated by loss of volition, and the central ganglion and other ganglia by the convulsions which supervene. When a person dies of epilepsy, it often happens no organic lesion can be found; under such circumstances death being caused by irritation, and ultimately, destruction of the organic nervous system.

In delirium tremens, the irritation is propagated from the organic nerves in the coats of the stomach, by the par vagum, to the brain; from the latter to the central ganglion; by reflex action, to the brain and spinal chord, to the intervertebral ganglia and organic filaments. Hence the delirium can be explained—the nervous twitchings of the muscles, the convulsions as well as the death of the patient—by the irritation and final exhaustion of the organic nervous system: here, too, post-mortem examination often fails to account for death. Thus, a man apparently and in truth possessed of great muscular strength, dies in an incredibly short time; perhaps by an attack of convulsions or syncope; thus showing the cessation of the heart's action depends on the destruction of the organic nervous system.

Every physician knows that hysteria can be almost always traced to irritation of the genital organs. The organic nerves of the uterus act consentaneously with the central organic ganglion through the connection of the hypogastric and sacral nerves with the uterine and vaginal nerves to the spinal chord, and thence to the brain; the phenomenon which succeeds does not now require explanation.

Epilepsy, produced by masturbation of the genital organs, can, in the male, be readily understood in the same way. Compression of the brain, followed by loss of volition, sensation and motion, as well as characterized by a slow pulse, stertorous breathing, and dilated pupils; here, recollecting the location of the central organic ganglion, and knowing that it can be compressed through pressure on the brain, it accounts for the condition of the patient.

A slice of the brain may be removed without disturbing the functions of organic life; because there is no pressure exercised on the central ganglion.

A man eats certain kinds of shell or putrid fish, and it is followed by cutaneous eruption; the connection here, between the organic nerves of the skin and the stomach, is the cause, by continuity of surface.

When a man gets concussion of the brain, he gets into a partial state of coma from which he can be partly made conscious; but it is well known that, even when his intellectual faculties are almost totally annihilated, he will get up and pass water; this fact shows how the organic nervous system presides over the protection of the body. In making post-mortem examination of persons who have died of concussion of the brain, no lesion of the brain, very often, can be discovered. Mr. Colles used to remark in his lectures, that the only thing that could be observable was, that the brain seemed to be compressed so as not to fill the cranium.

Here, it will be perceived, if the brain is thus circumstanced, it must necessarily compress the pineal gland, or central ganglion of organic life, and thus squeeze the vital principle out of the gland, and, consequently, the destruction of life itself.

In poisoning from lead, the muscular fibres of the intestines become spasmodically contracted, although not furnished with motor-spinal nerves, or apparently any nerves. The abdominal muscles become rigidly contracted after some time, showing that the same influence operates over them. If the irritation is kept up, paralysis of the muscles follow, particularly in the arm, showing the destruction of the organic nerves.

In caries of the vertebræ, the muscles of the lower extremity are rigid, and a man walks as if on stilts. Here the irritation is propagated to the intervertebral ganglia and organic filaments, proceeding from the latter to the muscles.

A man gets bad typhus fever; the abdomen becomes tympanitic; the pulse scarcely perceptible; the action of the heart extremely feeble; with involuntary discharges of fæces and retention of urine. Here the organic nervous system is on the brink of death. It has lost its power over the intestines and heart, and it cannot keep garrison over the bladder or rectum.

A man gets ileus, or invagination of the intestines; is followed by spasms of the muscular fibres of the part affected; the part of the intestines above the stricture becomes dilated, whilst the part below is constricted. When mortification sets in, the powers of life situated in the organic system quickly give way; recognized by the absence of the pulse; the intermitting action of the heart; the cold, clammy perspiration; the hiccup and hippocratic countenance, together with the relaxation of the bowels; thus showing that death has destroyed the barrier of obstruction.

When a man wishes to feel anything, he directs the mind to it; communication is thus had with the central ganglion, which acts by reflex action through the brain, spinal chord, and roots of the spinal nerves on intervertebral ganglia and organic filaments accompanying the brachial plexus; at the top of the index finger the branch of the median nerve and organic nerve inosculate, and thus the mind is made sensible of the nature of the part touched. Thus, the organic nerve acts as an afferent and efferent nerve.

When a young fellow sees a handsome girl he becomes enamored with her; the genital organs sympathize; here the optic nerve communicates the impression to the brain; the latter corresponds with the central ganglion, which, by reflex action through the brain and spinal chord to the sacral ganglia and plexus, the spermatic nerve inosculates with the organic nerves in the organs of generation, and here they act and harmonize with the brain.

John Hunter remarks, to perform the act of copulation well, the mind must be fully intent on the object. This proves that the brain must act through the central ganglion.

It therefore follows that the organic nerves act at all times consentaneously: I am satisfied the nerves in the foetal and maternal vessel form a ganglion in the placental lobule, thus keeping direct communication up between mother and child, and thus verifying the truth of the gospel: "And it came to pass that when Elizabeth heard the salutation of Mary the infant leaped in her womb."

When a man gets an attack of intermitting fever, the rigor is characteristic; the organic nervous system is all out of order, and the condition of the surface shows how much the organic nerves in the skin are implicated. Reflection will at once suggest what occurs.

Here let me observe, that God showed, by his own act, that air or breath was necessary for the life of man; for the moment breathing ceases, man is the same as when God formed him of the slime of the earth. Man is made of the elements of the earth, and how true it is: "Remember, man, thou art but dust, and into dust thou must return."

Having now demonstrated that the iris acts under the influence of the central ganglion, I am anxious to point out some practical hints: every person knows, when opium is taken in small quantities, it produces exhilaration of spirits, exciting the cerebro-spinal nervous system; but when taken in excess, it stimulates the organic system to such a degree as to induce fatal consequences; this fact is proved by the contraction of the pupils to a mere point. Drs. Corrigan and Graves have shown that belladonna and opium are mutually remedial, and, in the present number of Braithwaite's Retrospect, Dr. Benjamin Bell alludes to a case of poisoning by muriate of morphine, when belladonna had the effect of neutralizing the pernicious effects of the morphine. The belladonna has decidedly a sedative action on the central ganglion, as shown by the dilated pupil, so that its *modus operandi* can be readily understood.

In tetanus, chloroform should be administered, together with sup-

porting the system. Chloroform acts as a sedative on the organic nerves, and relaxes the muscles. Here I should state, I reported a
· case of traumatic tetanus, a few years ago, in *Reese's Medical Gazette*, in which the treatment just mentioned was attended with the happiest results, namely, the recovery of the patient.

The late Dr. Graves, in speaking of the treatment of typhus fever, said he wished to have inscribed over his tomb, "that he fed fever." The stimulants and restoratives enrich and enliven the blood, which acts on the organic nerves, lining the blood vessels, as well as the en- ' tire ganglionic system.

There is a case lately reported in the *Lancet*, where Dr. O'Reilly, of St. Louis, treated a case of poisoning by strychnine, by nicotine, with success. This case just proves, that as the strychnine causes spasms of the muscles, by its irritant effect on the organic nervous system, that nicotine produces relaxation of the muscles, by its sedative action.

In puerperal convulsions the organic nerves in the walls of the uterus (the branches of the hypogastric and sacral plexus) inosculate with the uterine and vaginal nerves; the disturbance is propagated to the spinal chord by the latter, to the brain and central ganglion, and by reflex action from the latter to the brain and all the nerves proceeding from the cerebro-spinal axis. That this is true, is witnessed by the frightful rolling of the eyes, showing the lenticular ganglion has no control over the muscles it supplies; by the grinding of the teeth; the strangulation and convulsive movements of the muscles. Chloroform here should be the remedy to be relied on; and I find that Dr. R. J. Tracy, Physician to the Melbourne Lying-in Hospital, (see *Braithwaite's Retrospect*,) has administered it in cases of puerperal convulsions with the most satisfactory results.

In hysteria there is titillation, or pleasurable excitement created in the organic nerves of the uterus, which is conveyed by the usual messengers to the brain and central ganglion, and, by reflex action, from the latter to the brain and other ganglia, to the filament proceeding from the latter. Here it must be remarked, that a female, laboring under a paroxysm of hysteria, will be conscious of what is taking place; showing that the cerebrum—the seat of intellect—is not interfered with. Turpentine destroys the tickling sensation of the nerves, and hence one of the best remedies in an attack of hysteria is a large turpentine enema, as well as the administration of the same medicine internally. Dr. Elliotson well remarks, it has no specific effect when it reaches the colon.

When a man gets a lacerated and contused wound of one of the extremities, and it is followed by mortification, some surgeons maintain that amputation should not be performed until the line of demarkation takes place, whilst others advocate a different practice. It is evident the destruction of the soft parts is the effect of the death of the organic nerves in the part, and that the entire organic nervous system is suffering in consequence of a part of it dying; this is clearly evident from the symptoms. As every inch the mortification extends cuts off a link of life, on true physiological principles it would be better to remove the diseased part at once. It may be, and is objected, that if the limb is removed before the line of separation sets in, that the stump will be attacked with mortification. When amputation is performed too near the dead part, there is no necessity for ligatures; the blood is found coagulated in the vessels; this clearly shows that the organic nerves in the internal coats of the blood vessels are contaminated, and that, as a matter of course, a return of the mortification is to be expected; under such circumstances, therefore, amputation should be performed at a very long distance from the diseased part.

Should chloroform be given to a person whose organic nervous system is so smitten? I think not. The vital power situated in the organic nervous system is almost extinct, and ready to depart at a moment's notice: chloroform, by its sedative influence, would probably annihilate it *in toto*. In such a case, French brandy and other stimulants should supplant chloroform, and prop up the drooping powers of life.

A man who falls from a height, on the top of his head, will be found laboring under symptoms of concussion of the brain; blood will be found flowing from his ears, and after some time it will cease and be replaced with serum—a certain sign, according to the late Drs. Dease and Colles, that fracture of the base of the skull has taken place; the man dies; extensive extravasation of blood may be found under the cerebellum. Why, it may be asked, are there not symptoms of compression under such circumstances? The answer is, because the central ganglion is not compressed, the tentorium cerebelli acts as its safeguard.

It seems strange how one man may get a depressed fracture, followed by all the symptoms of compression of the brain, and another may receive, apparently, a much greater injury of the skull without such complication. The explanation depends on the part injured, as well as the region of the skull; if pressure is not made on the ganglion, the symptoms are only indications of concussion.

It is a remarkable fact, that of a man who has got concussion of the brain will have a pulse ranging between 80 and 100, as long as he remains lying on his back; but on making him sit up, the pulse will rise to 120. How is this to be accounted for? When lying on the back there is more blood sent to the brain, as well as to the central ganglion; consequently, the latter has more power over the heart, through the par vagum and cardiac plexus. The principle that operates here is the same that guides the treatment of syncope when the person is placed on his back. When a person is exhausted from immense haemorrhage, as parturient women sometimes are, every person is aware that getting the patient to sit up in bed may cause instant death. The heart is a vital organ; it is presided over by a vital organ, and that vital organ is the central ganglion located within the head; and that it is so is manifested, inasmuch as it ceases to exist the moment the stimulus of the blood is withdrawn from it, by the patient assuming the erect position. When the organic ganglia lose the stimulus of the blood they suffer from irritation and exhaustion; hence the convulsions and death which ensue.

Sir Astley Cooper cautions surgeons not to have recourse to bloodletting in persons who have fallen on race courses, as by doing so they abstract the natural stimulus for the heart's action. This is quite correct; but it is clear it goes further—it prevents the heart from sending the requisite stimulus to the central ganglion. Here, again, I must reiterate, the brain has no influence over the action of the heart, as is proved by the vigorous state of the circulation in acephalous monsters.

Any oversight that I have been guilty of in writing this paper I hope will be pardoned, when I state it was written under a heavy press of professional business, *currente calamo*.

On the Bradycrote, or Abortive Treatment of Fever.

By THOMAS CLOSE, M.D., Portchester, N. Y.

Can fevers generally, without reference to the causes producing them, be arrested in their course, and healthy action completely established, in the short space of three to eight days?

A detailed account of the method I have pursued in the treatment of fever, for the last 8 or 9 years, will be the answer to this question.

It is well known that the tinctures of digitalis, veratrum viride and aconite all possess the property of restraining the frequency of the pulse, but the faculty in general do not seem to be aware that this property puts it in our power to arrest fever suddenly in its course, and thus curtail its duration in a most remarkable manner. Such, nevertheless, is the fact; *but it is essential to the success of this mode of treatment that the various materials from which these tinctures are prepared should all be the best of their kind, and that they should all be saturated alcoholic tinctures.* Digitalis is the most essential article, and that imported from England in one pound glass jars is far the best that I have been able to procure.

These tinctures may be variously combined, as the exigencies of individual cases seem to require. It is true, that as all the articles named possess the property of controling the frequency of the pulse, any one of them alone could be so managed as to arrest the progress of fever; but much experience has taught me that it is better to use them combined than separately, and any one who feels disposed to try the experiment will find, especially among children, that digitalis is too bitter, aconite too acid, and veratrum too prone to nauseate, to be used in large doses alone; and that by judiciously combining them, these inconveniences are in some measure avoided, and the desired result more readily attained. My usual prescription for adults is 5 to 7 drops of T. Digitalis, and 2 or 3 of Veratrum, to be repeated every second hour in severe cases, day and night; in milder forms, one or two doses may be omitted during the night, and if much pain be present, two or three drops of aconite may be added to each dose. In cases attended with little or no local inflammation, the pulse usually begins to diminish in frequency in 24 to 48 hours, and by the fourth, and sometimes by the third day, frequently falls to sixty, and sometimes to fifty in a minute; the heat of skin is found at the same time to have entirely subsided, and the whole phenomenon of fever is entirely brought to a close. I have frequently seen all this accomplished in three to five days. In cases of fever, complicated with, or depending on, acute inflammation of some important organ, two or three days of extra time are usually required to overcome the disease, and one or two drops of the sedative tinctures should be added to the doses, daily, to meet the resisting influence of violent inflammation.

The practitioner will soon learn, by his own observation, that children from 6 to 12 years of age will bear nearly the same doses as adults; often quite as large. The youngest child that I recollect treating with these remedies was an infant only two months old, laboring under a smart attack of fever, complicated with dysenteric irritation of the bowels. Two drops of digitalis, 1½ of veratrum, and one of morphine were administered once in two hours; the complaint ceasing on the fourth day.

In aggravated attacks of inflammation of the brain, lungs, bowels, &c., whether the patients are adults or children, it is usually desirable that they should lose blood; but I have never found it necessary in any case to bleed more than once, provided the sedative remedies have been used freely for three or four days, in doses adequate to the exigencies of each individual case. If the disease is not then found to yield, it will be proper to let blood freely, and the pulse will then soon—sometimes even within half an hour—rapidly abate in frequency and force; the skin becomes cool, and the whole aspect of the disease undergoes a most gratifying change. A little further perseverance with the remedies, and the fever ceases altogether.

The following case will illustrate the influence of the sedative remedies in the treatment of acute inflammation. A little boy, between three and four years old, was suddenly attacked with an ardent fever, commencing with prolonged chills. On seating myself by his bed-side, I found him constantly agitated with strong convulsive struggles, but totally unconscious of anything around him. His skin was very hot, his head intensely so, and his pulse full, strong and very frequent. The symptoms strongly indicated the necessity of bleeding, but the agitation of the muscles was so constant and so violent, that no part of him could be kept still for a moment. His mother was directed to dip a cloth in cold water, and to brush it over all parts of his head, within reach, and as soon as the rag began to feel warm in her fingers, to dip it again in the water, and renew the application. This process was continued constantly for an hour, during which time the temperature of the head was reduced several degrees. The convulsive struggles now began to abate, and a full dose of calomel was, with some difficulty, got down, after which 5 drops of digitalis, 3 of veratrum, and 2 of aconite were administered, with directions to repeat the dose every second hour afterwards. This treatment was commenced about ten A. M., and, when visited the next morning, his eyes were observed to be open, though he did not seem to fix them upon any object, nor did he make any attempt to speak. The heat

12

did not return to his head, the disease seeming to have left the brain to fix upon the lungs. Considerable cough came on, with mucous rattling and shortened and oppressive breathing. The pulse was a little softened, but still quite frequent. Leeches should now have been applied to the chest, but could not be procured in season, but a cantharides plaster was laid on, and the febrifuge treatment steadily persisted in. The calomel operated sufficiently, about 24 hours after it was taken. On the third day the influence of the sedative tinctures began to be manifest; the pulse was more softened and considerably less frequent, and the lung affection very much abated. On the fourth day there was still further amelioration of all the symptoms; pulse but slightly accelerated, and the patient was beginning to recover his mental faculties. The febrifuge was directed to be continued through the day, but omitted at night. On the fifth morning the pulse was found to be reduced below its normal frequency, and every vestige of febrile action had entirely ceased. There was slight cough remaining, but no other evidence of lung disease. As I had occasionally seen fever to kindle up afresh when the febrifuge was discontinued too soon, it was persisted in for a day or two longer.

The little fellow was now convalescent, but so entirely prostrated by the violence of the disease he had gone through with, that it was two or three weeks, even with a good appetite, before he recovered strength enough to bear his weight. I certainly had never before seen so young a child recover from so violent an attack, and there cannot be a doubt that his recovery is almost entirely to be attributed to the powerful influence of the sedative tinctures in controling intense vascular excitement, and that too without the loss of one drop of blood.

The case just described occurred last summer, in the month of June; and this winter (Dec., 1858,) a lad 13 years of age has just recovered from an attack in all respects similar, with the exception that the brain affection was still more intense, and the loss of consciousness more protracted. A nursing infant, scarcely twelve months old, has still more recently passed safely through the same form of disease, distinguished only by a few shades less of intensity.

For about eight years past every case of fever, with the exception of intermittents, that has fallen under my observation has been treated in this way, and with almost uniform success. Scarlet fever, measles, and several cases of natural small-pox have been treated in the same manner, without the loss of a patient. During the last two years, a period in which very many severe attacks of inflammatory fever have occurred, I can only recall two fatal cases of inflammation of the brain, both in persons far advanced in life, and three or four cases of infantile dysentery. All else have recovered. Can an immunity so remarkable be rationally ascribed to any other cause than the speedy and absolute control exercised by the sedative tinctures over morbid vascular excitement? Fever is effectually cured, irrespective of the causes which produce it, by reducing the action of the heart a little below the frequency of health, and holding it steadily there for a day or two. No sooner does the pulse lose its febrile frequency, and especially if it falls steadily below the frequency of health, than the heat of skin subsides, thirst ceases, the tongue assumes a more natural aspect, and all febrile action is found to have passed away.

The attentive observer cannot fail to notice the remarkable curtailment in the duration of fevers, and especially in their most aggravated forms, when thus treated; contrasting as it does so strikingly with their tedious and prolonged course when combated by the old method. So little evidence, indeed, is there of any material shortening in the natural duration of fever as generally treated, that many medical writers do not hesitate to declare it a self-limited disease, and wholly incapable of being arrested in its course by medical treatment. For myself, I certainly am not aware of having been more fortunate than the faculty in general, while treating fevers by the long-established method, either in respect to their duration or fatality.

During the first three or four years of my experience with the sedative remedies, I did not succeed in arresting fever as promptly as can readily be done now; having been too sparing in their doses, from an apprehension of doing mischief by reducing the action of the heart below the point of safety; but never meeting with anything in the slightest degree unpleasant in that respect, I gradually became bolder, and now do not hesitate to give doses twice as large as were then thought safe, whenever the resisting influence of intense disease requires such enlargement; and I now entertain a perfect conviction that there are few if any cases of fever that will not bear with perfect safety enough of the remedies to control them in the space of a week.

I cannot refrain from adverting once more to that feature of this most interesting process, that surprised me much at first, and still seems most wonderful; the so often noticed fact, that from the first time that the arterial pulsations are found steadily ranging below sixty in a minute; from that time not the slightest vestige of febrile heat remains, for fever itself no longer exists. This is a most significant fact, and shows unmistakably that the sedative remedies exercise as positive and certain control—though not quite as speedy—over continued fevers as the anti-periodics exert over intermittents. Years have passed away, and that pulse has never once deceived me; and it affords much pleasure to be able to say to anxious mothers, "dismiss your fears; that pulse has never disappointed me, and will not now."

The greatest inconvenience attending this mode of practice is, that we cannot send our prescriptions to the druggists, for their tinctures are too variable and uncertain to be trusted where such perfect accuracy is required. If we estimate two drops of the alcoholic tinctures to be equal to a minim, the following formula will show the most convenient method of preparing the febrifuge mixtures. Into a ℥iv. phial, pour from a minim glass 100 minims of tincture of digitalis, 36 minims of tinct. veratrum viride, ℥ss. sweet spirit nitre, ℥iss. of syrup of rhubarb or simple syrup, and fill up the phial with water. To adults, or large children, a teaspoonful should be given every second hour, day and night. If a lung case, attended with much cough, is prescribed for, syrup of conium should be substituted for syrup of rhubarb.

For grown persons I have administered the remedies very frequently in the form of pills, and with the most gratifying results.

R.—Pulv. Digitalis ℈iv., extr. conii. ℥ij.

Acet. extr. colch. and mass. pil. hydr. ää ℥i.

Tinct. verat. virid. and tinct. aconite ää ℥iiss.

Evaporate slowly in the mortar, with frequent stirring, to pill consistency, and divide into 120 pills.

One pill should be given every third hour, so that 8 are taken in 24 hours, and continued until the disease is found to be decidedly abating, after which 6 pills a day should be administered until the fever ceases altogether.

Any physician desirous of putting this mode of treatment in practice, by addressing a letter to Dr. Thomas Close, Portchester, Westchester Co., N. Y., will be informed where he can obtain the tinctures prepared as above directed.

Case of Meningitis scarlatinosa—Convulsions. Treatment with Ice-Bath. Perfect and rapid Recovery.

By Louis Bauer, M.D., M.R.C.S., Eng., Surgeon to the L. I. College Hospital of Brooklyn.

The little son of a German bootmaker, aged 2½ years, had been in the enjoyment of most excellent health up to the 28th of July,

1856, when he exhibited signs of scarlatina. The development of that exanthem proceeded kindly till 11 o'clock A. M. next day, when it turned pale, the child simultaneously becoming morose, irritable, and feverish. At 3 o'clock P. M. fever ran high, combined with drowsiness. At 4 o'clock I was sent for, the patient being then attacked with violent convulsions. On entering the sick room I met with a most oppressive and close atmosphere, produced by hermetical closure of door and windows, with a view to protect the patient from cold, the thermometer ranging then *only* 96° Fah. in the shade.

The little fellow was fearfully convulsed; there was hardly any remission; pulse innumerable; skin burning hot, and light red, as in erythema; respiration 75 in a minute; tongue parched; bowels distended and constipated; face hot and flushed; carotids pulsating violently; eyeballs highly injected, and pupils firmly contracted; the child, of course, senseless. There was so great a hyperæsthesis of the skin that the slightest touch would increase the convulsions.

Scarlatina had been at that period very malign, especially through brain affections, and the case before me indicated a fatal termination also. The antiphlogistic apparatus, with derivation upon the bowels, was the proper course of treatment, yet the disease was too violent and rapid to be reached by that. My impression was, that for the mere want of time I would fail in my efforts. I acquainted, therefore, the parents with my apprehension, and indicated a hopeless prognosis.

It was at that time that I had just read the excellent work of Prof. Virchow on Inflammation and Fever. Conclusive to my mind he has proven that both are but alienations of the nutritive process, that the morbid generation of animal heat is the only standard symptom of either, and that the reduction of it is tantamount to their cure.

Despairing of any relief by ordinary means, I considered myself justified in putting his opinions to a practical test. I fully realized the grave responsibility I should incur by so doing; I anticipated not only the objections on the part of the parents, based on the popular prejudice that cold temperature in any shape is unequivocally injurious to exanthematous diseases or their sequels, but also that of the profession, on the ground that repressing the circulation in an organ would necessarily increase the morbid supply of another already in a state of inflammatory engorgement.

On the other hand, I argued that there was nothing to be gained by other means, except the approbation of those practitioners holding other opinions; that in cooling down the entire body I would directly

ameliorate the febrile process, and self-evidently the existing inflammation; that this might even actuate the skin to resume its function, being obviously below par then. A number of other reflections crossed
my mind appertaining to analogy in natural science, as to the process
of combustion, fermentation, &c., all strengthening my position.

Before I had explained to the parents, the urgency of the case, my
views as to its treatment, and obtained their consent, some 15 minutes
had elapsed, during which time the little patient grew evidently worse.
A large tub was then procured, filled with well-water, and a good
quantity of ice was put in, to reduce still more its temperature. Into
this bath I placed the convulsed child. The very contact with the
ice water arrested at once, and almost magically, the convulsions;
the child seemed to feel perfectly comfortable and relieved.

The bath lasted 11 minutes, at the end of which the pulse had settled down to 135, and respiration to 40, which were the leading
points. The patient was then lightly covered with thin blankets, and
remained on the bed 10 minutes, by which time the pulse had risen
again to 160, and respiration to 55, when a new, but less violent
paroxysm set in. This was, as I thought, a signal to renew the bath.
Its contact arrested a second time the convulsions, and brought down,
within five minutes, the pulse to 125, and the respiration to 30. The
child, being again surrounded by dry blankets, remained for twenty-
five minutes perfectly quiet, and, literally speaking, without a stir,
whilst of course the temperature, pulse, and respiration rose again.
At the expiration of that time a faint convulsion commenced, passing
off in one minute, and after a clear remission of two minutes a stronger
one followed, with aggravation of all symptoms. A third bath was
then resorted to, which extended not over four minutes; the pulse
sunk this, time to 94, the respiration to 19, and the pupil dilated
slightly on shading the eye. Whereupon the child was surrounded
with a cold, wet sheet, and above that with a dry blanket. He remained therein perfectly quiet and comfortable. At 9 o'clock P. M. a
kind perspiration commenced, continuing till morning.

At 8 o'clock, A. M., on the following day, the child was sitting up
and playing, to all appearance perfectly well, though somewhat weak.
The scarlatina took henceforth a mild and regular course.

Almost at the same time, that is, on the 81st of July, Dr. Bleek
called me in consultation in a child's case, (daughter of a German
grocer, named Beine,) that had been a few days previously attacked
by scarlatina. The patient was about 8½ years old, and had been prior

of good health. The exanthem had taken a mild course up to that date, when it suddenly evinced symptoms of great danger. Dr. Bleek being called, fully realized the importance of the change, and invited my co-operation. We saw the patient together at 9 o'clock in the morning, and this attack was said to have commenced about an hour and a half previously. The following was the status morbi: innumerable pulse, and small; the body very hot and dry; whereas the extremities were cold and covered with profuse and clammy perspiration; all the maculæ scarlatinosæ livid, not suppressible; countenance presented the highest degree of anxiety; cheeks and lips cyanotic; the eye glossy; the patient seemingly conscious; all respiratory muscles in full operation, particularly those of the neck, and yet not succeeding to move the thorax, the child all the while gasping for air; no abnormal sound on either inspiration or expiration; no dullness or crepitant rale about the thorax; purely diaphragmatic respiration; over the region of the heart extensive dullness on percussion, without being able to notice its sounds on the walls of the thorax; slight pulsation and distension of external jugular veins.

I have to state in addition that there were no signs of poisoning, no dilatation or contraction of the pupils, no nausea, vomituration or purging.

Our diagnosis was pericarditis scarlatinosa acutissima with *effusion*, perhaps also complicated with *endocarditis*. The violence of the disease foreshadowed a fatal termination, and the inefficiency of any mode of treatment was fully realized. As the only feasible remedy I suggested ice-bath, which was accepted by Dr. Bleek, but very reluctantly by the parents. It was administered in the same way as in the previous case, and its effects perpetuated by an iceberg upon the cardiac region. No medicine was otherwise administered.

By this treatment the number of pulses and respirations, and the temperature of the body, were quickly reduced, whilst the extremities became warm, and of natural color.

All signs of cyanosis disappeared simultaneously with the other symptoms; the maculæ becoming red again and commencing to show detached epithelial scales (desquamated); angina pectoris and diaphragmatic breathing gave place to deep thoracic respiration; and, in fact, the child improved so rapidly as to require no further attendance beyond the fifth day. On the tenth day the patient became again subject for treatment of diarrhœa. On the 20th hypostatic pneumonia set in, and on the 24th it expired from that disease. We were permitted to open the pericardium, in which we found about five ounces of fluid, containing a large quantity of albumen, several fragments of fibrin, a few blood and granulated inflammation globules, besides some traces of pseudo membranes and a few adhesions with the heart.

In addition I may state, that another child of the same family, nineteen months old, was attacked in the very same manner and under the same circumstances; it died within two and a half hours, and before medical aid could be procured.

Since that time I have had no opportunity of repeating the ice-bath, and I make these communications for the sole purpose of exciting the attention of the profession, reserving to myself the continuation of my experiments in all cases that may justify them. As the water was but the medium of low temperature, I have no doubt that very cold air acting upon the body would produce the same effects if otherwise practicable.

Case of Syphilitic Ischias; Reflex Phenomena—Recovery.
By the Same.

Syphilitic affections of the nervous system are well-authenticated facts. Von Graefe has observed some instances of syphilitic amaurosis with rarification of the retina and atrophy of the optic nerve; Rayer, syphilitic ramollisement of the brain and gumatous tumor at the basis cranii; Ricord, paraplegia; Canstatt, epilepsy of syphilitic origin, &c. The number of exact clinical observations is, however, limited, and the following case may, therefore, be accepted as an interesting contribution.

A German tailor, from Elizabethport, aged 35 years, was admitted to the Long Island College Hospital on the 15th of January, 1858. For two years he had suffered from intense pain along the sciatic nerve of his left extremity, which was much attenuated. Several physicians had looked upon his disease as rheumatic, and treated it accordingly, though with no relief. When first applying to me as private patient, I was disposed to take the same view of his case, and prescribed some, chiefly narcotic remedies for him. Deriving a slight benefit from their use, he entered the hospital with a view of following up the results by a systematic treatment.

He was then carefully examined; rather decrepid in general appearance; bald scalp; face ashy; lips and gum red; appetite and evacuation tolerably good; urination normal. His posture was bent forward in order to relax the abdominal muscles; the latter being subject to spontaneous but periodical contractions. In assuming the erect posture, these spastic contractions immediately commenced so as to bend his trunk and cause noisy expirations. Left nates flattened; pain on pressing behind large trochanter and along the course of the sciatic nerve, seemingly very severe, for his pulse became accelerated and himself hot all over. No soreness along the spine, but some in the sacral region.

The sciatic neuralgy and the reflex symptoms were almost contiguous and without much change as to time and season, although wet and cold weather seemed to aggravate them. He felt himself otherwise free from pain, and denying positively that he had at any time been infected with syphilitic virus, the examination was not pressed in that direction. Furthermore, stating that prior to his present malady he had been subject to rheumatism, and that this was a common difficulty among the inhabitants of Elizabethport, no other diagnosis suggested itself than that of rheumatic neuralgia with reflex from the lower portion of the spinal chord. Within the first days of his reception into the hospital, it was, however, noticed that the patient very often used his handkerchief; that his nasal secretion was rather purulent and bloody, and that he diffused an oppressive odor from his nostrils, which thereupon were inspected, when a perforation of the septum and ulceration of the mucous membrane were ascertained. Admitting, then, that he had contracted the disease some three years previous, and been attended by a quack, who pronounced him cured, I altered my treatment accordingly, and in about six weeks he was discharged, completely relieved. Other syphilitic symptoms guiding diagnosis did not manifest themselves.

SELECTIONS.

ASTONISHING IMPUDENCE.

One of the most impudent things perpetrated on the scientific profession for a long time, has been witnessed in this city within the last thirty days. And what, good and unsuspecting reader, do you imagine it is? It is nothing else than that Drs. Newton and Bickley, *Professors in the Eclectic Medical Institute* of this city, have taken not only the contents of the *Edinburgh Medical and Surgical Journal*, but also the name, issuing it under the title of the *Cincinnati Eclectic and*

Edinburgh Medical Journal!! We really could scarcely believe our eyes, when we saw the first number. Only think of it: the names of Syme and Newton, Bennett and Bickley, side by side! Think of it, too, medical men, that this *Eclectic School,* this hot-house of steam, homœopathy, hydropathy, phrenology, "roots and yarbs," conducted in the past by men whose only cry against legitimate medicine has been "poisoners and butchers;" by men who were never heard of beyond the limits of a small country village until their sudden advent before the public on the foul stage of this so-called school; think of it, we say—of their appropriating, printing, and binding up the Journal which represents the great Edinburgh University with what they are pleased to call the *Eclectic Journal.* Faugh! Language fails us to express our disgust. Yet it is a fact.

It is, however, to expose these "wolves in sheep's clothing" that we have thus far condescended to notice even so glaring and striking a piece of medical impudence, in those latter days of brilliant humbugs and deceptions. At last, be it known, these pigmy leaders of a dirty and miserable foray on legitimate medicine find that their stock in trade is about giving out; that, like an old prostitute who has lost her charms, they find it necessary to assume a virtue which they never had, and never will have, solely for the purpose of sustaining a pitiful delusion.

Yes, plain *Eclectic Medical Journal* was proving a bad card. It had ceased any longer to delude; it had failed to establish for this small sect —sprung originally from two remedies, a hot bath and a lobelia emetic —any position in the regular scientific world; it had failed to make any headway, and the time had come for something to be done. Hence the appropriation of the *Edinburgh Medical Journal.* We shall expect at the end of the year to read the announcement of the course of lectures in the "Eclectic Medical Institute and University of Edinburgh!" Stranger things are happening every day. The "Eclectic Medical Institute and University of Edinburgh of *Cincinnati!*" This reads quite as well, and sounds as sweetly on the ear as *Cincinnati Eclectic and Edinburgh Medical Journal.*

The school which this Eclectic Journal represents is, we believe, well understood by all intelligent and reading medical men. It was removed to this city from Worthington, a small village in this State. No sooner was it removed here than its professors commenced a scurrilous abuse of the regular profession for the use of mineral medicines and for surgical operations. When they opened here they performed no operations; all diseases of a surgical nature being advertised as curable by *Eclectic remedies* or *Eclectic practice*. When the cholera made its appearance, they advertised in the daily papers the wonderful power of Eclectic practice to cure all cases of that terrible disease, at the same time loudly proclaiming that "old school practice," as they were pleased to call scientific treatment, saved no cases. They published their cases. No one ever heard of any patients dying under their treatment. In addition, they pronounced in the public papers that all mineral medicines were poisons. They blowed what they called Eclectic practice and themselves on the corners of the streets, and in all public places. Next, we find in the faculty the representatives of all known quack systems: homœo-quack, electro-pathic, hydro-pathic, electro-biological, *et id omne genus*—black spirits, green spirits, and blue; with their class made up of unsexed *women*, broken-down preachers, sickly school teachers, crazy mechanics, and sugar-loaf headed individuals who have but two ideas—terrible opposition to "mineral practice," and a profound admiration for " Eclectic practice." They graduated a large number from this intellectual set, with one year's attendance on their course of lectures.

More still: This Dr. Robert Newton has been a *professed cancer curer*, and for a long time had a *secret remedy* for its treatment.

And what now is their course? Still crying out against legitimate medicine, while using the very remedies they have so long vilified and abused as poisons. They have advanced, no doubt, from the reading and *editing* of the works of truly scientific authors. Newton gives mineral medicines; he has even given, as we have been told, that much abused remedy, calomel. He has edited *Syme's Surgery*, in which many wonderful and new ideas from *Eclectic surgical practice* have been introduced. He even admits now that he cannot cure all cases of cancer; that it will return after it has once been removed. He even finds that Eclectic practice and remedies fail to take a stone out of the bladder, and resorts to the knife.

Such is a brief history of this school and its most prominent man. It once had a fellow in it by the name of Sanders, who had the impudence to edit *Gregory's Chemistry*. O *tempora!* O *mores!* And last, but not least, to cap the climax of this grand Eclectic quack school, it has had the impudence, nay, more, has so far stultified itself as to print and publish the journal of all others which has, and does at present, support legitimate scientific medicine.

They wage a continual warfare against the *code of ethics*, and yet have the greatest disposition to be on friendly terms with the regular profession. The editorial department of the January number of this hybrid journal is full of protestations of friendship. Like all the quacks, they seek a corner of the great mantle of true medicine to cover them. They can fraternize with all sorts of quacks, according to their own account.

Some very respectable professional gentlemen, and even journalists, are ignorant of the position of this class of quacks in this city: Newton's school, and Cleaveland's school—the two eclectic quack concerns of this city, with whom no regular member of the profession has anything to do. If our space permitted our sketch would be much longer.

Before we close, let us give our readers the contents of the *Cincinnati Eclectic and Edinburgh Medical Journal*. It is nearly all Edinburgh. 1st, "An *Eclectic* treatise on the practice of medicine, by R. S. Newton, Professor of Surgery," in which he claims that Eclectics brought forward twenty-five years ago the anti-bloodletting treatment of disease! With the exception of one other article, on ptyalism, from a Dr. Woodruff, of Pittsburgh, Indiana, all the others are taken from the *Edinburgh Medical and Surgical Journal*. Even, too, they cannot write reviews of books, for, with the exception of a notice of Dr. Sanger's book on Prostitution, all the others (and there are several) are from the same source.

We are happy to be able to inform our readers that these two so-called schools are dying slowly. Their great effort to preserve a so-called position is mainly directed to appropriating the books and journals of scientific men, publishing them as Eclectic treatises, widely different from old school authors. In proof of this, Dr. J. King brought out an *Eclectic Dispensatory*, so full and glaring with wholesale *plagiarisms* from the *U. S. Dispensatory*, that Wood and Bache, its authors, sued out an injunction against its sale, so that Dr. King was forced to re-write his Dispensatory. So of Dr. Cleaveland, with his *Medical Dictionary*, whom Dr. Reese, of New York, charged boldly with plagiarizing from him. And last, but not least, Newton and Bickley have appropriated one of the first journals in the world, representing "old school medicine." The professors of these two schools have amazed the professional public, and even the unprofessional, with the number and variety of books *written* and issued by them. The truth is, not one of them is celebrated in any speciality of medicine in this city. We hesitated for some time before penning this article. We felt it to be our duty to say what we have said, in our capacity as medical journalists of true scientific medicine. We have not written for our friends and readers in this city, but more particularly for our readers and editorial brethren at a distance. We leave these people, their schools, and journals to time, which sooner or later will number them in oblivion, where so many worthless systems already lie, " unwept, unhonored, and unsung." We are not to be dragged into any discussion; our pages can be devoted to much more profitable matter.—*Cincinnati Lancet and Observer*.

DISCOMFITURE OF THE FRENCH HOMŒOPATHS.

Persons who possess a thin dermal covering are often found to manifest a want of caution, leading them to engage in conflicts the result of which is almost inevitably a severe punishment. The homœopaths in Paris have lately been in this predicament. They have brought an action for libel against our contemporary, *L'Union Médicale*, laying the damages at *fifty thousand francs;* and, after a three day's trial before a legal tribunal, they have lost their cause, and been sentenced to pay costs. *Voici les faits.*

In 1857, a Dr. Magnan published a book entitled *De l'Homœopathie, et particulièrement de l'Action des Doses infinitésimales.* The author forwarded a copy of the work to the *Union Médicale*, and himself called on the editor, to request a notice. It was courteously represented to him in reply, that the sentiments both of the editorial staff and of the readers of the *Union Médicale* were as one on the subject of homœopathy; that it was not probable that the review could be otherwise than inimical to the doctrine; and that, as the habitual readers of the paper were fully aware of the fallacies of the system, it would be better to leave the book alone. M. Magnan, however, reiterated his request in pressing terms; he " preferred criticism, however severe, to silence; and asked neither indulgence for the author nor complaisance towards the doctrine."

Accordingly, the work of M. Magnan was placed in the hands of Dr. Gallard, a well-known contributor to the *Union Médicale*; and a review, written by that gentleman, appeared in the number for October 24, 1857. This review is before us. To Dr. Magnan, individually, the tone is courteous; Dr. Gallard states, that he believes him to be "a man seriously convinced, and capable of acknowledging his error when pointed out." On homœopathy, the writer was more severe:

" Homœopathy is not a doctrine, and much less a science. It is a commerce carried on by some individuals, to the detriment of science and of humanity; and if there be a time when it has been possible to apply the Hahnemannic method without being an ignorant or miserable charlatan, it is certainly not the present. Dr. Magnan must be told, although he ignores the fact, that the most ardent followers of homœopathic doctrine have the good sense to abandon it in practice. Whenever they meet with a severe disease, they bleed, they purge, they give large doses of medicine, absolutely as if Hahnemann had never existed; but they proclaim on the house-tops what they have done by means of homœopathy. A short time ago, one of the most renowned homœopaths was called to a lady of rank, who, towards the end of an incurable malady, was attacked with anasarca and ascites. The homœopath gave her daily *fifty centigrammes* (nearly *seven grains and three-quarters*) of calomel; thereby producing a colliquative diarrhœa, which indeed diminished the dropsy for the time, but certainly hastened death. Nevertheless, the patient's friends could not see through this deception, but proclaimed in all the Parisian saloons *the happy results of homœopathic treatment.*"

Severe, but just, are these remarks, which are only a specimen of the tone of Dr. Gallard's article. And it is not surprising, therefore, that the Parisian homœopaths should have winced under the rod thus skillfully administered to them. This review, as we have already said, appeared on October 24, 1857. On the 29th of the same month, Dr. Amédée Latour, the editor, and Dr. Richelot, the *gérant* of the *Union Médicale*, received from two homœopathic practitioners, calling themselves the president and secretary of a " Central Homœopathic Committee," a request to make a public retraction! Of course, this very modest demand was not complied with; and thereupon twelve homœopaths brought a civil action against Drs. Gallard, Richelot, and Latour, for prejudice done both to their general reputation and to the practice of their art. For this double injury they demanded damages to the amount of fifty thousand *francs* ($10,000.)

To meet this charge, several plans might have been followed. That which was adopted by the defendants was to place the matter on scientific grounds. Personality could not enter as an element into the debate, because none of the complainants had been mentioned in Dr. Gallard's article; and the " Central Homœopathic Committee" had no legal existence.

Dr. Gallard therefore published a *Note scientifique sur la Doctrine dite homœopathique,* which was distributed to the president and judges composing the first chamber of the Civil Tribunal. The homœopaths issued a reply—unfortunately for themselves; for it fell into the hands of Dr. Béhier, president of the Medical Society of the first *arrondissement* of Paris, who, at the desire of his colleagues, published a report, in which he followed the homœopaths through every twist and turn of their argument, leaving no retreat but confession of their error.

The cause was tried before the first chamber of the civil tribunal on November 17, December 1 and 3, 1858. Messire Emile Ollivier was counsel for the twelve homœopaths; Dr. Gallard was defended by Messire Paul Andral (son of the distinguished pathologist;) and Drs. Richelot and Latour by Messires Bethmont and Victor Lefranc. On December 1, the prosecution against Dr. Latour was abandoned; and on December 3, M. Sallantin, acting for the *procureur impérial*, summed up in an admirable speech, which is published in the *Union Médicale* for December 11. We must make a brief extract. M. Sallantin has shown that Dr. Gallard mentioned none of the complainants by name, and cites the commencing sentence of the paragraph which we have above quoted from Dr. Gallard's article. He continues:

"And M. Love and each of the complainants cry: 'Hear you the blasphemy? He means me! A charlatan—it is I! an *illuminé*—it is I! a fool—it is I! Quick, let him be mulcted of 50,000 francs!' Really, messieurs homœopaths," (continues M. Sallantin,) "you have a very thin skin (*la fibre bien sensitive*). Why does that word 'charlatan' make you raise your heads? Have you a troubled conscience? Your conduct would really give one a right to think so! Let us be serious; you have but one argument. You say: 'We are homœopaths; but M. Gallard has attacked homœopaths in general, without exception, therefore the injuries wound us severely in full front. You are not named nor pointed out; and you have no right to complain. ... The attack of M. Gallard, inasmuch as it is general, cannot affect you. To admit the contrary, would be to interdict all criticism and all scientific discussion. Suppose, for instance, that any one courageous enough to express his opinions, good or bad, on some of our modern writers, were to draw a contrast between Molière, Corneille, and Racine, and those who . . . forgot that the theatre ought to be a source of instruction in manners, and not a place of corruption, and a school where the crowd may learn to applaud crime and to admire all the vices. . . . He would be ready to meet criticism; but must he undergo legal prosecutions without end? Must he have to defend himself against all the journalists and *vaudevillistes* in France, and pay 50,000 *francs* to each? The supposition is really absurd."

On December 10, the civil tribunal pronounced judgment. Dr. Latour was declared to be dismissed from the case, and the plaintiffs were sentenced to pay his costs. As regarded Drs. Richelot and Gallard, the court nonsuited the homœopaths (the plaintiffs), and condemned them to pay all costs.—*British Medical Journal*, December 25, 1858.—*Medical News*.

[From the American Medical Monthly.]

Report of the Committee of the N. Y. Pathological Society, appointed to examine the Case of Mr. E. A. Groux, affected with Congenital Fissure of the Sternum.

Mr. Groux has a congenital fissure of the sternum situated in the median line, and extending the entire length of the bone.

There appears to be no deficiency of the bony substance in this case, but a simple median fissure. The clavicles are articulated with the lateral halves of the sternum, and the costal cartilages join the bone on each side in the usual manner. The sternal attachments of the sterno-mastoid muscles are also in their natural position; but the sterno-hyoid and sterno-thyroid muscles, both right and left, are attached below to the left half of the sternum. The left half of the sternum is also situated upon a plane somewhat anterior to that of the right; so that, when the two edges of the fissured bone are drawn together by muscular action, the left edge projects slightly in front of the right.

When Mr. Groux stands erect, in an easy position, the fissure is one inch wide at its widest part, i. e., about the junction of its upper and middle thirds. By forcible separation of the two halves of the sternum, the width of the fissure at the same spot is increased to two inches. By forcible approximation, it is diminished to a quarter of an inch.

The space between the two lateral halves of the sternum is covered by integument, and apparently also by a strong subcutaneous fibrous sheet or aponeurosis which unites the edges of the bone, and prevents their separation beyond the limits above mentioned.

The respiratory sounds generally, over the chest, as perceived by auscultation, are natural in character. The impulse of the heart, also normal in character, is felt at or a little above the level of the fifth rib, a little inside the plane of the left nipple.

In the medio-sternal space, in the ordinary erect position of the body, there is visible to the eye a pulsating tumor, situated apparently just beneath the integument and subcutaneous aponeurosis. The pulsations of this tumor extend from the second to the fourth intercostal space, and from the median line to the left edge of the fissure. They consist of alternate dilatations and contractions, which correspond in frequency with the pulsations of the heart and arteries. The filling up of the tumor takes place from below upward, and from left to right; while its contraction runs in an opposite direction, with a rapid wavy motion, from above downward and from right to left.

The contraction of the tumor is synchronous with the impulse of the heart, at the level of the fifth rib.

A majority of the Committee perceive a slight interval of time between the contraction of the tumor and the pulsation of the carotids in the middle of the neck. All the members of the Committee are agreed that there is a perceptible interval between the contraction of the tumor and the pulsation of the temporal arteries.

If a stethoscope be applied to the tumor, the two cardiac sounds are heard very distinctly, and natural in character.

If the finger be pressed deeply into the medio-sternal space immediately above the tumor, there is felt, exactly in the median line, a rather firm, deep-seated, pulsating body, which is beyond a doubt the ascending portion of the arch of the aorta. By applying the stethoscope firmly in this situation, the double cardiac sounds may be heard quite as distinctly as upon the superficial pulsating tumor. The pulsations of this part of the aorta, as perceived by the finger, are synchronous with the impulse of the heart, at the level of the fifth rib.

When Mr. Groux takes a deep inspiration, followed by a long, slow, and forcible expiration, the pulsating tumor in the medio-sternal space disappears at the time of inspiration; but toward the end of the expiration it again shows itself, and gradually becomes very much increased in size. It enlarges from below upward, on the left of the median line, till it reaches, at its highest point, the level of the lower edge of the first rib, on the left side. It also enlarges from left to right; until, at the level of the third costal cartilage, it extends quite over to the right edge of the fissure, and thence occupies the whole width of the fissure, down to the level of the fifth costal cartilage.

If this experiment be tried while Mr. Groux lies upon his right side, the tumor becomes excessively prominent, and at the time of its greatest distension a band is seen extending across it in a nearly horizontal direction, and partially dividing it into two upper and lower halves. In the opinion of the Committee this appearance is probably due to an unusually prominent fibrous bundle of the intersternal aponeurosis, which produces a partial constriction of the tumor at this point. When respiration again commences, the tumor is reduced to its original size, and its pulsations for a few seconds are more hurried than usual.

This pulsating tumor has been considered by different observers to be—1st, the right auricle; 2d, the right ventricle; 3d, the aorta.

The Committee are of the opinion that it is not the right auricle; for the pulsations of the tumor, in its ordinary condition, are situated altogether to the left of the median line—at least they do not extend toward the right beyond this line. The right auricle, on the contrary, in the natural position of the heart, is seated altogether to the right of the median line. The body of the auricle is very deeply seated, and quite posterior to the plane of the ventricle; and the only part of the auricle which approaches the front of the chest is the appendix. This, however, is situated quite to the right of the median line, even when distended, lying sometimes behind the second costal cartilage and second intercostal space, sometimes at the third costal cartilage and sometimes at the third intercostal space. If the tumor in this case, therefore, be the right auricle, the heart must be considerably displaced toward the left. But the aorta can be felt, as above stated, in its normal position in the median line; and the point of the heart strikes the chest, also in its natural position, a little inside the plane of the left nipple. The Committee, therefore, regard it as certain that the whole heart is normally situated; and that consequently the pulsating tumor seen in the fissure cannot be the right auricle.

They are also of opinion that it is not the aorta; for if the superficial tumor to the left of the median line be the aorta, then the deep-seated pulsations above and in the median line must belong to the arteria innominata. But the characters of the two pulsations, which would be the same were they both arterial, are in reality very different. The deep-seated pulsations give to the touch the sensation of a firm, vibrating, cylindrical body, the tension of which does not vary very much at different times; the same sensation, in fact, which is communicated to the finger when placed upon the aorta of a living animal. The superficial tumor, on the contrary, is alternately hard and soft, and exhibits a very free pulsating movement.

Furthermore, when the superficial tumor is distended, as above described, in expiration, it extends upward, near the left edge of the fissure, toward the top of the sternum; so that this part of it is on the same horizontal level with the deep-seated pulsating body in the median line. The latter, therefore, cannot be the arteria innominata, unless it happens in this instance to take an abnormal origin from the side or the concavity of the aortic arch.

If the superficial tumor also be the aorta, it is not easy to understand why it should become distended during a forced expiration.

The Committee are of the opinion that the pulsating tumor in the medio-sternal space is the right ventricle.

First—On account of its situation. In the natural position the most superficial portion of the heart is the anterior surface of the right ventricle. The conus arteriosus lies to the left of the median line, at the level of the second intercostal space. The bases of the aorta and pulmonary artery are situated nearly upon the median line, at the level of the third costal cartilage, and the right ventricle lies behind the sternum, from this point down to the sixth or seventh costal cartilage. There is every reason to believe that this is very nearly the position of the ventricle in this instance. The only peculiarity of position, therefore, would be that in Mr. Groux the heart is placed a little higher in relation to the ribs than in the majority of instances. This is actually the case in him, since the point of the heart strikes the chest at, or a little above, the fifth rib. The pulsating tumor, therefore, corresponds in situation with the right ventricle, and with no other portion of the heart.

Secondly—The character of the pulsations corresponds with those of the right ventricle. They are wavy and peristaltic, and run from above downward, and from right to left. The contractions of the appendix auricularis, on the other hand, (the only part of the right auricle which could present anteriorly,) are different in character, and are directed from the point of the appendix, toward the body of the auricle, more posteriorly and toward the right.

Thirdly—The most striking proof is that derived from the appearances produced by a suspension of the breath in prolonged expiration. When the heart is exposed in a living animal, and the movements kept up by artificial respiration, if the respiration be suspended for a time, the blood soon begins to accumulate on the right side of the heart, producing a distension of its cavities. Under these circumstances, the right ventricle becomes swollen quite as soon, and to quite as great an extent, as the right auricle; and the swelling takes place from left to right quite as much as from right to left; so that the right ventricle extends much further beyond the median line, and occupies much more of the space just behind the sternum, than in the natural condition. The conus arteriosus also swells and becomes prominent from left to right.

Two of the Committee have found the same condition of things in the human subject after death, which has been preceded by distension of the right side of the heart. The right auricle, under these circumstances, though very full of blood, projects but little or not at all to the left of the median line; while the right ventricle extends beyond this line, to the right, for at least one inch.

When Mr. Groux suspends the breath in a long and slow expiration, the distension of the tumor, already described, corresponds exactly with that of the right ventricle. The swelling does not take place from right to left, but from left to right. The upper part of the distended tumor, corresponding with the conus arteriosus, comes prominently into view, to the left of the median line, running up to the lower edge of the first rib; while its lower portion extends over to the right edge of the fissure, at the level of the third costal cartilage, and thence downward, exactly in the position of the right ventricle, to the fifth costal cartilage. During this time the pulsations continue, but the contractions are incomplete, and the tumor does not disappear at any time until a new inspiration has taken place.

There are several other appearances, more or less connected with the fissure of the sternum in this case, which have some interest.

(1.) When Mr. Groux takes a moderately full inspiration, and then compresses the chest suddenly by muscular action, a portion of the lungs are forced out at the upper part of the fissure, forming a prominent oval tumor, highly resonant on percussion, which dispppears on again relaxing the muscles. The Committee are unable to decide whether this protrusion is formed by the right or the left lung, or by both together.

(2.) When Mr. Groux lies upon his right side, the heart falls a little over in the same direction, and the tumor then becomes more prominent, and passes a little beyond the median line. When he lies upon his left side, the heart falls away to the left, and the tumor slightly recedes.

(3.) When the heart has become very much distended by prolonged expiration, its pulsations may be felt on the left side of the chest, gradually extending from the fourth to the second intercostal space.

(4.) Mr. Groux has also the power, by making two or three quick inspirations and then forcibly compressing the chest, of stopping the pulse at the left wrist. This is perhaps due to the unusual mobility of the clavicle, by which the subclavian artery is compressed at the top of the chest.

JOHN C. DALTON, JR.,
JOHN T. METCALFE, } *Committee.*
EDMUND R. PEASLEE,

QUACKERY AT HOME AND ABROAD.

When our indulgent reader takes up this number of the Journal and sees the heading on this article, let him repress his inclination to turn to something more interesting than this well-worn theme. We would like to have a little familiar talk on medical topics, and would fain say something about quackery. Necessity compels us, however, to the course which some brilliant lights invariably adopt—that is, to do all the talking ourselves. We will then begin by asking the question: Are we especially favored by Providence in the distribution of quacks; or are we greater sufferers than our brethren on the other side of the water? We opine that, as a rule, the profession in this country suffers most; but occasionally we have accounts of such brilliant success ·of the gentry in Europe, that we feel almost inclined to yield the palm. An item has appeared in a late number of the Boston Journal, which gives us some idea how the Parisians are sometimes humbugged in the midst of their stringent regulations in regard to the practice of medicine. It has been said that the African race does not inspire the European with the same disgust which is felt for them by some of our philanthropic countrymen, and we therefore imagine that Paris would be an admirable field for the operations of a sable charlatan. We know that here, in the Southern States, it is not unfrequent to find old negroes who have quite a celebrity in the treatment of various diseases; such a notoriety as is sometimes enjoyed by our old women in the North, who have therapeutical tendencies and immense diagnostic intuition; but we have never before heard of a full-fledged black quack in successful practice. But for an example, see the following account of how Sambo is succeeding in the practice of medicine in Paris:

Quackery in Paris.—There is now at Paris a negro who carries everything before him as a quack doctor. He is a fine man of his race, covered with trinkets and diamonds, displaying great wealth in house, carriages, &c., &c., and obtains the most fabulous fees from the easily-gulled Parisians. Amongst his various feats, *L' Union Médicale* relates the following : He was sent for the other day into a very rich family, where a lady had for years suffered from very obstinate recurrence of fibrous tumors about various parts of the body. The best surgeons of Paris had failed in arresting the disease, and recourse was naturally had to wild systems of medicine; all these, however, including homœopathy, were powerless. Magnetism, necromancy, &c., &c., had their turn, but nothing succeeded. At last, the negro's turn came. When he had cursorily examined the patient, he exclaimed, "this lady is curable, and I shall get her well in fourteen days." " Well, then," said the husband, " undertake the case at once." " My fee is £800; £240 is to be paid at once, and £40 on every other visit." Much demur was made to such a demand; but as the quack threatened to leave the lady to her fate, he was allowed to pocket the £240, and has begun the treatment. The result is not known, but may easily be guessed at.—*Druggists' Circular.*

We have never thought of this before, but it now strikes us what immense natural advantages the black race has over the white in the field of quackery. Once out of the reach of the prejudice which would prevent success among *intelligent people* in this country, all his national characteristics operate immensely in his favor. First among the essential elements of his calling, is *unblushing* effrontery, and a mendacity which is sometimes almost incomprehensible. We do not desire to

---

* *Appropos* of quackery in Paris, some of our readers may have heard of the libel suit against the *Union Médicale;* we clip the following, which gives the result of this remarkable suit, from a daily paper :

A curious libel suit has recently come off in Paris. Twelve homœopathic physicians sued the Union Médicale for having asserted that "homœopathy was neither a doctrine nor a science, but a trade ;" and that "if an epoch had ever presented itself at which the method of Hahnemann could be employed by any one who was not abjectly ignorant—a crack-brained visionary, or a wretched charlatan—it certainly was not the present one." The editors and proprietors of the Union Médicale pleaded, by way of defence and justification, that what they had stated was only the truth. The tribunal before which the suit was brought, without passing any judgment on the rival claims of allopathy, yet held that the plaintiffs had no ground of action, and dismissed the case, with costs.

enter into any discussion as to the equality of the white and black races; but in making a comparison of their characters, we conceive that it will be generally acknowledged that the black are superior in the above respects. There are, of course, noble exceptions to the rule; but, in general terms, it is as much the physiological state of a negro to disregard the truth, as it is for an Indian to be uncertain in his ideas in regard to *meum* and *tuum;* the beautiful character of "Uncle Tom" to the contrary notwithstanding. Another element of success would be a profound ignorance which it would be impossible for a light-complexioned quack to attain. Strange as it may seem to the uninitiated, you know, kind reader, that this is a most important element of success. It is necessary for a person to be profoundly ignorant of the simplest principles of medicine, in order to take any stand in the ranks of the fraternity of quacks. Without that, how could the practitioner state that a certain disease in a child was due to "an absorption of calomel by the system from the flesh of an ox which had had a disease of the skin, for which, *perhaps*, mercurial ointment had been applied and had *struck in;*" or that an induration on the finger, produced by sewing, was "dependent upon a disease of the medium nerve?" This last *bon mot* was related to us by a patient only a few days since.

In both these qualifications, however, a white man might possibly equal the negro, though such a case would be only the rare exception; but there is a quality in which he would always be his inferior, namely, in external decorations. The natural admirable taste in dress of the black race, with which we are all so familiar, must have a tremendous effect upon the Parisian; and if the reader will return to the paragraph which we have quoted, he will see that this point is particularly mentioned. With all these qualifications, we will have to look no further than the Parisian negro for our beau-ideal of a quack.

This, we imagine, is nearly as hard a case as we ever have in this country, and we cannot but suppose that it is but one of numerous instances; but look for a moment how the profession of France rid themselves of such an evil, while we submit to it from a necessity which arises from a person's right, in this country, to do what he pleases with his life and health. We copy the following from the Nashville Journal, with the editorial comment:

Quackery in France.— The Physicians demand Protection of the Government.— Their Petition to the Emperor.

SIR—At an epoch in which the history of your benevolence is writ-

ten in ineffaceable characters on the face of France; at the moment
in which society, imitating your example, is striving to ameliorate the
condition of the poor classes, the medical corps deem it proper to call
the attention of your majesty to one of the social evils which paralyze
your generous intentions.

Sir, alongside of that medicine which consoles and cures, there boldly marches an ignorant, sordid, and illegal medicine.

If, in the cities, the instruction of the masses can sometimes coun-
teract its grievous effects, it is not so in the country, where, unfortunately, ignorance still predominates, and where it lavishes its scandalous and deceitful promises with unrestrained publicity.

Sir, there is in this a serious danger, which barrier constantly im-
pedes that impulsion which you so freely give to mortality and humanity.

Permit us to hope that your majesty, so careful of the children of
the poor, and so provident for the aged poor, will deign to pursue his
work by protecting the whole community by an efficacious *repression*
against the illegal practice of medicine.

Such, sir, are the wishes of the medical corps, so often called to the
honor of propagating the benefits of your touching solicitude for the
suffering, but too often fettered by prejudice in the accomplishment of
its mission of humanity.

We have the honor to be, with the most profound respect, the very
humble and the very devoted servants of your majesty.

[SIGNATURES.]

The above is a copy of the petition of the deputies of the Medical
Societies of the Seine to the Emperor, who received it with great
complaisance, and even with gratification. The Emperor expressed
surprise that the practice of medicine was not more effectually protected by existing laws, and inquired if it were possible that remedies
were advertised in the public journals, and sold to the public, without
having received the sanction of the Academy of Medicine; and he
promised that the petition should be sent to the proper Minister, with
special instructions to examine it and give it the attention that its importance demanded.

Such a measure is impossible in this country; we might petition the
Legislature year after year without any result; and should we succeed
in having any remedy attempted, we would, perhaps, be in as bad a
situation as the profession of Massachusetts, who succeeded in pro-

curing the passage of a law, by which irregular practitioners could not collect their fees in the courts. Quacks, however, still found their dupes, whom they compelled to pay in advance, saying, with a great deal of force, that it was absolutely necessary, as they could no longer collect by law. This gave this class of practitioners such an advantage, that the profession actually petitioned for the repeal of the law which they had formerly desired, and were content to let the matter rest as before.

We fear that it is impossible for us to put a legal check upon quackery in this country; even the abortionists are permitted to advertise their nefarious compounds, and, we fear, will continue to do so in spite of us. The articles in our September and October numbers, by which we, in our enthusiastic inexperience, expected to do some good, met with so faint a response from journals and societies, that we reluctantly have given up the battle. We cannot but hope, however, that though our feeble efforts did so little, the powerful influence of the American Medical Association will do much in behalf of the cause. The mind of the profession will be admirably prepared for the subject, by a series of articles which have been commenced by Dr. Storer, of Boston, in the "*North American Medico-Chirurgical Review.*" Dr. Storer was directed to prepare a report on this subject, at the meeting of the Association at Nashville, 1857, but has not been able till now to fullfil the task. We wish him all success, and are still convinced that a united action will do some good.

We have expended so much on the Parisian negro, that we have little space left for quacks in general. Where, by the way, do we draw the line? Are we not to regard the homœopathist in that light? We certainly are sufficiently abused, not only by homœopathic practitioners, but by those who employ them, to justify us, when speaking of them at all, to give the only rational view of their pretended system.

Yes, they are a variety of the genus quack, and should be regarded as such, and invariably treated as such by us! We are members of a noble and dignified profession; one which has grown, by the accumulated labors of great men, to a science, our reverence of which must increase with every advance we make in its mysteries. As members of such a profession, we must countenance in no way the insolent upstarts who seek to rob it of its glory, who traffic in death, and who grow fat upon the spoils wrung from the sufferer, deluded by their false promises of health and strength. It is undoubtedly the fact, that irregular practitioners derive most of their gains from persons whose minds, worn down by an incurable malady, and dissatisfied that they can extract no promise of cure from the conscientious physician, morbidly craving encouragement, will go to the quack who promises a perfect cure in a month, for $100, for example, *in advance.* This is the way in which money is extracted by our itinerant doctors, who find it necessary to migrate as soon as there is any danger of a falsification of their promises.

It seems to us that we have but one duty to perform in regard to irregular practitioners, and that that duty is due, not to ourselves, but to the profession which we have chosen—that is, never to countenance them in any way; never to consult with them, to satisfy a patient, for example; never to let the world say that there exists between us and any irregular, merely a friendly difference of opinion in certain points. We may differ in opinion with men with whom we are working for the advancement of a common cause, and acknowledge that we may be wrong and they right; but that is not the case with men who wish to throw discredit upon a profession which, I hope, we all love with our soul, and to decry the great names of those whom we cannot but revere. Let us guard our science above all things, and do nothing which can take from its dignity, whether we be influenced by the head or by the heart.—*Buffalo Med. Journal.*

MEDICAL SCIENCE AND COMMON SENSE.

[This is the title of a Lecture by Professor Linton, of St. Louis Medical College, from which we extract a few pages as a specimen, the whole being too good to be lost.]

I beg the attention of my audience whilst I pass in review some of the so-called axioms and principles of this new system; and, first, of the law that like cures like; or, as it is learnedly expressed, "*similia similibus curantur morbi.*"

The idea is, that what will produce a disease will cure it. Thus, quinine, says Hahnemann, causes intermittent fever when given to a healthy person, and this is the reason why it cures the same diseases. He lays it down as a principle, that we must administer in disease a drug which is known to produce symptoms like those of the disease itself. The regular physician, following the dictates of *common sense*, acts on the contrary maxim, namely, that the remedy should be opposed to the disease; thus, if a part be inflamed and irritated, the regular physician endeavors to soothe it, not to add to the irritation.

If an organ, as the brain, be engorged with blood, he apples cold water to the head and cupping-glasses to the temples to drive and draw away the congestion from that organ. If the patient be exhausted by long disease, or a sudden haemotrhage, he gives food and tonics destined to produce an opposite state. If a limb be dislocated, he brings it back to its joint; he does not push it further out. If a bone be broken, he adjusts it; he never thinks of pitching the patient from the top of a house so as to cure it by breaking it worse. If a patient be parched with thirst, he gives him cold water to quench, not salt, to increase it. Opposed to the regular practice and to common sense and nature, stands homœopathy.

According to the Hahnemannian maxim, the true homœopath must ascertain the symptoms of his patient, and then give a medicine or employ an agency that will produce similar symptoms. Very well. Let us look at this procedure. A patient is diseased from deficiency of food; he is weak, hardly able to walk; what will cause similar symptoms? Evidently, a little further starvation or a bleeding. The patient has swelling about the throat that renders breathing very difficult, he gasps for breath, his lips are blue. Just tighten his collar or tie a cord around his neck, and you will cure him if homœopathy be true. The patient has inflammation of the eyes—they are red and irritated; apply something that will cause sore eyes—say cayenne pepper, and a cure will be effected if homœopathy be not a humbug! The patient is deaf;—stuff his ears with wax—an accumulation of ear-wax will cause deafness: common sense and the regular physician take it out; the homœopath, to be consistent, puts more in. The patient has his head broken by a stone—"hit him again" with a brickbat, "*similia similibus*."

It is clear that this cardinal principle of the homœopath is false, not only in part but *in toto*. It is never to be followed in the cure of disease. It is true that the patient may recover after its adoption; that is, he may recover in spite of the fact that his disease has been aggravated by the ignorant administration of remedies. Evidently, the object of the physician is to induce a state of the system not similar to, but opposed to the disease.

As an example of homœopathic cure, we are told that snow is used as an application to a frozen limb. But keep the snow to a frozen limb and it will remain frozen forever. It is the rubbing with snow, which gradually re-introduces the heat, that cures; the limb must not be too *suddenly* heated. Hence it is best to commence the cure with but a slight degree of heat.

Another example insisted on, is the cure of delirium tremens by the use of alcohol; but the explanation is the same as that of the cure of the frozen limb. The system has become accustomed to the stimulus; the sudden cessation of its use causes the disease; and it is given in gradually diminished quantities to cure it.

It is also said that the vaccine virus produces in the system a disease similar to small-pox, and thus homœopathically prevents small-pox. But this is preventing, not curing disease. Take a patient with small-pox and vaccinate him. It will do no good. It would cure if homœopathy were not utterly false. If a person can have a disease but once, then, of course, one attack will prevent another attack. You might as well call death homœopathic, because a man cannot die a second time. In the annals of human delusion, there is nothing that surpasses in absurdity the idea that the cure of disease is to be effected by causing a similar disease; and if I did not suppose that I have said enough to demonstrate its absurdity to every reflecting mind, I might go on for an hour with the mere mention of its follies. The idea of curing disease by giving medicines to aggravate it, as Hahnemann says his remedies do, is equalled only by that of the quack who always endeavored to throw his patient into fits, for the reason that he was—skillful in the treatment of fits.

Another maxim of the sect is, that but one medicine is to be given at a time; that combinations of medicines are not to be used. Now, what reason is there for this? The human system is used, in health and disease, to being operated on by many agencies simultaneously, and but for these combinations it could not be sustained. The air we breathe is a compound; so of water; our food is obliged to be a compound to support life. Moreover, what is meant by *one* medicine? Most medicines are compounds in the state of nature. The precept to give but one medicine is vague, valueless, and unreasonable. Besides, Hahnemann violates his own precept by advising that medicines be used with alcohol. Alcohol itself is a compound.

Hahnemann's attempt at defining disease shows at once his want of medical knowledge and philosophical acumen. He defines it as a change in the vital principle. Then, as if not satisfied with this definition, he says that it is a change in the state of the organs. In this definition he stumbled on the truth. But, again, he says that the disease consists of the totality of the symptoms; and then, again, he defines *sensations* to be *states* of the system.

It is clear, at least to the medical portion of my audience, that these definitions apply to very different things; they confound the categories, as logicians would say. The symptoms of disease and disease itself, are as different as an entity and an action.

The definition, however, to which Hahnemann attaches the most importance, and on which he builds his system, is that which regards disease as a change in the vital principle. With him, disease is a change in the immaterial, not the material; a change rather in the spirit than in the flesh; and hence he contends that only immaterial or spiritual agencies can produce it, and only immaterial agencies can correct it; and hence, again, he endeavors to reduce the dose of medicine so low—so to attenuate it—so to manipulate it, that it shall be as near nothing as possible, hoping thereby to make it spiritual, and thus adapt it to the cure of his spiritual diseases. With him the disease is nothing material; and he wishes to render the medicine a nonentity, so as to cure it on the principle *similia similibus*. He could not avoid seeing that material substances cause disease. He saw that overeating and drinking, and the ingestion of poisons, and chemical and mechanical injuries, caused disease; but to make these facts harmonize with his favorite theory, he said that these things caused disease by their spiritual influences or properties ! !

According to this view it is the spiritual influence of the sabre that pierces the body, not its material form. It is the spiritual influence of the club that breaks the skull. It is the spiritual influence of fried onions that causes an attack of cholera morbus. Now, is it asserting too much to say, that this is *nonsense* ?

Physicians and everybody else recognize material and immaterial agencies in the cause and cure of disease. The material are our food, the air we breath, various poisonous substances, &c. The immaterial are the passions—as fear, hope, love, despair, disappointment, and the like. The distinction is clear to every one; but Hahnemann confounds these things. He confounds the moral with the physical—the material with the immaterial. With him food is as immaterial as fear; hot air is as immaterial as hope; gunpowder as immaterial as good news; cabbage and care act in the same way. Need I say that *common sense* repudiates all such stuff as this.

Hering, the commentator of Hahnemann, says that material substances cannot cause disease, because they create such a terrible disturbance in the system. He also says that this terrible agitation of the system casts off the offending matter. Then, again, he says that these material agents kill the patient; therefore they cannot cause disease. Oh no! They only occasion derangement and death, but never cause disease. This is more than contradictory—it is absurd—it is an outrage on the common usages of language. Hering is a worthy disciple of Hahnemann, whose "Organon" of Medicine, as he presumptuously calls it, is a tissue of unfounded assertions, contradictions, and absurdities, from the first to the last page. According to this "Organon" nature cannot cure disease, except by inducing another disease, *similia similibus*—which is exactly equivalent to saying that no one ever gets well without medicine; and as, according to the same "Organon," the regular faculty never cures a disease, except by accidently inducing a similar disease, there are no cures except those of the homœopath. Now, everybody knows this to be false. Everybody knows that diseases get well without medicine. Everybody knows that they get well under the treatment of the regular faculty. It would not be a more reckless assertion to say that no one dies without medicine, than to say that no one gets well without it.

But Hahnemann professes to cure disease by inducing a similar disease. How does the disease which he induces get well? Here is a gordian knot; but he cuts it, by saying that nature can cure the medicinal disease without inducing a similar disease. This is the idea—nature cannot cure any disease, except those which the homœopath induces. So he substitutes his medicinal disease for the natural one. Nature will cure his disease, but not her own. Now, we know that diseases induced by medicines are as difficult to cure as any others—as the palsy, induced by lead; the mercurial cachexia, &c. Medicines may kill as well as cure.

Let us vary our review with a few of Hahnemann's flat contradictions. He says that all chronic diseases are caused by three miasms, as he calls them; and contradicts the assertion, by saying, that the worst of chronic diseases are caused by the allopaths. He asserts that a disease is the totality of its symptoms; and then contradicts the assertion, by saying, that disease is a state of the system; and then contradicts it again, by saying, that it is nothing material but only a change in the vital principle. He asserts, that to extinguish the symptoms is to cure the disease; and then contradicts the assertion, by saying, that allopaths, and even nature, extinguish the symptoms without curing the disease. He asserts, that homœopaths cure disease by inducing a stronger and more powerful disease; and then contradicts the assertion, by saying, that the remedies employed are so weak, and the impressions they make so light, that nature cures them directly, and without any trouble.

We see that nature cures disease, allopathically, even according to the testimony of homœopaths. It is well it is so, otherwise there would be no cures; for nature cannot cure a natural disease except by inducing another disease, but she can cure the medical disease *directly;* so says Hahnemann. This is a happy circumstance, otherwise no disease could ever be gotten rid of.

Here is the whole secret in a nut-shell. Neither art nor nature can cure one single disease, except by inducing another; but when art has cured one by inducing another, then nature can cure the disease induced by art without inducing another. So two curative agencies are necessary in every case—that of the homœpath, to obliterate the natural disease by substituting one of his own make; and that of nature, that plays allopath, and cures the medicinal disease *directly.*

To hide the palpable error of his system, Hahnemann drew a broad distinction between medical and surgical diseases. His theory applied only to medical diseases. He did not pretend to cure any other. It is a remarkable fact that quacks rarely meddle with surgery. The results of bad practice are too plainly seen in surgery. They prefer the dark corners of medicine, where what they do is hidden from the view of the public; and where they can claim, as the effects of their nostrums, the healing operations of nature. Oh, no! Homœopathy applies not to surgical diseases. So says its author. Very well. If this be true, then it cannot apply to medicine; for, in a vast number of instances, medical and surgical cases differ not in kind but only in degree. Thus, an inflammation or a congestion, which is a medical disease, gives rise to a tumor or an ulceration, which is a surgical disease. The medical case of to-day is the surgical disease of to-morrow; and the surgeon uses in the treatment of surgical diseases the same remedies employed by the physician, and for the same reasons and on the same principles. Indeed, that which is a medical disease in the interior is a surgical disease on the surface. Inflammation of the knee-joint is a surgical disease—an inflammation of the lungs is a medical disease. But homœopathy does not cure an outside inflammation. It cures only an inside one. The reason why homœopaths do not pretend to cure surgical disease is, that these diseases will not, as a general rule, get well of themselves. They can do better with those nature can cure.

Most writers who have turned their attention to this medical delusion have dwelt at length on the absurdity of its small doses. I shall be brief with them. How much water do you suppose would be required to make a grain of medicine, mixed directly with it, as weak as it is in the 30th dilution? Do you suppose that a hogshead would dilute it sufficiently? not at all. All the water in the new reservoir? that would not be a beginning. All that is in the Mississippi? the northern lakes? the Atlantic Ocean? the Pacific? All the water in the world? Why, all this would be but a beginning. An eminent mathematician has calculated the amount for me. Here is what he says: A grain of opium, or anything else, dissolved in a body of water eleven trillions and five hundred and seventy billions of miles cube, would just be in the thirtieth dilution. At this rate, one grain of medicine would supply all men for all time. A body of water a million of miles deep and wide ought to make one grain weak enough. But it takes a thousand of millions to make a billion, and a thousand of billions to make a trillion, and we have seen that over eleven trillions cube are necessary for the thirtieth dilution; and this is not the highest dilution. What has common sense to say to this? What a mountain labor for this ridiculous mouse. How it outherods and surpasses every other "much ado about nothing," and casts into the shade even old ocean

> "———— into tempest toss'd,
> To waft a feather or drown a fly."

A body of water eleven trillions of miles cube to a grain of medicine! Here is an ocean across which no electric cable could ever be stretched. A hundred generations of ships, each generation lasting a hundred years and sailing five hundred miles a day, would all decay and rot, and go down before they reached the middle of this ocean. The rapid comet itself, flying 150,000 miles an hour, and doubling heaven's mighty cape in its wide sweep, would require more than 40,000 years to circumnavigate such a gulf as this! Were the earth itself drawn to wire, it would not reach across this wide, wide sea! Only the wild lightnings of heaven and the swift-winged arrows of light might essay to traverse the mighty cube!

Perhaps a better idea of the weakness of the thirtieth dilution may be afforded by the following statement : Put a grain of medicine into a hogshead of water; of this take one drop only; throw the rest away, and mix it with the waters of Lake George; then take one drop of the lake and mix it with Lake Erie; then take one drop of Lake Erie and mix it with the waters of Lake Superior—mix well—then take one drop of the lake and put it into a hogshead of water. I do not know that this would come up to the thirtieth dilution; but it would be weak enough for all practical purposes. One would suppose that the patient would be required to drink pretty largely of this attenuated dilution. Not at all. He is not allowed a glassful—no, not even a teaspoonful. What! is it to be taken in drops? No, not even a drop is allowed. One drop moistens three hundred globules, and one of these is the dose. Are they not taken very often? No! one in from ten to fifty days—though Hahnemann thinks it is often best not to swallow it at all, but only smell it—not with both nostrils, but only with one, and then only for an instant, and repeat in about nine days.

But leaving the absurdity of the higher dilutions, let us come to the stronger doses; such as a grain of chalk, dissolved in the Atlantic Ocean; or a grain of aconite, dissolved in the Mediterranean Sea; or even a stronger dose, such as a grain of sulphur, dissolved in Lake Michigan; and this would be strong enough to startle a true son of Hahnemann. But we will make it even stronger yet: say a grain of iron, dissolved in the reservoir here. Here is the strongest kind of a homœopathic dose. But I venture to say that even this could have no effect at all on the human system; it would amount to nothing in the treatment of disease; *and this* I can prove to the satisfaction of everybody. It is well known that a glass of water, moderately impregnated with lime, contains more lime than all the homœopaths in the world would give in a lifetime, even at the tenth dilution. What! do you pretend to believe that you are being cured by lime, administered homœopathically, when you are swallowing a thousand times as much of the same article in every drink of water you take? You may try to believe this, but you will not succeed; common sense will prevent you.

Every egg you eat has a thousand times as much sulphur in it as the homœopathist would give; and can you believe that his dose of sulphur is curing you, when you take a thousand times as much every morning, and when you have a million times as much in your system? Every morsel of meat you take contains more iron than the homœopathic dose. Is it his iron alone that produces any effect? Suppose that some one were to propose to quench your thirst with a drop of cold water, but took care to give it to you mixed with a pint of the same fluid; would you attribute the effect to the one drop, or to the pint taken along with it? Very evidently the system is not affected in any way by the homœopathic dose; and the man who can believe otherwise, after the facts I have stated, would be capable of believing that he was nourished by the incantations of a conjuror, instead of the food which he swallowed with the sorcery.

14

The fact is, that matters and things in general are mixed up with each other in this world in stronger than homœopathic doses. When you step into an apothecary's shop, you inhale more ipecac than a homœopath would administer. You breathe more lime from the dust of the streets than all the homœopaths would give in a thousand years. The odor from a drop of laudanum is more than a Hahnemannian dose; and were you so sensitive as to

"Die of a rose, in aromatic pain,"

you would still be too obtuse to be affected by even the stronger dilutions. But Hahnemann attempts to explain the efficacy of these small doses, by saying that their power is increased by shaking them; and Hahnemann guards his disciples against the danger of rendering the doses too strong by shaking the phial too often. He thinks that if the doctor were to jump out of his buggy with unbecoming agility, the shake given to the medicine in his pocket might endanger the welfare of his patient. If it be true that medicinal substances—and all substances are medicinal—can be thus potentialized by shaking, it is the greatest discovery ever made. The mariners' compass, the art of printing, the power of steam, the electric telegraph, are nothing to it. If this be true, cargoes of medicines need not be imported; one grain of each kind will do for a nation during its whole history, be that history ever so long, just shake it enough. Brandy and wine are medicines—let the grape fail—just shake what is on hand and increase its potency ten thousand fold. Broth is medicinal—shake a thimbleful, and it would nourish an army during a long march, if Hahnemann be not a humbug! Cease, restless mortal, your efforts to accumulate the goods of this world; sit down and shake what you already have; perhaps your dimes may become dollars, or even doubloons. If the alchymist could have succeeded in transmuting the baser metals into gold, the discovery of Hahnemann would still stand unrivalled.

It happens, however, that this assertion of the homœopaths is capable of a direct and overwhelming refutation. Were it asserted that the moon was made of green cheese, we could not refute the assertion. Of course no one would feel particularly bound to believe it, but he could not get at the moon, and thus prove a negative. But we can prove the negative of this monstrous proposition about shaking; every man, woman and child can test it for him, her and itself. Take a drop of alcohol, and see if, by shaking it all day, it can be made to intoxicate. It will do so if there be truth and virtue in homœopathic medication. Take a drop of paregoric, and see if, by shaking and diluting, and shaking again, you can put a patient to sleep with it. Potentialize the tenth of a grain of arsenic, and poison a dog if you can. Everybody can satisfy himself of the utter falsity of this cardinal principle of homœopathy, by direct experiment.

Independently, however, of this direct test, I should not be disposed to have much faith in shaking. I have known some persons to shake their heads very gravely, but I never thought they were the wiser for it. The shaking of an ague evidently weakens the patient. When houses are shaken by earthquakes, they sometimes fall down. A reed, shaken by the wind, is an emblem of frailty. · The Shaking Quakers are not a very strong sect. When one's faith is shaken it is certainly not strengthened, but rather weakened. But if any one is disposed to believe in shaking, let him shake for himself; and if he will not *shake*, why, let him *slide*.

Time will not permit me, on this occasion, to notice in detail all the unfounded assertions, absurdities and contradictions of Hahnemann. His "organon," which is the bible of homœopaths, is a mass of transcendental balderdash, at war with common sense. That common sense will be the victor there can be little doubt. No science, no philosophy, no religious creed can stand, which is opposed to the common sense of mankind.

I know that it will be still argued that, at any rate, contradictory and opposed to common sense as homœopathy may be, it still cures. This is the argument of its advocates, and they say, moreover, that the children take the medicine without wry faces. But it must be remembered that a vast majority of diseases get well of themselves. What are called homœopathic cures are evidently cures of nature; for we *know* that nature cures, and that homœopathic remedies are null and void.

Some years ago I tested the skill of a somewhat distinguished homœopath. I told him that his remedies would effect nothing in cases that would not terminate favorably without medicine. I assigned him, at his request, several cases in the hospital, which I knew would not terminate of themselves in health. His remedies had not the slightest effect. Andral had tested the system on a larger scale, with the same effects, long before. I have also tested these medicines on myself. I am almost ashamed to acknowledge it, but I did, some years ago, when I had time for trifles, try these medicines on myself. The doctrine is, that they will produce the disease which they cure.

I never could get sick with the little things Perhaps I took too many of them!

It may be argued, that if nature cures so vast a majority of diseases, why have any physician? I answer, that it is not necessary in all, or even in a majority of cases; but as the patient may not be a judge of what case needs a physician, or the contrary, he very rationally and properly calls on a man of science, in whom he has confidence, to decide the question for him. Moreover, in many cases in which the patient would get well without medicine, the physician can hasten the cure, and in some cases but for his aid the patient would die. This is more clearly seen in surgery than in medicine. No one will deny that in many cases the surgeon saves life; as in hernias, severed arteries, and the like.

But do homœopaths really stick to their own system? Not one of them, I suppose. I have known them to employ remedial agents just as the regular practitioner; applying powerful revulsives to the head in inflammation of the brain; giving large doses of quinine in intermittents; and, in short, using medicines as well as *they* knew how to use them. Some of them even profess to give medicine in allopathic doses. An idea seems prevalent that this new system is favored by the governments of Europe; that in Germany, especially, it is very popular. It would be very strange, indeed, if Europe, with its advanced civilization, endorsed such a system. It would weaken one's faith in the common sense of mankind. But the fact is otherwise. Dr. Ellsworth Smith, of this city, has taken the pains to correspond with European authorities on this subject. Through our ambassadors at the courts of France, Austria and Prussia, he has learned that homœopathy is merely tolerated in those countries. All the public hospitals are committed to the regular faculty; none, of course, are left for homœopaths. I may mention here, as well as anywhere else, that Hahnemann was engaged, in early life, in compounding and vending NOSTRUMS. One of his infallible powders was found, on examination, to be nothing but simple borax. I mention this fact to show that he was not a mere crazy philosopher; he was a true quack.

Reasonable men ought to be satisfied, even without investigation, that all new-fangled systems must be wrong. Would the great body of the profession be apt to ignore any truth which might be discovered by anybody? The motto of the profession is to seize the truth wherever found, and this it would do without caring whether the discovery were made by Samuel Hahnemann, Samuel Thompson, or Sambo, the African. The regular profession is the depository of the learning and investigations of all time.¹ It has ransacked all the kingdoms of nature for remedies. It extends all over the globe. It comes down to us in regular succession from the earliest ages. Its philosophers have adorned every century since the dawn of science; it has given to the world some of its most venerable names; its calendar of worthies is an honor to our race; its followers command the colleges and hospitals of the world; its history is the history of civilization and humanity; its stars of science decked the midnight skies that shrouded the empires of the past. And who are they who set themselves up as the rivals of this profession? A few insignificant sects of yesterday, contradicting each other, and agreeing only in their opposition to the great universal body of the regular profession. The hydropathist, with his wet sheets and water tubs, looking like the superintendent of a washing establishment; the steam doctor, with his cayenne pepper, and lobelia, and witch-hazel, reminding one of a retail vender of spices; the electropath, with his shocking machine, hardly distinguishable from the organ grinder; and the homœopath, with his cases of globules, suggesting the idea of a new Yankee invention in the way of food for canary birds. Common sense cannot be long gulled by such things. I repeat, that nothing can permanently command the faith of mankind that is not in accordance with *common sense.*

IMPOSTORS IN MEDICINE.

By T. J. COGLEY, M.D., Madison. Indiana.

That certain tastes—certain likes and dislikes—are inherent in human nature, does not admit of a doubt. That our perceptive faculties are more keenly alive to some objects than others, is equally indisputable. I must have an inherent dislike for pretenders in all departments of knowledge, more especially in Medicine. When yet a school boy, I remember feeling great disgust for a respectable farmer of Pennsylvania, who was the father of two delicate children, a son and daughter, for going several days' journey—this was before railroads were invented—into a neighboring State for the purpose of consulting a German doctor, *alias* a "water doctor." He carried with him a vial of urine from each of his children, both past the age of puberty. He was a simple-minded, well-meaning Pennsylvania Dutchman, and he had heard of this *German p*** doctor*—they even now receive that title in that region—and, from what he heard of him, placed implicit faith in his ability to tell all.about a case, no matter how distant or how obscure, by mere ocular inspection of the urine of the patient. Although I had not then thought of the study of medicine,.I felt that I knew intuitively that the " German p*** doctor" must be an impostor. In maturer years my intuitive opinion was confirmed by hearing related, by intelligent persons in his vicinity, many truly laughable stories about how he had been exposed by persons taking the urine of animals, or of persons in perfect health, to him, under the pretense that it was the urine of afflicted persons of certain age and sex. His diagnosis, prognosis, and treatment in many such cases, although most ludicrous, did not destroy the confidence of his superstitious and deluded patrons. From that early period to the present I have been a close observer of pretenders in medicine, and my observations have established some curious facts, which I consider worth recording, amongst the more prominent of which is the fact that at least nine-tenths of the charlatans, who have come within my observation, were Germans; the remaining tenth perhaps about equally made up of all other foreigners and native Americans.

Aside, therefore, from Homœopathists, Thompsonians, Eclectics, Mesmerizers, and such like, it is obvious that we have a very numerous class of charlatans, scattered, doubtless, through all the States, one or more in almost every important locality, whom their *elite* patrons call the German Doctor, the common people call them the Dutch Doctor, and those who are less respectful in their address not unfrequently denominate them Doctor Sourcrout, or the p*** doctor. Nor does this militate in the least degree against the honest, scientific physician from Germany; if there be any such in our land, he will readily perceive that the portraiture which we shall attempt to give of the Dutch quack does not suit him, and he will be unmoved. The kind of thing which we are going to portray may take offence, but it is probable the earth will continue to revolve.

So far, then, as they have come within my observation, they are extremely selfish, ignorant, illiterate, low, mean, ill-bred, worthless fellows; they make out most of their cases extremely dangerous, requiring unusual skill in their treatment; many of their cases are "pecoolar," differing from all the cases they have met with in " dis coontry," having seen but one or so of like character in " Sharmany," where, I believe, they never practice medicine, except in the capacity of leechers and cuppers. In Germany barbers are allowed, under the direc_ tion of physicians, to cup and leech; many of our German doctors were barbers in Germany, and this accounts for their expedients in some things, having, as it were, picked up many items of real value from regular practitioners. But it is exceedingly rare that the qualified German physician comes to this country. The class to which reference is made all find it very "*deficoolt to spic Anglish*," and whenever the ladies puzzle them with interrogatories they shield themselves behind "*Ih caunet forstha*"—I cannot understand. Another of their tricks is, that if there happens to be an old Dutchman in some obscure corner of the town—a Mr. Fogle, or a Mr. Hauversack—who has a few musty roots or " arbs," whenever a case becomes critical, and they are forced to add to their humbuggery, this old Dutchman has some medicine which he has imported from "Sharmany," especially for, and under the direction of the "German Doctor." I have repeatedly known these statements to be followed up, and in every instance the article was found to be in common use, kept everywhere, and of course never imported from "Sharmany."

Another trick to blind the patient, to stop all inquiries about the nature of maladies, and appear transcendently wise, is, "your disease, Madam, is in de great sympatetic narve;" "your affection, Sir, is in de membrauns of de prain;" "my dear Miss, you have disease of de heart; it is obvious to me dat de valves of your heart are affected, and you have but distinctly, Madam, de bruet de sooflay." In another case "dar is sarcumscribed inflammation of some of de peritoneum," and disease of the *pancreas* is of common occurrence in their practice. The case is always dangerous, more or less obscure, and generally rare; but it never is his fault if he do not perform a perfect "coore." With the German doctor all is "cure;" he has no use for the *vis medicatrix naturæ*, he desires none of that kind of assistance, and if the patient does not speedily and perfectly recover, it is always blamed on the nurse, the druggist, or his spoiled drugs, imprudence in eating, sitting up, or atmospheric vicissitudes.

A lady came to consult me about having nearly lost the hearing in one of her ears. She had been under the treatment of one of the "German doctors," who told her that he perfectly understood her case, (although I learned he had never examined the ear with a speculum,) and "if he was in Sharmany he could get some tings dat would cure her immediately." In this wooden country of ours he could not procure the desired remedy. A careful examination of the external ear, in a strong light, with the speculum, revealed a large perforation of the tympanum, doubtless from the bursting of an abscess, which was still discharging, incurable in almost all cases of long standing, but as curable in America as in Deutchland; and this was the case for which he could get a "coore in de ole coontry." A severe case of granular inflammation of the eyelids was presented to me, which had been under the care of one of these sourcrouters. The patient believed her eyes would have gotten well had not the "Dutch doctor's medicine gin out" The scoundrel induced her to believe that he had in his garden a vine—and there was but one like it in the United States —from which, at certain seasons of the year, their exuded a juice, which was a sovereign remedy in "sore eyes." This was his diagnosis for all the various diseases of the eyes. At a certain stage of the cure this fellow's vine ceased to furnish the so much desired remedy; he was very sorry, but he had to quit. In a vial which contained a few drops of the precious "fluid I found a solution of some Dutch drug.

To me it seems strange that such pretenders are often employed by those who think themselves the very elite of society, and who are aware of these tricks so peculiar to the charlatan. Such people often pass by well-educated, skillful American physicians, and employ these dangerous quacks, to gratify their inordinate propensity to be humbugged. Many of those thus slighted would, if encouraged by patronage, display extraordinary abilities; but seeing those vile charlatans encouraged and employed by those who should denounce them, become disheartened, and seek amusements, feeling that it is useless to try to obtain patronage by meriting it, when common Dutchmen can flourish without even brains. Many young gentlemen who have been well qualified to begin practice, upon seeing the Dutch impostor preferred, have left the profession in disgust. Thus we sometimes find men of superior education and fitness for the *most important and responsible station on earth*—that of the good physician—driven to engage in secular employment, which might be conducted by men of more ordinary ability—employments which even Dutch doctors would be competent to engage in. It is high time for the people to pause and reflect upon the true merits of these creatures, and upon the effect upon society and the profession of sustaining them. And I would urge upon all respectable physicians the importance of holding no sort of intercourse with them under any circumstances. By no means consult with them, or be consulted by them. Do they seem to be taking away from you some of your best patrons? Draw the lines of non-intercourse the tighter; the higher they rise for a brief period, the farther, simply, have they to fall, and the more will your friends be mortified by having had any connection with them. Their sole dependence is upon being successful in deception. The German physician who is thoroughly qualified for the practice of his profession, rarely, if ever, leaves his native country, where all such find ample employment and much better remuneration than the most distinguished physicians do in this country.

I have been told of a case where one of these beings attended a case in conjunction with a homœopathist. Whichever got to see the patient first in the morning prescribed, and some days the patient would take globules, and on other days the most nauseating drugs from the Dutchman. After a while they tapped the patient for dropsy, and drew off a little blood. The patient died, and I have no doubt a post-mortem examination would have revealed a perforated intestine, uterus, ovary, or kidney. The consequences need not be named. I have heard of one of these bipeds throwing buckets-full of water upon a lady, in a very fine bed, on account of incipient syncope from hæmorrhage after delivery. Upon seeing the ruinous effects of the water upon the fine bed furniture—the room literally flooded with the same—he exclaimed, "Oh, dat was one very good act of mine; dis will be recorded for me in Heaven." The slightest sprinkling of cold water upon the face, together with the proper posture, would have been amply sufficient. Thus in almost every case they strive to make the impression that the issues of life and death are solely in their hands. Heaven always frowns upon such presumption. I am informed that this class of quacks is unknown in those states where the medical profession is protected by law. In this state, unfortunately for the people, every man has a right to practice either medicine or law.

I could fill many pages with the sayings and doings of this class of "doctors," but if what I have said is sufficient to attract the attention of respectable and regular physicians, and enable them properly to appreciate the *genus*, it will serve quite as well as though I were to occupy one-half of your journal. I hold this to be a self-evident proposition: that if all reputable physicians will treat them as they merit, their prosperity in deception will be short-lived. I would not recommend open personal denunciations, which I believe would nourish them and promote their objects; but a firm, dignified non-intercourse. I have found that a well-timed, well-merited word of ridicule is far more potent in unmasking them than angry denunciations.—*Nashville Medical and Surgical Journal.*

EDITOR'S TABLE.

NEW YORK ACADEMY OF MEDICINE.

In our last number the introduction of the controversy, most indiscreetly obtruded into the Academy, on the subject of Mr. Whitney's death was given to our readers, together with the documents and speeches made by the parties concerned. A brief commentary on the facts of the case was prefixed, editorially, in which our own views were indicated. Since then, one entire meeting of the body has been wasted in the discussion, which, having been widely published by the secular press, renders any detail here unnecessary. Our readers all know, that the result reached by the action of the body was the almost unanimous exoneration of Dr. Horace Green from all participation in the death of Mr. Whitney, or any mal-practice in the case, as had been alleged both by Drs. Beales and Mott, and extensively bruited abroad by the public press. And yet they will perceive, by the published proceedings in the case, that the resolution of Dr. Sayres exculpating Dr. Green, who alone had been impeached, was so modified—after an earnest appeal from Dr. Mott and the retraction of his accusation explicitly made—by Dr. Gardner's substitute, which finally passed—that both he and Dr. Beales were exonerated from any improper treatment of the case after it came in their hands, which they and their friends feared might be implied, unless they were somehow included in the resolution.

We do not marvel at the sneers of the public press at this evasion of the true issue, which they style a "whitewashing resolution," and heartily concur in the lay-judgment, pronounced by high authority, that the reports of the Academy as published, from the inception of the case until its termination, are disreputable to the body, and will bring discredit upon the profession.

We should not be surprised if the sober second thought of the Academy at large, many of whom refrained from any participation in the debates, should lead to a motion to EXPUNGE from the minutes every record made in the case, and we believe such motion would prevail with a large majority of the body.

Our reasons are briefly these, viz.:

1. The objects of the Academy, as stated in its charter and constitution, render the introduction of this topic unconstitutional; and had the President not been a novice in the chair, he would have pre-

vented its introduction by declaring that the Academy could not entertain it.

2. The only constitutional way in which the Academy could have the case before them, is that provided for in our law, viz.., by the presentation of a "charge against a Fellow of the Academy," in a sealed envelope, and so endorsed; and even this could not be read, but must be referred to the Standing Committee on Ethics.

3. The precedent here established, if permitted to stand on record, will, in future, authorize the arraignment before the Academy in this summary way of any Fellow, whether surgeon or physician, when any error in diagnosis may be alleged, in any fatal case of disease or operation, on no other authority than an ex-parte post-mortem, or the allegation of an excited patient, or the clamor of survivors, or even the gossip of a newspaper. Are the members of the Academy content with this precedent?

4. The meetings of the Academy may henceforth be perverted into seasons of heated and profitless controversy, instead of occasions for the cultivation of medical science.

To *expunge* the whole proceedings in this case, and thus rebuke its introduction into our body, which ought to be a purely scientific association, and which will else degenerate into a bear-garden for mutual wrangling and strife, would seem to be the dictate of wisdom and policy; nor could it fail to elevate the character of the Academy, and wipe out this foul blot from our escutcheon.

That the presiding officer should have left the chair, and then, forgetful of the sacred maxim "De mortuos nil nisi bonum," take occasion to reflect upon the personal character, habits, and vices of the deceased, and this in a promiscuous assemblage, whether his strictures were true or false, was not only unprecedented and uncalled for, but aroused a feeling of indignation in and out of the body, which was with difficulty suppressed. It furnishes, however, another source of regret that the subject was ever brought before the Academy, and is a potent argument in favor of expunging all from the minutes. So mote it be.

MEDICAL POLITICS.

The medico-political offices of *Health Officer* and *City Inspector* continue *in statu quo*, both the incumbents holding over until their successors are appointed, from among a multitude of hungry expectants.

Meanwhile, the Legislature have two projects before them for a new organization of the Health Department of our city, having an increase of the medical element in our Board of Health. One of these, known as Dr. Griscom's plan, and the other, as modified by Dr. Watson. And though we predict that neither will ever be passed, for reasons obvious enough on the face of them, yet we cannot withhold an exposition of them both, which will occupy all the space we can afford to the subject.

Dr. Griscom's bill provides that the Presidents of our three Medical Colleges, and of the Academy of Medicine, should represent the profession in the Board, together with the City Inspector, who is to be a medical man, &c., all of whom are to be associated with the Mayor, &c.

Dr. Watson, in the Sanitary Association, stoutly opposed this plan, chiefly on the ground that the colleges were mere private associations, and their presidents do not represent the profession. Moreover, he maintained that they were not qualified for the duties required, and for the reason that the president of one college was, as usual, a superannuated man, physically unable to act—such being usually chosen for that post. He said the president of the second college was not a medical man at all, but only a *chemist!* and as to the president of the third college, he was a mere specialist, whose practice, he alleged, was opposed by the profession, and rendered him offensive. He left them to infer that *he*, as President of the Academy of Medicine, *did* represent the profession, and not merely the cliques and caucuses who elected him by a bare majority of those present, his votes being less than an eighth of the Fellows. He objected decidedly to the President of the Pharmaceutical Society, comparing him to the *mere cook of the Astor House*, in his relations to the medical profession. Whereupon sundry gentlemen moved to include the cook of the Astor House in the Board of Health, as important to the dietary and sanitary interests of the public; while others regarded a chemist, architect, and engineer as the most useful members of the Board.

Thus the matter stood before the Sanitary Association, when the Senatorial Committee's report brought up the subject before the Legislature of the State, where it is now pending. It is probable that some improvement in the constitution of the Board of Health will be made, although the personal motives of certain gentlemen we might name are so transparent, that an entire new Board of Health will be provided for, with power to introduce a medical element whenever any emergency may require it. But the introduction of the President of the Academy as such into the organic law of the State, is preposterous; for he may be an " old fogy," or an old woman by possibility; and hence unfit for the duties of the Board of Health.

We trust that the Mayor will be the only president hereafter, and that he may select the medical men for the medical offices irrespective of the Colleges or Academy, and beyond the veto of a faction in the Board of Aldermen, who may be bribed to prevent any appointment unless dictated by themselves.

"SLAUGHTER OF THE INNOCENTS."

Under this startling caption, several of the leading editors of the city press are belaboring the Governors of the Almshouse for the inhumanity of the system by which the foundling infants' and outcast children, thrown upon the public charity, are boarded out to " nurse" at a dollar per week, to the miserable and often profligate inmates of the wretched hovels, cellars and garrets of our tenant houses, who, for the most part, suffer them to die by neglect, or perish by starvation and drugging. The half has never yet been told, of the extent of infant mortality resulting from this abominable and cruel system; and we do not marvel at the ironical rebuke to its authors by one of our legislators, by proposing that the Governors be authorized to adopt the still more economical and less inhuman method of " poisoning by strychnine," to dispose of these infantile pensioners on their bounty.

An ample and all-sufficient remedy for these evils is only to be found in the proposed *Foundling Hospital,* or Infant's Home, so long and so often urged upon the public authorities by philanthropists; and the delay in the .opening of which by the Governors, now that it is sanctioned by our municipal legislature, is wholly inexcusable. The outcast children of unfortunate and even criminal parentage in this city are increasing in numbers annually; and, as is now notorious, they are farmed out in squads, only to die, thus relieving the city of their support by sending them en route to Potter's Field.

Why is not a building hired for the purpose of sheltering and saving these little ones ; a matron of sober habits and maternal instincts placed at its head, with cleanly and temperate nurses as assistants, so that this heinous and murderous waste of human life shall cease?

We trust that the Tribune, Times, Express, and other papers, will continue to "cry out and spare not," until they make themselves heard.

Dr. Griscom a PATENT-monger.

What next? If anything were needed to signalize the downward proclivity of the medical profession in these degenerate days, we find it here. A member of the American Medical Association and of our Academy of Medicine has taken out a PATENT! for his "improved system of ventilating buildings!" We suppose that we shall next have the *inevitable names* of Mott, Francis, Parker, Watson, & Co., certifying and recommending this *patent* nostrum in the newspapers, as they and others have been doing for the bogus *patent* of the honest Morton! for etherization; and our Code of Ethics is again to be trampled upon with impunity, and this by the very men chosen to protect their profession from such degradation.

Ours has heretofore claimed to be a *liberal profession*, and hence, whatever of invention or discovery we make in the science of health, is forthwith promulgated for the public benefit. Our fathers, such men as Rush, Chapman, Post, Hosack, and Warren, in their day, would have denounced any attempt to appropriate a scientific discovery for the promotion of the public health to personal emolument, by securing a *patent* therefor, as the most arrant quackery. What, then, are we coming to? If Dr. Griscom does not purpose the abandonment of his profession, he will repudiate this patent, or every member of the profession is bound to repudiate him: unless, indeed, our Academy and its ethics are henceforth to be justly stigmatized as a farce.

WELLS versus MORTON.

The County Medical Society of Hartford, Conn., has recently taken decisive action in relation to the claims of the late Dr. Horace Wells, as the discoverer of anæsthesia, by the inhalation of ether, nitrous oxide, &c., his experiments having been repeatedly witnessed by members of the society, *two years* before Morton pretends to have discovered anything. Hence they earnestly protest against the efforts made here, and elsewhere, to reward Morton for his piratical appropriation of what he learned from Dr. Wells; and they forcibly remonstrate against their medical brethren striving to uphold the bogus patent of Morton, when Dr. Wells had promulgated the discovery as free to all the world, and scorned to seek a patent.

That $1,500 voted to Morton by the Almshouse Governors has been by him assigned to Pudney & Russell, the printers of the book compiled by Dr. Rice, who have sued the Board to compel payment, so that the plunder may be divided between the parties. Not a ghost of a chance remains that they will ever see the money.

NEW YORK STATE MEDICAL SOCIETY.

The 52d annual meeting was held at Albany, Feb. 1, 1859—Dr. T. C. Brinsmade, President, in the Chair, whose inaugural address was highly spoken of, abounding in practical suggestions. Thirty-seven counties were represented, 115 members and delegates being in attendance. Governor Morgan extended the hospitalities of his mansion to the Society; the oration was delivered in the Capitol, the use of which was courteously extended by the Legislature, now in session; and in all respects the meeting passed off pleasantly and profitably. A large number of papers were read, resolutions adopted, &c., all of which will appear in the Transactions, soon to be published by the State. We regret, only on our own account, and those similarly situated, that the season of the year has always precluded the possibility of our being present, our occupations and the weather interposing insurmountable obstacles..

MEDICAL ASSOCIATION OF SOUTH CAROLINA.

This body met at the Roper Hospital, in Charleston, on the 2d of February The annual oration by the President, Dr. R. W. Gibbs, of Columbia, is an able and highly interesting discourse, and appears in the Charleston Courier, the editor of which, after reporting the proceedings in full, thus facetiously speaks of their finale, viz.:

"The members of the South Carolina Medical Association, not having the fear of dyspepsia before their eyes, and instigated by several propensities, and the best attractions of their noble profession, placed their locomotive limbs under the mahogany, in St. Andrew's Hall, on Wednesday evening, and submitted with commendable grace to sundry prescriptions which had been compounded from improved ingredients of the *Materia Alimentaria* by *Nat Fuller*, culinary manipulator. The Doctors had a most delightful consultation, but such affairs, of course cannot be well reported."

JEFFERSON MEDICAL COLLEGE.

The catalogue of this great school has been published, and shows the aggregate of 570 pupils for the present session! It also appears that 75 of these are graduates of some of the other colleges already, leaving still, however, 495, whom it is fair to presume are *bona fide* students; and this is a larger list than any other school in the country will be able to furnish. *Thirteen* of these hail from *New York*, but nearly 400 of the whole number are from States *south* of Pennsylvania, including the southwest. The prosperity of this school is unparalleled, and its march seems still to be onward, notwithstanding the rivalship of three other colleges in Philadelphia, all highly respectable, including the old University School, which is this year almost distanced in the race of competition.

DEATHS IN OUR RANKS.

The following eminent and worthy physicians have recently departed this life, viz.:

Professor Newton, of Augusta, Georgia.

Professor Gaillard, of Charleston, South Carolina.

Dr. J. C. Goble, of Newark, N. J., formerly President of the State Medical Society.

Professor Ellet, of South Carolina University.

Dr. Edward Hudson, Surgeon U. S. Navy.

All distinguished and useful men.

N. Y. STATE MEDICAL SOCIETY—OFFICERS FOR 1859.

President—Dr. B. F. Barker, of New York.

Vice President—Dr. D. T. Jones, of Onondaga.

Secretary—Dr. S. D. Willard, of Albany.

Treasurer—Dr. J. V. P. Quackenbush, of Albany.

PROFESSOR THOMAS D MUTTER

Has consummated his magnificent donation to the Philadelphia College of Physicians, and the splendid Museum and Lectureship he has endowed will henceforth bear his name, and posterity honor his memory.

ST. LOUIS MEDICAL COLLEGE

Has 135 students in its present class, as we learn from a correspondent.

Dr. Reese's Speech in the Whitney Case.

[We insert the following *report* of our own remarks at the N. Y. Academy of Medicine, by request of a number of friends—as we find it in the American Medical Monthly. It will serve to define our position in the late unfortunate attempt to crush Dr. Horace Green.]

Mr. President, I think I can demonstrate to any man of sound reason without a particle of anatomical knowledge, that there is no justifiable ground for any allegation against either of the gentlemen except what has grown out of this discussion, in which things have been said on both sides which ought never to have been said.

The critical position to which we have arrived in this discusssion prompts me to detain the Academy with a few remarks in advocacy of the action proposed in the resolutions just read. I am unwilling that the free and full expression of opinion in open Academy should be interrupted either by the *reference* or *indefinite postponement*, or any other form of *gag law;* nor can I consent to any *evasion* of the true issue by any measure short of a decision by this body upon the merits of the whole subject—such as the profession and the public expect and require, and such as Dr. Green demands, as his undoubted right.

Sir, I yield to no man in the respect I entertain for the venerable Dr. Mott, and, until this controversy commenced, my regard for Dr. Beales has been equal to that felt toward other brethren of the Academy. But the grave charge against Dr. Green, whom I esteem as equally worthy of his position here, and of the confidence of the profession and the public, constrains me to assume a position antagonistic to both of those gentlemen, because I am persuaded that the facts of this unfortunate case will not sustain them; but when justly considered, will not only exonerate Dr. Green from any, the least participation in the fatal result in the case of Mr. Whitney, but will prove that both Drs. Mott and Beales were more in error, alike in their diagnosis and prognosis, having been at first misled by the patient's censorious denunciations of Dr. Green, which referred all his sufferings to the treatment of the latter gentleman, in terms I care not to repeat.

Mr. President, is it any new thing in your professional experience or mine, to hear physicians accused of killing their patients, when sudden and unexpected death has followed their best exertions? Have we not often known surgeons whose patients have unfortunately died on the table, clamorously charged by surviving members of the bereaved families with butchery and murder? And this, when the duties of both had been performed with the utmost skill and humanity?

15

Has this Academy ever brought up before it any man on a charge
of that sort? Has it ever left its high position to inquire why a man
died, because his wife said, or the relatives said, or people said he had
been killed by one of its members? And are we to have every member of our body brought up here when an allegation is made by friends
or parties interested, implicating him in the death of an individual?
I conceive that the declaration of Mr. Whitney, that he had been
killed by Dr. Green, is unworthy of notice by the Academy, and deserving of utter contempt, [applause;] and I will say farther, that the
reiteration of that declaration before the Academy is worthy of equal
contempt. [Renewed applause.]

There is an ancient maxim which ought to be introduced into our
professional ethics, as it has been into every other kind of ethics, that
the most favorable construction possible should be placed on the most
unfavorable appearances.

This venerable maxim of ethics has been ignored by both Drs. Mott
and Beales in the present case. On learning from the patient that he
ascribed his sufferings to Dr. Green's use of the probang, they at once
adopted his asseveration, that Dr. Green had killed him; and this on
no other evidence than the occurrence of emphysema; and hence joined the outcry against their brother and equal in the profession, even
before the death of their patient, instead of suggesting, as they ought
to have done, that the patient's suffering and danger might possibly
turn out to have some other cause.

But, Mr. President, I propose to show, that had these gentlemen
waited for the post-mortem they anticipated, before committing themselves to the theory of the patient, that the trachea or larynx had
been "perforated by Dr. Green's probang," they might have escaped
the unfortunate dilemma in which they have involved themselves.

The gentlemen concerned must surely now perceive, since the revelations of their own post-mortem, that their theory and that of their
patient was disproved, when they not only found no abrasion or perforation in either trachea or larynx, but both organs a "perfect type of
health." I submit to the gentlemen themselves, whether they had not
then a fitting opportunity at once to proclaim the innocence of Dr.
Green of any violence inflicted by his probang, and fully to exonerate
him from any direct or indirect agency in causing the death of the patient, which charge they had previously countenanced if not authorized?

Mr. President, is it too much that Drs. Mott and Beales shall consent to this statement of fact—that when they discovered that emphy-

sema, in connection with the rumor that the wind-pipe had been ruptured by the instrument of Dr. Green, it was perfectly natural for
them, and would be natural for us to ascribe that emphysema to a
wound of the trachea?

Had they at this discovery of the error of their patient and themselves, finding no lesion of the air-passages by the probang, at once
acquitted Dr. Green, to the family and friends, of all participation in
Mr. Whitney's death, all the public clamor and all the agitation of
this Academy would have been prevented. Is it too much to ask
that they should admit this error and correct it now? Sir, I do not
despair even yet, that these gentlemen may review and retrace their
steps, and hence I proceed to remark upon the progress of their secret
autopsy; nor can they complain if I infer the *animus* which impelled
them, from their manifest purpose to implicate Dr. Green in whatever
causes of death they might find; and this after the larynx and trachea were found uninjured, and their anticipations in this respect were
disappointed.

Their next exploration was into the throat, to discover what caused
the protrusion of the thyroid body and prevented both deglutition
and respiration. Behind the larynx and under the deep cervical fascia, pus was observed to follow the scalpel, and they report an *abscess*
extending a little laterally and posteriorly to the pharynx, which was
" as large as a hen's egg. This was a large enough tumor, it seems, to
close the œsophagus and reach over to the glottis, and even to bulge
forward the trachea and thyroid body, and lead to the exclamation,
" the largest larynx and trachea we ever saw."

DR. MOTT.—The trachea did not bulge.

DR. REESE.—Then the protrusion was only an enlarged protraction!

DR. MOTT.—That is all.

DR. REESE.—That won't save the gentleman, because this man was
choked to death—he could neither swallow nor breathe. [Laughter.]
" His breathing was performed very imperfectly, and deglutition was
impossible." If they could not have found out what was the matter
while he was living, surely they ought when he was dead. But in the
post-mortem they find a cavity which they infer to be an abscess,
and deglutition, they say, was obstructed by it. Unluckily, " this abscess had a hole in it large enough to admit two fingers," out of which
the pus *ought* to have escaped by the *laws of gravity*. Nothing in it.
[Laughter.] It was a cavity containing filamentous tissue. But
surely if it was empty, the tumor as large as a hen's egg could not

have choked and suffocated the patient, as it undoubtedly did, unless it broke after death; or, as Dr. Sayre has shrewdly suggested, was opened during the post-mortem, by that hole of two fingers' width having been made by the scalpel—an inference which is authorized in the premises. The most uncharitable inference that could be invented was put upon that circumstance, viz, that that hole had been made by Dr. Green's probang. The abscess was just as much due to my cane as to the probang, and every man here understands it. If any man could be found who believed that an ordinarily prudent physician could, by introducing the probang, produce a rupture sufficient to cause the abscess or cavity that was found in Mr. Whitney, then I will surrender to him all credulity. The introduction of that probang could not by any possibility have produced an abscess in that direction. But as Dr. Green did not wound the larynx, he must have struck the pharynx, for as the doctors had committed themselves to the theory that the patient "died from Dr. Green's treatment," his probang must be the instrument of death. Now, I am persuaded that, except Drs. Mott and Beales, no other member of this Academy can believe this theory, and the profession at large will ignore such medical logic. The abscess was doubtless there before Dr. Green's operation, and accounts for the complaint of being hurt, in the unsuccessful attempt of Dr. Green to enter the fauces, on the morning before the patient's illness. It was not discovered then by Dr. Green, nor in two hours after by Dr. Beales, nor the next day by Dr. Mott, nor suspected by anybody until after the patient was dead!

May I now submit to the gentlemen themselves whether such abscesses do not often occur from *other causes* than the wound of a probang? Have they not seen them? (Dr. Reese here related a recent case and its result.) Is it, then, too much to ask them why they do not now correct their error, and admit that this abscess arose from constitutional causes, or some other morbid agency?

But now the thorax was opened, and behold, an abscess or "cavity" was found in the left lung, a nondescript affair, which, however, confirmed Dr. Green's diagnosis of a pulmonary lesion, made two months before. Both Drs. Beales and Mott insist that this anomalous "cavity" was not tuberculous, as Dr. Green regarded it, but yet it was found at the precise spot that the latter had detected and recorded it.

Then, again, in that anomalous cavity of the lung they found what they supposed was sloughing, which, as there was an *animus* in the matter, must of course have been produced by Dr. Green's nitrate of silver. An ulcerated degeneration had occurred through the pleura, and now for the first time the source of the mysterious emphysema was disclosed; and the idea was next started, that Dr. Green's injection into the lung of *one and a half grains of nitrate of silver in a drachm of water!* some 15 days before, had occasioned all this chronic mischief; for Dr. Green was to be made accountable for the cause of death wherever it might be discovered. Sir, I am persuaded that every member of this Academy, who has seen or heard the report of this post-mortem, will concur with me, that this pulmonary lesion must have existed for months, perhaps years before, and in a *depraved constitution* was all the while tending by a fearful proclivity to the result, which, by a contingent coincidence, developed itself with the formidable symptoms of collapse which Dr. Beales found on the 14th of Dec.

Now, was not this ridiculous? Then, again, we come to the certificate. Now, in all the courts of England and this country, the certificate of death officially given by the physician was invariably relied on. It is the legal and final record, behind which no judicial tribunal can go, given as it is, on our professional oath. Now, what did Drs. Mott and Beales do? It would not do to say that Mr. Whitney died of perforation of the trachea, for there was none. If it was an abscess, then the presumption was that it existed before. If it was rupture of the pleura, then these physicians were in the same position with Dr. Green. What then did they do? Why, they gave a certificate that I would undertake to say was not on record in the statistics of any sanitary office, either in this country or in Europe. I defy you to bring me, from the mortality tables of this or any other country, a single instance in which the cause of death was recorded as effusion into the lungs—and yet that is the certificate. Now, did Dr. Green produce this effusion into the lung? Was it caused by introducing the probang to cauterize the larynx, or was it rupture of the pharynx, or was it caused, if it existed, by that disease of the lungs which must evidently have been of longer standing, must have existed more than a week, a month, and even a year, from their own description? Such a morbid condition as they make out never existed since the creation, unless it resulted from chronic disease, as this undoubtedly did. The effusion of the lungs was, therefore, the consequence of that disease, with which the probang had nothing to do.

Now, they might have given a certificate which would have protected Dr. Green, honored themselves, and screened the profession and the Academy from public clamor and its consequences. Was it not in the power of these gentlemen to say he died of a complication of diseases terminating in abscess, which caused suffocation? For he died as everybody dies, for want of breath—suffocation. The proposition that he (Dr. R.) would make, was this: that Drs. Mott and Beales were perfectly justifiable in having attributed the emphysema to the rupture of the trachea, from the testimony then in their possession, until they made the post-mortem; and that, having made the post-mortem, they had been satisfied, and were satisfied now, that the man did not die from that cause. Indeed, neither have insinuated that he did. It followed then, inevitably, that if he died from any disease of the trachea, it was not from Dr. Green's treatment. Had they given a certificate to cover that cause, in truth, declaring the facts in the case, and which they could have constructed at their own pleasure, they could have framed it so as to prevent any of the clamor that had been raised; and he thought that they regretted, and saw cause for regret, that they did not take that course. Now, could not this matter be arranged in the Academy without having recourse to the offensive measures proposed in the resolutions? Why not adjust it in a way far more creditable to the Academy, making the resolution more specific, and implicating nobody? He thought it could. He thought it was not asking too much of Dr. Mott or Dr. Beales, to say that the man did not die of any perforation of the trachea. That would put a veto on the scandalous publications that were going through the country.

Now, these gentlemen should say that Mr. Whitney's death might have arisen from other causes. No man ought to say that his disease was only a week old, or ten days old. I have not met the man in the profession who entertains that idea at all. I assert, that the use of the probang is legitimate treatment, endorsed by the highest authorities in the world, both medical and surgical, and why not acknowledge it?

Now, Mr. President, my object is to be a pacificator if I can. The position is not an enviable one to which this Academy is tending. I desire to deliver it, if possible, from its impending danger. I have no preference for any particular form, but I want the Academy to state what it believes to be the truth, viz., that in regard to Mr. Whitney's death no blame can justly be attached to either of the medical men who had his case in charge; though as to the position respectively assumed by these gentlemen towards each other, he was obliged to declare his opinion, that Drs. Mott and Beales had considerably the worst of it.

DR. HORACE GREEN.

This gentleman, who had been censured by Drs. Beales and Mott, imputing to him mal-practice in the case of Mr. Whitney, as detailed in our last number, has triumphed over all his enemies, both in and out of the profession, in the *N. Y. Academy of Medicine*, before whom a full investigation was had, two entire meetings being devoted to the subject.

That body, with entire unanimity, adopted a resolution exonerating him from all the allegations, made in and out of the Academy, against his professional treatment of the case. Drs. Beales and Mott were acquitted of any mal-treatment of the patient, which was not alleged, but might be implied, and this was done in accordance with their wishes. We need scarcely say to our readers, that our sympathies have been with Dr. Green, not by reason of any personal relations or partiality to him, but singly and only because of our conscientious convictions that he was wrongfully censured in a case where no blame could justly attach. We rejoice that the sober second thought of those who opposed him has prompted to the general, if not universal persuasion, that the treatment he has received was unmerited. His fame and emolument will doubtless be increased by the notoriety of the case, a result at which we shall rejoice. Said Dr. Johnson, "When God Almighty has given a man wings, you may clip them as often as you will, but he will still *fly!*" Let those who would fain "*crush*" their more successful rivals by persecution, see the impotence of their efforts, and henceforth learn the wisdom of silence.

ORIGINALITY AND MERIT

have been generally awarded to Dr. Ayres' report of the cure of congenital exstrophy of the female bladder, by an autoplastic operation, which appears in our February number, with illustrations. In the present issue the same attributes will be found to characterize Dr. J. O'Reilly's paper on nervous pathology, his views being not merely ingenious and novel, but highly important and useful. We hope none will fail to read it.

LINDSAY & BLAKISTON,

of Philadelphia, have issued the last Half-yearly Abstract of the Medical Sciences, which is reprinted by them at $2 per annum in advance, with postage free. It is still ably conducted by Drs. Ranking and Radcliffe, of London.

Health Officer and Resident Physician of the Marine Hospital.

These two medical offices are still a part of the political spoils of the party in power in the State, and at the disposal of the Governor and Senate. Dr. Woodward, of this city, is the prominent candidate for the former, and Dr. Stirling, of Staten Island, for the latter; although there are a score or more of competitors. Dr. Thompson's term does not expire until late in April, and it is not probable any appointment will be made for some weeks to come. We are sorry that so many of the brethren are wasting their time and money in Albany, and annoying the Executive by their importunities, in view of the disappointment which is before them. These are political offices, made and used for political purposes, and no man will get either who will not pledge the spoils in liberal proportion to the party, to defray the expenses of the General Committee, &c. But for this, the extortions upon commerce and the poor sailors by the Health Officer would cease, by the abolition of the enormous fees at present exacted, and a fixed salary substituted therefor. But the party want money and must have it, and hence this great medico-political prize is in the market for the highest bidder. It is well worth bidding for, being a better office than the Presidency of the United States in its emoluments, even after paying the political tax annually. Moreover, the only qualification necessary is to be of the right stripe of politics, and available to the party, to whom belong the spoils, and who hold the office in their gift. If we are lucky enough to get good physicians, like Woodward and Stirling, into the bargain, so much the better; for we have had *quantum suff.* of inferior men at Quarantine.

DR. JOHN MILHAU'S

Reclamation of the original preparation of the "Elixir of Calisaya Bark," the name and the thing being alike his own, will be found in our advertising columns, and speaks for itself. We repeat our commendation of the article, as worthy of trial by those medical men who have not tested its efficacy.

DELINQUENT SUBSCRIBERS.

We have at length commenced the necessary work of retrenchment, by cutting off 125 subscribers from our list, who will not receive the GAZETTE hereafter, until they remit the amount due for 1858 and 1859.

Payment in advance is henceforth the rule, and the time is hereby extended until April 1st.

ARTIFICIAL ARM.

Dr. B. F. Palmer, of Philadelphia, having long since eclipsed all competition in the construction of artificial *legs*, has now introduced a similar substitute for the *arm, forearm, and hand*, which promises to increase his claims as a public benefactor. Our old friend, Professor T. D. Mutter, thus speaks of this useful novelty in a letter to the inventor:

"*Philadelphia, Dec. 14th*, 1858.

"My Dear Sir—I am really very much gratified to find that your ingenuity and perseverance have at length accomplished what the profession has so long waited for in vain—*a useful artificial hand and arm*. The models you showed me the other day appear to accomplish every indication, and are worthy companions to your *unequalled* "artificial legs." After many years' observation of the working of the latter, I am compelled to repeat, what I have already expressed in writing, that neither in Europe nor America is there an instrument of the kind, in my judgment at least, worthy of comparison with them.

"Trusting that you will continue your efforts to relieve your afflicted fellow creatures, I remain,

Very sincerely yours,

THOS. D. MUTTER.

"B. Frank. Palmer, Esq., etc., etc."

Sending Newspapers and Pamphlets to Europe.

Persons who send newspapers and pamphlets to Europe should be careful not to enclose them in wrappers, as it subjects them to letter postage, generally so high that the papers are refused by the persons to whom they are directed. A gentleman just returned from England informs the Philadelphia Ledger that he saw baskets of American newspapers and pamphlets in one of the English post-offices, which had been thrown aside on this account. If the newspapers are tied around with a piece of twine or cord they will go as well as if in a wrapper, and the postage is then the ordinary price for newspapers. The fact that many newspapers and pamphlets fail to reach persons in England and France, to whom they are directed, may be accounted for in this way.

OUR MICHIGAN CONFRERE.

Dr. "A. B. P." is advised to keep cool, and not to strike at three or four of his neighbors at once, who happen to differ with him in opinion, in reference to the status of the medical faculty of the Michigan University, and the relations they sustain to the great subject of medical education. This Journal belongs to the whole profession, and just "complaint" coming to us from our Michigan brethren will ever find a "willing ear and a ready hand" to state their grievances, correct their errors, and seek redress for their wrongs. For peace sake, we have withheld much on the mooted subject, and treated the "recusant professors" with kindness and courtesy, but it seems our forbearance is not appreciated. Brother P. had better endeavor to be quiet. We prescribe a dose of veratrum viride!

The Medical and Surgical Reporter.

This new weekly journal of Philadelphia, now conducted by Drs. S. W. Butler and R. J. Levis, has been enlarged and improved every way, and deserves the success it has achieved. Its illustrations of hospital practice are rich in variety and in practical interest, while its original articles are brief, and yet possess both novelty and merit. How our neighbors can afford to publish it at the low price of $3 per annum is a mystery only to be explained by a long list of paying subscribers, a blessing which they seem to have acquired, and deserve to retain. Success to their enterprise in the "medical emporium," as Philadelphia may still be called, so long as *twelve hundred students* are annually attracted to her colleges. May her shadow never grow less.

THE MEDICAL SOCIETY OF NEW JERSEY.

This ancient and honorable fraternity, who will soon celebrate their centennial anniversary, having been founded in 1766, held its 93d annual session at Trenton, on the 25th of January, 1859. It seems to have been an occasion of much interest, and among those present was our old friend, Dr. Lewis Condict, of Morristown, a graduate of the University of Pennsylvania, of the class of 1794, who has been 65 years a practitioner! and has always been eminent in the profession. This venerable patriarch, now more than four score years of age, by his *esprit de corps* is a living rebuke to the apathy of the medical men of this generation, so far excelling them, even now, in his attachment to his profession, although he has spent many years of his life in the Legislature of his state, and in the Congress of the United States. Still he journeys to Trenton annually to the State Medical Society.

CONSERVATIVE SURGERY.

Samuel W. Gross, M.D., of Philadelphia, reports a case of aneurism of the right femoral artery, cured by digital compression, which is a higher trophy of science and skill than that furnished by the most dazzling achievement with the knife. This is progress in the right direction. He also reports 22 other cases, all treated in the same way. We have not seen his pamphlet.

NASHVILLE MEDICAL COLLEGE.

We learn from a Western correspondent that the class of the old University School in Nashville numbers 434, which is an increase in the number of students beyond any former year in its history, and places this college numerically ahead of every medical school in the country, except the Jefferson College at Philadelphia, which still takes the lead.

LONDON LANCET.

The republication of this greatest of the British monthlies is announced on the cover of this journal. A portrait adorns every number, and that of the great Surgeon Syme, in the January number, is said to be admirably life-like. The clinical lectures are models in this department, and we still regard our files of the London Lancet more valuable than those of any other European periodical, for they constitute a library in themselves.

CONTENTS.

AMERICAN
MEDICAL GAZETTE.

Vol. X. **APRIL, 1859.** **No. 4.**

ORIGINAL DEPARTMENT.

ON THE UTERINE SPECULUM.

By ADRIAN T. WOODWARD. M.D.,

Professor of Obstetrics and Diseases of Females in Castleton Medical College.

The importance of uterine affections being now almost universally acknowledged, the question arises, By what means can the physician best acquire a knowledge of those diseases? Without discussing the propriety of ocular examination of the parts affected, and assuming that all reasonable medical men will at once admit the unfortunate necessity, I desire to call attention to an improved Speculum, by means of which all may be able, with much less embarrassment than usually attends examinations made with any of the numerous varieties now in use, to examine not only the *os* and *labia uteri*, but, with equal facilities, the entire vaginal cervix. Many of the numerous varieties of the speculum now in use have their admirers, and I should not attempt to introduce another to the profession, were I not perfectly satisfied, after a reasonable amount of experience, that it is superior in many points to any other instrument.

First—It is as easily introduced into the vagina as any other.

Secondly—The blades are *broader* than those of the ordinary bivalve speculum, which prevents the walls of the vagina from pressing in between the blades when separated, and thus obscuring the view of the parts beyond.

Third, which is the most important point, the anterior valve is one-half inch shorter than the posterior. The importance of this will at

16

once suggest itself to the operator.   At the junction of the vagina
with the uterus, is formed what may be called the *utero-vaginal angle*,
which gives a greater depth to the *cul de sac* of Douglas posteriorly.
Now the instrument which I have constructed and used for several
years, is a bi-valve speculum of the usual length, with the blades of

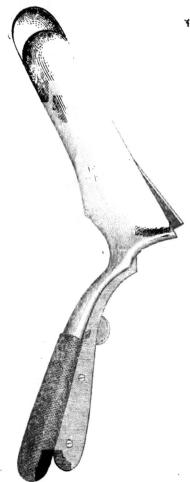

increased width.   The posterior
blade is of ordinary length, but
the anterior shorter by half an inch.
When introduced, the position of
the uterus being previously ascertained by touch, the 'longer or posterior blade is glided into the posterior or larger *cul de sac;* and as
the anterior is the shorter blade,
and rides its fellow, it strikes the
uterus as it glides upon the con-
cave surface of the posterior blade
and arrests the instrument, so that
when the handles of the instrument
are closed and the blades thus separated, the distal extremity of the
anterior glides over the *os* and
anterior lip of the uterus, bringing the whole vaginal cervix into
view.   Any one who has had much
experience in the use of the bi-
valve or hollow cylinder speculum
will hardly be able to give preference to either.   The common bi-
valve speculum will often pass
either behind or in front of the vaginal cervix, which necessitates its
withdrawal and a new trial. Or the
anterior valve may take its proper
position, (as it usually does, when
the uterus is normally situated,) and when the instrument is opened,
only the anterior lip of the uterus is visible. I know with the uterine
sound we can often raise the uterus up and set it upon the posterior
valve, and I know just as well that we often fail to liberate it from
its cramped position.

The converse holds good when the speculum passes into the posterior *cul de sac*, (which happens when the cervix is tilted forward.) When a speculum of the pattern I have described is introduced, these accidents never happen. The most important objection to the hollow cylinder variety is the cramped position which it gives to the uterus when carried up against it, preventing the possibility of raising it so as to exhibit the *os*, except by force exerted by the uterine sound sufficient to injure an *inflamed organ*. I understand perfectly that inflammation of the cervix has been successfully treated with every variety of instrument now in use, even when it has been subjected to all 'the violence necessary to raise or depress it in order to bring it into view; but that does not prove that any unnecessary injury should not be avoided, nor that patients improved as rapidly as they would have done had the uterus been more rationally handled. I know there are many men who can in almost every case expose the os uteri with any instrument without inflicting any injury. All I contend for in my speculum is, that such is the facility of its introduction that it can be done by any one with a tenth part of the trouble and perplexity which often attend the use of the other varieties.

For all ordinary examinations and for the use of the nit. argent., I use No. 2 Speculum, which measures, the long or posterior valve $5\frac{1}{4}$ inches, short or anterior valve $4\frac{3}{4}$ inches from the handles. The breadth of the valves at the uterine extremity, where in contact, $1\frac{1}{16}$ inch. No. 1, which is preferable to any tri-valve or multi-valve speculum in cases of loose and superfluous vaginal walls, measures, the long valve $5\frac{3}{4}$ inches, the short or anterior valve $5\frac{1}{4}$ inches, breadth of valves at point of contact at uterine extremity $1\frac{3}{8}$ inch. It will be borne in mind that there is just half an inch difference in length between the two valves: this I have proved, by many experiments in shortening and lengthening the anterior valve, to be the most convenient length; a sixteenth of an inch either way would make no great difference.

This instrument is manufactured by George Tiemann & Co., 43 Chatham Street, N. Y.

CASE OF SURGERY—A CLINICAL REPORT.

By M. EYRE FOY,

Licentiate Royal College Surgeons, Edinburgh ; Resident Fellow Academy Medicine, N. Y.

James P., ætatis 23, lymphatic temperament, applied to me for advice in March, 1856. Complains of pain, stiffness, and swelling

of left knee, which has existed more or less for nine years past.
When a lad of seven years old, he jumped from a height and hurt
his knee; inflammation ensued, but, under leeches, purgatives, and
antiphlogistic treatment, the inflammation was relieved.

Since then the knee has frequently become inflamed and greatly
swollen, but always amenable to treatment until last year, when the
pain became constant and more severe, accompanied by startings of
the limb at night.

Examination of the knee showed it to be one and a quarter inch
larger in circumference than the healthy one; hot, puffy, and intol-
erant of the slightest motion; general health good, but dullness in the
right sub-clavicular region, and prolonged, roughened expiration.

Ordered complete rest, cod liver oil, tinctura ferri muriatis, and an
evaporating lotion. He improved slightly, and, notwithstanding my
remonstrances, returned to business in April. In June he again came
under my care. General health bad; stomach irritable; dullness increasing over the right lung; cough; night-sweats, alternating with
diarrhœa; knee very painful; requires a full opiate every night; abscess
pointing under tu erosity of tibia. Startings of limb at night are
agonizing.

Opened the abscess. Ordered hydrargi bichloridi, gr. ij.; tinctura
cinchoni composit. ʒi. M; cochlear. parvum ter in die sumendum, cod
liver oil and generous regimen, with absolute rest.

Placed the limb on a double-inclined plane, and looked for anchylosis as possible and desirable. For three weeks he steadily improved,
and general health was much improved.

In August the pain returned with increased severity; great wasting
and night-sweats. Startings of the limb at night are intolerable.
Requires from six to ten grains of morphine every three or four hours.
MÉDICAMENTA CONTINUENTUR.

In November, a large abscess pointed about four inches above the
outer edge of the patella, which, when punctured, gave exit to about
three pints of fœtid, greenish, unhealthy pus.

Early in October I suggested the necessity of amputation. In
beginning of December, hectic, with colliquative diarrhœa, wearing
him rapidly away. I again urged amputation as a dernier resort.
To this his friends would not submit.

On 24th December his stomach became so irritable, that hydrocy-
anic acid, ice-water, morphine, were not retained an instant. Diarrhœa unchecked. I requested a consultation. I met Prof. W. Par-

her, who agreed with me that amputation afforded the only chance, and that a gloomy 'one. I administered suppositories of morphine and tannic acid, and got the bowels checked. On 4th January, assisted by Prof. Parker and three of his pupils, having the patient under the full influence of chloroform, I amputated the thigh six inches above the joint, (by circular method,) and laid open the abscess on the outer aspect of thigh, down throughout its whole length to the face of the stump.

I found the femur healthy, notwithstanding the suspicious abscess which occupied the thigh. I dressed the stump to heal by first intention.

The stump healed by first intention, except a mere speck on its outer angle. Hectic disappeared; he gained flesh rapidly. About four weeks after operation, the muscles on anterior aspect of thigh began to retract, causing great tension over the bone. I applied a fillet round the stump, to which I attached four tapes; these being united to a cord, it was passed over a pulley at foot of bed and a weight attached to it; this relieved the bone from pressure.

On 1st May he returned to his business, having been previously supplied with one of Palmer & Hudson's invaluable artificial legs. He gained flesh and strength daily. The tuberculosed lung is in *statu quo*.

The knee-joint presented ulceration of all the cartilage and incrustation; crucial ligaments almost destroyed; semilunar cartilages eroded and rough.

The cancellated structure in head of tibia was sound, but there was a large carious cavity about an inch below its tuberosity.

I am induced to publish the above case from its bearing on the fact, that constitutional diseases are frequently checked by local treatment. While the diseased knee-joint remained, tuberculosis was making fast progress in the lung. The removal of the diseased joint, destroying one source of irritation, gave power to the constitution to recuperate, and prevented the further deposition of tubercle. Thus we may suppose that where laryngeal and pulmonary phthisis coexist, the treatment of the laryngeal affection, by topical medication, may greatly alleviate, if not altogether arrest the pulmonary affection.

106 West 25th Street.

DR. JAMES BRYAN AND HIS STUDENTS.

At a meeting of the Class attending the Lectures and Catechetical instruction of Dr. James Bryan, held February 22nd, 1859, S. T.

Overstreet, of Florida, being called to the chair, and M. Lampen, of Pennsylvania, appointed Secretary, the following Preamble and Resolutions were unanimously adopted:

Whereas, The subscribers have had the pleasure of attending Dr. James Bryan's private courses of instruction during the present winter, and have been favorably impressed with the very excellent manner of communicating information by our teacher; having found him not only in manner and address a gentleman and a scholar, but thoroughly informed in all the branches of a sound medical education, with literary and teaching talents, and acquirements of the highest order; and joined to these qualifications, a warm and active desire to forward the professional interests of his Class: Therefore,

Resolved, That we cannot close our term of attendance in Dr. Bryan's lecture-room, without expressing our sincere thanks and deep obligations to him for the faithful, friendly, and eloquent manner in which he has filled the chair of a medical teacher.

Resolved, That his medical examinations bear the stamp of experience, practical utility, and a thorough knowledge of the subject passing under review, and are well calculated to familiarize the student with the great principles of his profession; while the happy facility which he possesses, in an eminent degree, of imparting information, is well adapted to make an indelible impression on the mind of the student.

Resolved, That we consider his instructions invaluable to every young man who desires to become proficient in his profession; as his experience, practice, and numerous advantages, enable him to arm the student at all points.

Resolved, That we will ever bear in mind the sound, scientific, and practical instructions of our late teacher.

Resolved, That these proceedings be published in one or more of the medical journals.

Attending Lectures at the Philadelphia College of Medicine.

Jefferson Medical College.

Pennsylvania University.

PHILADELPHIA, *February* 22, 1859.

S. T. OVERSTREET, *Chairman.*
M. LAMPEN, *Secretary.*
ALVIN SATTERTHWAIT, N. J.
PRESTON RAMSEY, M.D., Ky.
J. KOERPER, M.D., N. J.
A. MERRITT ASAY, Philadelphia.
WM. J. ADDISON, Md.
D. GRIFFITH, Philadelphia.
J. LAMBERT ASAY, "
AND OTHERS.

[For the Medical Gazette.]

VERATRUM VIRIDE.

Those who discover, or first introduce to the notice of the public, a new remedy for the cure of diseases, are very apt to overrate its therapeutic powers; at any rate, my hopes and expectations have been so often disappointed in my trials of new remedies, that had been lavishly extolled, that I now withhold my confidence from all such, until I have myself brought them to the test of experiment. Although specifics, in the strict sense of the word, do not probably exist, still, as remedies capable of fulfilling important indications, in the cure of disease, have been discovered and brought into general use, it is not improbable that many others may be so, of which at present we know nothing.

Whenever, therefore, a new remedy, supposed to possess such powers. is announced to the public, in common, I presume, with all practical physicians, I receive the intelligence with pleasure. I have, consequently, noticed with interest the various statemens that have appeared in the medical journals respecting the properties and curative powers of *Veratrum Viride*. Many who seem to have used it quite extensively assert that, by its use, inflammatory action can be as readily controlled as by the lancet, and even more so, and speak with great confidence of its efficacy in pneumonia, acute rheumatic affections, neuralgia, and inflammatory diseases generally. From the trials that I have made with it during the past two years, I have sufficient proof that it is a powerful sedative, and one that sometimes acts most unexpectedly with great and dangerous energy; and I am very much surprised that, of those who have used, and recommend it, no one, so far as I have noticed, says anything of its occasionally dangerous effects; and my object in this article is to call the attention of practitioners to these; for I can safely assert, that with no medicinal agent that I ever used, have I knowingly come so near killing my patients. It often exerts great and speedy control over the nervous system, and I have repeatedly seen it produce, after a very few doses, of the ordinary size—5 drops of the saturated tincture—vomiting, faintness, vertigo, and coma, to an alarming degree.

Dr. Norwood, of South Carolina, who, in the "*Southern Medical Journal*," seems to have been among the first to call public attention to this article, recommends it as useful, not only in inflammatory diseases, but also in *typhoid fever*. How an agent so entirely sedative as this can be beneficial in a disease in which the vital forces are already in a state of depression, is to me inexplicable upon any principle with which I am acquainted; and if Dr. Norwood, or any one else, has been successful with it in curing that disease, it must, I think, have been a very different kind of typhoid fever from that which I have been in the habit of recognizing under that name. From what I have seen of the effects of Veratrum, my inference is, that bloodletting would be a remedy quite as proper in typhoid fever, and, indeed, likely to do the least harm of the two. Dr. Norwood and some others seem to think that, with it, slowness of the pulse can be secured at will. This may be true; but it does not, by any means, follow that therefore it is a remedy adapted to the cure of those diseases in which rapidity of pulse is a characteristic symptom. In my opinion, it is an unsafe remedy in any disease in which debility is prominent. The slowness of the pulse that is gained by Veratrum is at the expense of the strength of the patient, and in typhoid fever this cannot be afforded without risk of serious injury. In many diseases of an inflammatory character, and those that may properly be denominated dynamic, in which I have employed it, it has often seemed to exert a favorable influence on the disease; but those very marked and conspicuous good effects, which some practitioners seem to have derived from its use, it has never produced in my hands. I, however, believe it to be a useful addition to the armory of the cautious physician. From the trials that I have made with it, the following are my conclusions:—1st. That it is a direct and powerful sedative, much more speedy in its action, and more potent than digitalis. 2dly. That its use should be confined to inflammatory and dynamic diseases. 3dly. That even in these, it should be prescribed with great caution, and its effects carefully watched, if we would avoid the unpleasant contingency of being sent for in great haste, perhaps in the middle of the night, with the unwelcome message that our patient is supposed to be dying.

From numerous cases of similar general character, I select a few, as illustrative of the preceding remarks:—

No. 1.—J. C., aged about 50 years, of sound and vigorous constitution, had catarrhal fever, with a firm, full, and somewhat accelerated pulse, but was not confined to his bed. I prescribed veratrum, 5 drops, every 3 hours. After the third dose I was sent for in great haste, the messenger stating that Mr. C. was a great deal worse. I found him in a state of great distress and agitation, but without pain. His sensations, he said, were indescribable, but very bad. He kept moving from one part of the room to another, and could neither lie nor sit still. There was a feeling of oppression in the chest, a tendency to faintness, coldness of the extremities, paleness of the face, and great weakness. The pulse was reduced from 80 to 46. Having at this time had but little experience with veratrum, I was in doubt whether to attribute these symptoms to it or not, but could not otherwise account for them. They subsided, upon the use of strong stimulants, in the course of two or three hours. The next morning I again prescribed veratrum, the same as on the previous day, 5 drops every three hours. In the evening I was again sent for to come to Mr. C. as speedily as possible, the same symptoms as on the previous evening having returned in an aggravated form, and the patient being very much alarmed. I was now satisfied that they were due to the veratrum. It was laid aside, and they returned no more. The patient soon recovered.

No. 2.—Mrs. W., aged about 60, had chronic disease, the symptoms of which indicating the propriety of a sedative, I prescribed veratrum, 5 drops, every three hours. The next morning, having taken in all five or six doses, I was summoned in great haste to the patient, as she was supposed to be dying by the neighbors, who had been called in. I found her in a state of great prostration, with coldness of the extremities, paleness of the face, and difficulty of breathing; and, although not in a state of coma, she was unable to speak, yet seemed conscious of what was going on around her. Her pulse was reduced to about 40. By the use of external warmth and stimulants, she was relieved in two or three hours. The veratrum was discontinued, and these symptoms returned no more.

No. 3.—Miss W., aged about 10 years, had pneumonic inflammation, with soreness in the chest, cough, and some fever, with rapid and moderately full pulse. I prescribed veratrum, 2 drops, every three hours. Three hours afterwards I was called in great haste, the messenger stating that the family feared the patient would die before I arrived. I found an immense change in the state of the patient. She had by mistake taken 3 instead of 2 drops, and in less than an hour this was followed by faintness, nausea, vomiting, profuse watery evacuations from the bowels, coldness of the extremities, with profuse sweating, and great prostration; indeed, she was in a state much resembling that of collapse in cholera; her pulse was reduced from about 100 to 60. From this condition she was relieved with great difficulty, in about four hours, by means of opium, ammonia, brandy, external heat, and sinapisms. At first everything was rejected from the stomach, whether medicines or cold water, until a powerful impression had been made over the region of the stomach with mustard. The veratrum was not resumed, and these symptoms did not return.

No. 4.—Mrs. S., aged about 70, of good constitution and previous good health, had erysipelas, with a full and strong pulse, fever, and much pain in the head. I prescribed veratrum, 4 drops, every three hours. This was in the evening. About two o'clock at night I was called, and found that after the second dose she became faint, had a feeling of oppression at the stomach and chest, with nausea, which was soon succeeded by vomiting, looseness of the bowels, coldness of the extremities, profuse sweating, great prostration, and profound coma. When I entered her room I really thought her dying: she was nearly pulseless, and could not be roused by any irritants whatever. Brandy, ammonia, and external heat and sinapisms were resorted to; but the coma continued for nearly twenty-four hours, and a number of days elapsed before she was entirely relieved. Of course, the veratrum was not resumed.

Other cases similar to the above might be related; but these, I think, are sufficient to show the grounds upon which my conclusions respecting veratrum viride are based.   P.

RHINEBECK, *March*, 1859.

PALMER'S PATENT HAND, ARM AND LEG.

Fig. 1 represents an arm to be applied above the elbow. The articulation, A B, is a ball and socket, connected by the steel plates, C C, and turning upon the pinion, D. The functions of the bones in the forearm (radius and ulna) are imitated by the conical shaft, E, which terminates in a ball at the elbow and wrist, J J. The wrist is articulated with a ball and socket firmly united by catgut tendons, F G H, tensely drawn over the convexity of the shaft, E, at the elbow. It has every motion of the natural wrist. The hand rotates on the forearm, being susceptible of pronation and supination, or any angle or degree of flexion and extension desirable. The extensor tendons, K L M N O, acting with the springs, 1 2 3 4 5, open the hand. The detached ball and socket joints of the thumb and fingers are indicated by the figures 1 2 and 1 2 3.

The fingers are articulated on steel rods and pinions imitating the bones, as seen in the thumb and the first and third fingers. The ex-

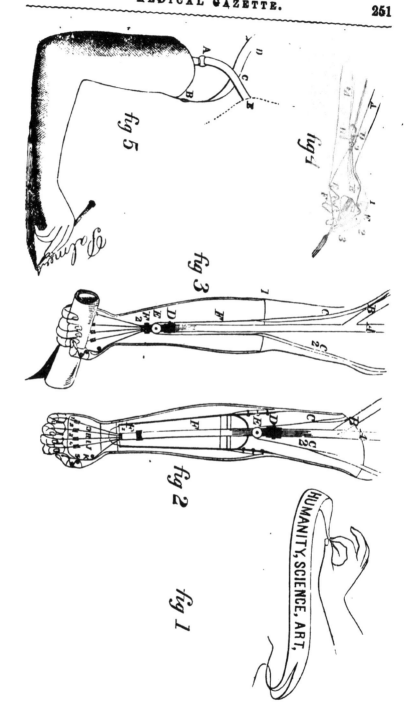

fig 5

fig 4

fig 3

fig 2

fig 1

HUMANITY, SCIENCE, ART,

terior is brought to a perfect imitation of the natural arm, (as shown in the outline, or in Fig. 5,) by a soft, elastic substance, which rotates around the forearm, preserving anatomical symmetry in every position. It is covered with a delicate skin.

Fig. 2 is the same arm extended, with the fingers semi-flexed. The belt, A, attaches the arm to the body. The small belt, C C 2, is connected by a tendon to a clasp and pulley, D E. The great muscle, F, is the continuity of the flexor tendons, G H I J K. These tendons pass sinuously over pulleys or fixed sheaves, 1 2 3 4 5, through the hand, to the end of the fingers and thumb. The principles of the lever and pulley are thus combined, and the maximum power retained at all angles of flexion or extension. A slight motion of the shoulders, with extension of the forearm, produces an incredible grasp, as seen in Fig. 3.

An object of any shape, such as a pen, a fork, or an apple, is held with facility. By a slight motion of the shoulders, the belt, A B, causes the great muscle, F, and its tendons, to contract powerfully, closing the hand. A movement easily and naturally made actuates the tendon, C C, and fastens the clasp, D, upon the muscle, so as to retain the grasp in any position or motion of the arm, when in use. This is regarded as invaluable for holding reins in driving, or carrying articles with safety. An easy counter-motion unfastens the clasp, relaxing the flexor muscle and its tendons, and the extensors open the hand. This principle performs most perfectly in an arm applied below the elbow, as in Fig. 3. In this are seen the belt, A B C, the great muscle, F, and its tendons, the clasp and pulley, D E, as in Fig. 2. A fixed eyelet, F 2, clasps the great muscle, F, and thus guides the flexor tendons of the fingers. The line, 1, shows the union of the natural with the artificial arm.

Fig. 4 shows a hand holding a fork. The tendon, A A 2, passes through the clasp, B, and around the pulley, C, to the side of the clasp, D, where it fastens or unfastens the clasp by movements before explained. The joints of the fingers and thumb are flexed upon the fork by powerful tension of the great muscle and its tendons. The sinuosity of the tendons passing over the pulleys or sheaves, E E E, shows the new and useful principle of effectually combining the lever and pulley to gain the utmost power, strength, elasticity, and adaptability to the various uses of an artificial arm and hand. They are easily adjusted by the wearer.

The articulations of knee, ankle, and toes, consist of detached ball-and-socket joints, A B C. The knee and ankle are articulated by means of the steel bolts, E E, combining with plates of steel firmly riveted to the sides of the leg, D D. To these side plates are immovably fastened the steel bolts, E E. The bolts take bearings in solid wood (properly bushed) across the entire diameter of the knee and ankle, being much more reliable and durable than those of the usual construction. All the joints are so constructed that no two pieces of metal move against each other in the entire limb. The contact of all broad surfaces is avoided where motion is required, and thus friction is reduced to the lowest degree possible. These joints often perform many months without need of oil, or other attention— a disideratum fully appreciated by the wearer.

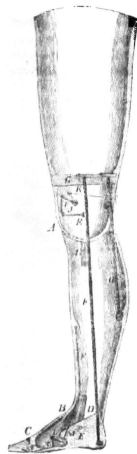

The Tendo Achillis, or heel tendon, F, perfectly imitates the natural one. It is attached to the bridge, G, in the thigh, and passing down on the back side of the knee-bolt, E, is firmly fastened to the heel. It acts throurh the knee-bolt on a centre, when the weight is on the leg, imparting security and firmness to the knee and ankle joints, thus obviating all necessity for knee-catches. When the knee bends in taking a step, this tendon vibrates from the knee-bolt to the back side of the thigh, A, (semi-flexed view) It descends through the leg, so as to allow the foot to rise above all obstructions in flexion, and carries the foot down again, in extension of the leg for the next step, so as to take a firm support on the ball of the foot. Nature-like elasticity is thus attained, and all thumping sounds are avoided. Another tendon, H, of great strength and slight elasticity, arrests the motion of the knee gently; in walking thus preventing all disagreeable sound and jarring sensation, and giving requisite elasticity to the knee.

A spring, lever, and tendon, I J K, combining with the knee-bolt, give instant extension to the leg when it has been simi-flexed to take a step, and admit of perfect flexion in sitting.

A spring and tendons in the foot, L M N, impart proper and reliable action to the ankle-joint and toes. The sole of the foot is made soft, to insure lightness and elasticity of step. The stump receives no weight on the end, and is well covered and protected, to avoid friction and excoriation.

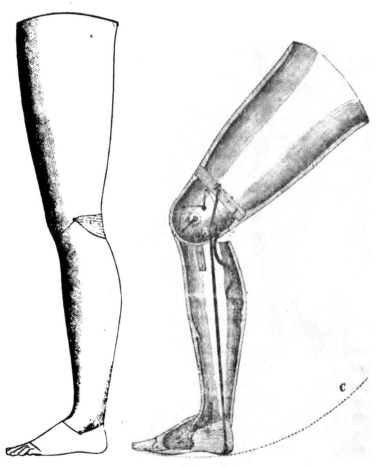

But the most ingenious piece of mechanism, and one that seems to us as likely to do greater service for humanity in relieving them from the deprivation of enjoyment and capability to work, which generally follows an accident, is the arm and hand, of which we present full drawings.

COMMUNICATIONS.

OUR PHILADELPHIA CORRESPONDENT.
No. 11.

Colleges, Professors, Students, et alia varia.

"Let us, my friend, in joy repine,
Bathe, crown our brow, and quaff our wine;
Short is the space of human joys;
What age prevents not, death destroys."—RUFINUS.

"When Magnus sought the realms of night,
Grim Pluto trembled for his right :
'That fellow comes,' he said, ''tis plain,
'To call my Ghosts to life again.'"—LUCILLIUS.

DEAR GAZETTE—Please excuse my apparent neglect to correspond with you during the last two months. The truth is, the winter campaign was coming to a close, and the forces-medical were converging to a focus, carrying all other forces and duties with them. The Students demanded extra examinations, the Professors had extra soirées, and with all it *was* the beginning of the year, when extra bills were to be made out, *collected*, and *paid*. Now is the winter of our discontent, &c., &c. So here goes for a gossip with the GAZETTE. I see in your last number, that your city has been convulsed with the Whitney case. Those whom I have consulted here about the matter, think it a very unprofessional series of movements to engineer a successful practitioner *out of the way*. But he has shown his usual skill in a rough-and-tumble fight, and it is very evident has come out of the skirmish the better of his opponents. *We* have been remarkably quiet. The Blockley gives out its usual weekly amount of corruption and vulgarity, in which the "Chief" comes in for a large share, as usual. The clinic has scarcely been successful. Better luck next season.

The great centres of attraction now are the Colleges; and how many students, how many graduates, how many rejections, &c., are among the questions of the hour! The Jefferson is the talk and envy of the town: her mammoth class, her fine clinics, her popular and skillful teachers, her fine salaries, and her general prestige. It is said that nothing less than the Academy of Music will do for her commencement; of course the old school will follow, as she has in everything during the last nineteen years. *Tempora mutantur*, my dear GAZETTE, since you and I were boys. The bully school is getting less than second. The faculty is redeemed by a *very few* names, otherwise she would not stand at all. As it is, the income to her professors must be very small, for some of them have to resort to private teaching, in all its forms, driving out the aspiring young men among them, in order to live.

The graduating classes this year will stand about as follows: Philadelphia College, 15; Pennsylvania do. 35; University, 130; Jefferson, 260.

The outside Colleges, Female, Eclectic, Homœopathic, &c., have smaller classes than usual. The popularity of the Jefferson will, I think, absorb them all in due time. The opposition of the old school brought them into existence at first, at least some of them.

There runs a report about town that the Jefferson is rejecting a large number of candidates, and producing thereby great trepidation among the aspirants for medical honors. The truth is, that many of these young men have been trusting to the unauthorized and inflated promises of some of the popular grinders for their passports to the diploma, and the faculty seem determined to show the young gentlemen and their teachers the fallacy of such proceedings. Many also come here to graduate, after attending one imperfect course in some provincial school, and thus find that one winter is not enough in which to fill up the many vacua left by such a course. Besides this, we do really believe that the requirements for graduation are gradually increasing. It is true that three years' study and three courses, with a competent knowledge of our own language, and of the dead languages, to understand technical terms and compose well, are not yet required. Yet the examinations are more rigid, and the gentlemen who have won for themselves so enviable a position as teachers and writers, are no longer willing to place their signs-manual on a parchment that certifies to the learned qualifications of a blockhead. Be assured, friend GAZETTE, we have many such, who come to Philadelphia to be *made* doctors. A thousand influences are at work to produce the desired result, but without effect, without the necessary acquirements. The old idea of belonging to the F. F. V. does not now have the charm it formerly had.

I have said, on a former occasion, that there is room here for another good school, and I repeat it. If a faculty, which I will name, could be induced to try their fortunes here, they could build up a noble institution among us. Philadelphia is the Paris of the United States, and it is to here that the first talent of the country ought to look for those rewards which are its due, and a recognition by Philadelphia, on the spot, should be sought by the great teachers of our country. We are flooded by young adventurers, who fill up the cracks and crannies of the profession. Different from New York and other cities, and different from other pursuits and professions among us, the Eastern mind does not succeed so well in medicine in Philadelphia as the native, Western, Southern, or European.

You will doubtless perceive that a terrible split has taken place in our County Society, and the seceders have taken up the charter of the good old Philadelphia Society. Several old Societies, however, monopolize the active and rising talent of the city, and many of the medical men will join none of them. They prefer peace, and professional and personal quietness, to the perpetual turmoil of these bodies.

The winter with us has been exceedingly mild, and the only general disease among us has been an influenza, or cold, affecting chiefly the throat, nasal passages, and head.

The election to the medical staff of the Pennsylvania Hospital has been made in the place of Dr. Pepper, resigned. The successful candidate—and there were some ten or twelve candidates, and over 30 ballots—was Dr. Meigs, the son of the Professor. He is considered a lucky man, and is fortunate in the appointment. The hospital will be well served by Dr. Meigs. This is one of the few appointments among us in which clinical and pathological investigations might be made the means of a great reputation. Dr. Meigs will, no doubt, fill the post to his own credit and the credit of the profession.

The terrible odor which the Board of Health and Guardians of the Poor have succeeded in surrounding themselves with, has induced our Legislature to attempt to put the appointing power of these bodies in the hands of the courts. Money and influence are, however, actively engaged—a consummation devoutly to be wished. No medical man who has any regard for his character can now belong to, or act under, these Boards; they are sinks of corruption. But my sheet is full, so adieu. Yours, truly,   SENECA.

PARAGUAY EXPEDITION.

U. S. STEAMER CHAPIN, *January 17th*, 1859.
CEIRA, COAST OF BRAZIL,
DR. JAMES BRYAN, *Philadelphia:*   *South America.*

Respected Sir—According to my promise to you, I give you a short detail of the incidents of our voyage, medical and otherwise.

We left the Capes of the Delaware on the 2d of December, and on the 17th dropped anchor in the Harbor of Barbadoes, after a run of sixteen days, without any incidents to make the passage remarkable or interesting as a sea-voyage.

But, sir, to you, as a collator of a Medical Journal, it may be interesting to have a short and concise description of the medical cases coming under my charge as surgeon.

To render the cases I shall describe more plain, it may be as well to give you a short description of our vessel and crew.

In the first place, then, our steamer is supposed to be the smallest craft of the kind that has ever crossed the line, her length being one hundred and twenty feet, and twenty feet wide, burden 240 tons; a screw propeller. Officers and crew, all told, between forty and forty-five. So far, then, you have a short, but to you perhaps a not very plain description of our craft.

I will now as well, and as plain as I am capable of, give you a description of the medical cases I have attended to from the time of leaving the United States; and here let me say, that though I have often been told that Jack Tars were a peculiar people, I had no *idea*, as the saying is, that there was so much peculiarity in the sailor.

But I am satisfied that they are something of the sea, and that something fishy; to be plain, they are a rough, devil-may-care people, whom you must hold at arm's-length, or they will take the advantage, and blame you for your kindness and civility to them. To attend to a people of this kind, in a medical point of view, requires tact in a physician of kindly feeling to the human family in general.

The first case of sickness on board our vessel was a well-defined case of low fever, running into typhoid. The patient was taken down on the third day out, and after finding that sea-sickness had nothing to do with the case, the patient was placed in my hands, and remained in a very low state until we reached Barbadoes, one of the most southern of the West India group of islands, and refused to yield to cathartics—hydra. clo. mit. in two-gr. doses three times a day, or other usual remedies—but in the end yielded to sul. of quinine in five-gr. doses three times a day. On landing the patient at Barbadoes, the disease assumed the peculiar feature general in this fever—delirium—which did not make its appearance as long as we remained at sea. Our stay at Barbadoes being limited by the direction of the Secretary of the Navy, we were compelled to leave our patient on that island. But I am happy to say a decided improvement had taken place in his case before we left, and no doubt he would return home perfectly convalescent. The other cases on board our vessel consisted of trifling complaints, viz., colds, indigestion, &c., yielding to simple remedies.

In Barbadoes, our sailors having liberty to go on shore, I am sorry to say, contracted disease in several cases. Of two cases coming under my notice, (both syphilis,) one I think worthy of particular notice. When my attention was called to this case the extremity of the penis presented one mass of purulent matter; so much so as to render it, in my opinion, the worst case that had ever come under my particular notice. In treating the case, after cleansing the bowels with saline cathartics, I adopted a practice in the emergency of the case, and which the circumstances partially rendered necessary, (the vessel being short of hands, and this patient a valuable and necessary hand to be on duty.) A flaxseed poultice was applied as a cleanser, to remove the matter and assist the sloughing off, and allowed to remain about six hours. Onr emoving the cataplasm, with a feather I applied *pure* creosote to the whole diseased surface; in twenty-four hours it had stopped sloughing, and with proper internal remedies the patient began to recover, and in fifteen to sixteen days was discharged from the list as cured.

I have other cases, but must defer until my next letter, which will be dated from Pernambuco, Brazil. The port in which we now lie at anchor, viz., Ceira, Brazil, we were compelled to enter for coals, having run short in coming from Barbadoes, and in trying to reach Pernambuco, our regular port to coal at on our way to Paraguay. This town looks prosperous and improving; the inhabitants are sociable for Brazilians, and one of their peculiar institutions is the fishermen's boats, called cattamarans, which consist of three or four round logs bound together, on which they go to sea for miles. Excuse my haste, bad writing, &c.

WILLIAM PENN LAMBERT, M.D.

DR. D. M. REESE: RHINEBECK, 14*th March*, 1859.

Dear Sir—I sent you, a day or two since, a communication on the subject of Veratrum Viride. I had not then read the article in the last GAZETTE on the "Bradycrote" (the inventor of this word should get a copyright) "or Abortive Treatment of Fever," by Dr. Close, of Port Chester. It would not, however, have changed my views of veratrum, as I must prefer my own experience and observations to those of another, let that person be who he may. I very much fear that the term "*abortive*" applied to the treatment of fever as recommended by Dr. Close, will turn out to be the appropriate term. Of one thing I am confident: that whoever prescribes those three potent sedatives—digitalis, veratrum, and aconite—in the doses, and in the manner he advises, if he should have many patients, will often have cause to regret it. For a boy between three and four years old, he prescribed digital. gtt. 5, veratrum gt. 3, aconite gtt. 2, every two hours, and the patient escaped. Now, with 3 drops of veratrum alone, I, not long since, *came very near killing* a little girl *ten* years old, which is case No. 3 in the paper sent you for the GAZETTE; and there can be no doubt that the symptoms were caused by the veratrum, for her pulse was reduced from about 100 to 60 by my watch. In my judgment, if she had had the misfortune to have taken the dose prescribed by Dr. Close for the boy, *it would most infallibly have killed her*. In another case, No. 4, in the paper, the subject of which was Mrs. William Schell, an aunt of Collector Schell, of your city, two or three doses of 4 drops each had like to have produced a fatal result. I prescribed it in the evening, her pulse being then full, strong, and frequent, with fever and heat of skin. I left her with no apprehension of danger, and at two o'clock the same night was summoned in great haste to see her; and on my entering the door her daughter, who was in great agitation and distress, exclaimed, "Oh! doctor! I believe my mother is dying." This fell upon my ears like a clap of thunder. I found her profoundly comatose, with slow and heavy breathing, extremities cold, nearly pulseless, and reduced from probably 85 or 90 to about 40 beats in a minute. From this state she was resuscitated with great difficulty. What would the result have been had she taken Dr. Close's doses?

Not ten days ago I had another, but not quite so bad, a case. I prescribed veratrum for a gentleman here—Mr. Cushman, late of Newburgh, and son-in-law, I think, of General Belknap—a very intelligent man, and capable of giving a correct account of his feelings and sensations. He had bronchitis, with fever, and a full, strong, and frequent pulse, cough, &c. I prescribed the veratrum in the morning, and then left to visit some patients in the country. On my return in the evening, I was told that Mr. C. had suddenly got a great deal worse, and I not being at home, they had called in another physician. I immediately called on him, but found him quite relieved; but he said that he had had for two or three hours a very bad time of it indeed. After the first dose of 5 drops, he felt that the medicine, as he said, did not agree with him. The second dose was soon followed by nausea, vomiting, faintness, great precordial distress, dimness of vision, vertigo, and difficulty of breathing. He felt, he said, as if his lungs were collapsed, and he and his family were much alarmed by this array of distressing symptoms, as was natural. The physician who was called in finding his pulse very slow, in connection with the above symptoms, concluded, and correctly, that he had taken veratrum, and that this was the result.

Occurrences like the above, every one, I think, will admit are anything but agreeable to the attending physician, or any of the parties; yet Dr. Close, *without a word of caution*, recommends the agents that produce them, as if they were not attended with hazard.

Your obedient servant,   E. PLATT.

[From the following, it appears that we have been "*sold*," and inadvertently inserted a smuggled advertisement. Thank you, Dr. Mead.]

ALBANY, *March* 10th, 1859.

DR REESE:

Dear Sir—I wish to notice briefly the article in the last number of your GAZETTE, on the "Abortive Treatment of Fevers," by Dr. Close. It purports to be simply his successful treatment of fever with the tinctures of digitalis, veratrum viride, and aconite.

The use of these nervous sedatives in inflammatory fevers, and in certain types of idiopathic fever, has been long advocated. Dr. Norwood has published on the use of the veratrum in these cases; and Baron Störk himself advocated the efficiency of aconite. Still, as these articles of the Materia Medica have not established a reputation for the value that is claimed for them by some, the profession will thank Dr. Close for his statistics, though they may smile at his enthusiasm in presenting a subject which he thinks so new. But the doctor has ulterior and more benevolent designs than this. We are all aware of the variable strength of the extracts and tinctures of the vegetable medicines; and Dr. Close urges, with all the strength of italics, that "*it is essential to the success of this mode of treatment, that the various materials from which these tinctures are prepared should all be the best of their kind, and that they should all be saturated tinctures.*" We understand the force of this passage when, at the close of his article, we read, "Any physician, desirous of putting this mode of treatment in practice, by addressing a letter to Dr. Thomas Close, Port

Chester, Westchester County, N. Y., will be informed where he can obtain the tinctures prepared as above directed."

Now, whether for the sake of the information or something else, I leave you to infer, I have written to Dr. C., and have received a prompt reply, containing the requested information. I am also informed that many physicians in New York have made the same request that I have.

It has occurred to me that it is a needless trouble for every one wishing this information to write to Dr. C. and wait his answer. The world should at once know where they can procure these invaluable preparations; and therefore I wish, through your columns, to spread the information I have taken the trouble to get.

Dr. C. says, " I have refered (referred) them all to Geo. C. Close, No. 106 Fulton Street, Brooklyn. He is a son of mine; a thorough-bred druggist and chemist, and has long prepared the tinctures alluded to, as well as many other choice articles, for me. Enclose a one-dollar bill," &c., &c. Certainly it is very praiseworthy in this venerable father to make public the merits of his erudite son, who, though so long and successfully engaged in this difficult department of art, is yet, it seems, unknown to fame. Hereafter, especially after this public announcement, the laboratory at No. 106 Fulton Street will be throng-ed, and it may be advisable to establish a branch in the metropolis for the accommodation of those " many physicians" who are inquirers after this great new thing.

But, Mr. Editor, jesting aside, is it not beneath the dignity of our profession to resort to any *such* means to secure private advantage? It is too much like the widely-spread message of the retired clergy-man, whose sands of life have been so long running out.

It is our boast that we make known all truth that can tend to the perfection of medicine as a science, and those who selfishly refuse to do this we declare to be without the pale of our fraternity.

If the young Dr. Close prepares a superior tincture, let him tell the members of the profession so, and they will be ready to- test it; much more ready-than when he gets his father to speak a good word for him in what assumes to be a scientific essay.

Yours, truly,　　　　M. L. MEAD.

KAPPA LAMBDAS—WHO ARE THEY?

Mr. Editor—I am a native of an adjoining State, and have recently taken up my abode in New York City for the purpose of practicing my profession. During my sojourn here, about ten months, I have visited the various medical institutions, in order to make myself acquainted with the general run of matters appertaining to the profession. I have recently listened to the several addresses, delivered at the Commencement exercises of the three colleges.

At one of these, delivered by an eminent member of the bar, Mr. Brady, I heard, although not for the first time, of the existence of a secret society in this city, composed of medical men, who are leagued together for the purpose of monopolizing, as far as in their power lies, the benefits and profits of the profession. The words used by Mr. Brady were, as reported in the *Daily Times*, as follows: " He recommended the graduates to be generous towards all who were of the profession, and condemned a *secret society* existing in this city, the object of which is to exclude from the honors and emoluments of practice, by combination and clandestine organization and action, all the other members of the profession not included in its aristocratic schedule."

This is a matter of serious import to myself, and I suppose equally so to other parties similarly situated. Moreover, the learned orator proceeded to state that this secret society, besides planning and plotting to secure the rich fees of business, combined also to degrade and slander their professional brethren; thereby endeavoring to crush any rising man, who might disdain to play toady to them, or refuse to unite with them against others.

I am aware that a secret society called the Kappa Lambda was in successful operation about the year 1830, and that a libel suit was brought against Dr. Anderson and others for telling the truth, and exposing the nefarious doings of the worthies who were thus associated.

I am also acquainted with the names of the seventeen physicians who were thus hunted out of their warrens, and who will ever remain branded and exposed in the pillory of public opinion.

Now, sir, I solicit of you, as an Editor devoted to the interests of the profession at large, to inform me, a comparative stranger here, whether the secret society alluded to in the address I have quoted be the Kappa Lambda Society, or whether it be a society organized under another name, but having for its aim the same ignoble and traitorous purposes? One of the Profession.

VARICOSE VEINS AND THE SILVER SUTURE.

Letter from Professor ARMSBY.

ALBANY, *March 8th,* 1859.

My Dear Doctor—I am treating varicose veins with the silver suture, and like the plan of treatment very much. I have introduced
as many as twenty-eight in one leg·at the same time. All the cases
(seven or eight in number) have been successful.

I pass a common curved needle, armed with the silver thread, around
the vein, including the skin and considerable substance with the vessel, and twist it up tight, so as to obstruct the circulation. The inflammation is slight, and easily controlled. Plastic lymph is deposited
in and around the vessel, and when the obstruction is complete the
wire may be removed. I have passed the wire through and through a
mass of tortuous and varicose veins without serious inflammation,
and with the most satisfactory results. My operation for hernia is
also succeeding well.

Our Observatory war has been ended by the acceptance of Prof.
Mitchel. Mrs. Dudley united with us in the invitation.

Truly yours,   J. H. ARMSBY.

SELECTIONS.

[From the New Orleans Medical and Surgical Journal.]

Wonderful Effects and New Application of the "Ready Method" of Marshall Hall.

By HUMPHREY PEAKE, M.D., Arkadelphia, Ark.

On Tuesday evening, August 23d, 1858, between eight and nine
o'clock, I was called to see William A. Dickinson, of about the age of
twenty-two years, a resident of this place. The messenger, a negress,
came to me in great haste, saying that Billy was dead; that they had
found him so in the garden. Suspecting that there might be some
mistake, I ran with all my might to the house of his brother, a distance of three or four hundred yards, where the patient was. I was
informed, as I entered the house, that he was not dead; and on going
to the room in which he was, I found him tossing wildly about the
bed, apparently in the very greatest agony, uttering cries and groans
indicative of the most intense suffering. The report of his condition
having spread rapidly, a number of persons had collected at the house.
He seemed conscious, but returned no answers to my questions. His

feet and hands were very cold, the coldness extending a considerable way up his arms and legs. The pulse was feeble, and beating about one hundred in a minute. I gave him half a drachm of McMunn's elixir of opium, with two drachms of aromatic spirit of ammonia in a draught of brandy, which he swallowed, it seemed, with some difficulty. I ordered his legs and arms to be rubbed with flannel cloths wetted in brandy containing Cayenne pepper; sent immediately for mustard, and had a hot bath prepared. I noticed that he had cramps in the muscles of his feet and legs. I now got the following history of the case:—He had been in the river seining during the whole of the afternoon, exposed to a very hot sun. The day was a very warm one. He came home in the evening after dark, and ate his supper alone, the balance of the family having already eaten. Nothing unusual was observed of him. Shortly after eight o'clock, on the family's retiring to bed, his absence was noticed. Nothing, however, was thought of this; it was merely supposed that he had gone down town, which was nothing unusual with him. Shortly after this a negro woman happened to go in the garden, where she found him lying upon the ground—speechless, senseless, and, she thought, dead. This negress was dispatched for me, and a general alarm given.

I regarded the case as one of pernicious fever. The rubbings seemed to afford little relief; when, the bath being ready, he was put in up to his hips, and his hands immersed; mustard was added to the bath. This soon afforded relief, and he now answered my questions. He complained of great pain in the head, epigastrium, and hypochondriac regions, more particularly the left one. He was taken out of the bath and rubbed with dry cloths. His sufferings, although relieved, were still intense. I began immediately to prepare sinapisms for the arms and legs. They were being put on him as I prepared them in an adjoining room. The last one made, I went in the room where he was. I had noticed a minute or so before that his moaning had ceased. The room was full of persons, some of whom were applying sinapisms. I approached near enough to observe him as they were making the applications, for convenience in which, they placed him crosswise on the bed, his head being towards the wall, against which the bed was placed. I looked at him for some time. He seemed very calm, and watched to see him breathe, but could not. All this must have taken up the space, at least, of more than a minute. I then told those at the bedside to get away, and I took hold

of his wrist, to which the plaster had not yet been applied. The
pulse was gone. I then felt the temporal artery, but could not feel it
pulsate, he still not breathing the while. Then said I to those
around. "He is dead." I now straightened him out in bed, placing
him lengthwise in it. He was as limber as a wet rag. I re-examined
the pulse, but could discover none. A thought of the "Ready
Method" passed through my mind, and at once, without any explanation, put it in execution. I continued my efforts as directed by
Marshall Hall for at least four or five minutes—bystanders thought
longer. Then, thinking that those around would consider it foolishness to be thus handling a dead man, I was about desisting, and said,
"Poor fellow, he is dead; I don't believe I can do anything for him;"
still, however, continuing the turning, etc., when a man at my elbow,
who seemed to understand my efforts, said, "Doctor, keep on a while
longer—don't quit." Somewhat encouraged, I still continued the
turning. In something over a minute more he made a feeble inspiration, while in the supine position. I continued the turning, and in a
few seconds this was succeeded by another of considerable depth.
They became more frequent as I continued the operation, and in the
course of about ten minutes the breathing was fully re-established,
and the senses had returned. He spoke a few words in answer to
questions loudly propounded, and moaned piteously. I got him to
swallow some brandy. The pulse, which was very feeble when I left
off turning, became more full, and gained strength. I now had the
sinapisms applied to the forearms. All seemed to go on well for about
half an hour, when the breathing became suddenly feeble and frequent, and in less than a minute ceased altogether. I did not take
time to feel his pulse, but began immediately the posturing. At the
least calculation, five minutes must have elapsed before my efforts
were rewarded by his gasping feebly while supine. This was soon
followed by others, and the breathing, the posturing being continued,
was gradually re-established, with partial return of the senses, and
evidently of great suffering.

To cut a long, and to me astonishing story, short, he *died* and was
brought to life *six times.* I say died, because I know no other word
to express his condition. It sounds badly, I know, but I use it for
want of a better word. If I had left him when I said he was dead first,
no one would have doubted that he "died." I know that he would
have been buried the next day. So say twenty witnesses who saw
what took place.

But to return. Until he had "died" the fourth time, I had not the faintest hope of his ultimate recovery. It then occurred to me that if he could, by any means, be kept alive during the night, or until reaction should take place, that he might get well. I now determined to try electricity, with, I confess, no very clear idea of how it was going to effect any good; and, in the absence of anything better, I had procured, in a few minutes, a plate electrical machine. For this, and much kind assistance, I am indebted to Professor Samuel Stevenson, of the Young Ladies' Institute. A Leyden jar was charged, and the contents passed through myself and the patient. The charge was a moderate one, yet lightning could have had no more instantaneous effect—the breathing stopped at once. The machine was immediately put aside, and "Marshall Hall's Method" resumed. In about four minutes, it was supposed, an inspiration took place; this was followed by others, and the breathing was, for the fifth time, restored. Still regarding the case as one of pernicious fever, I had been thinking all the while about giving quinine, but had thus far foregone doing so. I determined now to do so at once, and accordingly fourteen grains of the disulphate were given at a dose. My father, who is a physician, and was distant one mile, was now sent for. Before he arrived the breathing again ceased—the sixth and last time. I did as I had done before, and persisting, even after we had all given up hope, was rewarded with like success. It most certainly was eight minutes from the time he ceased to breathe until he made the first effort at inspiration. It was a very feeble one, and it was a long time before the breathing was satisfactorily re-established. I was completely tired out.

My father now arrived, and I told him what had taken place, and what I had done. On examining him now, we found the pupils somewhat contracted, and insensible to light. The light of a candle, however, seemed to hurt his eyes, from which tears flowed freely, though the pupils did not obey the stimulus. My father regarded the case as one of the forms of *coup de soleil*, named, by Dr. Bennet Dowler, of New Orleans, *solar exhaustion*. He proposed that he should take fifteen drops of tinc. opii., and have sinapisms on the back of the neck. Both were immediately complied with. I had sent and got my apparatus, intending to cup him, but had deferred doing so. It was now, however, thought proper, and, as preparatory, to shave the temples. He seemed to be getting better, and wanted to know what was going to be done. When told, and I ready to do so, he objected stoutly and jocosely. He did not like the looks of the scarificator; he had seen persons cut with them, and thought he could get along without it. Said he wanted to go to sleep. After much persuasion, he still objected; and, as he seemed so much better, it was concluded not to cup him.

He was soon in a sound sleep. This was about three o'clock, A. M. I remained with him until 5, when I left him, still asleep, and doing well.

At six o'clock he began taking the disulphate of quinine, in four-grain doses, every hour. This he continued until 12, M.; after which time, he took two grains every hour until night. He also took, during the day, some fluid extract of senna, to move the bowels. He slept nearly all day, and generally had to be waked to take his medicine. At bedtime he took eight grains of blue pill and six grains of quinine. He slept well during the night, and when he awoke, generally called for water. This he also did the previous day.

On Thursday he took two grains of the disulphate of quinine every hour during the day, and until bedtime at night. On the Sunday following, I met him on the street well. There was a complete blank in his memory from the time he ate his supper on Tuesday evening, until the following morning.

REMARKS.—Whether the foregoing case was one of pernicious fever, as I regarded it, or one of *solar exhaustion,* or whether it was either one, I leave to the readers of this paper to determine: It may not have been either one. Possibly it was a complication of both. To describe the various forms in which this cousin-german of Proteus, pernicious fever, may appear, would transcend the contemplated limits of this article

These remarks are appended mainly for the purpose of offering a suggestion in the treatment of *ictus solis, coup de soleil,* or sun-stroke. All standard works, so far as I know, are meagre as to information on this subject. The only paper on this malady of any value, in my estimation—and that is a really valuable one—is from the pen of Dr. Bennet Dowler, of New Orleans. This may be found in volume xii. of the *New Orleans Medical and Surgical Journal,* page 474, *et seq.,* to which I beg to refer the reader. Dr. Dowler, in his pathological investigations on this disease, has shown no lack of that indefatigable industry which characterizes all his labors. The result of his inquiries proves conclusively that the theory which regards *ictus solis* as a cerebral apoplexy, is an erroneous one, and that the organic lesions are found in the lungs.

In regard to the cause of death, Dr. Dowler says: "Be it what it may, the cause of death begins, continues, and ends in the breathing apparatus." But the most remarkable fact which his investigations have developed is the post-mortem circulation of the blood. He says: "After the death of the lungs, or the cessation of respiration, the heart and arteries will, in some instances, continue to act." Again he says: "Mr. C. died of solar asphyxia on the evening of the 24th of July, 1836. About an hour after he had been laid out, two messengers called upon me to visit the corpse, which was supposed to be alive. I found the body as warm as at death, though it had since been washed. I found a slight pulsation at the wrist, and a feeble motion of the heart."

The suggestion which I set out to offer is, the application of the "ready method" of Marshall Hall to the treatment of *coup de soleil* in its worst form, *i. e.*, the *solar asphyxia* of Bennet Dowler. The remedy is so simple and easy of application, under all circumstances, that it seems unnecessary to urge its trial. An argument in its favor, however, may be found in the fact that, so far, no other remedy has effected any good.

There is one important fact, I admit, as noticed by Dr. Dowler, that would rather lead to the conclusion that this means must fail. From his observations, it would seem that congestion or hæmorrhagic infiltration of the lungs, always present, precedes death. But from other important facts noticed by the observer, may it not be possible that in some cases, at least, this condition is the effect of the post-mortem circulation or exudation of the blood? Does it not seem probable that the "ready method" of Marshall Hall would have restored to life the man seen by Dr. D., in whom, an hour after death, there was a slight pulsation at the wrist and a feeble motion of the heart?

ARKADELPHIA, *September* 25, 1858.

[From the North Carolina Medical Journal.]

MEDICAL ETHICS.

Much discussion has recently taken place upon the subject of Medical Ethics. Volumes have been written in exposition of it; codes have been promulgated, pregnant with all the learning of the Nestors of the profession, and appealing to the most honorable principles of human nature for sanction and approval. Clauses have been continually inserted, providing against every contingency in which the interests of practitioners can be brought in conflict, and so arranged as to serve, under all circumstances, as sign-posts, to direct those interested out of the wrong way and into the right one. But, unfortunately for medicine, no practical and permanent advantage has resulted from this protracted excitement, and instead of fraternity and friendship, ill feeling and hostility exist, in too many instances, among the followers of Æsculapius. The elements are yet in a condition of confusion and disturbance. The angry waters are boiling and surging as of yore. The disagreement of doctors is still a source of amusement to others, and of disgrace to themselves. No Solon or Justinian has arisen to establish laws so just, equitable, and imposing, as to recommend them immediately to the cordial admiration and entire approval of the medical world. No "brighter day" has dissolved the mists of selfishness and prejudice which have so long hung heavily upon the profession. Physicians can be readily found who are ready to pander to the prejudices of the multitude; to use the most disreputable articles for their own advancement, and to detract from a professional brother without shame or compunction, for the sake of a little ephemeral distinction, or a few dollars and cents Some of the fraternity will scruple at nothing, however mean, low or contemptible; will practise the most shameless and disreputable arts; will cringe, and fawn, and vilify, just so far as their pusillanimity permits them to go, or opportunities present themselves for the cowardly stabs of such miscreants. Professional success—that is, securing patients—is considered the *summum bonum* of existence; and for it honor is sacrificed, the most sacred obligations despised, and tricks attempted which would disgust the "lowest juggler who ever threw his balls." The rich are flattered and caressed; the poor courted and petted; the virtuous treated with reverence and respect; the vicious approved and smiled at; and every popular breeze wooed with such adroitness, that not a breath escapes the distended sail which flies before it—perhaps to its own destruction. But this is not all; a regular war is made upon rival practitioners, in which no civilized law is observed, and whose watchword is, "every advantage, and at any cost." We might notice in detail the means employed by these persons to effect their purposes; the appliances by which the eye of the community is dazzled; the arts used to publish marvelous successes to the world; the schemes invented to injure professional brethren, and all the machinery by which

pretension and meanness seek to advance themselves in public estimation, not to mention the flatteries exhausted upon twaddling crones, or
the hypocritical cant invested in religious demonstration; but the task
is too disgusting to be attempted by a decent man for respectable
readers.

This condition of things results from two passions, which, unfortunately, find but too genial an atmosphere in the human heart; we
mean avarice and vanity. The Scriptures have long since declared,
that "money is the root of all evil;" and the experience of mankind
has amply confirmed the truth of the maxim. For it men are willing
to sacrifice the ties of blood and kindred; to stifle every generous sentiment and ennobling principle within their bosom; to despise honor,
truth, and justice; to trample upon the laws of God and man; to forget the endearments of home, and to drive the plowshare over the
graves of their fathers; to spend long years of dreary toil amid the
snows of Siberia, the fervid heat of India, or the lonely wilds of California; to brave the dangers of the ocean's traitorous waves, and the
mysteries of its hidden caverns; and to count no sacrifice too great,
no labor too onerous, and no crime too appalling, in the accumulation
of its golden treasures. Avarice feeds upon every acquisition; grows
with each indulgence, and strengthens upon the very longings it in-
spires. It enters the heart a helpless infant, but is speedily transformed into a giant, whose heavy heel crushes out the virtuous sentiments implanted there, and compresses all beneath it to the consistency of iron. It first closes gently the too generous hand, and then
binds it with such unyielding cords, that not even the strongest appeals of poverty and wretchedness can break them. In a word, it
takes possession of a man's soul, reduces his highest powers to a state
of abject servitude, and tyrannizes over his entire nature.

When this passion actuates a physician, it unspheres him, places
him in an orbit whose centre is *self*, breaks the link which bound him
to a more elevated destiny, and paralyzes his usefulness as a member
of the profession. He graduates his sympathy and attention by the
prospect of gain. He only enters the sick man's room to thrust his
hand in his purse. He hears but the chink of the dollar in his "aus-
cultations." His "explorations" are all after gold. His "percus-
sions" have the ring of the *real metal* about them. And his prescriptions are redolent of *mint drops*, suggestive of *heavy draughts*, and are
put up more for the benefit of the doctor's pocket than the patient's
stomach. In fact, his mind is nothing but a ledger well posted; his

heart an iron chest with money in it; his degree a false advertisement, and his profession his stock in trade; whilst the contempt and enmity of every respectable brother is the sure reward of the miserable passion which has so depraved him. He may succeed in accumulating money; but death finally closes the scene ! And he goes to his last account without carrying with him the consolation of a good conscience, or leaving behind an honorable name for his children.

We can but quote the words of the poet:

" May his soul be plunged
In ever-burning floods of liquid gold,
And be his avarice the fiend which damns him."

All have vanity to some extent, but we are convinced that physicians possess more of it than any other class of men. All have their admiring friends, who esteem them more learned than was Hippocrates himself. Each one is an autocrat within his particular sphere. So many cures are effected through the benignant ministrations of nature, and in despite of doctors and drugs, that the veriest tyro imagines himself the embodiment of all the skill and attainment known to the profession. The lawyer's effort is made in public, before bench, bar, and jury, so that an accurate estimate of his talents and qualifications immediately obtains, before which he sinks or rises until his proper level has been reached. The minister of the Gospel is constrained to submit to the same searching ordeal, and soon learns to graduate his self-esteem by the general estimate of his abilities. But the physician struggles with disease in private, with no competent spectator of the scene, under circumstances which render his will absolute, and his slightest word the voice of destiny; surrounded by those whose anxieties make them credulous and confiding, and assisted by an overruling Providence, which comes to his rescue in an extremity, either by restoring the patient to health, or consigning the victim to that narrow resting-place which covers up all errors and utters no accusation. His vanity feeds upon the pabulum which this accumulated responsibility supplies. His self-love expands under the stimulus thus afforded. His ideas of his own dignity and importance increase with each trial to which he is subjected. And he finally becomes that inflated, supercilious, and pedantic specimen of professional development, by whom the rights of others are invariably despised, and medicine brought so frequently to an open shame. Such a man grieves over the loss of patronage as a calamity and a wrong. He weeps bitter tears at the grave of friendship, not from real sorrow at the bereavement, but because of an apprehension that in failing to effect a cure, his reputation may suffer in the estimation of the community. He can never be induced to mention a fatal case, save for the purpose of an egotistical explanation, or a sly insinuation that his medicines were improperly administered, and that he was called too late. He hates a funeral procession, bribes the sexton to toll the bell as quickly as possible, and pays "the devil" to omit all obituary notices of the patients who have died under his charge. He avoids consultations with his professional brethren, treats all physicians habitually as inferiors, and when forced into contact with them at the bedside, takes particular pains to whisper into the ear of some one interested in the result of the case, that but for his timely intervention, the sufferer would have been hurried to another world with the speed of lightning and the certainty of fate.

This picture may seem overdrawn, but we are confident that its original can be found within a stone's throw of any man who will seek for it; and we only hope none of our readers may discover in it their own counterpart.

We are so far from having that confidence in the perfectibility of human nature, which has distinguished the Utopian philosophy of these latter days, that we utterly despair of the complete moral regeneration of the race. The evils which we have mentioned originate in that natural source of depravity upon which the seal of corruption has been impressed by the hand of Divinity itself. They are the fruits of that forbidden tree which tempted and depraved our first parents in the garden. They are the legitimate offspring of those base passions wherewith humanity was cursed at the fall. Their complete eradication can only be effected by revolutionizing man's entire being, by elevating and purifying his nature, by destroying that selfish principle which possesses his heart, and by inaugurating that glorious millennium of virtue and happiness, whose coming has been proclaimed by the voice of inspiration. But, though perfection be impossible without the special interposition of Providence, improvement is always within the compass of human effort. If the profession cannot be entirely purged of its impurities, it may be made better than it is. Much can be done towards the elevation of its members, if it be attempted judiciously and persistently. Many of the abuses by which it has been disgraced may be corrected, if those interested in the maintenance of its dignity will make a united and disinterested effort in its behalf. And we now propose to sketch, hastily, the plan by

18

which these most desirable ends can be effected promptly and effectually. A few preliminary observations, however, will be necessary to a proper elucidation of our ideas, and an introduction of the subject. This is a fast age. Haste is the grand characteristic of the times. The value of everything is measured by the celerity of its attainment. Society is only a *rush* and a *scramble.* The minds of men have become so habituated to the annihilation of space by steam and electricity, that they die of ennui unless time can be destroyed with the same rapidity. Youth does not wait for "its beard to grow," but is a man in taste and vices, when the rod of the pedagogue should be " teaching the idea how to shoot." Manhood courts the cares of age and assumes its dignity, when the *toga virilis* is still an unfamiliar novelty. And old age, forgetful that it is appointed for man to die, occupies itself in devising expedients for the consumption of the few remaining hours of life. Medicine has felt this baneful influence, and yielded to it sadly. A physician's qualifications are determined by the rapidity with which his diploma was obtained. Schools have sprung up, whose only object seems to be to enrich themselves by striving to turn out the greatest number of doctors, and in the shortest possible time. They scramble for students as boys for marbles or ginger-cakes. They pounce upon a fee with the rapacity of a hawk after its prey. They hurry through their courses and examinations with the speed of an "express train" They stuff their matriculates with such a mass of heterogeneous materials, that no intellect is cormorant enough to digest them. And they send forth crowds of graduates, invested with all the dignity of the doctorate and privileged to prescribe for the sick, but who have not one moral or intellectual qualification for the work, before them. Their only ideas of the responsibility of their calling, or of the ethics of the profession, are derived from the well-thumbed valedictory of some superannuated professor; whilst the medical knowledge with which they are to combat disease and make a name for themselves, is nothing more than that superficial smattering crammed into them by a quizer, or picked up at that *last* of *humbugs*, a public clinic.

These men go forth to the world as exponents of the dignity of medicine, without understanding the meaning of the term; to sustain its honor, without feeling more than a selfish interest in it; to be brought in contact with other physicians, without knowing their rights, or estimating the importance of such knowledge; to be tried by a code of ethics, without the least familiarity with them, or the ability to appreciate their signification; and to involve the profession in the disgrace attendant upon their shameless acts, without compunction or regret. It is hardly necessary to assert our sympathy in those measures which have been attempted so unsuccessfully, for the prolongation of scholastic terms, the extension of the curriculum, and elevation of the standard of graduation in all institutions where medicine is taught. These things would secure more knowledge of the science, and a greater success in the practice of physic; but they would conduce in no material degree to an observance of the ethics of the profession, or the inculcation of more elevated sentiments among its members. We propose, for the accomplishment of this end, the establishment of separate chairs in every school of the country, devoted exclusively to the great subjects of medical ethics, literature, history and jurisprudence. We would have professors appointed for the purpose of teaching all that relates to these important branches of a physician's education, so that he might meet the multitudinous responsibilities of his calling, properly prepared for them. We would have candidates for the degree examined searchingly as to their motives for desiring it, their ideas of its dignity, their acquaintance with its literature, their knowledge of its history, their ability to solve the complex problems of medico-legal science, and their acquaintance with those practical amenities and duties which should engage the attention and study of every cultivated practitioner. The good thus accomplished would be incalculable; and we trust to see the day when this plan will be perfected in North Carolina.

In the next place, we would have boards of examiners appointed, delegated with ample powers to inquire into the moral as well as intellectual qualifications of those who come before them, and privileged to ostracise all against whom charges of professional impropriety could be substantiated by their peers. We would have them scrutinize the lives, habits, and bearing of every aspirant, so that the question of his respectability might be satisfactorily settled. We would have them determine the motives actuating him, the principles acknowledged as his guides, and the views entertained by him of professional honor and dignity. In a word, we would have them ascertain whether he be a *gentleman* or not, and to reject him promptly if the slightest doubt existed on the subject. Those to whom certificates might be granted, and, indeed, all in the ranks of the profession, should be amenable to this board, to be tried faithfully by those composing it, and sentenced, if a proper case be made out against the accused, to an ignominious expulsion from the society and fellowship of more honorable practitioners. This idea of continued responsibility on one part, and of constant surveillance on the other, will doubtless prove distasteful to some—for

> " No wretch e'er felt the halter draw
> With good opinion of the law."

But we are well assured that it would act as a most salutary restraint upon many, whose daily practices are a disgrace to their vocation, and who can be reached in no other way. The third plan we would suggest for the improvement of medicine, relates entirely to the *morale* of those who are disposed to inveigh against the evils complained of, and who desire their eradication. They should despise everything that bears the slightest semblance to unfairness or meanness. They should discountenance those who are continually disgracing the vocation and dishonoring their titles; they should frown down quackery in every guise, expose pretension wherever it raises its specious form, and hold the derelict up to public scorn, without exhibiting a fear or demanding a favor. They should remember that the profession is a common brotherhood, bound together by links of sympathy and interest, and so delicately organized as to respond in every part to whatever affects a single member. They should protect the rights of a rival as zealously as those of a friend, and defend his character and reputation with as much cheerfulness as their own. They should reverence their vocation, and diligently endeavor to qualify themselves for its high and holy offices. And, though jealous of their individual honor, and mindful of their legitimate interests, they should look beyond the contracted horizon of mere selfishness; scorn the allurements of every groveling passion, and live for the honor and glory of that calling which, when properly pursued, is perpetual incense to heaven

But as no creed yet promulgated by ecclesiastical prerogative has ever received the sanction of a people, unless it appealed directly to their religious sentiments; as no system of laws, however seemingly wise, salutary, and equitable, or by what authority sustained, has succeeded in commanding obedience, unless addressed immediately to the ideas of right and justice pre-existing in the minds of those for whom they were designed; so no code of medical ethics can secure the permanent support of the profession, unless its members possess the moral attributes requisite for their appreciation.

To sum up, the alpha and omega of the whole matter is this: the evils which disgrace our calling in these latter times can be most surely abated by a rigid cultivation and practice of those cardinal virtues which constitute the character of a gentleman. And to all who desire the elevation of medicine; who mourn over its fallen greatness; who deprecate the ungenerous spirit which characterizes but too many of its followers, and who are really anxious tô aid in regenerating, purifying, and ennobling our beloved profession, we would say in conclusion, begin the work at home; cleanse your own bosoms; regulate the evil spirit of your rebellious hearts; prostrate that altar whereon the idol of selfishness has been so ardently worshiped, and let virtue be your guide, honor your friend, and truth your polar star.

> " Above all, to thine own self be true,
> And it will follow as the night the day,
> Thou canst not then be false to any man."

[From the New Orleans Medical and Surgical Journal.]

LYING-IN HOSPITAL, DUBLIN.

October 11th, 1858.

DR. STANFORD CHAILLE:

 Dear Doctor—I have been intending for some time past to send you some account of the practice, etc., of the Dublin Lying-in Hospital, but have been prevented by various circumstances from doing so before this. This hospital was founded more than a century ago, and is the largest of the kind in the United Kingdom. It contains one hundred and thirty beds, fifteen of which are reserved for chronic diseases of the uterus and its annexes. About two thousand women are confined here annually, making an average of five per diem.

The medical staff consists of a master, Dr. McClintock, and two assistants, all of whom reside in the hospital. The master is elected by the Board of Governors, and holds his office for seven years. The assistants each pay five hundred dollars per annum for the privileges they enjoy. The interne pupils pay one hundred dollars for six months, or half that amount for three months, besides their board. The advantages here are very good, though not as much so as could be wished. Students are not permitted to perform operations, however well qualified they may be, but can only look on while they are performed by the master or his assistants. At Vienna, I am told, students enjoy the privilege of applying the forceps, or making version when necessary.

The ventilation of this hospital is very good, and every attention is paid to cleanliness; but notwithstanding every precaution, there are occasional epidemics of puerperal fever. In each ward is a couch on which the patient is delivered, and two hours afterwards, she is removed to her bed. A purgative is usually given on the second day after delivery, and if the patient goes on well, she is allowed to sit up on the fifth day, and is discharged from the hospital on the eighth day. Prolapsus uteri appears to be very common among the lower classes of Dublin, which is doubtless owing, in many cases, to getting up too soon after confinement.

Dr. McClintock lays great stress upon the use of the binder after delivery, to keep the uterus firmly contracted, and to diminish the size of the abdomen. In the Paris hospitals, the binder is considered useless, and is not usually applied. The patients here are always delivered on the left side, not only in natural labors, but also in all operations. In Paris they are always delivered on the back. In natural cases I think the side position is preferable, but when an operation is to be performed, I think it is much more convenient to place the patient on her back, with the hips drawn over the edge of the bed.

In all obstetrical operations here, chloroform is usually given, unless there is some special contradiction. It is especially useful when it is necessary to make version, or to introduce the hand to bring away a retained placenta.

An interesting case occurred a few days since, showing the advantages of chloroform. It was a case of retained placenta caused by spasmodic contraction of the cervix uteri. After waiting four hours without result, Dr. McClintock decided to administer chloroform, and to introduce the hand; gradually dilate the os uteri and bring away the placenta. The patient was with considerable difficulty brought under the full influence of the chloroform, and on introducing the hand into the vagina, the os uteri was found to be dilated, and the placenta extruding, so that it was easily extracted, without introducing the hand into the uterus, which may justly be considered one of the most dangerous operations in obstetrics.

The only forceps used in this hospital are the straight forceps, but with longer blades than the ordinary short forceps. The following are considered indispensable conditions in order to render the forceps applicable: 1st "That the child be alive, or at least that there is no reasonable ground for supposing it to be dead." When the child is ascertained to be dead, the perforator and crotchet are used, being considered as less dangerous to the mother than the application of the forceps. The stethoscope renders most valuable aid in ascertaining the condition of the fœtus. If the fœtal heart is heard in the early stage of the labor, and afterwards the most careful examination fails to detect it, the death of the fœtus may be considered as almost certain, if not absolutely so. Hence it is an established rule of the hospital to ascertain if the fœtal heart is audible, when the patient enters, so that if the labor becomes difficult, and instrumental aid is required, it can be ascertained with almost absolute certainty whether the child be alive or dead. 2d. "That the head has remained stationary within reach of the forceps, for six hours at least." This rule, of course, is not adhered to, when there exists any pressing complication, such as hæmorrhage or convulsions, etc. 3d. "That the membranes be ruptured and the os uteri fully dilated." 4th. "That the head of the child be so circumstanced that the ear can be distinctly felt, without the use of any force or violence on the part of the examiner. Dr. Rigby, of London, does not approve of this plan of feeling for the ear. In his "System of Midwifery," he very justly remarks: "The blades should always, if possible, be applied one on each side of the head, the position of which must be determined by the direction of the fontanelles and sutures, *not by feeling for the ear*, as is usually recommended in this country. The ear can seldom be reached without causing a good deal of pain, even under the most favorable circumstances, &c. &c. 5th. "That the state of the soft parts be such as denotes the absence of inflammation; in other words, that they be free from undue heat, dryness, tumefaction, or morbid sensibility." These views are extracted from Hardy and McClintock's report of the hospital practice.

When the above conditions are absent and instrumental aid is necessary, craniotomy is performed with the perforator and crotchet. The cephalotribe is never used—it being considered a dangerous and unnecessary instrument. The ergot of rye is used with great caution during labor, as experience has shown that it exerts a very injurious influence on the fœtus, unless it be born soon after the ergot has been given. In cases of inertia uteri, when the head presents and the os uteri is fully dilated, and stimulating enemata of salt and water have failed to excite efficient contractions, ergot, 3ss., is given, and the dose repeated in twenty minutes if necessary. But if the child is not born within *two hours* after the administration of the ergot, the forceps is applied and the child speedily extracted, as the experience of this hospital has been that the child was generally still-born, if not born within two hours after the ergot was given. Dr. McClintock is opposed to the administration of ergot during the third stage of labor, to produce the expulsion of the placenta. He says that if the placenta should happen to be morbidly adherent, the ergot might cause hour-glass contraction, render the operation of introducing the hand into the uterus to detach the placenta much more difficult, and, consequently, more dangerous to the patient. It is the common practice here to push out the placenta by grasping the fundus uteri and making considerable pressure, which is generally effective, if the placenta is detached.

We have recently had quite a number of cases of puerperal fever. The usual treatment consists in local depletion by means of leeches to the seat of tenderness; mercury and opium internally, and mercurial inunctions to the abdomen. I cannot say that this treatment has been more successful than many others that have been recommended for the cure of this terrible malady. The muriated tincture of iron has recently been very much in vogue in London, as a remedy in puerperal fever. It was tried in several cases here, with varied success. Two cases appeared to be much benefited, while two others died. I have not seen a sufficient number of cases to judge of its efficacy. It was not thought much of here, and was soon abandoned for the old treatment. One of the cases that appeared to be benefited at first, died after a month's illness from exhaustion, produced by a phlegmonous inflammation of the calf of the leg. Twenty-four leeches were applied in the commencement of the attack, and then the muriated tincture of iron (ten drops every two hours) was given. The other case appeared to be convalescing, when she was attacked with arthritis in the wrist. She was removed from the hospital by her friends before convalescence, so that I am not able to say whether she recovered or not.

To give you an idea of the advantages a student has for seeing obstetrical operations, I will mention that during three months that I have been *interne* in this hospital, there have been eight forceps cases, three craniotomies, and two cases of version.

A very unnatural and interesting case of complicated labor occurred a few weeks since, the details of which may interest you: B. B., æt. thirty-seven, primipara, was admitted into the hospital at noon on the 14th of September. She stated that at 9, A. M., on the 12th, she had been delivered of a dead child, at a village seven miles from Dublin. Her medical attendant discovered that there was another child in utero, and after waiting two days for its expulsion, advised her to come to the hospital. Accordingly, she was placed in a cab and brought in.

On examination the os uteri was found to be half dilated, the membranes unbroken, the breech of a second child presenting, and the cord of the first hanging out of the vulva. In a short time the second child was born alive, and apparently of eight months' development. It was now discovered that there was a third child presenting also by the breech. There being some hæmorrhage, it was deemed expedient to bring down the feet and hasten the delivery. The third child was also born alive. The uterus contracted, and the hæmorrhage ceased; but commenced again in about fifteen minutes, and the placentæ were still retained. There was no time to be lost; if the hæmorrhage was not speedily arrested, the patient would bleed to death. Although she was very much exhausted, it was deemed necessary to introduce the hand and bring away the placentæ without delay. This was accordingly done, giving her, at the same time, stimulants. There were two placentæ, both of which were partially morbidly adherent. The uterus now contracted firmly, and all hæmorrhage ceased; but in spite of all efforts to sustain her vital powers, she sank rapidly, and expired in a few hours after delivery, from the combined effects of exhaustion, arising from the protracted labor, the shock of delivery, and hæmorrhage. The pulse continued perceptible to the moment of dissolution. The great error committed by the " village doctor " in this case, was in not rupturing the membranes of the second fœtus, soon after the birth of the first, and before the os uteri had time to contract. Had this been done, the patient would have stood a much better chance of recovery, although the adherent placentæ and hæmorrhage would have rendered the prognosis very unfavorable.

The most remarkable feature of the case, however, was revealed at the autopsy: The uterus was very large, and on its anterior surface was an *enormous fibrous tumor*, seven or eight inches long and four or five wide. The woman stated on coming in, that she had perceived a tumor in the abdomen for about two years. This shows conclusively that organic disease of the uterus does not prevent conception; and it is not a little remarkable, that utero-gestation should have gone on almost to the full term with triplets, while at the same time, there existed such a large amount of organic disease in the body of the uterus.

The children were in a healthy condition when taken from the hospital.   Yours, very truly,

                                        W. A. McPheeters, M.D.

WESTMINSTER HOSPITAL.

Epilepsy for Thirty-two Years in a Man, aged Forty-four, with Discoloration of the Skin from Nitrate of Silver. Operation of Castration.

(Under the care of Mr. HOLTHOUSE.)

Amongst the causes of epilepsy mentioned by various writers, extreme sexual excesses are considered as not the least important. They would appear to have much influence on the frequency of the fits, as is shown in the narrative of the following case, the notes of which were taken by Mr. H. Ponsonby Adair, house-surgeon to the hospital. There are cases on record in which castration has been resorted to as a means of relief. In one reported by Mr. J. P. Frank, the *aura epileptica* began in the testicle, and it is asserted that a permanent cure followed castration.

This operation is much practiced at the present day amongst the Eastern nations, for the sole purpose of depriving their slaves of manhood; and Mr. Curling informs us, in his work on the "Diseases of the Testis," that in Italy it was once frequently performed on account of its effects on the vocal organs.

Eli B——, aged forty-four, widower, native of the United States, bookseller, was admitted into Luke ward in the above hospital, on the 4th of January, under the care of Mr. Holthouse, in order to have the operation of castration performed for the cure of epilepsy.

The patient is one of fourteen children, of whom eleven are living and healthy; his father is alive, aged eighty-four, and his mother died at eighty. There is no insanity in his family, nor is any member of it afflicted with epilepsy. He was a healthy child till he was ten years of age, when he commenced to practice masturbation, and soon after had an epileptic fit, in which he bit his tongue. This was followed by severe pain in the head, and incapacity for exertion the next day. The fits recurred every three or four weeks. They came on suddenly, without any premonitory symptoms. During the first two years he took "skullcap tea" without effect; his diet was also regulated. He still continued to practice self-abuse, and did not finally relinquish it till he was twenty-two, about the time when he began to take nitrate of silver. For two years he tried homœopathy, the fits increasing in severity. He was at school up to the age of fifteen, when he tried a sea-voyage, but without benefit. Having returned, he sailed for South America, where he remained two years, the fits being as frequent as before. While at New York he contracted gonorrhœa, having been accustomed to frequent sexual intercourse from the age of sixteen, in addition to the habit of self-abuse. He remained in New York for a few months, trying various remedies, amongst them sulphate of zinc, but without relief. He went again to the South for a few months, and upon his return he placed himself under the care of Dr. Kissam, who prescribed nitrate of silver, in doses of one-eighth of a grain, three times daily, and in two months it was increased to half a grain. Very soon after he began to take this remedy the severity and frequency of the fits began to decrease, and he was so convinced of its efficacy, that he continued its use for about eight months, against the advice of Dr. Kissam, who feared it might affect his skin, which, indeed, it did to some extent, giving it a blue tint. At the end of this time, the fits left him for a period of two years, having gradually decreased in frequency under the use of the nitrate of silver. From the time of his contracting gonorrhœa till his marriage, he abstained altogether from sexual intercourse and the habit of self-abuse, so that during the whole time that he was taking the nitrate of silver he had no extraneous sexual excitement; yet during this period he says that he was constantly troubled with nocturnal erections, and frequent seminal emissions. Being now twenty-four years of age, he married, shortly after which he again became addicted to sexual excesses. He left his wife and his business for several months, and traveled; the fits, however, recurred every three or four weeks, and were very severe. On his return his wife died, and he remained a widower six years, abstaining altogether from sexual excesses, although frequently troubled with erections. During the six years he broke his arm, several fingers, and his leg twice, whilst in the fits. At the age of thirty he married a second time, the fits having increased in number and severity. He was often compelled to send his wife into the country for a day or two, in order to avoid sexual excitement. The fits now recurred daily. His wife died a year after marriage. After this he again abstained from sexual excesses. Dr. Horace Green, of New York, now cauterized his larynx daily with nitrate of silver, and at the end of three or four months he would be free from fits for nineteen days; when they did recur, they were so slight that he scarcely lost consciousness, and did not fall down. This plan of treatment was pursued for two or three years, at the end of which time he became attached to another young woman, which revived all his old amatory feelings, and the fits began to increase in frequency, recurring at intervals of fourteen days, when they would continue daily for a week, and then cease for fourteen days more. Galvanism was now tried, with some slight beneficial effect. Next arsenic, in the form of Fowler's solution, which he continued till the fits recurred daily, and he became so prostrate that he was confined to his bed. For a long time he took iron to neutralize the effects of the arsenic, but for months he was compelled to walk on crutches. He came to England two years ago, to have tracheotomy performed by Dr. Marshall Hall, who had advised it when he saw the man in America. Dr. Hall died soon after the man's arrival, and he went to Paris, and was under the care of M. Nélaton. Afterwards he placed himself under M. Trousseau, who gave him belladonna, which affected his vision, but not his fits. Dr. de Lasiauve next treated him with camphor for four months without effect. He returned to England, and was under Mr. Simon, at St. Thomas's Hospital, in order to have castration performed, in which he had great faith, for he attributed his fits chiefly to sexual excitement, which still troubled him much; but his wish was not acceded to. He took bromide of potassium without any benefit, and then the nitrate of silver for two or three months, in half-grain doses, three times a day. The skin became darker than before, and the fits recurred daily. He next went to Germany, and was there sounded for a stone in the bladder on account of frequent micturition, which he has had since infancy. No calculus was present. He was an inmate of the hospitals of Vienna, Prague, and Dresden. He left the latter in October, 1858, and was admitted into the Westminster Hospital, under Dr. Radcliffe, on the 30th of the month, and remained in two months, during which period he took quinine and iron, and camphor, but without avail. Since his second wife's death, he has entirely abstained from sexual intercourse, though he has been constantly troubled with nocturnal erections, and occasionally seminal emissions, and these continued up to the time when he came under the care of Mr. Holthouse, to whom he applied to perform castration, which, after much deliberation, he consented to do, and it was performed upon both testicles on the 4th of January, 1859, under the influence of chloroform. Two or three hours afterwards there was considerable hæmorrhage, which was checked by the application of cold. He had one fit during the hæmorrhage. His face has a bluish-slate tinge, which pervades the body, but the color is darkest on the face. His fits are of the rotatory kind, preceded by a sudden scream, and lasting not more than a minute, and when over, he is quite himself again. In the fit which he had while in bed after the operation, he did not scream, but merely strug-gled violently.

Jan. 5th.—He had another fit this morning.

6th.—The fit recurred early this morning.

7th.—At four this morning another fit occurred. He says that after his second marriage, the fits frequently followed immediately on the act of connection.

8th.—Has had no fit at all to-day.

9th.—Had a very slight attack this morning, scarcely more than a giddiness for a minute. Altogether, since the operation, the fits have been exceedingly mild.—*London Lancet*.

Transfusion in Yellow Fever—A Successful Case.

By N. B. BENEDICT, M.D., of New Orleans.

MESSRS. EDITORS—In consequence of the pressure of indispensable engagements, I am able to furnish you only a brief outline of the cir-cumstances attending the case of transfusion which was successfully practiced in this city, on the 25th of October last.

The patient, Miss J. B., was a young lady whose life, until early womanhood, was passed in Northwestern New York, whence she re-moved, in 1845, to Mississippi, and thence, in 1854, to New Orleans, where she has constantly resided during the past four years: never having suffered any serious illness within the last fourteen years.

On Monday, October 11th, she was exposed to a drenching rain, but felt no alarm at the sensations which followed, (supposing them to be merely those of a bad cold,) until the evening of the following day, when she was seized, at 9 o'clock, with a violent chill. The symptoms of yellow fever—the pains in the head, the back, and the limbs, the flushed face, the fiery-red eye, and the rapid pulse—could not have been more characteristic than in this case. It proved unu-sually obstinate—the treatment exerting little influence upon any of the symptoms, during the first stage of the disease. My near rela-tionship to the patient induced me, on the third day, to request the assistance of Dr. C. B. White. On the 5th day the counsel of Dr. Wm. E. Kennedy was requested, and both those gentlemen continued their attendance, daily, throughout the course of the disease. On the fifth day, there was some bleeding from the mouth; but the flow was moderate, and occasioned no alarm. On the sixth it continued, but was so slight as to be regarded as marking a favorable tendency.

The average pulse, on these two days, was 86—ranging from 80 to 92. On the morning of the seventh day, the eye presented an appearance as if a drop of serum had collected in the outer canthus; the bleeding from the mouth had increased, and the appearance of the napkins employed to absorb the blood agitated her excessively; but at the mid-day visit, although the hæmorrhage was unabated, yet so much had the complexion improved, that the impression on the minds of the medical attendants was, upon the whole, favorable. The hæmorrhage increased until a late hour in the evening, being aggravated by the uncontrollable perseverance of the patient in wiping away the clots. It suffered a slight check during the night, but returned on the following morning. Throughout the eighth, and most of the ninth day, it continued without abatement; and her efforts to clear the mouth by hawking, rinsing, spitting, and wiping, not only increased the flow, but occasioned great fatigue. To prevent these efforts, except by a resort to unjustifiable force, was impossible. The effects of such protracted hæmorrhage were apparent in the blanched complexion, the colorless lips, tongue and gums, and the pinched features; and serious alarm began to be felt at a loss which resisted all the measures employed to restrain it. Some estimate may be formed of the quantity lost, from the fact that, in the single night of the eighth day, the blood, diluted with saliva, saturated two sheets, so that no part of them remained unsoiled. Added to all this was the hæmorrhagic tendency manifested by other mucous surfaces besides those of the mouth, during these two days. Toward the close of the ninth day, the hæmorrhage from the mouth was several times interrupted for short intervals; but owing to the discomfort caused by the clots, she provoked its return by removing them. About 8 o'clock, P. M., she had a sudden imperfect syncope. Thence forward the bleeding became very slight, and although nourishment and stimulants were retained, the complexion was much blanched, and the mental condition was that of utter despair as to recovery. The rate of the pulse was steadily accelerated; the average for the seventh day being 98, for the eighth and ninth days 104, for the tenth day 115, and for the eleventh and twelfth days 120.

On the tenth day there was much complaint of soreness of the throat, the tongue, and the inner surface of the lips, (which were found to be invaded by small superficial ulcers;) of severe pains in the sides of the head, at the tops of the ears; of morbid sensations— at one time, as if ashes filled her throat; at another, as if the feet were much more elevated than the head; and there was uncontrollable desire to talk of affairs and of interests the most foreign to a sick-room; yet, all was perfectly rational. In the course of this night, the hæmorrhage ceased, and did not again return. The eleventh and twelfth days were characterized by a continuance of those nervous vagaries, and by the increased frequency of the pulse to 120.

At 3 o'clock, in the morning of the thirteenth day, she had profuse perspiration, and a paroxysm of hysterical weeping The general surface, as well as the extremities, were cold and clammy to the touch; the pulse so feeble and so rapid as not to be counted; and the restlessness and desire to toss about the limbs were excessive. Under the use of stimulants, this condition was relieved, the natural warmth was restored, and she fell asleep. At 7, A. M., the pulse had receded to 112, and was regular, though feeble; and nearly every portion of the surface—the limbs as well as the trunk—was found to be covered with sudamina. At 10½, A. M., the apparent amendment was so marked, that the medical attendants were more hopeful than on any previous occasion. The pulse had fallen to 103. From the sixth day to this time, nourishment and stimulants had been taken in quantities such as to encourage the belief that the terrible waste of blood would be repaired by the ordinary process of assimilation. At 11½ o'clock she awoke from a quiet sleep, complained of strange and bad sensations, and said she thought she must be dying. She presently turned upon her side, and was suddenly seized with vomiting, which continued throughout the day and part of the following night. Nothing was retained by the stomach, with the single exception of brandy, and even that only occasionally. After mid-day an enema of mustard and water was given, but did not return. It was followed by other enemata of warm water, with no result except distention of the abdomen. The sinking and prostration were excessive; the pulse was scarce perceptible, yet its frequency was not found, at any time, to exceed 108; and she exhibited a constant tendency to lapse into stertorious slumber. Over the whole region of the aorta was distinctly heard the bellows-sound so characteristic of anemia. Injections of beef-tea, brandy, and carbonate of ammonia were repeatedly given, only to be rejected; but the action of the bowels seemed limited to the rectum. At every movement of the body, distressing hiccough occurred, convulsing the whole frame, and lasting on each occasion about a minute. A sinapism applied to the spine was succeeded by arrest of the vomiting, at 10, P. M., but there was no other improvement throughout the night of the thirteenth day.

On the morning of the fourteenth day, a stimulating enema was followed by discharges resembling coffee-grounds, and by relief of the distention, but there was no amelioration of the symptoms, which steadily tended towards the fatal close. The mortal restlessness increased, the pulse became but the merest flutter, and was, much of the time, inappreciable, and its number could not be ascertained.

At the morning consultation, Drs. Kennedy and White declared their conviction that she could not possibly survive for more than three or four hours. I then said, "It is an old saying, that 'drowning men catch at straws.' For the past twenty-four hours, I have been in torture with the thought of such a straw, and I cannot refrain from naming it: I mean transfusion ; these fatal symptoms being occasioned by the loss of the last few ounces of blood. I cannot persuade myself that it is not a serious duty to inject into her veins a few ounces of fresh, healthy, living blood, as nearly as possible identical with that which she has lost." Both those gentlemen promptly embraced the suggestion that it was the only remedy that could save her life; but thought it impracticable, for want of persons experienced in the operation, and a suitable apparatus. Having, in 1853, prepared a report on transfusion, (which was read before the State Medical Society, and a part of which was printed in *the New Orleans Medical and Surgical Journal* for that year,) I had become imbued with the conviction that the operation is one which, on 'certain occasions, cannot be withheld without criminality; and I had obtained from England the apparatus for the purpose, which was approved by the father of transfusion, Dr. James Blundell, formerly "Lecturer on Midwifery and Physiology at Guy's Hospital." The possession of such an instrument at once gave form to the proposition, and it was determined that if a person could be found who would undertake the most difficult and delicate part of the process—that, namely, of preparing the vein of the patient— the operation should be attempted A little past the hour of noon, there were assembled at my house, Drs. Wm. E. Kennedy, C. B. White, C. C. Beard, D. W. Brickell, and L. Greenleaf. The apparatus was examined, its use described and illustrated, and every part of the process was fully explained and discussed. The task of preparing the vein was undertaken by Prof. C. C. Beard. An incision about two inches in length was made over the median vein in the left arm. A director was passed beneath the vessel, near the lower part of the incision, in order that it might be held under perfect control, and the loss of any blood from its distal extremity be prevented. An incision was then made into the vein, immediately beyond the director, to receive the beak of the syringe It is due to Prof. Beard to say, that nothing could exceed the skill and steadiness with which this operation was performed. The blood was obtained, by the assistance of Dr. Greenleaf, from the arm of a young gentleman who exhibits a remarkable example of perfect health, and who had experienced yellow fever during the epidemic of 1853.

It was my purpose to use the apparatus myself; but as the moment approached, my near relationship to the patient made me distrust my firmness, and I requested Prof. Brickell to take my place. He consented to do so, but substituted for the syringe belonging to the apparatus one of simpler construction, into the beak of which he absorbed the blood as it flowed into the receiver of the transfuser. By inverting the syringe and pushing upward the piston, the last bubble of air was expelled. The beak was then introduced, by Dr. White, into the orifice of the exposed vein of the patient, and Prof. Brickell, with consummate care, passed the blood into her arm, before it had time to cool or even to repose for more than a few seconds. All the apparatus employed was immersed in warm water, or wrapped with heated cloths, so as to prevent any reduction of the temperature of the transfused blood. The operation was commenced at a few minutes before one o'clock, and was finished safely and satisfactorily, in all respects, a few minutes past that hour.

Another person who was constantly with her, writing to a distant friend, used the following language: " There is no doubt that Death had begun his work before this took place. Her extremities were cold; she swallowed with difficulty; her nose had the pinched look of death; her lips were depressed and bloodless, covered with a yellow, dry, parched skin; and her distress was very great. The effect of the transfusion was immediately apparent in the calming of the nervous system The next morning, her lips were full and red; I picked off the yellow parched skin, and found them as natural as health, and she had no subsequent bad feelings except dryness of the mouth, and stiffness of the muscles of the throat. She was like a new creature, and was saved."

I will merely add to this statement, that the pulse, which at half past 12, under the influence of medical excitement, became once

19

more appreciable, numbered 136, and immediately before the operation, 125; at its termination it was 120; and three hours later it
remained the same, but had acquired more fullness and strength.
The voice recovered its natural tone, the face acquired color, the extremities grew warm, all nausea and hiccough ceased, and ordinary
drinks were perfectly retained. From the time mentioned to the
present hour, her recovery has been uninterrupted. Her health has
long since ceased to be a subject of any anxiety.

It was not doubted, at the time of the operation, that the quantity
of blood injected was equal to three and a half ounces. It was afterwards ascertained, by accurate measurement of the syringe, that its
capacity was not quite equal to two and a half ounces. Small as the
quantity was, it yet sufficed to turn the scale in her favor.

I have thus, Messrs. Editors, endeavored to give a plain statement
of the facts as they occurred. I have been the more particular in these
details, because I am informed that an erroneous impression has, to
some extent, prevailed that I was the sole operator. The error is
attributable to ignorance of the complicated nature of the operation,
and to misconception of the flattering notices which appeared in a
daily paper of this city, shortly after the event. Transfusion was
not adopted without the consent of men who are among the first in
the profession; and I venture the assertion that it never will be safely
performed, on the human subject, without the assistance of four medical gentlemen at least. Nothing could be more mortifying to me than
the acquiring of professional distinction by any means but such as are
recognized by the medical profession as legitimate, unless it should be
the acquiring of distinction which is unmerited. I trust that you will
appreciate, therefore, the propriety of these explanations being made
in your journal, inasmuch as justice required details which are improper in a newspaper.

Were the true nature and statistical results of the operation of
transfusion generally known, its performance would be demanded in
many cases which are now consigned to a remediless doom. There
is no fear that it will ever come to be employed as one of the common remedies. It is applicable to no pathological conditions, save
that which is commonly called "collapse," induced by hæmorrhage,
by certain exhausting discharges, or by utter inability to receive or
retain nutriment; and the only transfusion now sanctioned, either by
physiology or by common sense, is that of *human venous blood into
human veins, identical, as nearly as possible, with that which has been lost,*

and in quantity just sufficient to arrest the tendency towards death.
Prior to the year 1853, the total number of recorded cases, practiced
under these conditions and restrictions, amounted to twenty-one. Of
these, but two died—or, less than one case in ten!

If I have any merit in this affair, it is, that I have been, for many
years, the earnest advocate of transfusion, in those cases where alone
it is proper; that I have labored to make it binding upon the con-
sciences of medical men to practice transfusion whenever it is justifiable; that I have proved my faith in it by submitting to it, as the first
instance which I am apprised of in America, a person whose life is as
dear to me as my own; and that before it was attempted I seriously
declared to those professional friends, heretofore named, my willingness to take upon myself all the odium that might attach to a failure.
I feel that I can never sufficiently thank those gentlemen for what
they did for me in this the bitterest trial of my life; and that they
have thus laid upon me new obligations of fidelity to the principles
of our noble profession.—*Ohio Med. and Surg. Journal.*

NEW ORLEANS, *November 27th*, 1858.

[From the Boston Med. and Surg. Journal.]

THE WOMAN WHO LIVES WITHOUT EATING.

MESSRS. EDITORS—Having seen several notices of the above case
in newspapers, and hearing still more from persons who had seen this
"living miracle," I made her a visit a few days since, for the purpose
of learning more fully and accurately her real state.

Her name is Betsy Hays. She lives in the town of Horicon,
Warren County—some sixty miles from our village, (Saratoga
Springs.)

I found her lying upon her back, with her head drawn so far over
that I could only see her chin, her face looking back towards the
walls of the room. The first impression, on seeing her, was such as
one gets from a severe case of hysteria. She seemed generally convulsed, tremulous, and rigid. She had been in this condition for a
long time. I learned from those who often see her, as well as from
her husband, that she usually presents the same appearance. She
looks fresh, and is not emaciated. Her body is warm, and the skin
very clear and soft. Her respiration is very irregular. The pulse
was small and threadlike, but I found it difficult to ascertain accurately its frequency, so constantly were the muscles moving. I

should think it something over a hundred. Her husband (who seems a simple, honest-minded man) told me her age was 28, and that she had never been sick—until about four years ago, when her present illness commenced—except at her confinements. She is the mother of four children.

Four years ago, she was taken with pain in her back and hips, inability to walk; in fact, with all the symptoms of falling of the womb. This was in November. In June following she became worse, lost her eyesight, and in July was taken with spasms. These increased in violence. They would sometimes last for weeks; then she would recover consciousness, converse, take some light food, and again relapse into the same state.

For the space of two years from last June, she has not taken any food of any kind or description. She took a table-spoonfull of cold water once in a few days, until February, *two years* ago—since which time she has *neither ate nor drank*. Her respiration, which I said was irregular, is at times apparently suspended for an hour, and even more than that, often for fifteen or twenty minutes. Her face and neck become very livid at such times, and there is a choking sound in the throat. During the spasms, she sometimes raises herself up in bed, her head still thrown backward, and then down again on the pillow with great force.

She has had no dejections from the bowels, nor any secretion of urine, for the *last two years.* Her feet are cramped, and most of the time the left foot rests upon the instep of the right. Her toes are drawn under and imbe'ded in the flesh, and her feet are drawn under to such a degree that they present almost the appearance of club-feet. The left hand, with the fingers tensely flexed, is pressed against the left side, where it permanently remains. It required great strength to raise it an inch from her body. The right hand is cramped and the fingers flexed, but she is continually striking her stomach with it, when the spasms are violent. At such times her jaw is dislocated and thrown into its place with great rapidity, making a noise that can be heard across the room.

Such is the state of this extraordinary woman. We can dispose of the case very easily by saying that it is one of " successful fraud and deception," as the State Medical Society have just done at their annual meeting in Albany.

The Society, no doubt, came to such conclusions by the evidence placed before them; but, as one of your best jury lawyers in Massachusetts said, " he wanted to *see* the testimony as well as hear it," so, in this case, one cannot tell all about it. You want to see it; you want to see the room, the husband and children, and talk with them, the neighbors, and those who have seen the most of this wonderful woman; you want to put your hands on those rigid muscles, and then watch the suspended breath, with the whole body quivering with the tenseness of the convulsions, until you are obliged to turn away for your own relief. I say one wants to see all these phenomena, and then learn that there can be no motive for the deception, no reward for all this suffering, no object, no inducement. One wants to see all this, and he will be strongly inclined to call it *no fraud.*

An article in *Blackwood's Magazine,* and republished in the April number of the *Eclectic Magazine,* on the " Phenomena of Hunger and Thirst," relates several such cases, some of which lived from four to eight years. They were mostly reported in the *Philosophical Transactions.* The writer disposes of them in this manner:—" It is rather startling to find so learned a physiologist as M. Bérard recording such cases, and trying to explain them. The possibility of deception and exaggeration is so great, that we are tempted to reject almost every one of these cases, rather than reject all physiological teachings " But, M. Bérard says: " Admitting that there has been deception in some of these cases, and that the love of the marvelous has presided over the narration of others, we cannot refuse to believe that some are authentic. Every year such case are registered."   L. E. WHITING.

SARATOGA SPRINGS, *February* 22. 1859.'

QUACKERY.

It is, in spite of philosophy, a humiliating circumstance to the true and honorable physician, to witness the extent to which arrant quackery is patronized by our people; and New Orleans is every winter the especial scene of their depredations Here the real physician toils on from one year's end to another, through rain and sunshine, through yellow-fever epidemics, through every vicissitude incident to the most arduous of all avocations, with too often a remuneration scarcely sufficient to defray the actual expenses of his family; while during a few winter months there comes flocking in a horde of lung doctors, pile doctors, corn doctors, biologists, phrenologists, electricians, etc., etc., etc., who fill their pockets through the miserable credulity of mankind,

and as soon as our spring sun begins to shine too warmly on their fair
skins, off they go to the North or West to invest their ill-gotten gains,
and await the next harvest-time. Instead of these harpies being
frowned on by all honest men, and forced to betake themselves to
some honest avocation, they are applauded for their iniquity, and
honest men are let to starve. But there is no use inveighing against
them; rather let us amuse ourselves over

THE LATEST QUACK ADVERTISEMENT.

Homœopathy, hydropathy, *et id homne genus*, must now hide their
diminished heads. Mr. Gayetty, of New York City, has found that
the public mind is prepared for anything whatever in the shape of
humbuggery, and he at once, with true Yankee readiness, administers
to their rapacious appetites in a manner to be admired—if humbuggery is ever admirable. Inasmuch as this idea of Mr. Gayetty is
strictly a fundamental one, it must be valuable, and we cannot resist
the temptation to "give him a lift" in our pages. We, therefore, insert his advertisement in full, as we clip it from the *National Intelli-
gencer* (!!), with one suggestion, viz., that he not only places his au-
tograph on each sheet of his invaluable paper, to prevent counterfeit,
but that he furnishes his millions of patrons with his photograph in
like manner. More, we suggest that the photograph be taken with a
bland smile on the face. We are really anxious to see the face of
the man who is going to eclipse even homœopathy in the inestimable
benefits he thus rubs into mankind; and then, again, it would be such
a capital idea to be thus cheering up the sufferer by smiling on the
very seat of his troubles. The cheerful countenance of Mr. Gayetty
would be worth the small price of the paper. *Oh, tempora! Oh, mores!*

"*Misery Obviated.*—The greatest blessing of the age is J. C. Gayetty's Medicated Paper for the Water-closet. It is endorsed by the
press, the clergy, the bar, the school-teacher, the merchant, the family,
and the public generally. To use the language of one of the New
York dailies:

"'It is beautiful pure Manilla paper, as delicate as a bank-note,
and as stout as foolscap, entirely divested of the poisonous chemicals
of so-called pure white paper, and of printer's ink, and is medicated
so as to cure and prevent piles. The medication is perfect, acquired
by a processs for which the discoverer has taken out a patent.

"'It is harmless to healthy persons, and a luxury into the bargain.
It is warranted, let us repeat, to cure and prevent piles. It is a house-

hold comfort. It will become a popular necessity. It is cheaper than all other paper, retailing at the rate of $1 per thousand sheets.'

"It is sold by druggists throughout the world. Depot, wholesale and retail, at No. 41 Ann Street, New York City. It will be sent anywhere, by express, upon receipt of the price.

"N. B.—The name of J. C. Gayetty is water-marked on every genuine sheet."—*N. O. Med. News.*

Convention of College Professors at Louisville, Ky.

[The Editors of the *Medical News*, of Louisville, offer the following programme for the consideration of the Convention of College Professors on Medical Education and its Improvement, in May.]

Firstly: We regard it as important that the period of attendance upon lectures should be lengthened. We propose, to this end, that certificates of attendance upon three full courses, each of four months, and only one annually, shall be made a uniform requisite for graduation.

Medical schools may readily prove that, in the adoption of such a rule, they are not actuated by purposes of self-emolument, but only by an earnest desire that students should be better perfected in all branches of the profession before being admitted to its honors; by admitting such students as have paid for two full courses to the third without additional charge for fees.

Secondly: We strongly urge the repeal of that rule under which some schools have regarded a term of years' engagement in practice as equivalent to a full course of lectures. That this measure has been an important aid to many deserving practitioners, we doubt not; but, at the same time, we do not hesitate to express a conviction that its general working has been to hold out an inducement to students to commence the practice of medicine without adequate preparation, so as to obtain the benefit of this clause.

Thirdly: In the feelings of rivalry which have prevailed between medical schools, some faults have been introduced into the beneficiary system. We recommend medical schools to instruct their representatives to institute careful scrutiny into the workings of this system, to ascertain if the abatement of certain features now practiced would not be promotive of the interests and success of medical teaching and of the profession generally.

Fourthly: As this Convention of Teachers is assembled in obedience to a call from the whole profession through their representatives in the General Association, they should, after having answered the expectations of the profession by adopting some positive measures of reform, move the National Association to support their efforts to elevate the standard of medical education, by recommending physicians not to admit students to their offices whose primary education is deficient, and to give closer personal supervision to the course of study of those whom they consider as proper to be admitted.

We leave these propositions to the reflection of our readers. We doubt not they will be received as they are offered—as a manifestation of an earnest intention to join in every measure of genuine reform. Although we entertain them now as propositions the most conducing to the ends to be attained of all others occurring to our minds, we shall not hesitate to abandon them for the support of those which may hereafter strike us as being preferable, from whatever source derived.

EDITOR'S TABLE.

TO CORRESPONDENTS.

"Anglo-Saxon" complains without reason; for, with all the faults of the profession in New York, foreigners who come hither to settle among us are under no disability or prejudice to hinder their success. The fact that a regular *John Bull* presides over our University School, and a *native Irishman* has been made President of the Academy, and *Germans* have been chosen Coroners, are only a few of the proofs which might be cited in refutation of his charge of "Know-Nothing"-ism being in the ascendant. His reference to Dr. Mott's course in the Academy is equally unfortunate, and is a perversion of his Inaugural. Even the "unnaturalized foreigner" to whom he alludes fared better than he deserved, for which he was indebted to the forbearance of Americans. We cannot insert his groundless charge, lest we should admit, even by implication, any nationality in science, or aliens among regular physicians, because of the accident of birth.

"Secret Societies" is reminded that it is only while the secrecy is preserved that these are potent for mischief; and the fact that he would expose through our columns the old K. L. still lingering among us, proves that he, at least, is possessed of their secrets. The late Dr. John Stearns "scotched the snake" many years ago, by his pamphlet; and if our correspondent will send us a copy, we will publish it anew, rather than insert his long article; for this latter might be actionable, if its facts and names are disputed. If any member of any "secret society" now refuses to meet the writer or his friends in consultation, let them combine to refuse to meet him or his clan, and the *lex talionis* will soon annihilate the conspirators.

MEDICAL EDUCATION.

This vital and all-important subject promises to be the engrossing one at the approaching "Medical Congress" at Louisville, in May. The convention of delegates from all the schools of the country are summoned to meet on the Monday preceding the session of the Association on Tuesday, as elsewhere announced. They are expected to crowd all their action into a single day, so as to be prepared to report; and hence the delegates will need to be instructed by the colleges as to the reforms, improvements, or concessions they are prepared to make to the wishes of the profession at large.

In this Journal we have so frequently and at so great length discussed the subject in all its bearings, that our interest in the results of the approaching session cannot be doubted. And though not hopeful, because of our past experience, that anything will be done, yet we cannot forbear to repeat our well-settled conviction, that no reform can be worthy the name, unless it provide for the *utter separation of the teaching from the licensing power*, so often urged in the Association, and in the Journals all over the country. This may, and doubtless will, be resisted by many of the schools; for, as has been well said of irresponsible power, "its march is ever onward, and its tremendous tendency to accumulation." But we predict that the "moral power" of the Association will ere long constrain the colleges to discover the short-sightedness of their policy, and the profession of the country will rise in their might, and take the authority in their own hands to decide who shall, and who shall not, be admitted as their peers. Let there be a large representation at Louisville.

THE BLUE MAN—CASTRATION FOR EPILEPSY.

Our readers will remember the case of a Mr. B., formerly of this city, whose skin became discolored under the use of nitrate of silver, employed in the treatment of epilepsy, of which he had long been a victim. He was literally a "blue man;" and his case became the object of very great professional interest, and awakened very general sympathy.

About three years since, he read the article in the GAZETTE from a Southern physician, reporting several cases of the cure of epilepsy by castration. He called on us for consultation, and, by our advice, on Professor W. Parker, of this city, and proposed to submit himself to this operation, despairing of every other remedy. We concurred in advising it, as he was suffering fearfully from a repetition of epileptic paroxysms, traceable to a morbid excitation of the genital organs, and one of his testes being much diseased at the time. A day was fixed for the operation, but it was postponed for a renewed trial of the water-cure, electro-magnetic bath, &c., until we learned that he had suddenly left for Europe. The next we heard from him was from St. Thomas's Hospital, London, where he wrote to us, at the request of Dr. Simon, to whom he had applied for castration, and who declined until he could hear from us on the subject. Our letter to Dr. S., and the cases in the GAZETTE, did not induce that gentleman to operate. Since then, the patient has found his way to Westminster Hospital, where, at his urgent request, he has been emasculated; and an interesting report from the *London Lancet* will be found in this number of the GAZETTE, detailing the operation and its encouraging results thus far, although time has not elapsed sufficient to render it certain as to his permanent relief. We sincerely hope he may be cured of his terrible malady.

DR. HORATIO R. STORER, OF BOSTON,

Is furnishing the *North American Medico-Chirurgical Review* with a series of articles on *Criminal Abortion*, which do honor alike to his philanthropy and scientific attainment. The subject is by far the most important one before the profession, and in its medical as well as moral bearings appeals alike to our patriotism and humanity. In a brief Report we had occasion to make to the American Medical Association on the causes of "Infant Mortality in Large Cities," we alluded to this source of increase, and characterized the accursed trade of abortionism in the Anglo-Saxon terms of reprobation it deserved. Indeed, we have been writing and speaking on this abomination for many years, impressed as we are with its heinous enormity and incredible frequency.

Dr. Storer deserves the thanks of the profession, and the public gratitude for the thorough exposure he has made, and continues to make, of this giant iniquity, as it exists in our country, as well as in foreign lands; the statistics of criminal abortionism, the world over, having been cited by him in these valuable contributions to Medical Jurisprudence. We honor him for the manly and fearless independence he manifests, in denouncing as murderous, and worthy of the highest penalty known to our laws, every principal or accessory to criminal abortion. The demonstration he makes of the frequency of this crime, and this among every class of our population—by facts and figures, as shown in our bills of mortality—exhibits proof that the "slaughter of the innocents" in our own country exceeds, in cruelty and extent, any records of this crime in ancient or modern history. When will legislation and reform arrest this terrible iniquity?

DEATH OF PROFESSOR TULLY.

This distinguished gentleman, eminent scholar, profound and learned physician, whose fame as a medical writer, teacher, and practitioner, for the last thirty years, has given him a historic prominence throughout the New England States, died recently at Springfield, Mass., in advanced years, a martyr to his professional studies and toils, to which he was devoted with all the vigor of youth, down to the period of his decease. He was formerly a professor in the medical department of Yale College, at New Haven, Ct., where his remains are deposited, and where his memory will be long cherished by his colleagues and the alumni of that eminent seat of learning. He was a physician of the old school, a class now nearly extinct among us, in these degenerate days. His latest years were diligently employed, amid failing health, in his great work on Materia Medica, which has been long in course of publication; and in this work he has been essentially aided by his attached friend, Dr. Church, of Massachusetts, without whose earnest and prolonged efforts his book had never been forthcoming, and who merits, for this labor of love, the gratitude of the profession.

We are without the full particulars concerning the cause and circumstances of his death, but we learn that it was occasioned by exposure to the wintry blasts and snows of the Green Mountains, while visiting a patient, some thirty or forty miles from his home; so that he literally "died in the harness." Such a man deserves a memorial and a monument; though we fear that he, like most of us who survive him in the ranks of the working men of the profession, can have no other epitaph than this, viz.: "He lived well, worked hard, and died poor."

THE ANNUAL COMMENCEMENTS

Of our several Medical Colleges have recently been held in this city, as elsewhere.

That of the New York Medical College was the first in order, on the 1st of March. The valedictory address was by James T. Brady, Esq., one of the Trustees, and the degrees were conferred by Dr. H. Green, President of the Faculty, upon 25 gentlemen. The audience was large and brilliant, and the music excellent. The oration and the distribution of prizes were warmly applauded.

The University School followed next, on the 4th of March, when the Chancellor conferred the degree of M. D. upon 128 gentlemen, and President Draper gave the valedictory. The chapel was crowded; the Mott and Metcalfe prizes were adjudged, and Dodworth's band enlivened the exercises.

The College of Physicians and Surgeons held its Commencement on the 10th of March. The President, Dr. Delafield, conferred the degrees on 39 gentlemen; the valedictory was pronounced by Dr. Rufus Mason, of the graduating class, and an address to the Alumni by Dr. H. A H. Stevens. A list of 18 who graduated in October last was read, and two prizes awarded. The next evening, the Society of the Alumni was instituted, at the mansion of the President, on the Fifth Avenue; Dr. Mason, of Brooklyn, being in the chair, and Dr. Sands Secretary. A large representation of the profession was present.

The Medical Institute of Dr. Aylette closed with a public ceremonial: address by Professor Bedford, its President; and another service of plate by the class to their teacher, whose diploma they have received.

The *new College*, that is to be, at Bellevue Hospital, terminated its clinical teaching with addresses by Drs. Mott, Francis, Wood, and Elliott, and the distribution of diplomas and prizes.

DR. HORACE GREEN

Can need no other vindication than the masterly article in the last number of the *Nashville Journal of Medicine and Surgery.* Professor

Bowling comes up gallantly to his defence, and reads a homily to both Drs. Beales and Mott, which makes an appeal to both heart and conscience. He treats the subject ethically, pathologically, surgically and professionally, in his best style. We only wish that every member of the New York Academy of Medicine could read it, when they would all become clamorous for the *expunging* resolution we suggested in our last number. Dr. Green might prefer that the record stand, faulty and erroneous as it is; but we opine that both Drs. Beales and Mott would vote for expunging all. *Nous verrons.* Those of us whose names and remarks were *suppressed* in the minutes, will luckily escape going down to posterity as having participated in the disgraceful proceedings, and are personally indifferent to the fate of the expunging resolution. Not for our own sakes, but for the credit of the Academy, we would fain blot out every vestige of the proceedings by the Academy in the Whitney case, and for the reason that they are irrelevant and disreputable. Let black lines be drawn around. "Let those nights be solitary, and let no joyful voice be heard therein."

THE ATLANTA MEDICAL COLLEGE, GEO.

This young and thriving school renews its announcement, in this number of the GAZETTE, of the *Summer* Course of Lectures, commencing in May. Now that the old Harvard University is spreading abroad its circulars for a *Summer* Course, we presume the outcry of certain parties against our Atlanta brethren for this innovation will cease. And as there are three colleges in Georgia, having each a *Winter* Course, we commend the delicacy of the Faculty at Atlanta, in giving their course at a season which cannot interfere with those of their neighbors. Their success, thus far, would seem to show that their course is appreciated by the profession, and is likely to attract students. From our knowledge of the Faculty, we are not surprised to learn that their school is flourishing, as it deserves to be, with such enterprising and able teachers.

DEATH OF PROFESSOR MUTTER.

We had scarcely time to chronicle the noble and munificent generosity of Dr. Mutter to the Philadelphia College of Physicians, before we are called upon to record his death, which, we regret to say, occurred a few days since, at Charleston, S. C.

NEW YORK ACADEMY OF MEDICINE.

At the last meeting, on a motion for leave to print that paper of Dr. Corson, on the gymnastics of the shoulders in physical exploration of the thorax, with which a former meeting had been bored, Drs. Detmold and McNulty brought out the fact, that it had already been printed, without leave, in the *New York Journal*, with "picters to match;" and it might have been shown that, "twaddle" as it is, copies have been bound in book form, for *popular* circulation, especially, among clergymen, lawyers, &c., and it is already widely circulated. So transparent a device for seeking a specialty in practice is ludicrous enough, if it were not palpable that the paper contains nothing either new or useful. Its pictures will forcibly recall to memory the old school-books on elocution, in which the various attitudes were depicted by plates; or the recent cuts, showing the exercises of infant schools, "hands behind," "hands before," "hands overhead," &c. We are ashamed that any journal could be induced to insert it by any amount of importunity, or even by "paying for the illustrations;" and it is still more humiliating that the "Academy" should stoop so low as to give it even a *quasi* endorsement. But, alas! our profession in New York seems to be doomed, and there is no telling what we are coming to.

This topic being disposed of, Professor Dalton read a physiological and statistical paper, and Dr. Batchelder finished his Essay on Compressed Sponge.

A NEW MEDICAL SCHOOL,

In embryo, was announced by Dr. James R. Wood, at the close of the clinical lectures in Bellevue Hospital, a few days since. He announced that a necessity was now apparent for founding a regular medical college in connection with the Almshouse Hospital; and added, that in that event, some of the medical colleges in New York would have to "shut up shop." As we have only *three* in this great city, they are all thrown into "exercise of mind" as to the identity of the two lesser lights which are to be extinguished by this rising luminary at Bellevue, of which Dr. Wood is to be the bright particular star in the east, by whom the Bellevue school is heralded. We bespeak a place in the new school for certain worthy brethren, who are growing gray with aspirations for professorships somewhere, and will gladly take them even in the Almshouse.

BELLEVUE HOSPITAL.

There seems to be another screw loose among the doctors, in which the Governors and their hopeful Warden are mixed up. The cause of the row, as in most other cases, is RUM! Governor Anderson, shortly before his death, declared that hospital to be "an immense grog-shop," and at his instance the Board stopped the grog of the doctors and their patients. One of the doctors ordered Bourbon whisky for a patient, which the Warden furnished from his private stock, until his jug was empty. But, strange to tell, the poor fellow died, and notice was served on the Warden and Governors, that his death was caused by the want of whisky in the hospital, of which fact the doctor gave his certificate. Whereupon the Warden fired up, and the Governors were "frightened from their propriety," until the Medical Governor interposed professionally, and the matter was referred to the Committee having charge of the hospital. By the way, we have not learned whether all the tinctures are proscribed from use in the practice of the hospital; for if not, we should infer that stimulus enough might have been furnished by the apothecary to prevent a man dying for want of whisky, unless, indeed, the Medical Board have resolved that whisky is a necessary of life. It is a rich quarrel, as the matter now stands; and when settled, we shall probably learn which kills most people in and out of the Almshouse— the want of whisky, or too much of it.

Professional Appointments and Changes.

Dr. E. Geddings has been recalled to the Medical College of South Carolina, and takes the Practical Chair, formerly filled by Professor Dickson, and more recently by the lamented Dr. Gaillard.

Dr. Sandford Eastman, as Professor of Anatomy, and Dr. Austin Flint, Jr., as Professor of Physiology and Microscopic Anatomy, are the recent additions to the Faculty of the University of Buffalo, which, we are happy to learn, has had a prosperous session, with an increased class.

"UNIVERSITY OF THE PACIFIC."

A new medical school opens in May next at San Francisco, California. Its present Faculty consists of Drs. Morrison, Rowell, Cole, and Cooper, with the Hon. Geo. Barstow, for Medical Jurisprudence.

UNIVERSITY OF NASHVILLE.

The medical department of this prosperous school has announced a summer course of lectures, commencing on the first Monday in April, and continuing four months. No fee is required of those who attend the subsequent preliminary and winter course of five months. The collegiate course, therefore, for each year, will include nine months' lectures. The summer course is optional with the students, the winter course of four months being alone obligatory. Students attending the summer course only, pay a fee of fifty dollars on entering; and if they remain for the winter, they are charged $55 additional, which makes the usual fee of $105 for the full course. In brief, the Professors work nine months for the usual fee of a four months' course. It is probable that the other great schools of the country may find it necessary to "go and do likewise," for competition is the life of business.

FIRE-PROOF SAFES.

On the cover of this Journal, Silas C. Herring & Co., of Broadway, announce their claims to superiority in the manufacture of these useful and indispensable articles of office furniture, a business which they are prosecuting with the most extraordinary success, and to an extent which bespeaks their purpose to defy all competition in this department, and to supply any demand for their safes, in our whole country, as well as in foreign lands. For our profession, the protection of our books of account and other evidences of debt, valuable papers, surgical instruments, &c., from the destroying element, his Fire-proof Safes are invaluable. We recommend a call at their elegant establishment in Broadway, and their immense manufactory, 14th Street and 9th Avenue, as among the attractive curiosities of this great city.

APPARATUS FOR FRACTURED THIGH.

The signal success of Dr. Burge's admirable contrivance for the comfort of the patient and the convenience of the surgeon, in these severe casualties, which are ever recurring, is now so well established in hospital and private practice, as to give it a claim to superiority over every other apparatus. In the New York Hospital, and in the Brooklyn City Hospital, it has secured the preference, after actual trial and comparison. See advertisement, on another page.

Statistics of Medical Colleges for the Session 1858-9.

We have inserted the following statistical table, which includes all the schools we have heard from. It is necessarily incomplete, but we shall keep the table standing, and add the reports from other colleges which may reach us before our May number. Information from every school in the country is respectfully solicited, that we may perfect our list in the next number of the GAZETTE. If any errors occur, we shall be thankful for corrections from any quarter.

	Students.	Graduates.
Jefferson Medical College	570	256
University of Nashville	442	—
University of Pennsylvania	410	140
University of New York	350	128
University of Louisiana	306	—
College of Physicians and Surgeons, (N. Y.)	180	39
Medical College of Georgia, (Augusta,)	165	58
Pennsylvania Medical College	150	33
University of Michigan	143	—
New Orleans School of Medicine	140	—
Harvard University	139	30
St. Louis Medical College	135	40
Philadelphia School of Medicine	130	17
New York Medical College	107	25
University of Buffalo	67	13
University of Vermont	80	20
Shelby Medical College	53	—
Dartmouth Medical College	——	9
Albany Medical College	——	48
Medical School of Maine	50	—
Missouri Medical College	—	23
Rush Medical College	——	——
Cleveland Medical College	—	—
Atlanta Medical College	—	—
Ohio Medical College	—	—
Starling Medical College	——	—
Ogelthorpe Medical College	—	—
Savannah Medical College	—	—
Memphis Medical College	—	—
University of South Carolina	—	—
Medical College of Virginia	—	—

20

University of Virginia............. .... —   —
University of Maryland..................... —   —
Yale Medical College..................... —   —
Castleton Medical College.... .... —   —
Berkshire Medical School................... —   —
University of Iowa...................... —   —
University of Louisville.................. —   —
Kentucky School of Medicine............... —   —
Pennsylvania University................. —   —
Woodstock Medical College.......... .... —   —
Geneva Medical College................... —   —

DR. GEORGE SUCKLEY,

Our young fellow-townsman, formerly of the New York Hospital, and more recently surgeon in the U. S. Army, has been complimented abroad, in the Parisian hospitals, by no less a personage than M. Nelaton, who, having been taught by our young countryman the method of extension and counter-extension, by adhesive straps, in fractures of the thigh, &c., so successfully pursued in the New York Hospital, has not only adopted it, but given it the name of the SUCKLEY *Plan of Treating Fractures*, by which it is designated in the hospitals, where it has been found more useful in preventing deformity by shortening, than any of the complicated apparatus heretofore employed. The correspondent of the *N. Y. Times*, "Malakoff," understood to be Dr. Johnson, of Ohio, had an interesting letter in that print on the subject but a few days since.

AXES TO GRIND AT LOUISVILLE

The approach of the May meeting of the American Medical Association for 1859 begins to develop certain favorite projects, which their authors hope to effect at the Louisville meeting, or at least put on file for action in 1860. Some want the profession, at the place of meeting, to have no precedence for the office of President, as heretofore. Others of us think this change should not commence at Louisville, but be postponed until the session is held in Philadelphia, where there have been two sessions and two presidents already. Our brethren of the city of brotherly love, moreover, are clamorous for a *permanent secretaryship* for the association, for which office they doubtless have the man. Why not have a *permanent* President and *permanent* place of meeting where the *permanent Secretary* lives, and thus localize and sectionalize the association? Other plots and counter-plots are among the gossip of the day, but whether the ethical questions of the last annual meeting are to have a resurrection in another phase we are not informed. It is rumored that *patents*, and the relation of the profession to these, will come before that body, at the instance of a voice from Connecticut, having reference to the discovery of anæsthesia, the fictitious patent thereto, and its anti-ethical endorsement!

INFANT MORTALITY.

The annual mortality of children under 10 years of age is reported as exceeding 25,000 in the city of *London!* This paragraph is going the rounds of the public press, as though such a number of children perishing in a single year in the metropolis of Great Britain were a fact worthy of special wonder. And so it is, for such a waste of human life is a disgrace to civilization, and should bring the blush of shame to the faces of a Christian people. But before we express our astonishment or reprobation at the inhumanity and neglect, and abuses of sanitary laws, which produce this result in the great transatlantic city of the Old World, let us pause to inquire why it is that the infant mortality in New York should be 13 *per cent.* greater than that of London? Let us not forget the beam that is in our own eye, before we busy ourselves with the mote in the eye of another.

NAVAL MEDICAL BOARD.

A Naval Medical Board for the examination of assistant surgeons for promotion, and of candidates for admission into the medical corps of the navy, will assemble at the Naval Asylum, on Monday, March 7th. The Board will consist of Surgeons W. S. W. Ruschenberger, President; L. B. Hunter, J. M. Foltz; and Passed Assistant Surgeon George H. Powell, Recorder.

THE OBSTETRICAL SOCIETY OF LONDON,

For the promotion of knowledge in all that relates to obstetrics and the diseases of children, has just been inaugurated. A similar organization in New York would indeed be a desideratum, which we hope soon to see realized, and is indispensable if we would secure the *prestige*, as a school of obstetrics, to which New York is entitled.

AMERICAN MEDICAL ASSOCIATION.

The twelfth annual meeting of this Association will be held in Louisville, Kentucky, on Monday, May 3, 1859. The secretaries of all societies, and other bodies entitled to representation in the Association, are requested to forward to the Secretary, S. M. Bemiss, at Louisville, correct lists of their delegations so soon as they may be appointed. The Convention of Teachers, invoked by a resolution of the National Association, for the purpose of a general conference upon the best means of elevating the standard of medical education in this country, will meet in .the same city on Monday, the 2d of April.

Medical Journals throughout the United States are requested to insert the above. S. M. BEMISS, M.D.,

Sec'y Am. Med. Assoc.

OUR JOURNAL.

We beg to remind a few of our contemporaries that we do not publish a Medical Journal with an eye to them. That while we should like to please everybody, it is no part of our ambition to please them. Our great object is to please ourself, which we find the most difficult undertaking of our life. In this attempt we have incidentally succeeded in pleasing a list of subscribers in every way entirely satisfactory to us.—*Nashville Med. and Surg. Journ.*

[Ditto, Dr. Bowling.—ED. AM. MED GAZETTE.]

VERATRUM VIRIDE.

We direct special attention to the timely and much-needed cautions of Dr. P., of Rhinebeck, N. Y., in relation to the dangers of this potent drug. We wish we could be persuaded that certain cases of sudden fatality of which we have heard were not precipitated by its use. Dr. P's cases and suggestions are eminently practical and important. His letter, subsequently written, on the same subject, is also in this number of the GAZETTE, and replies to Dr. Close, as does another correspondent, Dr. Mead, of Albany.

MEDICAL POLITICS.

Since the issue of our last number, the rumor came from Albany that the candidates for *Health Officer* had been increased, and among the new names on the Governor's slate, Drs. Alexander H. Stevens! and

Gurdon Buck! were reported. We now learn that the latter of these gentlemen, Dr. Buck, has received the nomination of Governor Morgan, and his friends, in view of *his high character for integrity*, confidently predict his confirmation by the Senate.

Much surprise is expressed that the Quarantine restrictions of this great port should be intrusted to a *surgeon* instead of a physician who has tact and experience in discriminating disease, and this when some forty such were among the hungry expectants. Dr. Buck is, however, well known as a surgeon in the New York Hospital for twenty years, and since in the Eye and Ear Infirmary, and may be presumed to know more about the diagnosis of diseases of the throat and eye than either of cholera, yellow fever, or small-pox. As, however, he has long served the public for nothing, we congratulate him on now being likely to be well paid, unless the Legislature shall cut down the fees and salary for his special accommodation. But as he is of the right stripe in politics, this will hardly be done.

The nomination of Dr. S. C. Foster for *City Inspector*, has been withdrawn by the Mayor, with Dr. F's consent, and, as we predicted some three months ago, in the GAZETTE, all the doctors are laid on the shelf, and the " old war-horse of the Democracy" has been nominated, who knows no more about the health department than " a horse knows about holy water;" and yet he will be appointed!

At *Bellevue Hospital*, the Medical Board and the Governors are again at issue. A vacancy has occurred in the corps of visiting surgeons, and seven nominations have been sent in; but the Board of Governors have resolved to secure further nominations, by adding four new members to the Medical Board, thus creating five vacancies. In this way, Dr. Meier, Dr. A. B. Mott, and others of our neighbors, may possibly be introduced into the Medical Board, *nolens volens;* unless like Dr. Corson, they can be induced to back out. We shall see.

Meanwhile, the " Sanitary Bills" are tinkering at Albany, and we hear that an " entangling alliance" is projected between the State and certain private corporations, to introduce their officers or representatives into the new Board of Health. This feature will defeat the practical working of the reform promised, the selections not being made as they ought to be, in view of the qualifications of the medical men in sanitary science; but because of their accidental positions in colleges or societies, even if physically and mentally incompetent. We cannot be hopeful of any salutary reform.

MISCELLANEOUS ITEMS.

Professor W. P. Seymour addressed the graduating class of Castleton Medical College, at the late Commencement, in a highly felicitous manner. His subject was, "The Two Ways"—viz., to medical renown, or to the degradation of quackery; both of which are before the young doctor.

The Albany Medical College has changed the time for opening its next session from November to September, as will be seen by the announcement; for which, see our advertising columns.

Dr. Charles D. Smith has resigned his post as Surgeon to the Bellevue Hospital, and has sailed for a European tour.

The Belmont Medical Journal is still published at Bridgeport, Ohio, by Drs. Conahey and Afflick. It is refreshing to find so much fearless independence and sprightly criticism in our little neighbor. To those who complain of its stature, the Editors may say, with Pope,

> "Were I so tall to reach the pole,
>   And grasp the ocean with a span,
> I must be measured by my soul:
>   'Tis not the *size* that makes the *man*."

Dr. John F. Meigs has been chosen on the Medical Staff of Pennsylvania Hospital, in place of Dr. Pepper, resigned.

The New Hampshire Journal of Medicine has been discontinued.

COMMUNICATIONS.

LETTER FROM VERMONT.

DR. REESE: BURLINGTON, VT., *March 14th,* 1859.

Dear Sir—I have just learned from the Dean of our Medical College at *Burlington,* that we *have eighty* (80) *bonâ fide students now,* who are attending the lectures of the present course here. The College edifice is new, and the arrangements for the comfort and advantage of the students are unsurpassed. The museum is large, and well filled with preparations of great value and utility to the students. The lecture-rooms are spacious, and well lighted and ventilated; one containing 110 arm-chairs, and the other 135 seats, upholstered, with iron arms. The dissecting-room is commodious, and well lighted. In fact, the building is a model in every way. The town of Burlington is unsurpassed in the beauty and picturesqueness of its scenery, situ. ated upon a gentle slope towards the beautiful Lake Champlain. On the top of the hill are the College buildings for the literary and medical departments, and from the cupolas of these two buildings can be seen the waters of the lake for nearly one hundred miles. On the north, with a good glass and a clear day, Montreal is distinctly seen; in the west, the noble Rock Dundar, in the lake; then the Juniper Island; still farther in the distance, the beautiful islands, the Four Brothers; while bounding the lake, which is about twelve miles wide at this point, we see the long range of mountains, the Adirondacks, covered with wild forest trees, and sheltering wild game in abundance—such as deer, bears, leverets, otters, foxes, wolves, and any quantities of lighter game. And the sun-sets are not surpassed in the world—not even in the wild mountainous scenery of Switzerland. Now, let us turn back and look eastward, and we see the long range of the Green Mountains, whose towering eloquence has given Vermont its beautiful name. Slightly to the north of east, eighteen miles distant, we see the snow-capped summit of the noble Peak of Mansfield, and a little south of east we see the Camel's Hump. Though these may not advance the student in his medical studies, yet they lead one's mind from Nature up to Nature's God, and tend to generate that reverence in the soul which every true physician should possess for the works of the Great Artist of Nature.   e.

ANÆSTHESIA AGAIN!

The voice of the profession in Brooklyn in favor of Dr. Horace Wells.—Repudiation of Morton by Dr. Isaacs, and others, whose names have been cited in that book of N. P. Rice. Now let 300 New York physicians follow this example!

BROOKLYN, *March 15th*, 1859.

We, the undersigned, some of whom were induced, in company with many other medical men, to sign a paper endorsing the claims of Dr. W. T. G. Morton, of Boston, as the original discoverer of the means of producing complete insensibility to pain, during surgical operations, by the inhalation of gaseous substances, and especially of sulphuric ether, and, therefore, entitled to all the honor and reward resulting from such a discovery, beg leave to state:

1. That since signing that paper, we have had the most abundant and conclusive evidence presented to us, testified under oath, by many of the most respectable citizens of Hartford, Ct., and other places, that

Dr. Horace Wells, of Hartford, in 1844—nearly two years before Dr. Morton announced his discovery of the anæsthetic properties of sulphuric ether—did use, by inhalation, the nitrous oxide gas for the purpose, and with the effect, of annihilating pain during surgical operations.

2. That he fearlessly allowed himself to be placed under its influence, and while in a state of insensibility had a tooth extracted without pain, and that he was, therefore, so far as is known, the first human being upon whom a surgical operation was ever performed, while in a state of complete anæsthesia from the inhalation of gaseous substances. That he immediately proclaimed his discovery to the world, and that he, and his friends in Hartford, continued to use the nitrous oxide for anæsthetic purposes for nearly two years before Morton announced his discovery of ether, and that these facts were publicly known in Hartford and its vicinity.

3. From sworn and indubitable evidence, it appears that in 1844–5, and in the early period of his discovery, Dr. Wells and his friends had turned their attention to the inhalation of sulphuric ether, and had performed surgical and dental operations under its influence, and without pain, but that they preferred the nitrous oxide gas, on account (as they believed) of its superior safety. (See the work lately published, entitled " Anæsthesia," page, 77.)

4. The practicability and safety of producing anæsthesia by the inhalation of the nitrous oxide having been clearly and conclusively established by the experiments of Dr. Wells, the idea would naturally suggest itself to others to try the effect of other gases, or of volatile fluids, in order to obtain similar results. After the discovery of potassium by Sir Humphrey Davy, other chemists easily followed in his path.

5. In conclusion, we think that whatever may be the merits of succeeding discoveries, to Dr. Wells belongs the immortal honor of being the true discoverer of anæsthesia, and the first who ever applied it successfully for the relief of human suffering.

C. E. Isaacs, M.D.,	J. J. Swalm, M.D.,
C. S. Goodrich, M.D.,	Wm. C. Betts, M.D.,
D. E. Kissam, M.D., Brooklyn,	D. S. Landon, M.D.,
De Witt C. Enos, M.D.,	Purcell Cooke, M.D.,
L. C. McPhail, M.D.,	Samuel Boyd, M.D.,
Otto Rotton, M.D.,	Chas. A. Van Zandt, M.D.,
H. J. Cullen, M.D.,	Geo. J. Bennet, M.D.,
A. N. Bell, M.D.,	Charles Rowland, M.D.

BOOK NOTICES.

HARPER'S WEEKLY.

This Journal of Civilization was never better employed than in reprobating the inhuman and cruel system by which the Governors of our Almshouse are multiplying the waste of infantile life, which disgraces our bills of mortality. For a series of years we have diligently sought to expose and reform this "slaughter of the innocents," but alas, these poor foundlings and abandoned little ones are "only paupers, for whom nobody cares." To all our appeals for a "foundling hospital" in our city, we have been, until lately, only answered by the stereotyped objection to all such institutions, that their effect may possibly be demoralizing. But can any immorality be worse than the wholesale murder of the thousands who annually perish under the present iniquitous trade, of hiring these infants out to nurse at a dollar a week, to the ignorant, intemperate and profligate women, who thus eke out for themselves a subsistence in the squalid abodes of penury, while starving and drugging to death these abandoned little ones, who are thus perishing in multitudes which no man can number?

We urge the opening of the foundling hospital, now provided for and promised, not merely for the preservation of infant life, now recklessly sacrificed to so appalling an extent by the present system; but to prevent the almost nightly waste of adult life, by the suicide of unhappy mothers, who are "found drowned" often, with their unborn infants, or die by poison or other fatal device, for no other or better reason than that no provision is made, by a foundling hospital, for those children whom they dare not own, or whose guilty fathers have abandoned them to the fate of their unhappy mothers. Man's inhumanity to *woman* makes countless thousands mourn.

NATURE IN DISEASE, illustrated in various Discourses and Essays; to which are added, Miscellaneous Writings, chiefly on Medical Subjects. By Jacob Bigelow, M.D., &c. Boston: Phillips, Sampson & Co. 1859. Second edition, enlarged.

This volume comprises a series of pamphlets, which the author has written within the last quarter of a century, at intervals, on medical and non-medical topics, and are here brought together in a sort of "*omnium gatherum.*" Very few of them relate to "Nature in Disease," although this is the taking title, but refer to subjects of diverse character, giving the book the merit of variety.

In regard to the author's theory of self-limited diseases, we have elsewhere taken occasion to express our dissent, regarding the doctrine as wholly fabulous, and the facts cited in its support are perverted, into what Sir Gilbert Blane, in his medical logic, denominates "false facts," and with all these we are at issue. His "limited" estimate of the powers of medicine and the resources of the medical art are quite as objectionable as the exaggerations he deplores as indulged formerly by himself, and still confided in by the "majority of physicians." His narrow views on medical education, and his plea for limiting the colleges to a "four months' course," are only to be tolerated on the theory he holds, that "nature" is the blind source to wh'ch we are to look for disease and for its cure; and to follow nature is the limited province of medical science and art; in which case, medical education, as conducted in the schools, would be a mockery and farce. The other papers in the volume possess far more merit than we can discover in those which pertain to medicine.

CONTENTS.

RECEIPTS for 1859—Continued.

Drs. Culbert, Henderson, Vanvliet, Grammar, Downes, Stotesbury, Shearman, Richardson, Bibbins. Vanderpool, Rockwell. S. Griswold, Armsby, Whittelsey, Hamilton, Burdge, J. F. Eve, Arnold, Skilton.

ATLANTA MEDICAL COLLEGE.

Annual Announcement of Lectures.—The Fifth Course of Lectures in this Institution will commence on the first Monday in May next, and continue four months.

FACULTY.

ALEXANDER MEANS, M.D., Prof. of Chemistry and Pharmacy.
H. W. BROWN, M.D., Prof. of Anatomy
JOHN W. JONES, M D., Prof of Practice of Medicine and General Pathology
T. S. POWELL, M D., Prof. of Obstetrics.

W. F. WESTMORELAND, M.D , Prof. of Principles and Practice of Surgery.
J. P. LOGAN, M. D., Prof. of Physiology and Diseases of Women and Children.
J. G. WESTMORELAND, M.D., Prof. Materia Medica and Medical Jurisprudence.

Practical Anatomy under the immediate direction of the Professor of Anatomy. The Dissecting Room. supplied with good material. will be open by the 15th of April.

Fees.—For the course of Lectures, $105; Matriculation, (taken once,) $5; Dissecting Tickets, (required once only,) $10; Graduation, $25.

Good board can be had at $3 or $4 per week. For further information, address,

J. G. WESTMORELAND, Dean.

ATLANTA, GA., March 4th, 1859

UNIVERSITY OF VERMONT.

Medical Department.—Lectures commence on the last Thursday of February, annually, at Burlington, Vt , and continue 16 weeks.

Fees.—Matriculation, $3.00, Lecture Fee, $50.00; Graduation, $18.00; Third Course Students, $10.00.

BOARD OF PROFESSORS.

S. W. THAYER, JR , M.D., Anatomy.
W. CARPENTER, M.D., Theory and Practice, and Materia Medica.
J. PERKINS, M.D., Obstetrics and Diseases of Women and Children.

D. S. CONANT, M D., Surgery.
R C. STILES. M.D., Physiology and Pathology.
EDW HUNGERFORD, A.M., Chemistry and Pharmacy.

S. W. THAYER, Jr., M.D.,

February 28.   *Burlington, Vt.*, Dean of the Faculty.

THE DRUG STORES,
510 Grand Street and 32 Catharine Street.

EDWARD C. PASSMORE

Begs to intimate to his friends and the public generally, that he continues to carry on the business of

Apothecary and Retail Druggist,

in the above locations. and he desires respectfully to solicit a continuance of their patronage to these Stores, to which, as he is in no way connected with any other, he gives his undivided attention.

It is gratifying to EDWARD C. PASSMORE to know, that, in his business relations hitherto, he has always given satisfaction, and he trusts that this result of his efforts in the past will be accepted by his numerous medical friends and patrons as the best guarantee, which he can offer to them, that he will not fail of meriting their continued confidence.

The compounding of prescriptions, he wishes to say, receives his especial attention, and in both his Stores is himself assisted by apothecaries of proved competency and experience.

☞ Physicians will please to remember that the number of his Store in GRAND STREET is 510.

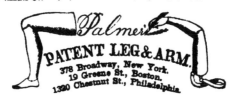

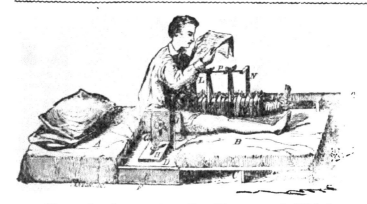

Burge's Apparatus for Fractured Thigh,

INVENTED BY

J. H. HOBART BURGE, M.D., of Brooklyn, N. Y.,

AND

WM. J. BURGE, M.D., of Taunton, Mass.,

has been thoroughly tested in actual practice, and has produced the most gratifying results. It is remarkably simple in its construction, easily applied, comfortable to the patient, adapted to fracture of either limb and to patients of any size. It is free from all the objections to which the ordinary straight splint is liable, and possesses other new features of great practical utility. By it the counter-extending pressure is confined to the nates and tuberosities of the ischia, and does not at all impinge upon the front of the groin, by which means one of the most frequent sources of annoyance and danger is obviated. No part of the body is confined except the injured limb and that to which it is immediately articulated, viz., the pelvis; thus the chest is left entirely unrestrained, and entire freedom of motion granted to the whole upper part of the body, which tends greatly to the comfort and health of the patient.

The pelvis is so secured as not to be liable to lateral motion or to sink in the bed.

Provision is also made for facility of defecation, thus insuring the greatest possible cleanliness, and preventing the necessity of disturbing the patient when his bowels are moved.

☞ Members of the profession may obtain this apparatus, complete in all its parts and nicely packed, by sending THIRTY-FIVE DOLLARS by mail or express to the address of

GEO. TIEMANN & CO.,
63 Chatham St., New York,

C. E. BORDEN,
Taunton, Mass., or

HIGBY & STEARNS,
162 Jefferson St., Detroit, Mich.

For further particulars see Transactions American Medical Association, Vol. X., and New York Journal of Medicine, May, 1857, and September, 1858.

HOME INSURANCE COMPANY
OF NEW YORK.
OFFICE, Nos. 112 and 114 BROADWAY.

CAPITAL STOCK, (all paid in)...........:. $1,000,000.00
SURPLUS,   1st Jan., 1859................ 477,990.40
LIABILITIES,   "   " 35,558.68

The capital of this Company having recently been increased by an additional *cash* subscription of $400,000, the attention of merchants and property holders generally, is called to the increased security afforded thereby. All kinds of property insured against loss or damage by fire, at rates as low as the nature of the risk, and the security of the Company and of the insured will warrant.

Losses equitably adjusted and promptly paid.

Agents in all the large cities and towns.

DIRECTORS.

CHARLES J MARTIN ....PRESIDENT.
A. F. WILLMARTH ....VICE-PRESIDENT.
WILLIAM G. LAMBERT.............Firm of A. & A. Lawrence & Co.
GEORGE C. COLLINS.... .... "   Sherman & Collins.
DANFORD N. BARNEY............. "   Wells, Fargo & Co.
LUCIUS HOPKINS...............Pres't Importers' and Traders' Bank.
THOMAS MESSENGER.......... ....Firm of T & H. Messenger.
WILLIAM H MELLEN.............. "   Chaflin, Mellen & Co.
CHARLES B. HATCH .... "   Hatch, Hiller & Mersereau.
B. WATSON BULL.................. "   Haskell, Merrick & Bull.
HOMER MORGAN ....
LEVI P. STONE..... .... "   Stone. Starr & Co.
JAMES HUMPHREY................. "   Barney, Humphrey & Butler.
GEORGE PEARCE .... "   George Pearce & Co.
WARD A WORK................... "   Ward A. Work & Son.
JAMES LOW...................... "   James Low & Co., of Louisville.
ISAAC H. FROTHINGHAM.......... "   I. H. Frothingham & Co.
CHARLES A. BULKLEY .... "   Bulkley & Co.
CEPHAS H. NORTON, .,.......... "   Norton & Jewett.
GEORGE D. MORGAN.............. "   E. D. Morgan & Co.
THEODORE McNAMEE...... ... "   Bowen, McNamee & Co.
RICHARD BIGELOW .... "   Doan, King & Co., of St. Louis
OLIVER E. WOOD.......... ... "   Willard, Wood & Co.
ALFRED S. BARNES........ ... "   A. S. Barnes & Co.
GEORGE BLISS.... .... "   Phelps, Bliss & Co.
ROE LOCKWOOD................. "   R. Lockwood & Son.
JOHN G. NELSON .... "   Nelson & Co.
LYMAN COOKE..... .... "   Cooke, Dowd, Baker & Co.
LEVI P. MORTON.............. ..... "   Morton, Grinnell & Co.
CURTIS NOBLE .... "   Condit & Noble.
JOHN B. HUTCHINSON............ "   J. C. Howe & Co., of Boston.
CHARLES P. BALDWIN............ "   Baldwin, Starr & Co.
AMOS T. DWIGHT............ ...... "   Trowbridge Dwight & Co.
HENRY A HURLBUT .... "   Swift, Hurlbut & Co
JESSE HOYT.......... .... "   Jesse Hoyt & Co.
WM. STURGIS, JR....... .... "   Sturgis, Shaw & Co.
JOHN R. FORD.................. "   Ford Rubber Co.
SIDNEY MASON.................. "   Mason & Thompson.
GEO. T. STEDMAN .... "   Stedman, Carlile & Shaw, of Cincinnati.
CYRUS YALE, JR.................. "   Cyrus Yale, Jr. & Co., of New Orleans.
WM. R. FOSDICK .... "   Wm. R. & Chas. B. Fosdick.
DAVID I: BOYD.................. "   Boyd, Brothers & Co., of Albany, N. Y.
F. H. COSSITT .... "   Cossitt, Hill & Talmadge, Memphis, Tenn.
SAM'L B. CALDWELL,............. "   Brewer & Caldwell.
LEWIS ROBERTS................ "   L. Roberts & Co.

CHAS. J. MARTIN, *President.*

J. MILTON SMITH, *Secretary.*   A. F. WILLMARTH, *Vice-President.*

AMERICAN
MEDICAL GAZETTE.

| Vol. X. | MAY, 1859. | No. 5. |

ORIGINAL DEPARTMENT.

An Address to the Philadelphia County Medical Society,
ON MEDICAL HEROISM.

Delivered Feb. 24th, 1859, by John Bell, M.D.

Our Society requires that its President shall deliver a public address at the close of his term of office. He is, of course, free to select his subject. It may be treated in a strain of advice or encouragement, of warning, or even of reprehension; provided, always, that it be clothed in the language of sincerity and good-will. The science, the art, the literature, and the ethics of medicine, furnish numerous themes for copious and learned, and even eloquent discourse. It has fallen to my lot, during a tolerably long and not idle life, to glean something from the various fields in our professional domain; and I might, perhaps, without presumption, make an offering to you at this time of some of these gatherings. But why should I attempt to indoctrinate those who are, as their title implies, already *docti*, learned men; or to penetrate into the mysteries of science, and to portray its diversified aspects and relations to those who, with microscope armed, can see through and through an object, and enjoy the additional privilege of afterwards reasoning round and round about it? Who shall say where the homologous ends and the heterologous begins? Some histologists are now inclined to question the correctness of the sentence of outlawry pressed against certain diseased textures, just as some historians would plead an arrest of judgment on certain personages who have always been spoken and written of in terms of execration. We are told, for example, that the terrible cancer itself, which

21

but yesterday, as it were, was declared to display its virulence, not only on its face, but in its ultimate cells, is, to-day, alleged to have no such special characteristics, and that its cells are merely deformed homologous ones. So, in reference to some historical names—Tiberius, Richard III., and, just now, Henry VIII.—we learn, the result of more careful investigations, that these much abused gentlemen were full of good intentions, not, in truth, well understood, and which had, somehow or another, gone astray. We are everywhere met by contrasts which, in the self-sufficiency of half-knowledge, we call contradictions. Bile and sugar are now found to keep company together, and even to be elaborated by the same organ, so that the old comparison—bitter as gall—must henceforth be qualified with the addition—and a touch of the saccharine. It must have been by a psychological analysis, conducted in a similar method, that the sweet part in the character of the tyrants just named has been discovered by their respective apologists. A history of the functions of the human organism would show almost as many changes and revolutions as general history does of successions of dynasties and overthrows of empires; both of them have their mythical as well as their proper historic periods. Scarcely, for example, have we become accustomed to hear of pepsin and the part which it is assumed to perform in digestion, as well as that other, by which it is made to figure in the advertisements and placards of lying quacks, who could not tell the difference between pepsin and pepper, when we are now presented with pancreatin. Hitherto the pancreatic juice was believed to be analogous to saliva, and to hold quite a subsidiary office in digestion. Now, through its active principle, pancreatin, it is invested with properties by which a common eater, who takes a dose of it, will be able to rival the gastronomic feats of a London alderman, or that more diminutive, but not less decided glutton, the hydra, which is all stomach. If the luxurious and degenerate Romans, under the empire, had known of the existence of this little polype and of its wonderful powers, they would have deified it, and placed its magnified image at the head of their supper-table. They endeavored to renew the pleasures of eating by taking an emetic, and thus making room for a second repast immediately after the first. The hydra can, as you know, do this and more besides; not only can it disgorge itself of its prey, but, if turned inside out, as you would the finger of a glove, what was before skin becomes stomach, and is as eager for food and as ready to digest it, as was its legitimate predecessor, which is now metamorphosed into skin.

When we speak of changes and transference of attributes, our minds immediately turn to the nervous system, and especially to the spinal marrow and the great sympathetic, which, although it is by no means a *terra incognita*, is still to physiologists what Central Africa has been to ethnologists and geographers—a wide field of discovery and no little speculation. For a while, we were allowed to settle down into a belief in the conclusions reached by Sir Charles Bell and by Magendie, on the functions of the spinal marrow; but we are all again at sea, watching the pilotings and soundings of men of another generation, who are as busy and industrious, and quite as confident of the truth of their views, as were their immediate predecessors.

Progress, change, reform and improvement, are the watch-words of the day, saving and excepting always in as far as medical education is concerned. Our medical schools constitute no exception to the universal experience, that corporations never reform themselves, are never the leaders, but always the opposers of innovation, which in their ears sounds like revolution and anarchy. Nearly a century has elapsed since the first medical school in the three British Provinces of North America was founded, (1765,) in the city of Philadelphia, by Dr. John Morgan and Dr. William Shippen, with whom were associated ere long Dr. Adam Kulin, Dr. Thomas Bond, Dr. Benjamin Rush, and at later dates Dr. James T. Hutchinson, Dr. Samuel Powell Griffiths, Dr. Caspar Wistar, and Dr. Benj Smith Barton, and at the early part of the present century, (1805,) Dr. Philip Syng Physick. During all this time the curriculum of medical studies has undergone little change, and this not always for the better. There have been more curtailments of the original scheme of instruction than additions to it. The chair of clinical medicine, filled first by Dr. Bond, and afterwards by Dr. Rush, has, since then, been thrust to one side; that of natural history and botany was never occupied except by Dr. Barton, before he was transferred to the chair of materia medica and botany. All the additions made to the first plan have been, not of branches, but of separate chairs for different branches, which used to be taught from one chair. The medical schools which, in succession, have been organized in different parts of the United States since the creation of that of the old Philadelphia College, afterwards merged in the University of Pennsylvania, have taken it as their model, and now, forsooth, in the entire length and breadth of the land, we are to content ourselves with a course of medical instruction, as measured by subjects or branches in the middle of the nineteenth century, which was not deemed to be more than what was thought to be barely requisite in the middle of the eighteenth. Branches of medicine which were then merely sketched have been filled up since to the extent of a hundred-fold, and new ones have been opened out; but still, all practical acknowledgment of the fact is made by a proportionately increased number of teachers, and scarcely by an increase of the period in which they are to lecture. With a hundred-fold more positive facts pertaining to every branch of medicine, and a hundred-fold more experiments for their illustration and enforcement, the collegiate term allowed for the introduction and arrangement of these facts, and the making of these experiments, is, with a very few honorable exceptions, as brief as ever. The inference from this state of things is obvious. They who wish to reach the full, or rather a liberal measure of medical attainments, must prosecute their studies outside of college walls. . Within these walls they cannot expect to receive methodical instruction in hygiene, public and private botany, pathological anatomy, pathology in its large and recognized meaning, medical jurisprudence, medical biography, including the history of medicine; finally, in medical bibliography. As far as collegiate instruction goes, we are quite unprepared to appear before the courts of law, and to give our testimony clearly and with understanding on questions which affect the reputation, the fortunes, and the lives of our fellow-citizens—questions which belong to medical jurisprudence, or legal medicine, as it is often termed. It would be thought strange for a politician, who aspires to figure in public life, to be ignorant of the history of his own country, or even of general history. What shall we say of the alumni of our medical schools being sent abroad into the world in ignorance of the history of medicine, its successive improvements, and the causes which at different times retarded its progress, as well as of the distinctive merits of those eminent men who have enlarged the boundaries of medical science, or made improvements in medical art? It may be grating to our national vanity, which certainly is not small, for us to be told that, in the matter of medical education, Young America has yet much to learn from Old Europe; but yet, unfortunately for us, the averment is undoubtedly true.

All honor and renown to those noble men who forego the distinctions conferred by office and the emoluments from practice in the eager search after and discovery of new facts, and the developing of accordant principles. They dig the gold, leaving it to others to convert it into crowns for kings and current coin for the people; they find the rich material for others to decorate themselves with. The world would hold of small account the common sense of those who, calling themselves utilitarians, should cry out to the patient delvers and miners of the precious metals, "We do not want your gold-dust or your lumps, or even ingots; give us something we can apply to purposes of use and ornament—vessels of various sizes and shapes, rings, broaches, clasps, chains, chased work, not to speak of plate for the table." The medical philosopher might ask, "Is there more wisdom in the cant of the, day among many practitioners of medicine, who are continually calling for the practical, not as the crowning capital of the column of medical science, but rather, according to their notion, as a separate block, almost as rough as when taken from the quarry, but whose surface has been hacked by random strokes of common workmen, each leaving his mark, and calling it his experience in architecture?" What long and patient delving into the interior of the human frame! What careful observation of the structure and connections of the several parts of which it is composed! What nice induction was exercised before an approach could be made to a knowledge of the uses and combined action of these several parts! Observation, experiment, hypothesis, theory, were invoked in turn before the meaning of what passes in the interior could be read on the surface, before the elaborated vital manifestations could be appreciated by and made serviceable to the practical physician. The practical man may be heard to boast that he contents himself, in the treatment of disease, with noting the symptoms and prescribing the remedies which experience has shown to be most available for the removal of those symptoms. But during this time he seems to forget that he is not dealing with separate phenomena, ultimate facts, which have no special connection with or relation to one another, and which require no chain of theory to unite them together. That of which the senses take direct cognizance is indeed a matter of fact, such as the color and coating of the tongue, the physical qualities of the pulse, &c.; but the meaning, semeiologically considered, of these appearances and states, is a question of theory respecting which we cannot speak with certainty, inasmuch as the precise relation between the phenomena observed and the state of the internal organs, of which the former are supposed to be the representation, the symptoms, in fine, is not equally demonstrable to the senses, is not a matter of simple legitimate experience. A practical physician, so called, will say, that a yellow and loaded tongue indicates bilious disorder, and that such is his experience; that is to say, that he was taught this symptomatology, and continues to believe it. From this belief, he deduces his practice of giving a mercurial purgative.

But may not more careful observation show that all this so-called experience, this alleged dealing in matter-of-fact, is false reasoning—is false theory; and that the stomach, not the liver, is in fault, and that a day's fasting, and the use of diluent drinks, may well be substituted for purging? There is not a single symptom to which a practitioner of medicine attaches any value that does not call on the intellect to trace in it a cause and an effect, and to deduce from this connection, be it real or be it supposititious, a new condition of things; in fine, a theory. How much more than theoretical, how purely speculative must be that so-called experience which rests on conclusions from obvious phenomena, the inner or remoter causes of which are conjectured or unknown! Your mere practical man feels, for example, the pulse of his patient, with a desire of ascertaining whether the latter has fever, and thinks he is no theorist if, at the same time, he avoids all discussion or inquiry into the proximate cause and nature of fever. It does not occur to him that in the very use of the term fever, he gives in to an abstraction, and deals with a theory of the most complex kind. But waiving this point, he may, perhaps, assure us that the pulse, whose beats, and their force and regularity, or intermission, are matters of certainty, furnish him with most reliable indications of the force and the degree of the fever. He has no doubts on this head; he confidently rests his belief on experience. But, to what does this experience amount? It is neither more nor less than a repetition for a lengthened period of a theory which supposes that certain physical characters of the pulse are caused by, or indicate those complex and unknown changes in the functions of the organism designated by the abstract term fever.

During the long period of nineteen centuries, or from the time of Herophilus of Alexandria, who was the first to speak of the arterial pulse, and of Praxagoras, who first gave it diagnostic value, down to the date of the discovery of the circulation of the blood by Harvey, physicians, practiced ones, too, spoke and argued with confidence of the diagnostic and prognostic value of sphygmology, although they were long ignorant of the very first step in the real process of causation—viz., the anatomical connection between the arteries and the heart, and of the pulsations of the former being the effect of the contractions of the latter organ acting on the contained blood circulating in elastic vessels. Galen, coming four centuries later, than

Herophilus taught that pulsations were caused by the vital forces, and that the heart, through the *pneuma*, communicated the pulsatile faculty to the arteries. He supposed the pulse to be an index to the vital forces, and, as such, that it pointed out, not only the character of the disease, but its probable termination, either in recovery or in death. He went further, and invested the pulse with the function of preserving the animal heat, of drawing in cold air, and of discharging effete matters from the blood. Galen wrote a complete course of sphygmology, divided into four sections, each including four books, besides several monographs on the same subject. In his first book he enumerates more than sixty varieties of pulse, each having its distinct or diagnostic character, and indicating a particular disease. Hence, there was assumed to be a pleuritic pulse, a suppurative pulse, a phthisical pulse, an hepatic pulse, a splenic pulse, &c. In these refinements, the teacher of Pergamos has found imitators among the moderns, and especially among the French physicians of the last century. For the next fifteen hundred years, or nearly until the discovery of the circulation of the blood, the Galenical doctrines of the pulse were taught in the schools, and received by practitioners of medicine as their guide in semeiotics. When Harvey appeared, and the true mechanical cause of the pulse was ascertained to be the contractile power of the heart and elasticity of the arteries, which last were no longer believed to contain vital spirits or air, in addition to blood, the practical men of the day thought themselves aggrieved at a discovery which would require them to begin their experience anew, and to reach conclusions so different from those which had previously satisfied them.

With the predominance of the iatro-mathematical school, and the forced reduction of the circulation of the blood and other fluids of the living body to the laws of hydraulics, the pulse came to assume new and different significations from those that had been attached to it by the fallacies of Galen.

Although called an eclectic, the eminent Boerhaave belonged to this school, and through his teaching its doctrines, during a considerable part of the last century, were disseminated, and generally adopted throughout Europe and in English America, as far as this country possessed at the time educated physicians. When, afterwards, by the labors of Stahl, Frederick Hoffman, and, above all, the horrid prelections of Cullen, vitalism, and with it solidism, obtained the ascendency, how many wise doctors shook their heads, and readjusted their wigs, and planted their gold-headed canes on the floor with additional en-

ergy, while relating their experience in the Boerhaavian views of
mechanical obstruction and *error loci*, and of tendon and viscidity, and
of the fluids being the cause of fever and inflammation! And the
pulse—did not all experience, they might be heard to exclaim, confirm the indications, in this sense, which it furnished? Boerhaave
himself, repeating the language of Hippocrates, had said, *experientia
fallax*, and the fallacies of the great professors of Leyden themselves
furnished abundant evidence of the truth of the aphorism.

There were other important phenomena in which the heart performed
a conspicuous part, and of which the pulse gave notice, but which
were not explicable by a knowledge merely of the mechanism of the
heart, and of the circulation, as furnished by routine experience. It
was necessary to look for remoter agencies, by which this mechanism
underwent such great and sudden transitions in its movements; as
when it was disturbed by fever and jarred by strong emotion, or the
irritations of other viscera. The pulse, under these circumstances, indicated great cardiac disturbance, but its revelations of more remote
disorder were not always read in the proper sense. Something more
than the blood, the normal stimulant of the heart was to be studied;
it was necessary to discover the connecting links between the heart,
the central organ of the circulation, and the brain, the material organ
of the mind, or great ganglionic centre of intellectual and emotional
life, and also between the heart and the ganglionic centres and plex-
uses of nutritive organic life. The nerves are these connecting links;
and now, when we feel a pulse in a case of fever, we ought to
be aware that we seek in the number and character of its beats an
index, not only to the momentum with which the blood is impelled by
the contractile power of the heart, but also the possible mental disturbance, and, still more certainly, the irritation or inflammation of a
viscus, or it may be of several viscera or tissues, which, by a continual
teasing, as it were, of the heart and the brain, keep up what we
call fever. But the blood itself, in the vessel beating beneath our
fingers, has also its share in modifying the character of the pulse, not
only by its quantity, but also by the varying proportions of its fibrin
and blood globules; and also, in fevers, especially in typhus and the
eruptive ones, by the introduction of a new and poisonous element, which
displays its effects in sometimes exciting, but more frequently weaken-
ing the contractile and propelling power of the heart.

It is impossible, therefore, for the most exacting advocate of experience, and of reliance on simple facts as our guide in practice, to

deny, while his fingers are on the pulse of his patient, laboring under fever, the necessity of passing in mental review the antecedent phenomena—hurried contraction of the heart, increased innervation from the nervous centres of animal and of nutritive life on the heart, the probable change in the viscera or the tissues exciting these nervous centres; and finally, the altered properties of the blood, and, it may be, modification of the cellular coat of the vessel itself, by the changes in its reticulated nervous tissue. As a practical man, he is bound to carry in his mind all the facts, and if he draws inferences from them, he must reason on them, must form certain notions respecting their relations to each other, and their bearing on the subject immediately before him; in fine, he must theorize, not indeed at random, but according to the rules of sound medical logic. How little did experience, during the many centuries of the rule of Galenical doctrines of sphygmology, add to the diagnostic value of the pulse in organic diseases of the heart! What strange experiences must have been recorded of the meaning to be attached to the feeble and exiguous pulse, and sometimes its entire absence in dilatation of the heart, with accompanying disease of the valves! What weakness of the nervous forces was inferred! What an amount of stimulation practiced, at a time when the organ was laboring with double, but ineffectual power, owing to the derangement of its mechanism! Let us, then, be ever ready to receive with an impartial and a kindly spirit any new fact of an experimenter, and not turn away from the plausible suggestions of a studious theorist, although they may conflict with our daily routine of observation, which we choose to dignify with the name of experience. But, in advocating the claims of science in medicine, as opposed to routine and empirical experience, and as combining doctrines and propositions which enable the practitioner to found upon them his rules for the treatment of his patients, we must not forget our legitimate line of study and logical argumentation. This will not be found in undue attachment to the opinions of men of general scientific enlightenment and over-estimation of novel acquisitions, fallacious semblance of positivism, or exactness, which has crept, as if it were an integral part of medicine, into the train of microscopical and chemical methods of investigation.

But it is time that I should pass from these topics, which have come up incidentally to the main subject of this address. I would here make a remark, in anticipation of some objections that may be brought to the strain of praise in which I shall be thought to have indulged

when speaking of the dignity of our profession, and the true nobility
of many who have toiled in it. In our regular professional meetings
we seldom indulge in mutual adulation. Our habit on these occasions
is to scrutinize the real value of the facts and suggestions which are
brought before us for the melioration and cure of disease, or for the
preservation and promotion of health. We are more anxious to keep
up the standard of medical ethics and to enrich practical medicine
than to elicit the plaudits of the multitude. Disguise it as we may,
toil, incessant toil, and anxiety from first to last, are the fate of all
who are engaged in the practice of medicine. It cannot, therefore,
be deemed amiss, or if it be an error, it is an excusable one, to make
occasionally a commemorative address a vehicle for words of encouragement and gratulation at the bright passages of our history, in
order that we may with patience bear our inevitable trials, and, at
the same time, be incited to emulous effort in the path which lies before us. The laurel is not gathered in fertile fields or flowery mead-
ows, but on the broken heights of rough ascent.

The present is an age in which not only the people of one nation,
or even race, but mankind, the universal man, is vexed with the
"love of change." It is an age not only of progress, but of transition,
in which old ideas, like old armor and old tapestry, have become
obsolete, and new ones are springing up in new and often, it must be
confessed, fantastic forms,—not susceptible of classification, according
to any known, or even conceivable system of psychology. But it is
enough for the thoughtful and the benevolent to be aware that great
changes are going on, and will go on, so that they may both protect
themselves against extremes and excesses, and contribute their efforts
towards giving a safe and useful direction to the new mental machinery, for the good of their fellow-men, whether of their own order or
members of the great body politic.

Medicine, both in her scientific and professional aspects, is also being subjected to remarkable changes; but amid all of them, it becomes
the duty of us who are votaries and worshipers at her altar, to see
that no impious forms, no witches' mummery shall take the place of
the simple yet solemn rites which the faithful in every successive age
have always performed.

In forms we have conceded, or rather abandoned, a great deal.
Let us not, in a too ready spirit of yieldingness, give up essentials. No
longer is the physician recognized, in his daily round, by peculiarity
of garb, manner, or language. The formal suit of black, the full

ballooned wig, the shining knee and shoe buckles, and the gold or ivory headed cane, have disappeared, and with them the solemnity of manner, the measured and aphoristic fashion of speech which used to characterize our predecessors of the olden time. Something more has been given up besides. We are now content, as was said of Shakspeare, with a *little* Latin and *less* Greek, in place of the deep draughts which were quaffed by all who wished to be regarded legitimate members of the schools of Hippocrates and Celsus.

But, although we may be less fluent in the language of Greece and Rome than even our immediate predecessors, let us not forget, for a moment, the histories of those men who, from him of Cos down to a Jenner, a Rush, and a Pinel, have adorned the profession, and illustrated and ennobled humanity. If, proudly, we claim to be professionally descended from the Father of Medicine, and believe the language of an eminent writer, when he asserts that "the duties of a physician were never more beautifully exemplified than in his conduct, or more eloquently described than in his writings," we must be careful not to discredit the family in failing to follow the example set by its illustrious founder. How much stronger still ought to be the desire to imitate our sires, when we know that every successive age, down to the one we live in, has sent forth from our profession its heroes of humanity and dispensers of the richest lore! The elevated position assigned to us by an eminent scholar, when he says that "in erudition, in science, and in habits of deep and comprehensive thinking, the pre-eminence must be awarded, in some degree, to physicians," imposes on us correspondingly lofty obligations to continue to merit the praise thus spontaneously given. If, at this time, we are unable to erect pyramids which might excite the wonder of remote generations, let us at least build houses of shelter, in which fountains are introduced for the refreshment of the weary pilgrim and the traveler across the deserts of ignorance, and the thorny and briered wastes of prejudice and superstition.

Not only ought we to have the consciousness of our own strength, of the unbroken succession of great names, illustrated by great deeds, and of the dignity of the order to which we belong, but we must, also, for the sake of giving greater scope to our own well-meant efforts, impress our fellow-men, in all the walks of life, with our true position and aims. One of the first steps to accomplish our purpose will be to diffuse, and to render popular and familiar as household words, that portion of our rich and teeming literature in which are recorded the discoveries of the means of preventing diseases, and the disinterested and devoted efforts of those who have either periled or laid down their lives to stay the march of pestilence, and to save their frightened fellow-citizens, and apparently doomed victims, from its merciless assaults.

We do not study enough our own history; we are not familiar, as we ought to be, with the great deeds, the true heroism of our professional ancestors. They ought to form an integral part of the history of mankind, and find their place in the brightest passages of the history of every civilized people. The first dawn of civilization reveals the respect paid to medicine and to those who practiced it, and with the advance in general knowledge, science and refinement, there has always been an increase of this estimation. The Greeks, like the Egyptians, believed medicine to be of divine origin. Its humanizing and softening influences were typified in its tutelary deity, Apollo, being also regarded as god of poetry and of music. Gratitude for the numerous and extraordinary cures of disease performed by Esculapius did not stop short of his apotheosis, and of causing temples to be erected to him. Orpheus, the priest-poet, was also a physician. During this, the heroic age of Greece, we find mention made of the name of Ex, who was of the school of Chiron the Centaur, and physician and surgeon to the expedition of the Argonauts, which we are afraid must incur the imputation of having been somewhat of the filibustering character, similar to that of the restless and buccaneering spirits of the present day, or to that of the age of Queen Elizabeth, as represented by Sir Francis Drake and his associates. Another and more celebrated pupil of Chiron, and also one of the Argonauts, was Hercules, who is more thought and spoken of for feats of great bodily prowess than as a reformer of abuses and ills, which interfered with the safety and the health of the people of the different countries which he visited. Viewed in this light, he is among the earliest of our medical heroes, and a great sanitary reformer. In fact, we must look on him as the symbol of the history of Grecian civilization; more particularly in its physical aspects, as in his draining of morasses and lakes, digging of canals, extirpating of forests and of the wild beasts that infested them. The story of Hercules destroying the Hydra, the many-headed monster, near Lake Lerna, is an allegory intended to show that he, or rather the first authors of civilization personified in him, cleared and drained the Peloponnesus, and so exposed the previously marshy soil to the sun as to cause a thorough desiccation. In another of his twelve labors, the cleansing of the Augean stable, we see the symbolic representation of accumulated filth, and at the same time a resort to the most judicious means for abating the nuisance. If Hercules had been the representative of mere animal strength, as he is too commonly regarded, he would have set about the task imposed on him by Eurystheus, in scavauger fashion, by digging up and shoveling out the accumulated filth in the stables of Augea. But the demigod, endowed with the higher qualities of mind, had recourse to a more complete and rational process, which consisted in turning the river Alpheus, or as some say the Peneus, through the stable, and thus carrying off the accumulations of thirty years, and at the same time thoroughly cleansing the receptacle of so many abominations. How many cities at the present day have their foul corners, worse than the Augean stable, without, however, a Hercules or even any of the Heraclidæ, his descendants, to cleanse and purify them! An entire river cannot often be diverted into a new channel for the purpose, but a portion of its water ought always to be distributed in minor and artificial streams, so that the streets should be washed by hose irrigation, and the contents of the sewers carried off by flushing, if a perennial flow can be obtained for this purpose.

The separation of history from myth took place in the persons of Machaon and Podalirius, reputed sons of Esculapius. They were the last of the heroic age who figured both as warriors and physicians, for such was their part at the siege of Troy. Thus Homer, in his Iliad, Book II., when giving a catalogue of the Grecian ships, tells,

> "In thirty sail the sparkling waves divide
> Which Podalirius and Machaon guide ;
> To these his skill their parent god imparts
> Divine professors of the healing arts."

Henceforward we are to meet with medical men in their true and appropriate relations to the world, as heroes of humanity, as men who peril their lives, but it is always to save those of others : they combat not their fellow-men—but unseen, often unknown enemies, and are led into ambuscades from which are discharged more fearful and destructive missiles than man's devilish ingenuity has yet devised. In the philosophic and scrutinizing age of Greece, which succeeded the heroic, Plato is heard to say that a good physician is only second to the Deity himself. This was the age of Hippocrates,—that in which Pericles bore mild sway in Athens, and when philosophy, poetry, history, and the fine arts found their teachers and representatives, who have ever since been regarded, and to all appearances ever will be, as models for all time.

The opinion of Cato the Censor, and the strong prejudices of the Roman people during the first centuries of their history, against physicians, are often cited by those who would detract from the usefulness and merits of medicine. The enmity would seem, however, to have been directed more against the persons who practiced it than against the art itself. The Romans were jealous of the intruding Greeks, and Cato kept no measures with the philosophers, orators, and physicians from Greece, while accusing them of corrupting the manners of the Romans. This rigid and rough moralist carried his animosity so far as to procure an edict for the expulsion of the two first-mentioned classes; but the physicians were spared. Something of personal and even professional rivalry may have had its share in Cato's persecution of the physicians, shall we call them the regular faculty? then in Rome. He was the author of a work on domestic and veterinary medicine; and in the habit of dosing with equal readiness and impartiality, and probably with equal success, his farm and house servants and domestic animals. He prepared the remedies himself; they were, we may presume, simples culled from his garden and fields, and were doubtless represented by him to be much more congenial with the patriotic stomachs of his countrymen than the exotic drugs brought and administered by the exotic Greeks. Unfortunately, however, for self-taught doctors, even of the Cato mould, there was a story at the time that the wife of the Censor fell a victim to his original and Roman method of medication. Pliny the elder, at a later period, was less consistent in his declamations against foreign physicians, inasmuch as he wrote a *Materia Medica* made up entirely from the works of the Greek authors. This early specimen of nativism may excite a smile of derision ; but is it not of quite a mitigated character when compared with the exuberant manifestations of our own people in this way a few years ago?

In Philadelphia they seemed to forget that a Girard, and in New York they were equally oblivious that an Astor had ever lived among them; the first to endow a paternal college for orphans,—the second a library rich with the productions of the genius and learning of the natives of every country under heaven. Voltaire pithily remarks, in reference to the obligations of mankind to physicians: To preserve and repair is almost equal to making. The Roman people let five hundred years pass without physicians. They were only occupied in destroying, and cared little for preserving life. How, adds this witty writer, did they make out at Rome, when a person was seized with a putrid fever, or had a fistula, or a pulmonary affection? He died. With the progress of civilization and of letters, the Romans acquired juster ideas of medicine and of its professors; a striking evidence of which is furnished in the language of the eloquent philosopher, Cicero, that nothing brings men nearer to the gods, than by giving health to their fellow-creatures.

But why should we seek to emblazon our escutcheon, by bringing on its field the symbolical figures of the mythology of Grecee and Rome? Receiving humbly our shield from him who has been called the Great Physician, and taking him as our head and guide, let us rather enrich its scroll with mottoes from sacred writ, than care to decorate its mantling crests or supporters, the creations of a truant fancy. The medical hero in Christian lands is not to be sought for in courts or in camps, nor in the busy and crowded haunts of the wealth-seeking; he is not in the Rialto or the Exchange, nor prominent at the polls; he is neither a demagogue, inflaming the passions of the multitude, nor a parasite, flattering the prejudices of the rich, or ministering to the caprices of those in power. He seldom finds a place in pageant or in festival; seldom is called upon to add his voice to the praises of victory. He passes through the crowd often unknown, uncared for, unless indeed it may be when he meets the face of one radiant with smiles, whom he had visited but a short time before, prostrate on the bed of sickness, or hears his name uttered by another in a tone which is equivalent to saying "God bless him!"

Where, then, shall we find our medical hero—what are his attributes, what his exploits? We shall soon see his fields of action, in which hundreds are gazing at him as a superior being, whose fiat determines their fate, either for recovery or for death. Unselfishness, sympathy—friendship, are words ever grateful to the ear of humanity; they represent feelings dear to our common nature ; and although genius may sometimes not know them, and the intellect fail to appreciate their intrinsic value, yet they must always form a part of a truly great and noble character. They are in continual exercise among physicians, and are the chief constituents of medical heroism. I shall now proceed to this averment, and begin by adducing a rare instance of self-abnegation and friendship derived from common or extra professional life.

A Frenchman of some literary celebrity, whose name I cannot

recall, was seized with a violent, and, as he rightly believed, a fatal disease. His cherished friend coming into the room, in which, at the moment, there were several visitors, was called to his bedside, and addressed in a low tone of voice, in the following words: " Send away these people, and come and nurse me yourself. You know that my disease is contagious, and you alone, as a true friend, are the only one entitled to expose himself for me." The request of the sick man was complied with, the many inquiring visitors retired, and the privileged friend took his post at the bedside, and remained there until the death of him who had given such unusual proof of his confidence. This friend soon after sickened and died of the same disease.

Sentiment and song might be, probably have been, enlisted to celebrate so touching a proof of disinterested and devoted friendship. I would not detract from its merit by the remark that a *true* man is bound to risk fortune and life, ay, reputation itself, for his friend. In the present warmth of his own feelings, in the reminiscences of past confidential intercourse and of innumerable kind and loving acts, he forgets himself, he sees no danger and hesitates at no sacrifice in the service of his friend. If he reason for a moment, he will say to himself: "I, too, would be sure of receiving from him, when the occasion requires it, a like proof of regard for me and forgetfulness of himself."

But in what terms, by what epithets shall we designate him who, without any such genial incentives, without any expectation of possible reciprocity, or hope of applause, and certainly without any of the returns for self-exposure which men expect from men, goes about from day to day, and often too in the silent watches of the night, in a spirit of self-sacrifice of ease, comfort, health, and life itself, ministering relief to the pestilence-stricken and fever-tossed fellow-creature; the inmate, it may be, of a garret or a cellar of some wretched tenement, in an infected court or alley, the approach to which is by a narrow passage, obstructed by accumulations of all kinds of refuse and impurities? Is this man a soldier, inured to scenes of carnage and death, whose vocation makes him regardless of danger, and who, although he is detailed on the forlorn hope, knows that if he fall, his name will be recorded in the Gazette, and his wife and children receive perhaps a pension ? Or is he a salaried official, who for a certain pecuniary return and perquisites is dicharging a prescribed and covenanted duty? O, no! This simple-minded man, who goes about his duty for duty's and humanity's sake, is only a *doctor*, one of a class at whom every witling is privileged to fling a sarcasm, and whom every venal quack may accuse of selfishness, and greediness of gold.

" During the famine fever of 1847 in Ireland, one hundred and seventy-eight Irish medical practitioners, exclusive of medical pupils and army surgeons, died, being a proportion of nearly seven per cent., or one in every 15 medical practitioners, in a single year." Some persons may say that physicians who thus expose themselves, and who pay the penalty of death for their exposure, are encouraged by the expectation of pecuniary advantage in the shape of fees. We must all wish that they had such inducements; they could readily afford to forego a part of their reputation for benevolence and disinterestedness, in consideration of their receiving that by which they could support their wives and children, or an aged parent, or a lone sister. But it so happens that in all epidemic and pestilential diseases, the chief privations and dangers incurred by medical men are in their attendance on the poor, the needy and the destitute, and not seldom the dissolute, who have no claim on them from prior acquaintance or the most trivial service, and from whom they receive no fees, and often no thanks, or the slightest token of gratitude.

The greater part of the mortality among the Irish physicians was caused by their attendance on hospitals, and on the poor and half-starved occupants of the cabins and hamlets, the air of which was often in such a state of concentrated virulence as to strike on the nervous system with almost the force and suddenness of the electric aura. And shall no page in history, no lines in poetry, celebrate the heroic deeds of these devoted men, who must have battled with a stouter heart against an unseen enemy than Leonidas and his Spartan band against the Persian host, or the Light Brigade in its daring and rash charge on the serried Russian lines at Inkerman ? These heroes of humanity ought to be honored with a monumental inscription, even though it were couched in as brief phrase as that over the remains of the Athenians under Miltiades:

" They fought at Marathon."

Some years back many physicians of the city of New York lost their lives in their attendance on the newly-arrived emigrants—strangers, who might indeed claim the rights of hospitality, but not at the cost of the lives of their benefactors.

Two of the most memorable and destructive pestilences on record occurred, the first in the early part, the second near the end of the

22

last century. I refer to the plague at Marseilles in 1720, and the yellow fever of Philadelphia in 1793, in both of which the medical profession furnished more than its proportion of martyrs to the cause of humanity. History has done justice, but not more than justice, to the apostolic labors and devotedness of the good and pious Bishop of Marseilles, M. De Belzunce, during the entire period of the plague in that city. It has failed, however, as usual, to record in appropriate terms the labors and services, without fee or reward, of its physicians; and still worse, it has been falsified, so as to make it appear that the city had been deserted by these, the guardians of her health, and her defenders against disease. Doctor Bertrand, author of the "History of the Plague at Marseilles," and one of the devoted band on that occasion, bears the following emphatic testimony to the courage and zeal of his colleagues: " Far from following the opinion of those who held that all attendance in case of plague should be left to the surgeons, to whom the physicians should be reserved as counselors alone, they never shrank from personal attendance on the sick, but exposed their lives in endeavoring to give them succor, with the most undaunted courage and generosity. They were the first to face the danger of the contagion, going from street to street, from house to house, examining into everything, approaching the patients, feeling their pulse, examining their tumors, even dressing them with their own hands, if it appeared necessary; attending them, in short, with the same assiduity as could have been shown to a wealthy person, who was laboring under a common malady, and from whom they had expectations of a great reward. They never refused any service required of them, either in the hospitals, the city, or the country; and all without any charge, except when they were obliged to go into the country, when some expense was unavoidable; but they never made any charge for their own trouble. All the recompense they received was contempt, and often insults, on the part of the people." This last sentence requires some explanation. It seems that the people became prejudiced against the physicians of the city, because these latter had declared the disease to be plague. But it was stupidly forgotten that, in dealing frankly and honestly with the public, the interests of the latter alone were consulted. The physicians knew well that their announcement of a terrible fact would at once drive away the wealthy from the city, and of course deprive them of the class of patients who would be able to pay them for their services, and none but the poor would remain to receive medical attention. Had they, to humor the

popular wish, concealed the nature of the disease at first, they would
have been subjected, and with good reason, to public indignation, for
concealing the truth, and lulling the people into a feeling of false security. The surgeons, who constituted a separate body, also acquitted
themselves nobly, with the exception of a few deserters. Human
nature is not always equal to the exigencies of time and place, even
under the strongest appeals of humanity. Among the members of the
community, outside of the professional ranks, it too often shows itself
in a most cowardly fashion, under the plea of self-preservation. In
the beginning of the plague at Marseilles there were only four physicians, independently of the surgeons, to attend the sick in the different
quarters of the city. Of these four, Mons. Bertrand had two attacks
of the disease, from both of which he soon escaped; but, worn out
with fatigue, and depressed by the loss of all his family, the members
of which fell victims to the disease, in their endeavors to relieve
and nurse the sick, this benevolent man was for some time disabled
from resuming his professional duty. Let us add, that during the
remainder of his life he was always regarded and treated with the
greatest veneration by his fellow-citizens. Another of the small band
died of the disease; and a third, exhausted by fatigue, and left without a servant, and almost the necessaries of life, was obliged for a
while to go into the country. The surgeons were also reduced to a
very small number, four or five only surviving out of thirty. Truly,
then, was it said by the historian of the Marseilles plague, in reference to the situation and conduct of the professional men of the city:
" And if, in the end, we were obliged to demand further assistance from
other parts of the kingdom, it was not because those whose duty it
was particularly to remain in the city had deserted their posts, but
on account of the excess of the ravages made by the disease." In
order to be able to appreciate in the smallest degree the services and
exposures of the Marseilles physicians and surgeons at this time, we
ought to have before our minds the frightful features of the disease,
and the destitution and abandonment to which the people were reduced; the breaking up of every social tie among persons of all ranks,
and the scenes of individual and family misery and suffering which
everywhere met the eye of the medical and religious visitors. During
a season, these were almost the only persons who dared to quit their
own abodes to solace and relieve their pest-stricken fellow-citizens.

There must be not a few still living in Philadelphia, among whose
early reminiscences are some of the scenes of the memorable year of

1793, in which the city was so grievously afflicted with the yellow fever. Like the plague at Marseilles, this fever has had its historians, who described what they themselves saw, and actively participated in. If their pictures want the high finish which was imparted by the pen of a Thucydides to his description of the plague at Athens, they offered the largely compensating qualities of statistical and personal details. During the prevalence of this fatal epidemic, when all the bonds of society were loosened and the affections became cold and repellent, less concern, to use the language of an instructive chronicler of the disease, the late Matthew Carey, was felt for the loss of a parent, a husband, a wife, or an only child, than on other occasions could have been caused by the death of a servant, or even of a favorite lap-dog. "Acquaintances and friends avoided each other in the streets, and only signified their regard by a cold nod. The old custom of shaking hands fell into such general disuse, that many persons shrank back with affright at the offer of the hand; a person with a crape, or any appearance of mourning, was shunned like a viper." In this worse than beleaguered city—one more suffering than if it had been a prey to domestic strife, or than if gaunt famine had stalked through its streets unchecked—where were the medical soldiers, they who are always expected to be ready armed to combat disease in all its forms? With few exceptions, they were at their posts. How they battled with the raging pestilence, how they suffered, and how many of them fell in the struggle, is related in the pages of Rush, himself among the most distinguished of the devoted band. Within the short period of six weeks, during which this fever raged with the greatest violence, no less than ten physicians were carried off, and scarcely one of the survivors escaped an attack of the disease. At one time, as Dr. Rush relates, there were but three medical men who were able to do duty out of their houses—not counting, we must suppose, the French physicians, lately arrived from St. Domingo. Medical students also in imitation of their preceptors, and animated with a youthful zeal, which mastered the instinct of self-preservation, applied themselves devotedly to the relief of their suffering and dying fellow-citizens. Had the physicians of Philadelphia in 1793 consulted their own safety, and availed themselves of the plea of its being their duty to follow the majority of the families of which they were the regular medical advisers, it were easy for them to have left the city with these latter, and others who fled, to the number of 17,000 persons, or more than a third of the entire population. In the history of the war of the Revolution, Dr. Benjamin Rush, as one of the signers of the Declaration of Independence, and Physician-General to the army, will always figure with the other worthies of that momentous period. But in the history of Philanthropy he will occupy a still higher place as one of the medical heroes who won his honors and enduring fame in the trying year of 1793, and in the other epidemic invasions of the yellow fever during the next twelve years. The fever of 1798 renewed the terrors and the mortality of 1793, and, at the same time, gave opportunities for a display of heroic devotedness on the part of the physicians similar to that manifested in the latter year.

The outbreaks and fearful ravages of the yellow fever, which have occurred in other cities in the United States, down to the recent catastrophes from the same cause by which Norfolk and Portsmouth, in Virginia, were so sorely afflicted, have been met by the same devotion to the public welfare, the same abnegation of self, and the same sacrifices, on the part of the physicians, wherever found.

Surprise is more frequently expressed at the escape of so many medical men from seizure and death, than at their falling victims during the prevalence of epidemic and malignant diseases. We are often asked, what are the means of prevention, what the charm by which we are able to walk abroad often unhurt, when death's arrows are flying in all directions around us If some who thus wonder at the escape of physicians would sally out daily with stout hearts and determined good-will, and visit the sick and the heavily laden, and administer to their necessities and wants in the way of little delicacies in food and drink, and of clothing when it is deficient, and, better perhaps than all, proffer pleasant words of encouragement and hope, they would readily understand the talismanic influence by which a physician is sustained in the consciousness that he is discharging a duty both to God and man. He is nerved to an exhibition of almost superhuman efforts, while he is continually risking his own life to save that of others. He ventures more than the bold swimmer, who plunges fearlessly into the rapid stream of the surging sea to save a fellow-being from a watery grave. Without his going through the imposing forms of initiation and taking the vows of the knight-errant of former times, the physician pursues his vocation quietly and unostentatiously, succoring, not only the distressed of the fair sex, but also the poor, the distempered, the outcast of his own sex, who are often as forbidding in their persons as in their minds. There are attractive histories of Chivalry. What restrains from writing a history of Medical Philanthropy? Why, for example, should not the discovery of vaccination, by Jenner, be as familiar a fact in school history as the invention of gunpowder by Roger Bacon, or the monk Scwarty? Had it been so, the women of England would have erected at least one other statue before that one which they did raise to the conqueror at Waterloo. They would have been taught to dwell on their obligations to Jenner, who had found the means of saving them and their children, and their children's children, to future generations, from a loathsome, disfiguring, and constantly, in large proportion, a fatal disease. In dwelling on this picture, they would have been less prone to glorify Wellington, who had led their husbands, their fathers, and their sons to battle, to carnage, and to death. Why, under any aspect, should women give a preference to the destroyer over the conservator, even though that destroyer should be the victor in a hundred fights? No history has yet told us that the celebrated French surgeon, Ambrose Paré, ought to share with the Duke of Guise the honor of the successful defence of Metz, when that town was besieged by the Emperor Charles V. At a time when the garrison was nearly exhausted by continual fighting, and the scant supply of food, the French king sent word exhorting it to hold out a little longer, and promised, as encouragement, to send them Ambrose Paré. The announcement had an electric effect, and the great surgeon was received within the walls of Metz with extravagant demonstrations of joy, as if he had come at the head of a powerful army to raise the siege. The soldier no longer feared wounds when he knew that he could procure Ambrose Paré to dress them, or even to direct their dressing by others.

Still more animated must have been the feeling of the whole French army in Egypt under Napoleon, or, as he was then more commonly called, Bonaparte, towards the chiefs of the medical and surgical staff. The troops, after witnessing the ravages of the plague, became alarmed and disheartened; and men who had never feared an enemy in the field of battle, now shrank with horror from the touch and breath of a sick companion in the quiet tent. To the general such a state of things was worse than the loss of a battle. In vain were the soldiers told that their fears were without foundation; in vain were they addressed in the language of encouragement and hope. Something must be done, either to change their belief or to appeal strongly to their imagination. Accordingly, Napoleon himself conversed freely with the patients who were stricken with the plague, and touched their bodies, and even sometimes performed the part of a nurse, by raising them up and supporting them in their beds, in order to prove that there was no danger, and that the disease was not contagious. These traits of cool courage are recorded by every historian of the wars of the French Revolution; but few have thought it worth while to notice the more daring exploit of Desgenettes, one of the physicians of the army of Egypt. He not only touched and handled the bodies of those who had sickened with the plague, but he inoculated himself with their blood and other fluids. On another occasion, after Berthollet had expressed his belief that the poison of the plague was conveyed into the body by means of the saliva, a patient, dying of this disease, begged that Desgenettes would take half of what was left of the draught which had been prescribed for him. Without hesitation, or betraying the slightest emotion, Desgenettes took the glass from the sick man, filled it up, and drank its contents entire.

If we believe that the design of the two—the military leader and the physician—was the same at this time, viz., to infuse confidence into the minds of the soldiers, it is not difficult to decide to which of them should be awarded the palm for disinterested exposure of his life. Napoleon felt that all his prospects of conquest and fame would be clouded unless he could restore the sinking courage of his army; and hence he readily incurred some danger to secure so important an end. Desgenettes was buoyed up by no such aspirations. His incentives were humanity and a search after truth.

Why not make this fine trait of the physician more prominent than that of the soldier in a school history? A small volume, consisting of incidents of this nature, might be prepared and introduced into the public schools. I would offer some additional facts and reflections, in the way of contribution to a chapter in a work of this kind.

While French medicine was thus represented in Egypt by the calm and self-possessed Desgenettes, who was at the head of the medical staff, French surgery shone with, perhaps, still greater lustre in the person of the eminent Larrey, who, by his invention of the light ambulance for carrying off the wounded from the field of battle, won the affection of the soldier, and by this act alone became entitled to honorable mention in the annals of philanthropy. From the burning sands of Egypt, to the ice-bound rivers and snow-covered plains of Russia, in Poland, in Prussia, in Saxony, in Austria, in Italy, in Spain, and in France itself, Larrey not only encountered all the vicissitudes of climate and season, and the hardships incident to camp-life, but he was constantly engaged in the discharge of his arduous duties as field and hospital surgeon, fearless of personal risk, and intent only on affording the promptest relief to those placed under his care. He did not wait at a safe distance from the field of battle for the wounded to be brought to him; he was found in the midst of the wounded, the dying and the dead, ready and resolute, and always self-possessed, operating with equal promptitude and skill on those whom he could first reach or who were most in need of his services, and not caring for the rank of the prostrate man before him. Instances are recorded in which Larrey and his assistants, carried away by their professional, and shall it be said in part, also, their national enthusiasm? were seen giving their attentions to the wounded near "the imminent and deadly breach" itself, amid a shower of destructive missiles which were carrying wounds and death to those around them. Larrey was exposed to the same fire under which Caffarelli, Lannes, Arrighi, Beauharnois, and many others fell, either wounded or never to rise again. After the long-contested and bloody battle of Eylau, in Polish Prussia, between the French and Russians, the Emperor Napoleon found Larrey standing in the snow, under a slight canopy of branches of trees, engaged in dressing the wounded; and on his passing by the same place, at the same hour, on the following day, he saw the indefatigable surgeon still occupied as before. In this way did Larrey spend twenty-four hours uninterruptedly, except in the few minutes snatched for a hurried repast. We have all heard or read of displays of zeal—religious, fanatical, patriotic and amorous, but seldom has there been recorded a finer example of benevolent zeal spent on so good and useful a purpose.

Larrey was with the Grand Army, which, under Napoleon, invaded Russia, and occupied Moscow. It has been said that the burning of that capital brought with it the extinction of the French empire as such. From that epoch the star of Napoleon began to be dimmed, and continued to give a flickering light, until, in a short time, it set forever behind the rock of St. Helena. Larrey participated in the sufferings of the terrific retreat from Moscow, in which all discipline was forgotten, and soldiers, losing even the semblance of men, were changed into livid spectres, or trembling shadows, decked in fantastic rags, following gaunt famine as their leader. But even at such a time as this, when the better sentiments of human nature seemed, like all the objects of external nature, to be frozen up, the soldiers did not forget their friend, their oft-tried benefactor. A river had to be crossed by a detachment of the army, for which two bridges were constructed. But not alone were the troops hurrying over. With the soldiers, and horses, and artillery, crowded on unhappy fugitives from Moscow, with their wives, and children, and baggage. In the advancing multitude Larrey was recognized; and immediately a thousand voices exclaimed: "Let us save him who has saved us. Let him come forward." All stop at once in their wild rush. Larrey is allowed to reach the bridge, and he is suddenly raised in the arms of the nearest soldiers and passed from hand to hand, until he is, in this manner, carried entirely across the river. He is saved just at the moment when the bridge gives way, and a crowd of human beings, of both sexes and all ages, together with horses, and cannon, and military wagons, are precipitated into the half-frozen stream beneath, most of them never to reach its banks, never to breathe again. Among these was a young mother, who held up her infant above her head, as a mute but touching appeal to save it. A soldier took it when she was about to sink in the water, and her last struggles were soothed by the consciousness that her child was saved.

Larrey, ever faithful to Napoleon, for whom he cherished a feeling of strong personal attachment, followed him to Waterloo, where he was wounded, and made prisoner by the Prussians, and was on the point of being shot by his exasperated enemies. He was, however, happily recognized by the Prussian surgeon-major, who was about to put the fatal band over his eyes, and he was then conducted to General Bulow, and afterwards to Marshal Blucher, whose son he had formerly saved from almost inevitable death. Larrey was soon set at liberty, and was sent at first to Louvain, whence he repaired to Brussels, and made the first use of his returning strength in visiting the hospitals, crowded with the wounded of both the victors and the vanquished, to whom he gave equally his services. At the solicitation of the commanders of the allied armies in Paris, he is recalled to that capital, and is once more restored to his family, which for many days had believed him to be dead. Under the Restoration he was deprived of his pension and the decoration of the Legion of Honor, but still preserved his post of surgeon-in-chief at Gros Caillore, the hospital of the Royal Guard. On the last of the three days of July, 1830, in which the troops of the line had suffered so terribly from the fires behind the barricades and from the houses, his hospital was surrounded by an exasperated crowd, uttering all kinds of threats. Larrey made his appearance, and addressed them in the following terms: "What do you mean? Whom do you dare to threaten? Know that these sick men are mine; that it is my duty to defend them, and yours to respect yourselves in respecting the unfortunate." This timely firmness put a stop to further attempts at violence, and the noisy troop withdrew, taking with them the arms from which they had no longer anything to fear. This brave and good man retained all his energies to an advanced age. In 1842, when he was in his seventy-sixth year, he made an official tour of inspection of the hospitals of Algeria, and at Bonn he performed the operation of amputating the arm of an Arab. Can we better terminate these brief notices of Larrey, as exhibiting him in the light of a true hero of humanity, than by a mention of the bequest of Napoleon of $20,000 dollars to him as the most virtuous man whom he had ever known?—a higher eulogy even than that paid by the Roman emperor to Galen, when he sent a medal with the inscription: IMPERATOR ROMANORUM IMPERATORI MEDICORUM.

We change the scene, and this time it opens in the Crimea, after the battle of the Alma, in which the Russians were defeated by the allied troops of France and England, in 1854. You have read of the feats of valor displayed on both sides on that bloody field—the sweeping fire of the artillery, the daring charge of cavalry, the deadly encounter of the columns of infantry, when men met men with bayonets crossed, in the mixed excitement of animal passion, national rivalry, and the thirst for honors and distinction. The names, St. Arnaud and Raglan, the victorious generals, were suddenly sounded, and sung in both hemispheres, and they took at once their places in history. But the real hero, the saviour, not the destroyer, appeared on the day after the battle, unheralded by drum or trumpet, a devoted, and to all appearances a doomed volunteer in the cause of humanity. The allied forces were under the military obligation of advancing rapidly on Sebastopol in pursuit of the retreating Russians, and in doing so to leave 750 of the wounded of the enemy behind them on the field of battle. "Who," to use the words of an English medical journal, "is that single individual who, of all the host that is marching away from the scene of its late triumph, is still to be found upon that blood-stained field? And what is the errand on which he is engaged, thus alone among his enemies, watching the retreating forms of his friends, his countrymen, and gathering up his courage as best he may, to undertake those duties which, in obedience to the dictates of humanity, it had become his duty to perform? This most painful and desolate duty was imposed on himself by Dr. Thomson, of the 44th Regiment, a native of Comarty, in the northern part of Scotland, the birthplace also of Hugh Miller, of the Red Sandstone fame. Provided with some rum, biscuit, and salt meat, he was left with his charge; his only companion a private soldier, acting as his servant. This was indeed a forlorn prospect. Could he escape from the savage assaults of the marauding Cossacks, a party of whom had ruthlessly destroyed a villa not many miles off, on the road to Balaklava, the residence, too, of a Russian country surgeon or physician, who had been obliged to make a hasty retreat? Even the patients themselves, whether under the influence of fever, caused by their wounds, or by mere brutal ferocity, had fired at or stabbed the humane individuals who were then dressing their wounds. Five days, however, did Surgeon Thomson pass in the midst of such a people, whose language was unknown to him, without any companion but his soldier-servant. Often were these two Englishmen obliged to extricate the wounded from beneath the dead before their gashes could be healed, and also to bury the dead because of the pestilential smell arising from the mutilated carcasses. Their scanty supply of food was about to fail them. On the dreaded approach of a swarm of Cossacks, 340 wounded men, who five days previously lay in helpless agony on the ground, walked away with Surgeon Thomson to the shore, and, after overwhelming their deliverer from death with expressions of gratitude, sailed for Odessa. The surgeon himself escaped from the Cossacks, and reached the English head-quarters on the 4th of October, but died of cholera the next day, worn out by the hardships he had undergone. Surely," adds the English journalist, "James Thomson, of the 44th Regiment, has earned a monument, for in his own noble character were united the physician's skill, the soldier's courage, and the Christian's humanity."

Of the strange events by which the present century has been distinguished—long and devastating wars, revolutions, pestilence, and famine—none have been so unexpected and sudden in its inception, and followed by atrocities beyond human belief, and, until then, beyond all that imagination could picture, as the Sepoy mutiny and rebellion in India. The numerous medical officers belonging to the British armies in that country furnished their full quota, not only in their own persons, but in their wives and children, to the victims of that horrible outbreak. They did more: they furnished at one hour a contingent of brave soldiers in battle and siege; and in the next, showed themselves as heroes of humanity, who disregarded danger and fatigue in the exercise of their legitimate vocation—the saving of lives, and the cure of the sick and the maimed. General Whitlock makes honorable

mention of Surgeon Bradley, who attended his wounded under a heavy
fire. The Victoria Cross, the highest reward of the brave, was conferred on Surgeon Antony Dickson Horne, of the 90th Regiment, "for
persevering bravery and admirable conduct in charge of the wounded
men left behind the column, when the troops, under the late Major
General Havelock, forced their way in the Residency of Lucknow, on
September 29th, 1857." The escort left with the wounded were forced
into a house, in which they defended themselves till it was set on fire.
They then retreated to a shed, a few yards from it, and in this place
continued to defend themselves for more than 22 hours, until relieved.
At the last only six men and Mr. Horne remained to fire. Of four
officers, who were with the party, all were badly wounded, and three are
since dead. The conduct of the offence during the latter part of the
time devolved, therefore, on Mr. Horne, and to his active exertions previously to being forced into the house, and his good conduct throughout,
the safety of any of the wounded and the successful defence are
mainly to be attributed. Assistant Surgeon Bradshaw received, also,
the Victoria Cross for acts of bravery of the same date and place, and
as associated with Surgeon Horne in the same gallant services.

In the massacre at Cawnpoor, one of the many terrific scenes by
which the Indian muntiny was marked, a number of medical men fell
victims to the savage fury of the Sepoys. Surgeon Kirk was shot in
the presence of his wife, who pleaded, with true womanly devotion, to
give her life for his. At Cawnpoor the high-tiled roof of the General
Hospital was the only mark open to the enemy, by reason of which
all their guns and mortars were directed against it. An assistant
surgeon, writing from that place after the siege, says: "Three round-
shot passed through my hospital roof, but fortunately, although bringing down plenty of tiles and dirt, no one was injured. Bullets continually pattered against the hospital walls; but all high up, as the
earthworks protected the lower part." During the first of the six days
in which this surgeon was in the intrenchments, he amputated eight
limbs, and dressed more than eighty wounded men, he himself scarcely
knowing night from day, and eating beef and biscuit, and drinking tea
and water, when he could get a chance. The siege of Lucknow by
the rebel Sepoys is full of instances of heroic fortitude and bravery,
in which medical men largely participated, acting the double part, as
occasion called for, of combatants and surgeons. Assistant-Surgeon
Henry Bartram was shot dead at the gate of the Residency, within
a few hundred yards of where his poor wife was expecting him. At

a subsequent date, Dr. Durby died from a gun-shot wound, received in action, in the advance on Lucknow, under Sir Colin Campbell, now Lord Clyde

It was indeed time for the English Government to awake to a sense of the real position and services of the medical staff, in both the military and maritime forces. Intelligent men, not warped in their opinions by the prejudices of routine and old customs, must always have been at a loss to discover any reasonable argument, or even a plausible pretext, for the indignity with which the medical officer was so long treated in both branches of the service, not only in England, but in the United States, by their being refused equivalent rank with other military and naval officers, and the same official privileges as these latter. I will not argue the question at this time, for fear of being betrayed into expressions which might savor of that arrogance for which those in the army and navy, who have opposed the demands of justice to our profession, should be pointedly rebuked. There are military officers, however, of high station and widespread fame, who have learned to appreciate, at their true value, the services of medical men in the public service. Conspicuous among these advocates is Sir de Lacy Evans, than whom no man stands higher in the British Army, for his gallantry, bordering on rashness, his long and brilliant services, and his strategic skill. General Evans made a speech in the House of Commons (June 21st, 1849,) at the conclusion of which, after pointing out the losses that the British troops suffered during the last long war with France, and the hardships and exposures to all the chances of war, including loss of life itself, by medical officers in active service, and of the distinctions and praises awarded to them by Napoleon, he submitted a resolution with a view of affirming:

"That the sanitary efficiency of armies must, in a great measure, depend on the ability, energy, and zeal of the medical officers attached to them.

"That the history of every war proves that this class of officers have been killed, wounded, or made prisoners, the nature of their duties unavoidably exposing them to these casualties.

"And that, as they share in the dangers and fatigues of war, as well as in some of its most essential responsibilities, it is not expedient or just that they should be excluded from a share of honorary distinction or reward, in proportion to their relative rank and the relative importance of their respective services."

General Evans, in the course of his speech, dwelt more particularly on the losses encountered during the Peninsular War. The general result proves, as we learn from him, that during the six years' contest about 500,000 men were successively sent back, restored to efficiency from the hospitals, to resume their duties in the ranks. "Can it be possible," asks the speaker, "to adduce stronger evidence of the weighty and fearful responsibilities, labors, and anxieties which devolved on medical officers in the field? A disciplined soldier, when brought before the enemy, has already cost the State a large sum. However adequate be the original numerical strength provided for a service, the preservation of the lives, health, and efficiency of the troops, so far as within the reach of art, must always, in contests of importance, intimately affect the combinations of the general, the termination of wars, and the national resources. For the adequate execution of such duties, science, courage, energy, and an ardent devotion to the service, must obviously be requisite. Money alone will not suffice for these qualities; a generous and honorable ambition must also be satisfied; but with this a treatment of indignity or contempt is incompatible."

Sir de Lacy Evans stated that, although he was more familiar, of course, with the case of the army medical officers, and that the motion he should submit referred verbally to the military department, yet substantially the cases of both services rest on the same basis.

Let us hope that the American Government will not be backward in placing the medical officers of the army and navy on a permanent footing of rank, nor niggardly in awarding them their proper share of honorary distinction or reward.

Any record of the feats of the benevolent daring which enters so largely into the composition of medical heroism would be incomplete, and want its brightest page, which did not include a notice of a professional brother and a countryman, and yet more, a fellow-citizen—a Philadelphian, whose name and whose fame are now world wide, while his remains rest on the banks of our own Schuylkill. Need I mention Dr. Elisha Kent Kane? His noble deeds, his chivalrous philanthropy, his Christian faith, buoying him up amidst dangers and privations at which the stoutest hearts might have quailed, are too fresh in your memory to require any commemoration of mine. Happily, there is no room for engaging in this pleasing duty, did it even lie more directly in my way, now that the world has the benefit of Dr. Elder's appreciative and well-written volume.

Another passage for the records of Medical Heroism, and I have done:

The name of Howard is everywhere celebrated, and praised in terms of warm gratitude, as the reformer of prison abuses and prison cruelties. It has obtained a place in the history of the world's progress. The name of Pinel is not, I am afraid, familiar, even to the medical world; and it is still less so to the world at large, as that of a physician, who, both by personal services and earnest teaching, brought about a reform in the management and discipline of Asylums for the Insane, which is now spoken of as one of the strongest proofs of advanced civilization. If a proper sympathy and sentiment for humanity and justice have been enlisted by the benevolent Englishman, in what light ought we to regard the services of the equally benevolent Frenchman, who reminded men of their duties to the Providence-stricken, but irresponsible insane? Excuse might be found for vindictive harshness to the criminal who has made war on society; but where is the extenuation for more deliberate cruelty, practiced so long and so generally on those unfortunate beings, bereft of their reason, many of whom, but a short time before, were the delight of the social circle, and cherished members of the family?

When we think of the old Bedlams and Hospitals for the Insane, in which not only the raving maniac, but the melancholy monomaniac was confined, and in which the only sounds were those of the clanging chain, the echoing lash, and the mingled cries and vociferations of the brutal keepers and the infuriated inmates; and then look abroad over the better portions of the civilized world, including our own favored land, and see the many noble edifices erected for the reception and treatment of this class of our unfortunate fellow-beings, we feel that we live in an age not only of progress, but of real improvement; one in which humanizing influences are more active and diffused than they ever were before. The contrast between the present and the past in this particular, while it should prompt all to the liveliest manifestations of gratitude, ought, undoubtedly, to find a place in general history, in which proper credit would be awarded to our profession, so many members of which have imitated, in their official position as medical superintendents of Insane Asylums, the noble example set by Pinel at the Bicêtre and the Salpétrière.

That was indeed a critical moment in the life of Pinel, and in the history of benevolent trials for the mitigation of human suffering, when Pinel resolved to test the correctness of his principles of non-restraint, by holding direct personal intercourse with a violent maniac, whose chains and fetters he had previously directed to be removed.

The trial was entirely successful. After an eager gaze and a movement, as if preparatory to a tiger-like spring on his visitor, who had
just entered his cell, the unfortunate being saw eyes looking at him
with kindness, and placid features, expressing benignity and good-
will. Soon his own countenance underwent a change; the mere brute
was once again a human being; and when the tones of affectionate
inquiry reached his ear, and the hand of greeting was extended towards him, he could only answer and reciprocate by shedding tears,
the fountains of which had long been dried up by the fiery furnace of
maddened feelings, wrought to fury by angry menace and brutal punishment. From this moment the cure of the poor maniac, which had
been before regarded as hopeless, was begun, and terminated in entire
restoration to health and reason.

After the inquiring visitor has been taken through a modern Lunatic Asylum, and traversed its spacious corridors, and looked into the
neat and cheerful dormitories, and is then taken to the Saloon and
the Lecture-room, and the rooms for social meetings and amusements,
and is then shown, out of doors, the extensive grounds for exercise
and recreation, all under the direction of the medical superintendent,
the presiding genius of the place, he gives utterance to his conviction
by exclaiming: "After all, madness is not so dreadful an infliction,
when it is met, controlled, and so often conquered by the harmonious
union of medical science, philanthropic vigilance and ingenuity, and, at
fitting times, the soothing balm of religious counsel and exhortation."

In the vestibule of every modern Lunatic Asylum, the visitor might
naturally expect to see a statue of Pinel, unless he should think at the
moment of the inscription on St. Paul's Cathedral, London, in allusion to its celebrated architect, Sir Christopher Wren: "If you ask
for a monument, look around you."

May I ask you to indulge me while making a few remarks in connection with the name of Pinel? We hear a great deal in these days
of specialties, and of the necessity of a physician or surgeon, as the
case may be, devoting himself to the study and practice of a particular branch, if he looks to doing the most good to others, and the most
benefiting himself, in a pecuniary point of view. Without engaging in a discussion of the question, I feel myself authorized to assert,
that a specialty ought, like the shaft and capital of a column in a building, to rest on an enduring and highly finished support, such as would
allow of our raising on it the final and more distinctive part in a
great variety of styles. Thus, for instance, as the atticurgic base is

the favorite one in architecture for columns of the Ionic, Corinthian, and Composite orders, so ought an accurate knowledge of the several parts of medical science, at least of their essential features, be the base for raising on it a specialty. Wanting this support, the practicer of any specialty is reduced to the level of a small literary artisan, who is unable to see the application of a general law, or the relations of his branch to the other branches of science. It is an exceedingly equivocal compliment, something like the knocking a man down with a hearty slap on the back as a friendly salutation, to say of a physician he is a good doctor, or he is famous for .curing diseases of the eye or the ear, but he is ignorant of everything else. Not in such language dare men speak of those distinguished members of our profession, who were accomplished scholars in general literature and science, and at the same time rich in medical lore, and ready with all the resources of medical practice.

Of this number was Pinel. Soon after his arrival in Paris from Montpelier, where, and at Toulouse, he had prosecuted his medical studies, he became a contributor to the *Journal of Paris*, and wrote on medicine, natural philosophy, moral philosophy, and political economy. His attention was also directed to anatomy and surgery, on which he wrote interesting papers. A little later we find him contributing to the *Encyclopédie Méthodique*, translating Cullen, and editing Baglivi. He was not content with being a teacher in these ways; he was also a learner, still adding to his stores of knowledge, by attending the lectures of his friend, Desfontaines, on Botany, and of D'Arcet and Fourcroy on Chemistry.

Was the mind of Pinel distracted by these various studies and labors? Did he continue to be a mere man of books, a book-worm, unfitted to make a direct and practical application of his powers and attainments to higher purposes, or, at any rate, to some useful specialty? Let not your men of mere facts without method, and of observation without reflection, triumph in anticipation of such a result. Pinel had undergone an intellectual training which fitted him for the active discharge of the most responsible duties, just as gymnastic exercises and field sports prepare a man to endure the fatigues of a campaign, and to win honors by his courage and presence of mind in the hour of battle.

When a man is thus trained, as Pinel was, by prolonged, and at the same time various study, a slight circumstance will give direction and application to his future labors. Grief for the loss of a dear

23

young friend, who wandered into the woods in a fit of mental derangement, and was torn to pieces by wolves, fixed the attention of Pinel
on the subject of insanity; and to its elucidation, and the treatment of
those suffering under this dread malady, he devoted the best part of
his subsequent life.

Here we may be allowed to pause for a moment, and ask, whether
Pinel would have been better prepared for the discharge of his duties
as superintendent of an insane asylum, by his having spent the years
of his noviciate in a similar institution, and become wedded to a routine
of hardships and cruelty to the inmates, in ignorance of mind, except
in its deformities, than by the prior exercise of all his intellectual
faculties in the manner already pointed out. The answer might, I
think, be left with a jury of practical, which most of the time means
practicing physicians, even though they may have had only a slight
sprinkling of human letters, and a very elementary knowledge of the
philosophy of mind. But Pinel's labors and learning were spread
over a wide field of medical science. For many years his *Nosographie
Philosophique* was the standard work in France on Pathology and
Therapeutics. In its perusal Bichat found some of the germs of his
doctrine and division of the tissues, which were expanded into their
full measure and harmonious proportions in his celebrated " General
Anatomy." Pinel's Treatise on Mental Alienation was of a subse.
quent date. In addition to the merits of this work in its facts and
lucid arrangement, it is pervaded by a vein of pure morality, full of
valuable suggestions to parents and teachers for the guidance of youth,
and for protecting them against temptations which, if yielded to, un-
seat Reason from her throne.

OSTEO-ANEURISM OF THE PELVIS.

Case of Ligature of the Right Primitive Iliac Artery.

Taken from the Minutes of the Medico-Chirurgical Society of German Physicians in New York.

F. H., born in Germany, 59 years of age, workingman in a jewelry
shop in Newark, applied last June, 1857, for relief, on account of a
painful and pulsating tumor in the right hip and inguinal region, that
prevented him from walking. He states that he never suffered under
any serious disease, with the exception of a syphilitic ulceration of the
penis about nine years ago, not followed by secondary symptoms. In
regard to the previous history of the present disease his statements

were very vague. He says that since the last two years, he felt great pain from the right groin downward to the knee. On applying for medical aid, various liniments and electricity were recommended to him, his disease being considered as a rheumatic affection. A year ago he noticed a swelling in the groin, and was treated for inflammation of the inguinal glands. Since that time he could only walk with a stick. Last December, (1856,) he fell in his room on the right hip, and since then he could not support himself on his right leg, and had to use a pair of crutches. A week ago, in stepping out of a bathing-tub, he made a misstep, and was then entirely unable to make use of his right foot, or even to move it.

When I saw the patient, in the latter part of June, 1857, he was lying on his left side; both thighs were flexed, and he could not extend his right lower extremity. On turning the patient on his back, I found apparent shortening of the right leg, and a pulsating tumor in the right iliac fossa, and over the right hip. On account of the great pain suffered at the examination of this tumor, I preferred to put the patient under chloroform the following day. I then found shortening of the right lower extremity, the trochanter nearer to the anterior spinous process than it was on the left side, and crepitus could be very distinctly felt, and heard over the trochanter. The right iliac fossa was entirely filled by a large, somewhat yielding, pulsating tumor, over which the pulsation of the external iliac artery could be traced. The hip from the crest of the ileum down to the fold of the nates, and from Poupart's ligament across to the os sacrum, was much enlarged in all its dimensions. This enlargement of the hip, compared with the left hip, amounted to nearly two inches in its different circumferences; passing a string from the anterior spinous process round the tuber ischii up to the posterior spinous process, from the middle portion of Poupart's ligament horizontally to the os sacrum, and so forth. The hip, on being pressed firmly, was found to be very painful at various points, particularly at the external surface of the os ileum. The swelling had nowhere a definite boundary. The rest of the ileum could be traced distinctly, but was twice as large as in the normal condition, its internal border passing over to the tumor in the iliac fossa. At some points over the external surface of the os ileum, some, but very obscure, fluctuation was perceptible, but the elasticity felt over the ischiatic notch was very distinct. The skin over the enlarged hip was everywhere movable, of normal appearance, and only on the anterior part of the ileum some superficial veins were discernible. On firm pressure in the iliac fossa, the finger resting on the external surface of the os ileum was raised up. The most prominent feature of this swelling was its pulsation, synchronous with the beat of the heart. This pulsation was very strong from Poupart's ligament and the iliac fossa externally in all dimensions of the os ileum, and from the crest of the os ileum downward to the tuber ischii. To the same extent these pulsations were distinctly apparent to the sight at every systole of the heart. When the hand was laid flat over the ischiatic notch a sort of friction would be felt, as if some liquid, pushed against a rough and hard substance, was slowly rolling under the hand; yet this friction was not always very distinct. On applying the ear or stethoscope, there was, synchronous with the heart's systole, a loud bellows-sound in the whole tumor, the most marked over the ischiatic notch; at one time there was perceptible at the same point a filing sound. The femoral artery could be felt below Poupart's ligament, and the external iliac traced some way up over the tumor in the iliac fossa, as these arteries had a stronger pulsation than the tumor in the iliac fossa. Pressure over the iliac artery, as high up as possible, diminished the bellows-sound, but did not cause it to disappear entirely; pressure over the femoral artery, a little below Poupart's ligament, increased the bellows-sound. The form of the whole hip appeared the more abnormal in consequence of the thigh being emaciated. The temperature of the right lower extremity was lower than that of the left. The heart on, examination, showed nothing abnormal; the appetite was good, patient slept well, and complained only of a sensation of formication in the diseased hip.

The diagnosis of this case presented some difficulties. In the first place, there was fracture of the neck of the femur, which dated probably from the last week, when the false step from the bathing-tub had occurred.

In regard to the pulsating tumor, there were different pathological conditions to which the apparent symptoms could be ascribed. The first idea was, that there existed an encephaloid tumor in the pelvis, or in the walls of the os ileum, the pulsations of which were produced by the large arteries of the pelvis. Opposed to this view, there were the resistance, and want of softness of the swelling, the great intensity of the bellows, and the occasional filing sound. The physical phenomenon of the friction, which was felt by the hand, could only be produced by a liquid forced by the action of the heart over a rough and unyielding surface. All the last-mentioned symptoms indicated decidedly an aneurism, and the next question arose as to what arteries were involved. The presumption that vessels of the second or third order were the seat of the aneurism was excluded, on account of the enormous circumference of the tumor. The vessels next in question were the external, the internal, or the primitive iliac artery. The external could be traced up a long way in the iliac fossa, and an aneurism of that vessel would probably have had its greatest development in the iliac fossa. Opposed to the supposition of an aneurism of the internal or primitive artery was the fact of its first appearance in the inguinal region, and the great circumference of the tumor, involving the whole right pelvis and hip, even below Poupart's ligament. From the circumstance that all the osseous portions of the right pelvis, and even the head of the femur, were involved, I was led to presume an aneurism of the nutritive vessels of the bones of the pelvis, although the charateristic parchment-like rattle of the broken-up osseous lamina could not be distinguished, on account of the great thickness of the soft tissues which covered them. But there was already a perforation of the os ileum proved by the fact above mentioned, that on firm pressure in the iliac fossa the finger resting on the external surface of the os ileum was raised up. I proposed to tie the primitive iliac artery, in case it should be found, during the operation, that the disease was confined neither to the external nor internal iliac, as this was the only means of cutting off the supply of blood to the bones of the pelvis, since the nutritive vessels come both from the internal and external iliac artery, i. e., the ileo-lumbar, the circumflex artery of the ileum, etc.

The process of such an operation was certainly very doubtful, particularly on account of the difficulty with which the collateral circulation would be kept up, (the collateral arteries being: the mammaria with the epigastria, the sacralis media with the sacralis lateralis, the lumbares with the ileo-lumbalis, and finally branches of the internal iliac artery of right side with the branches of the same vessel of the left side.) I could not rely much upon the development of that collateral circulation; but as it appeared that in no other way than by such an operation the further destruction of the parts involved could be prevented, I thought it justifiable to give the patient this, his only chance of saving his life. The case was fully stated to the patient, and he then very willingly submitted to the operation. The 15th of July, 1857, was the day fixed for the operation. Drs. Tellkampf, Gurdon Buck, Jones, Lee, and other medical gentlemen, were present, and very kindly assisted me. The patient was laid on a table, and brought under the influence of chloroform. An incision was made somewhat obliquely from about two fingers' breadth above and within the anterior spinous process, terminating half an inch above the middle of Poupart's ligament. After dividing the fascia superficialis and the internal oblique muscle, the fascia transversalis was cut into, and the peritoneum a little detached at the inferior angle of the incision. Then the third muscular layers of the upper portion of the incision were dissected, and the peritoneum detached from the iliac fascia, which required some care, as there were cord-like adhesions between these two tissues. The external iliac was found making a great curve, with its convexity towards the pelvis. On turning the patient towards his left side, the peritoneum was kept back by a broad hook, and it was necessary to dilate the upper angle of the incision, for the purpose of bringing to view the biformation of the primitive iliac artery. Nothing abnormal could be found on the internal iliac artery. By compression of this artery, as well as of the external iliac artery, and by the stethoscope applied at the same time over the hip, it was found that the pulsation of the tumor and the intensity of the bellows-sound were diminished, but could not be made to disappear entirely. The compression of the primitive iliac artery, however, caused both those indications to disappear. This seemed to justify the ligature of this latter vessel. The sheath of the vessel was opened and separated, the corresponding primitive iliac vein was lying just below the artery, and with the aid of an obliquely bent aneurism-needle carried under the vessel from its external side, the artery was tied about three-fourths of an inch above the bifurcation. The patient expressed a great deal of pain at the moment of tying the knot. Immediately after, not only the pulsations in the tumor ceased entirely, but the swelling of the whole hip diminished to about half its former circumference, and had the feel of an empty bag. Patient had, during the operation, lost not more than about an ounce of blood. The wound was united by ten sutures, and the thigh afterwards supported by a double-inclined plane.

Extract from my journal:

Evening.—Patient feels pretty comfortable; pulse 95; temperature of the right leg lower than that of the left.

16th.—Slept well; pulse 100; tongue moist; some bloody discharge from the wound; bluish appearance of the leg and foot; complete loss of sensation of the leg, which was cooler than the left, but the upper portion of the right thigh felt warmer than the corresponding portion of the left.

17th.—Slight tympanitic swelling of the abdomen; pulse 100, hard; patient complains of thirst, and is in a profuse perspiration; bluish discoloration on separate spots of the thigh; complete loss of sensation of the lower third of the thigh; no pulsation of any artery of the limb could be detected.

Evening.—Patient is very quiet; the borders of the wound show an erysipelatous redness; some discoloration at the lower angle of the wound, where the epidermis was raised.

18th.—Slept well; pulse 110; discoloration increasing; sensation limited to the upper third of the thigh; serous liquid discharged abundantly from the lower half of the wound; the abdomen somewhat tympanitic, but without pain.

Evening.—Pulse 120; temperature of the whole extremity higher than yesterday.

19th.—The lower half of the wound darkly discolored; the neighboring tissues around the wound red, hard, inflamed; discoloration of the thigh increasing; the toes and sole of the foot black; sensation only at the upper third of the thigh.

20th.—Pulse 100, soft; tongue moist; the lower half of the wound gangrenous; fœtid discharge; the right leg and thigh give the hand applied to it a hot, burning sensation. On the outer aspect of the leg is a large gangrenous spot, with crepitus, (emphysema.)

21st.—Sleeping, with a tendency to stupor, but is easily aroused; his look is dull; voice harsh; pulse 90, feeble; cold sweats; some dysuria towards evening; borders of the wound gangrenous; gangrene is increasing on the leg, only the popliteal space and a portion above the patella being free from it; toes and foot exhibited a dry gangrenous condition, which we might call mummification; temperature of the leg lower than on the two previous days, although the thermometer gave 94° in the popliteal space, and only 92° in the corresponding place of the left extremity, 95° at the upper third of the right thigh, 92 at the same place on the left thigh, 89° at the instep of the right foot. I am sorry that I did not before test the temperature by the thermometer; the right leg would have doubtless by this instrument shown a higher degree of heat than the left one.

22d.—Although the gangrene was increasing, patient seems to feel better; pulse 108, stronger; his voice, his look, more natural; secretion from the wound very copious and fœtid.

23d.—Patient is again falling back to a state of stupor; gangrene extends to the hip, but just below Poupart's ligament is a line of demarcation to the extent of two inches; no change in the aspect of the wound.

24th.—Patient talks incoherently; pulse 120; the circumscribed line of demarcation continues.

25th.—Patient dozes continually; deglutition difficult; the size of the limb has much increased; emphysematous crepitus all over the leg.

26th —The same condition.

27th.—Died in the morning, at 5 o'clock.

Autopsy seven hours after death.—The whole right extremity up to Poupart's ligament and above the trochanter major was destroyed by gangrene. There was circumscribed recent peritonitis in the neighborhood of the wound only, and slight adhesions between the intestines. The ligature was yet firmly attached, and above it was a strong and firm thrombus. The large arteries of the pelvis in a normal condition; some of the veins of the pelvis, for instance, the obturator vein, extremely enlarged. Some of the smaller branches of these arteries could not be followed up, on account of the gangrenous destruction, and others were finally lost in a spongy or cavernous tissue, which constituted the principal portions of the morbid structure. At a point over the ischiatic notch a branch of the ischiatic artery could be traced up in entering in one of the ducts, met with in the above-mentioned spongy tissue, which I will hereafter describe. Following the arteries within the tumor, they led into small ducts of the cavernous tissue, of the size of very small arteries, partly communicating one with another, resembling enlarged capillaries, partly giving off branches, which increased gradually in size, and would finally be lost in some larger cavities or alveoli. The interior of these ducts contained mostly coagulated blood, the removal of which caused them to become flattened. The internal surface was perfectly smooth; the external surface was entirely grown together with the surrounding tissue. These ducts were traced within a cellulo-fibrous tissue of new formations. Separate membranes could not be distinguished. The ducts, together with the alveoli or cavities and the cellulo-fibrous tissue, constituted the spongy or cavernous tissue.

The external portions of the tumor of the pelvis, covered by thickened periosteum, was of this spongy tissue. After removing the right half of the pelvis, together with a portion of the os sacrum and of the femur below the trochanter, it was found that this portion of the pelvis was completely involved in the disease. Both rami of the os pubis and os ischii consisted partly of the residui of the original bony tissue, but mostly of the above-mentioned cavernous tissue of new formation, in which were imbedded a great number of loose bones, pointed, rough, and perforated by small openings. Instead of the acetabulum were also only a few bony residui. To one of these was attached the ligamentum teres. This ligament had also retained its natural attachment to the head of the femur. The cartilaginous covering of the head of the femur was destroyed, and the head itself converted into a mere shell, with a few bony partitions. The neck of the femur was gone, the thickened periosteum only remaining. The spongy portion of the femur below the trochanter was hyperæmic, reddish and softened, so that a probe could easily penetrate. The os ileum was expanded, and the crest of this bone thickened. The external surface could be cut into by a knife, and consisted principally of thickened periosteum here and there, in a state of ossification. Two or three incisions brought to view a number of alveoli and cavities from the size of a pea to that of a walnut, which communicated with each other in a labyrinthic form. These cavities contained dark blood and firm fibrinous coagula at the bottom. An incision of the internal surface, in the region of the iliac fossa, showed the same pathologic condition as that of the outer portion of the os ileum, i. e., firm fibrous covering, ossified at different points, and four or five cavities larger than those of the external surface. These cavities were also filled with blood, separated by membranous partitions, containing bones of new formation of various forms, and communicated through others with the cavities of the external portion of the os ileum. The partition-walls between the cavities consisted partially of osseous lamina, terminating in very thin, flexible points, which, under the microscope, presented the usual bone-corpuscles.

Some portions of the soft tissue, particularly the alveoli, in which the bone-spiculæ were imbedded, were of a brown-yellowish color and gelatinous appearance. When brought under the microscope, it consisted of fatty substance and contained margarin-crystals. The so-called cancer-cells existed nowhere. The larger cavities contained fluid fat and fat-cells. The loose cellular tissue contained some small conglomerated cysts, also filled with fatty substance and margarin-crystals. Gangrene had proceeded so far as to prevent a more minute examination. No permission was given to make a further dissection of the body.

Remarks.—According to the foregoing statements, it is evident that my diagnosis was a correct one, and that the disease was the so-called osteo-aneurism, or *tumeur pulsative des os*, according to the French authors. I found a new structure in the bones, consisting of fibro-cellular tissue, as stroma for newly-formed ducts, tubuli, alveoli, and cavities; these alveoli containing fluid fat, fat-cells, and margarin-crystals. At some points arteries could be traced up to where they were entering into ducts and alveoli. Thus we have a similar condition here as we find in the erectile tumor of the soft tissues. I say a similar condition, since another distinction is to be made between the ordinary erectile tumor, (enlargement of the capillaries,) and the pulsating tumor in this case; as here I found a newly-formed structure, arranged in a similar way as the corpora cavernosa penis, and therefore called by German pathologists cavernous tumor.[*]

The pulsating tumor of the bones is a very rare disease, the principal seat of which is one of the epiphyses of the long bones, particularly the head of the femur. Some authors of the greatest reputation, as Dupuytren, have strongly sustained the opinion that in all cases of pulsating tumor of the bones there was encephaloid disease.

Breschet, Chelius, and others, maintain that in many of such cases there exists in the bones a somewhat similar pathologic process as in the erectile tumors of the soft tissues. It is only since the last six or eight years that, by the investigations of Rokitansky, Schuh, Virchow, and Robin,[†] the nature of the cavernous tumor has been studied. The ordinary erectile tumor and the teleangiectasis is an enlargement and increase in number of the capillaries; but in this case the tumor consisted of a newly-formed fibro-cellular stroma of a particular arrangement, with newly-formed ducts and alveoli containing blood, and therefore called, with great propriety, the cavernous tumor. Schuh, of Vienna, gives a very full description of the disease, points out its various forms, and the difference between it and the ordinary erectile tumor, and is of opinion that all the differences in the various forms of the cavernous tumor are principally owing to the various stages of development through which they have to pass. According to Schuh, the most common seat of the cavernous tumor in the soft tissues is the liver; then follow the lungs, the pia mater, and lastly the sub-cutaneous cellular tissue. It has a similar appearance as the ordinary erectile tumor, but grows more slowly. He considers it to be

---

[*] Rokitansky. pathologische Anatomie dritte Auflage, erster Band, page 191, etc.

Schuh.—Pseudoplasmen. Wien, 1854, page 164, etc.

[†] Ch. Robin, Mémoire sur l'Anatomie des Tumeurs érectiles, (lu à la Société de Biologie.) Gaz. Méd., 1854, pp. 22 et 23.

of a benign character. In the bones it is found in the head of the tibia, in the bones of the skull and of the pelvis. He mentions that he had seen it in one case only in the bones of the skull, originating from the diploe. Although many investigations are yet to be made before the nature of this morbid structure will be definitely and fully understood, yet I think that, by the publication of this case, I have somewhat contributed to show that there exists a pulsating tumor of the bones, which is not encephaloid, and presents a similar structure as the erectile tumor, i. e., is the cavernous tumor in the bones so called by Rokitansky, Schuh, and others.　　　　C. TH. MEIER, M.D.,

Surgeon to the Bellevue Hospital.

REPLY OF DR. CLOSE TO DR. PLATT.

EDITOR OF THE AMERICAN MEDICAL GAZETTE :

Dear Sir—Please permit me, through your columns, to reply to Dr. E. Platt, of Rhinebeck, who, in noticing my article on the treatment of fever, in your March No., seems to think my doses dangerously large; and notwithstanding my assurance that they have always proved safe in my hands, says, " he must prefer his own experience and observations to those of another, let that person be who he may." Dr. Platt is certainly right in this, but at the same time he will doubtless accord to me the same privilege of judging of the effect of remedies by my own careful observation. The veratrum that I have used has always been that put up by the New Lebanon Co., and seems very uniform in strength; but from the fact of its having required in my hands rather larger doses than those prescribed by Dr. Norwood— from whose notice of the article I was first induced to try it—I came to the conclusion that the root from which I had prepared my tincture was probably not as strong as that from which Dr. N. made his. This may in part, perhaps, account for the discrepancy between us, but the fact that Dr. Platt's doses were larger than mine is probably the principal cause of the difference of results. I have never prescribed over three drops of veratrum at a dose as a febrifuge, and rarely more than two; and these doses, to prevent vomiting, have often been accompanied by a drop or two of morphine. Dr. Platt's doses, he informs us, were four and five drops, and it is precisely because such doses cannot usually be borne alone without vomiting, and other distressing symptoms, that I have placed my principal reliance on digitalis as the means of restraining the force and frequency of the pulse in fevers.

Sulphate morphine, (15 grs. to ℥i.,) given drop for drop with veratrum, completely controls its nauseating effect, but does not in the least diminish its effect upon the pulse; and morphine is probably the best means of counteracting the effect of over-doses. And here I beg most truly and solemnly to assure Dr. Platt that, during the period of nine or ten years in which I have been treating fevers with these remedies, I have never met with one instance where any effects were produced causing the slightest alarm to myself or to the families of the sick. I have always been on the look-out for some over-action, and perhaps the reason why I have never met with any is because I have never used the remedies singly, but always in combination, placing my principal reliance upon digitalis, and giving the other articles in doses too small to cause any special disturbance.

With the word "Bradycrote" I am not better pleased than Dr. Platt seems to be; but finding it used by Southern and Western physicians in the sense of a shortening method of treating fever, I adopted it for want of a better. Drs. White and Ford, of Charleston, addressed a communication, the last year and the year before, to the Charleston *Medical Journal and Review*, the one headed, " Bradycrote Treatment of Yellow Fever by Veratrum Viride," and the other, "Bradycrote Treatment of Yellow Fever by Gelseminum Sempervivens." In both cases they claim for these remedies the effect of not only curtailing the duration of the fever, but of rendering it much milder, and very much less fatal; and the statistics they adduce fully sustain their claim.

Any country physician who may desire to give the sedative remedies a trial, I should advise to furnish himself with a percolator, which can be made at any tin-shop, and he will then be enabled to make his own tinctures in the most speedy and perfect manner. It will be important that the digitalis should be the kind imported from England in glass jars, as it is nearly twice as strong as the leaf, gathered and put up in the ordinary way in papers. With the percolator, a perfectly saturated alcoholic tincture can be made in twenty-four hours, by drawing off and pouring back several times.

THOMAS CLOSE.

PORTCHESTER, *Westchester Co., April 12th*, 1859.

New Medical College in Chicago, Ill.

DR. REESE :   CHICAGO, *March 18th*, 1859.

Dear Sir —As some changes have taken place in professional matters in this city of more or less general interest, I have thought it not improper to give you a correct account of them. Prof. N. S. Davis and Prof. W. H Byford have just resigned the chairs they occupied in *Rush Medical College*, and have accepted the same chairs respectively in a new institution organized in this city. The movement has *not* originated in any *quarrel* among the old school; but Dr. Brainard insisted on adhering to the old routine of college instruction, consisting of *sixteen weeks* lecturing on all the branches of medicine heterogeneously; while Drs. Davis and Byford were in favor of material changes. In the mean time, the Lind University, of this city, offered to a competent medical faculty all the necessary accommodations for a medical department, to be organized on just such a plan as might be desired, and it was thought that the true interests of the profession would be subserved by accepting the offer. The plan they have adopted embraces an annual college term of five months, with twelve professorships, divided into a *junior* and *senior* department The first 'includes the chairs of, 1st. Elementary and Inorganic Chemistry; 2d. Descriptive Anatomy ; 3d. Physiology and Histology; 4th. Pathology and Public Hygiene; 5th. Materia Medica. Also, Dissections, under direction of a demonstrator.

. The second, or senior department, embraces the chairs of, 1st. Surgical Anatomy; 2d. Organic Chemistry and Toxicology; 3d. Practical Medicine; 4th. Surgery; 5th. Obstetrics and Diseases of Women; 6th. Medical Jurisprudence; 7th. Clinical Medicine and Surgery.

Students attending their first course will be expected to take the tickets of the junior department only; while those attending their second course will take only those of the senior department. And all who can be induced to attend a third course will be permitted to select such branches from both departments as they may deem most necessary. The student may thus keep his attention restricted to such limited number of branches as is adapted to his stage of advancement, and make his two courses of college attendance progressive in their natural order, instead of repetitional and herterogeneous. The continued connection of Professors Davis and Byford with the Mercy Hospital will give ample facilities for *clinical instruction;* and it is believed that this new College will mark a *new era* in the system of

... . :n our country. The following named gentlemen
. ..... accepted appointments in the faculty, viz.:

   i. Hollister, M.D., Prof. of Descriptive Anatomy.
   t. L. Johnson, M.D., Prof. of Physiology and Histology.
   ...... Andrews, M.D., Prof. of Surgery and Clinical Surgery.
   '.. N. Isham, M.D., Prof. of Surgical Anatomy.
   W. H. Byford, M.D., Prof. of Obstetrics and Diseases of Women.
   N. S. Davis, M.D., Prof. of Principle and Practice of Medicine,
and Clinical Medicine.

The remaining chairs will be filled, and everything in readiness for
the first term, to commence on the second Monday in October next.

                                               R.

SELECTIONS.

DR. HENRY G. CLARK VERSUS LONDON "LANCET."

Extracts from the Records of the Boston Society for Medical Improvement.

By F. E. OLIVER, M.D., Secretary.

June 28th.—*Execution of Magee. Post-mortem Appearances.* Reported by Dr. HENRY G. CLARK.

The prisoner, Magee, was a healthy and very muscular man, but
of small stature, and weighing about 130 pounds. Age, 28 years.
He was executed in the rotunda of the Jail, at 10 o'clock, June 25th.
He was dropped a distance of from seven to eight feet. There was
not the least perceptible struggle or convulsion, but the urine was
passed immediately. At the end of seven minutes, all the sounds of
the heart were distinctly audible, and the number of beats 100 in the
minute. At nine minutes, the number was 98. At the end of twelve
minutes, the number was 60, and the pulsations fainter. At fourteen
minutes, the sounds had disappeared.

The body was lowered at 25 minutes past 10, at which time a careful examination of the chest revealed no perceptible sound or impulse
of the heart. A small space under the left ear seemed to have escaped active compression, so that some circulation might have been
continued through the carotid and jugular of that side.

The face was purple, and the pupils dilated, but there was no protrusion either of the eyes or tongue. The cord had taken just above
the thyroid cartilage, and had left a deep oblique wale or indenture.

along its whole course, excepting at the part before mentioned, the knot, which was over the mastoid, having lifted it off from this point.

At 10.40 the cord, and the straps with which he had been pinioned, were removed. After this, the body, the face especially, became gradually paler.

At a few minutes past 11, Dr. Ellis commenced the autopsy, at the House of Reception. The body was pale, and the skin mottled. A small ecchymosis was noticed just above the line of the cord on the right side. The right sterno-cleido muscle was ruptured through one-half of its thickness. No lesion was discovered in any of the other soft parts of the neck. The os-hyoides was somewhat broken, but the spine was entirely uninjured. Dr. Shaw examined the clothing, to determine the presence of semen, but none was found.

At 11.30, a slight but irregular pulsatory movement was observed in the right subclavian vein. Upon applying the ear to the chest, this was ascertained to proceed from the heart itself, which gave a distinct and regular *single* beat, with a slight impulse, 80 times in a minute. The chest was then opened, and the heart exposed, without in any way arresting the pulsatory movements. The right auricle was in full and regular motion, contracting and dilating with beautiful distinctness and energy. At 12 o'clock, the spinal cord having been previously divided, the number of contractions was 40 per minute, having continued with only a short intermission regularly up to this time. Dr. Ellis furnishes the notes of his own and Mr. Tower's minutes after this hour.

" The peculiar movements of the anterior wall of the right auricle gradually but occasionally recurred, either spontaneously, or excited by a passing current of air, until 1¾ o'clock. They could at any moment be excited by the point of the scalpel."

Dr. Ellis being obliged to leave at this time, the remainder of the record concerning the heart was furnished by Mr. Tower, one of the medical house pupils of the hospital. It is as follows:

" At 1.45, the movements still continued, without stimulus. Five were noticed in a minute, with corresponding intervals. At 2.45, all automatic movements ceased, but the part still responded to the stimulus of the knife. At 3.10, deep irritation of the same kind was followed by slight movements. The irritability was most marked at the lower part, where the venæ cavæ enter the auricle. At 3.18, all movements ceased. On opening the heart, it was found to be perfectly normal. The left ventricle was contracted; the right, not. No coagula were found."

Brain healthy.

Both lungs collapsed completely, and were in every respect normal.

The liver and spleen were darker colored than usual, owing to the presence of an unusual amount of blood.

The stomach contained a whitish pulp, like softened bread. The mucous membrane had a pinkish tinge, particularly in the neighborhood of the pylorus. In the large extremity, for some distance below the cardiac orifice, were numerous whitish glandulæ, about a line in diameter.

The upper part of the small intestine contained much green, bilious fluid. The mucous membrane was of a pinkish color. Peyer's patches were very distinct. No lacteals were seen.

The other organs were examined, and found healthy.

Dr. Jackson asked if any motion of the intestines was observed—to which Dr. Ellis replied in the negative. Dr. J. alluded to the case of a tumor removed from the shoulder, some fibres of muscle attached to which contracted under the stimulus of the knife, some time after its removal. He also alluded to the muscular contractions which were manifest after death in many cases of cholera, during the epidemic of 1833.

The absence of cerebral congestion, Dr. Gay thought probably due to the adjustment of the rope, which allowed circulation in the left carotid. He thought death might have been owing to the sudden shock.

Dr. Clark alluded to the three modes in which death takes place by hanging, viz: apoplexy, asphyxia, and fracture of the spine, and attributed death in the present instance to asphyxia.

Dr. Ainsworth remarked, that all the appearances usually observed in cases of hanging were here wanting, and thought that the first effect of the sudden fall was a powerful concussion of the brain, which paralysed the body, as in cases where a blow or fall is received upon the extremity of the sacrum, and that death occurred afterwards from strangulation.

Dr. H. J. Bigelow considered the motions of the heart to be solely due to local irritability.

Dr. Clark, in this connection, alluded to the unfortunate incident in the life of the celebrated Vesalius in consequence of which he was banished from his country and died in exile. Not allowing a sufficient time to elapse after the death of his patient before proceeding to the examination, the muscular irritability remaining in the body caused a pulsatory movement in the heart, which led to his arrest and punishment for murder and impiety.

Dr. Clark expressed the opinion that, as there was no lesion of any important organ, resuscitation might possibly have been accomplished by artificial respiration, &c., if efforts to that end had been made immediately upon the lowering of the body from the scaffold—that is, within half an hour after he fell. Strong shocks of electricity or galvanism would, in cases of accidental apparent death, destroy the little remaining vitality; and if these agents are used at all, they should be administered with great care.

The following is the article referred to, which is copied from the *London Lancet* for August 28, 1858, p. 230, and is entitled

"AN EXECUTION IN THE HOUSE."

" A thief unhung is a sorry sight for honest men; but we know no spectacle more painful than an execution in the house of a medical man.* An eager zeal for physiological science has more than once betrayed anatomists into positions of painful dubiety; but we have never seen a more equivocal recital than that which has this week gone the rounds of the newspapers touching the proceedings of some American surgeons in the examination of a criminal who had been delivered into the hands of the hangman, and upon whom they subsequently performed what would appear to be little less than a vivisection." "The appetite for hoaxes is so strong in America, that it might, perhaps, be hoped that some deception was practiced in this instance; but the details are given with scientific truthfulness and accuracy."

Here follow the only passages which the *Lancet* has copied from the report, and which are reprinted to show how ingeniously an extract, apparently fairly made, may be unfairly used.

"At half past eleven, a slight but regular pulsatory movement was observed in the right subclavian vein. Upon applying the ear to the chest, this was ascertained to proceed from the heart itself, *which gave a distinct and regular single beat, with a slight impulse, eighty times a minute.* The chest was then opened, and the heart exposed, without in any way arresting the pulsatory movements. The

[* The *insinuation* is, that the autopsy was done *privately*, or *surreptitiously*.—o.]

right auricle was in full and regular motion, contracting and dilating with beautiful distinctness and energy. At twelve o'clock, the spinal cord having been previously divided, the contractions were forty per minute, having continued with only a short intermission regularly up to that time."

The *italics* are *not* those of the report.

"Finally," the *Lancet* says, "in the discussion that ensued, Dr. Clark expressed the opinion," &c., (which is here quoted.) It thus concludes, in these words: "That opinion is amply justified by the details given. It amounts, however, to the most serious condemnation of the proceedings adopted. The man was not dead, but in a state of 'suspended animation.' How, then, characterize such a vivisection? Every man must shudder at the thought of what is implied, and we do not trust ourselves to speak out the deserved censure."

It will be perceived that the *Lancet* does not emphasize or even refer to the material fact, that *the motions were not interrupted by a division of the spinal cord*, because that would have disproved its charge. It also ignores the fact that my *theoretical opinion*, which it tortures into an implied censure of my friend, Dr. Ellis, had no reference whatever to the heart's motion, but was suggested upon entirely different grounds.

The Boston *Medical Journal*, commenting on this article, says:

"That this phenomenon was not caused by any remaining vitality in the system, is evident from the simple fact that the pulsations continued after the spinal cord was divided, showing that this phenomenon was owing to the inherent irritability of the muscular structure of the heart, which still responded to stimuli, as is well known to be the case for a considerable length of time after death, and which is often witnessed in cases where the autopsy is made soon after death. Opportunities are not very frequent for observing this in the human subject, since it is customary to wait many hours after death before making an examination; but any one may see it in animals that have been recently killed. We had occasion to make an autopsy soon after the death of a patient, and found so much irritability remaining in the heart, that it would contract powerfully when pricked with the scalpel, for a considerable length of time after it had been removed from the body. Contractions of the voluntary muscles, sometimes to a remarkable degree, are also witnessed in the bodies of those who have died of cholera, especially when the limbs are smartly struck. In many cases, however, these movements take place spontaneously, and sometimes to a remarkable extent, so that all the limbs are in motion, and continue so for the space of half an hour. The same thing is witnessed in patients who have died from yellow fever.

"In addition to the well-known instances of the persistence of muscular irritability not only after life was extinct, but after the removal of muscles from the body, Bernard, in his late work, 'Sur la Physiologie et la Pathologie du Système Nerveux,' furnishes us with facts which prove that contractility is a property belonging to muscular fibres as such, independent of the nervous or any other system. Having first shown conclusively, by experiment, that the poison 'curare' destroys the power of the motor nerve, he establishes the fact that portions of muscle, taken from animals destroyed by that poison, will contract with as much energy, when the proper stimuli are used, as under ordinary circumstances. He afterwards states distinctly, that 'the independence of muscular contractility is a fact well established experimentally;' and adds, after further researches, that 'the contractile property of the *involuntary* muscles does not differ from that of the muscles under the influence of the will.' "

In allusion to the statement that the criminal was alive when dissected, as circulated by various newspapers, the Boston *Traveller* of the 2d inst., in the course of a long article on the subject, remarks as follows:

"The professional report, however, gives no color for such a statement. On the contrary, it states expressly that when he was cut down all signs of life were absent. The fact that automatic motions of the *right auricle* of the heart, for they were confined to that, continued for some hours afterwards, goes for nothing, because it will be observed that they were not interrupted by a division of the spinal marrow itself; for no one will pretend that this man, as the legend says ST. FRANCIS was, could be alive after he was *beheaded*. The supposition that he might 'possibly have been resuscitated immediately after he was lowered from the scaffold,' was predicated simply upon the fact that there was no apparent injury to the structure of any important organ, and that he was in precisely the condition of a drowned or asphyxiated person; and, it might be added, had not the slightest reference to this peculiar irritability of the heart."

We believe that, under the circumstances, it would have been as impossible to resuscitate Magee, after he was removed to the House of Reception, as it would be to restore to life a patient dead of cholera, who exhibited the phenomena of muscular contraction. Vol. lxix., p. 46.

In Kirke's "Handbook of Physiology," published in *London* in 1851, we find the following observations: "The heart, especially in amphibia and fishes, will continue to *contract and dilate regularly* and in rhythmic order, *after it is removed from the body* and completely emptied of blood." "*Sudden destruction of either the brain or spinal cord alone, or of both together, produces immediately a temporary interruption or cessation of the heart's action;* but this appears to be only the effect of the *shock* of so severe an injury; for, in some such cases, the *movements of the heart are subsequently resumed,* and if artificial respiration be kept up, may continue for a considerable time." "The persistence of the movements of the heart in their regular rhythmic order, after its removal from the body, and their capability of being then re-excited by an ordinary stimulus after they have ceased, *prove that the cause of their movements must be resident with the heart itself.*" Pp. 98, 99.

My friend, Dr. S. L. Abbott, has called my attention to an article in the *Gazette Médicale* for July, 1858, and has been good enough also to furnish me with the following translated synopsis of it. It is the substance of a review of a work entitled "Recherches sur la durée de la Contractilité du Cœur après la Mort, (communiquées à la Société de Biologie, Février, 1858,) par M. Valpland."

"In a field-mouse," the reviewer says, "under his experiments, $46\frac{1}{2}$ hours after death, pieces of both auricles and venæ cavæ inferior, showed undulations of muscular fibres. The animal had died from a severe operation. In a dog that had been hung, a very decided movement of the right auricle was observed $93\frac{1}{2}$ hours after death; the heart and lungs having been removed for 22 hours after death, and placed in a dish exposed to the open air."

M. Valpland himself says: "I have not been able, as yet, to make any observations on man; but I am fully persuaded that, by employing the various processes which I have made use of to detect the amount of contractility after death, results analogous to those I have arrived at would be obtained: that is, that in certain cases, undulatory, spontaneous movements in these parts might be seen, by the aid of the microscope, persisting for more than 48 hours. And it would be interesting to study the influence of different kinds of death on these phenomena. The systolic movements *may continue in man more than 24 hours,* as appears by a fact observed by M. Emmanuel Rousseau, of which that learned anatomist has furnished me with this note: 'The following appearances I saw in company with my colleagues of the School of Anatomy at Rouen, in 1808. The observation was made on a woman who was executed about March or April of that year, and in whom the right auricle beat 24 hours after death, at the moment the chest was opened; and the movements lasted 5 hours after the pericardium was opened.' "

He mentions as witnesses MM. Lanmomier, Flaubert, Hippolyte, and Jules Cloquet.

I have also been informed of a similar case by a very intelligent and respectable gentleman of this city, which he himself witnessed in Paris, in the spring of 1850. He went, between 7 and 8 o'clock in the evening, with an English medical man, to the *Morgue*, and there saw and examined the body of a man *who had been guillotined some* 10 *or* 12 *hours before*, in whom these motions of the heart were still observable. The fact was witnessed, he assured me, by numerous medical men.

These extracts and cases prove conclusively that the case of Magee was of precisely the same character. That is to say,

1. That the death was complete before the body was opened.

2. That the motions of the auricle were automatic, and not vital.

3. That the same motions would have continued for a certain length of time if the heart had been entirely removed from the body.

These cases, and others which might be quoted, must have escaped the observation of the editors of the *Lancet*, or they would never have ventured the opinion that the *post-mortem* examination, as it has been proved to be, was a *"vivisection;"* or if they do not confess their ignorance on this point, they must plead guilty to the charge of willfully perverting "a plain and unvarnished tale" for the purpose of throwing an undeserved odium upon the medical profession of this city. The whole temper of the article, and the subsequent conduct of the editors in neglecting to take the slightest notice, so far, of an explanatory note addressed in respectful terms to them more than three months ago, by Dr. Ellis, than whom a more candid and humane gentleman does not exist, evince anything but the "*entente cordiale*" which should characterize the intercourse between members, however distant geographically, of a profession so noble as that of medicine, or of that courtesy which we have a right to expect from the conductors of a scientific journal which has a wide circulation in this country as well as in Great Britain.   H. G. C.

TWO PERIODS OF QUACKERY.

An American medium of considerable notoriety—a Dr. Randolph—
who has figured prominently in all the clairvoyant and spiritual manifestations of modern transatlantic philosophy, has given to the world
his revelations. He has shattered the idols, and opened the arcana
of the temple to the profane. He was a medium for eight years,
during which time he made three thousand speeches, and traveled far
and wide, proclaiming the new delusion. He confirms previous statements as to the frequency with which insanity follows the mental excitement produced by these manifestations. Five of his friends committed suicide; he himself attempted it. At the Zurich Hospital there
have been thirty cases of insanity attributed to such causes. Dr. Randolph winds up his confession thus: " Experience has taught me that
sixty-five per cent. of the medical clairvoyants are arrant knaves, humbugs, and catch-penny impostors, and that they are no more clairvoyant than a brick wall."

It is almost a relief to turn from the quasi-scientific jargon of the
spirit-rappers, the globulists, and the kinesipathists; dealers in senseless adjurations of the unknown, the doubtful, and the mysterious;
blasphemers against nature, who press into their mercenary service the
common reverence with which mankind are wont to regard the spirit-
world and the finer essences of dynamic physiological force; lying philosophers, who mouth about the unseen, and prate of invisible agencies, in the hope of leading the multitude by the nose. It gives a
mental refreshment to revert to the laughable orations of the more
honest mountebanks of bygone days—men who avowed themselves
quacks, cut their ridiculous antics to the sound of a drum, and with
visible glee extracted from the laughing chaw-bacon a groat in fee,
rather for their oratory than for their medicines. Mr. Morley has
just recalled to-day some admirable specimens of the mountebank oratory of the seventeenth century, from a little undated book published
about the year 1690, entitled, " The Harangues or Speeches of several
Famous Mountebanks in Town and Country." Here is an inimitable
specimen of candid self-glorification and witty abuse of his contemporaries—an address by one of the cleverest, Tom Jones: " Gentlemen
and ladies—You that have a mind to preserve your own and your
families' health, may here, at the expense of a twopenny-piece, furnish
yourself with a packet which contains things of great use and wonderful operation in human bodies against all distempers whatsoever.
Gentlemen, because I present myself among you, I would not have

you to think that I am an upstart glister-pipe apothecary. No, gentlemen, I am no such person; I am a regular physician, and have traveled most kingdoms purely to do my country good. I am not a person that takes delight, as a great many do, to fill your ears with hard words, in telling you the nature of turpet mineral, mercuri, dulcis, balsamum capiviet, astringents, laxations, heart-burnations, circulations, vibrations, salivations, excoriations, scaldations. These quacks may fitly be called soliniates, because they prescribe only one kind of physic for all distempers; that is, a vomit. If a man has bruised his elbow, take a vomit, says the doctor. If you have any corns, take a vomit. If he has torn his coat, take a vomit. For the jaundice, fever, flux, gripes, gout,—nay, even the distempers that only my friend, the famous Dr. Tuff, whom you all know, knows as the hocognicles, marthambles, the mooupauls, and the strongfives,—a vomit; tantum. Gentlemen, these impostors value killing a man no more than I do drawing an old stump of a tooth that has long troubled any of you; so that I say they are a pack of tag-rag, asafœtida, glister-pipe doctors. Now, gentlemen, having given you a short account of this spurious race, I shall present you with my cordial pills, being the tincture of the sun, having dominion from the same light, giving relief and comfort to all mankind. They cause all complexions to laugh or smile in the very taking them: they presently cure all dizziness, dullness in the head, and scurvy. In the next place, I recommend to you my incomparable balsam," and so forth. So that the world then, as now, was full of "one-idea men," and the rogue had the wit to laugh at them. His oration reads like a satire, by Swift, upon the quackeries of the present day. His men who " take delight to fill the ears with hard words;" his " tincture of the sun, having dominion from the same light;" have not the quacks of the present time their congeners openly puffed, day by day? have they not their infallible pills, their nervo-arterial essences, their dynamized sugar-of-milk, their spiritual revelations, their magnetic sympathies; and are not these of the same school?—*London Lancet.*

Yellow Fever.—Dr. Fenner reports, that he has used both chlorine and veratrum viride in yellow fever, and that he has found them of decided benefit. The terrible mortality of the late epidemic furnishes a most telling commentary on this statement, however.—*Med. Jour. of N. C.*

COMMUNICATIONS.

(For the MEDICAL GAZETTE.)

MR. EDITOR—In your last number " one of the profession" broaches the subject of the Kappa Lambda Society, a conspiracy long known to have existed in this city, and to include many of the older and more prominent physicians and surgeons of this metropolis. For many years this secret conclave have been ignored by the medical press, nor have any of the present generation of medical men attempted to expose the arts by which they have sought self-aggrandizement at the expense of abler men, and better physicians, who have patiently endured the proscription they have suffered, while in moral worth as well as in social position and professional status, they have been every way the equals of the best, and superior to the most of this clandestine organization, and which the public have not been slow to perceive·

The late Drs. John Stearns, A. Sidney Doane, and other of our departed worthies, were wont, in their day, to denounce and repel this and all other secret societies in the profession, as the source and exemplar of all quackery; and by their public appeals and exposure of the iniquitous combination, publishing the names and titles of the conspirators, they succeeded in driving these Kappa Lambdas into their dens, whence until lately they have been wont to hide themselves, and ever since they have been working in the dark, shunning recognition, and courting secrecy.

The occasion which has now brought out the faction from their dark concealment has been the indiscreet appearance of one of their number, at the late meeting of the American Medical Association in May last at Washington City. Most unluckily, his name is obtrusively recorded among the delegates as representing " the *Kappa Lambda Society of Hippocrates! !*" This egregious folly on his part, and consummate impudence on the part of those who sent him, would have been rebuked on the spot as it deserved, but that the physical and mental. imbecility of the quasi delegate was so notorious in New York, that the brethren shrank from taking a step which it was alleged by his friends might develop a relapse in his infirmity, and precipitate the necessity of the medical and moral treatment which his own safety and the impulses of humanity had so often rendered imperative. But the fact that *he* was delegated, betrays the character of the conclave, who thus sought to disarm the resentment, which their first appearance in public would occasion, by placing an " innocent" in the position of delegate, whom nobody would strike. It was the first time this secret society ventured into the light; and having thus evoked the coming storm, it is safe to predict that it will be their last appearance on any stage.

In the records of the Medical Society of the City and County of New York, nearly thirty years ago, your correspondent may find the Report of an able committee, of which Dr. Felix Pascalis was the head, in which the nature, history, character, and mischiefs of this secret society are fully exposed, and their names published to the world. I hope to see this Report in the GAZETTE, for although many of them have passed away, yet several of them still live, and their sons are members now; for the dark sessions of the Society are still held, and the conspiracy as rife as ever. In this Report, the *modus operandi* by which the Mutual Admiration Club monopolize consultations in their exclusive clique, at the expense and sacrifice of the character and pecuniary interests of their rivals and superiors in practice, is fully detailed; and if it could now be republished for indiscriminate circulation, and the names of the present members be added, the profession and the public would not marvel at the degraded rank of medical men here, as compared with other cities, where so dishonorable trickery would not be tolerated by any reputable member of the fraternity. The reason why quackery, in its most loathsome forms, has so often supplanted science, would be apparent. Many of the finest specimens of nature's noblemen in the profession of New York have fled from our ranks on the discovery of the intrigues and scandal they must encounter, if they remained in competition with these cliques of monopoly and mischief. Some such turned away in disgust to other professions, rather than enter the strife with those whose motto is, "Strike l but conceal the hand."

The Hon. Mr. Brady did himself honor in his late valedictory before the New York Medical College, by alluding in terms of reprobation to the present existence of this secret society of Kappa Lambdas. In his profession such a conspiracy would be scorned by all honorable men. It is found nowhere but among medical men, and only in New York.

Its origin some forty years ago, it is said, was ascribed to the ignoble object of putting down no less men than Dr. David Hosack and Dr. Valentine Mott, who at that time were worthily the leaders in our ranks, and whose reputation excited envy. The former of these great men continued to shine as a star of the first magnitude, despising and defying the conspirators. And the latter has lived to triumph over this pigmy combination, literally riding over these self-styled magnates of the profession, who have been wont to crawl into his shade, for he has been the Sun, in whose presence none of them could shine. So did Dr. Stearns, after long struggling against the clandestine conspiracy, break their power by exposing them, and the profession honored him by making him the first President of the Academy, when thàt body had not yet been conquered by this secret society, who now fill its offices with its members and tools, and control its downward degeneracy. In like manner, Dr. A Sidney Doane reached the position of Health Officer, in which he lived and died, by making war upon the Kappa Lambdas, who claimed then, as now, a monopoly of all the offices in the State and city. And the time is again at hand, if the rank and file of the profession *will* it to be so, when every member of this Kappa Lambda Club will be hurled from the high places they have usurped without merit, by unhallowed and secret combination in the dark; for, in the language of Kossuth, " *nothing is impossible to him that wills.*" Single out the conspirators, old and young, and " let no trigger be pulled until we see the whites of their eyes." SENEX.

A Case tending to show the Effects of Climate in California upon the Healing of Wounds.

By E. S. COOPER, A.M., M.D.,

Professor of Anatomy and Surgery in the Medical Department of the University of the Pacific.

The astonishing facility with which wounds heal in California has become proverbial among all classes of community.

In fact, the Pacific coast can already boast of some of the most extraordinary recoveries belonging to surgery. The following case in which the end of the thumb was sawed off, and afterwards united, and made the thumb almost as good as ever, is well worth recording.

Case.—Mr. Jesse ——, foreman in the steam saw-mill of Metcaff, corner of Fremont and Mission Streets, had the end of the right thumb detached by a circular saw, passing through the last phalangeal articulation.

After receiving the injury, Mr. J. started for the Pacific Clinical Infirmary, for the purpose of having his wound dressed, and had proceeded nearly a square without the detached fragment, when he conceived the idea of returning for it, to see if it might not still be attached and become useful. When I saw him some twenty or twenty-five minutes afterwards, the separated fragment was blue and cold as the cadaver.

It was shockingly lacerated, and I had little hope of securing its adhesion to the part where it belonged, and but for the astonishing recoveries which have so frequently occurred in California after injuries, I would not have attempted it.

After attaching it to its original place by three silver sutures, placed at equal distances from each other, I applied cold dressings, and gave him liq. ammon. acet. to take internally.

The patient did well, suffered no pain, and the detached portion grew fast, and bids fair to become useful as ever. The joint which was sawed through has a freedom of motion almost equal to that of the opposite thumb. The portion which was detached is still a little shrunken, and a part of the integument sloughed from the under side during the first four weeks after the reception of the injury; this, however, I am disposed to attribute to my having used a little too much pressure, since it looked perfectly healthy in color at the end of two weeks, at which time I began to use pressure to improve the slope, which was somewhat distorted by exuberant granulations. The bones were shattered by the saw, and two small fragments been cast off, which rendered the recovery more tedious.

It is now two months ago since the injury was received, and the wound is almost entirely healed.

SAN FRANCISCO, CALIFORNIA,
February 20th, 1859.

BOOK NOTICES.

ON POISONS IN RELATION TO MEDICAL JURISPRUDENCE AND MEDICINE. By Alfred Swaine Taylor, M.D., F.R.S. Second American from the Second and Revised London Edition. Philadelphia: Blanchard & Lea. 1859

The author of the well-known "Treatise on Medical Jurisprudence" is sufficiently familiar to our readers, by the wide popularity of that able work. This new book of Dr. Taylor on Poisons was welcomed on its first appearance as a valuable contribution to our knowledge in this special department. The present new edition, revised and almost re-written by the author, will be doubly welcomed by the physicians and lawyers of our country, especially as the last 10 years have very largely increased the interest of the whole subject, by new discoveries and improvements in Toxicological science. Moreover felonious poisoning has now become a trade, and its frequent practice in America of late years for murderous purposes, gives the subject of poisons and their antidotes very great importance to our profession, in view of the grave matters of investigation before our courts of justice, which such cases render imperative.

The work is eminently discriminating and practical, freed from the extraneous and obsolete matter which deformed the first edition, and devoted only to those poisons, and their antidotes and tests, a knowledge of which is most commonly required in cases of attempted homicide and suicide, and the analogous inquiries in this department of medical jurisprudence. It makes a noble volume, and is issued in the publishers' best style. That it is without a Philadelphia outrider, deserves the special thanks of the author and readers.

EDITOR'S TABLE.

TO OUR SUBSCRIBERS.

Those of you who have promptly responded to our call for the payment of the subscription for 1859—and they are many—are all gratefully remembered, and all such are in the receipt of the GAZETTE monthly, *free of postage.*

Those who find themselves still taxed for *postage*, have thus a perpetual reminder that they are still DELINQUENT on our books, and may relieve themselves by remitting their dues, for which the bills have been sent out. The amount is so small for each, that it is *forgotten*, as we suppose; for we cannot believe of any, that they purposely withhold payment so long, when the GAZETTE is furnished them at so low a price. If there be any such, they will confer a favor if they will *remail* this number, which will enable us to strike their names from our list, as we have been obliged to do in many cases, until the *two dollars* for 1859 are received, with which to *pay the printer.* Unless we hear from such soon, the paper must be stopped, which is our mode of collecting bad debts, and which has in many cases brought us apologies and the money, with the order for the missing numbers invariably. No subscriber who fails to mail the two dollars for 1859, before the next number is issued, can hereafter receive the GAZETTE.

We have greatly enlarged the Journal, and its improvement, in all respects, is avouched by the congratulatory letters which are reaching us daily from all quarters of the country. Our march is onward, under better auspices than ever, and with a few more paying subscribers, to take the place of the few who do not pay, we shall soon enlarge again, and be able to *pay more liberally* for original articles—a consummation devoutly to be wished—for our home circulation now extends from Canada, to California.

"THE KAPPA LAMBDA SOCIETY OF HIPPOCRATES"— WHO ARE THEY?

In our last number, we inserted a letter from an unknown correspondent on this topic, leaving its inquiries to be answered by others. The communication of " *Senex*," in the present issue, has supplied our lack of service. We recur to this subject now, because we find on our table a pamphlet, bearing date 1831, though obviously reprinted for present circulation. It contains the "Report of a Committee of the Medical Society of the City and County of New York, appointed to investigate the subject of a secret Medical Association." This report was adopted by that body of some three hundred physicians, and published at that time, nearly thirty years ago, with the signatures of five members, all of whom are now dead, except one, and he has been driven into Homœopathy, by the proscription of this Kappa Lambda Society, as have many others who once stood higher than he in the fraternity.

From this document we learn that this *Secret Society* of physicians was founded about the year 1820, and included in 1831 an unknown number, only twenty-six of whom are named. Many of these are dead, and of them nothing should be said but what is good, however great their error in this regard. Of the twelve who are now living, we may safely say that they include many of the *strongest*, and several of the *weakest* men in the medical ranks; a strange and incongruous medley of intelligence and stupidity, who could have been united by no other bond than pecuniary interest, the almighty dollar—which then, as now, too often assumes aristocratic airs, and puts on dignity, without either education or merit in its possessors.

The following card is prefixed to the present edition of the Report, viz.:

" *The secret society, Kappa Lambda, with additional members, is still in active operation in this city, and continues to make the effort to control the Medical Institutions, and has become bold enough, by its success, to send, in* 1858, *a delegate to the National Medical Association, at Washington City."*

No "additional members" are named, although we have received anonymously a list of some forty of our medical neighbors and friends, young and old, who are reputed to be Kappa Lambdas; and if truly such, there is the same mixture of intellect and imbecility, of enlightened and ignorant doctors, which characterizes the older members who are named in the Report. A few of them are men who have made their mark, and gained reputation and practice; but a majority of those included in this later list are men who, despite of the influence of the secret combination, do not feel a pulse in a month, and whose reputation has never extended beyond the North and East rivers, between which our city stands.

It cannot be denied, however, that this Kappa Lambda Society, by its members and those in league with it, have succeeded in securing and retaining the exclusive monopoly of most of the medical offices in the N. Y. Hospital, and other of our prominent public institutions; to effect which, their secret combination and mutual obligations afford great facilities, for they not only help each other, but oppose everybody else who does not come into their clique, or belong to their clan. Of this, there are notorious examples, in which able and gifted men, whose claims on the score of merit were paramount, and acknowledged to be such, have been defeated by these secret conspirators, and the positions they sought were given to others, not only their inferiors, but whose only fitness consisted in their being Kappa Lambdas, and having the support of this club, which artfully gains the ear of the appointing powers. Many such there are, whose manifest mediocrity dooms them to be mere ciphers and drones, a burden to the public charities, and who find their positions powerless in gaining them either practice or reputation. They have obtained the control of the Academy by their intrigues, and for many years have nearly monopolized the presidency, anniversary orator, and other prominent offices, as they do at present, some of them holding three or four offices at once, and having a majority in the Council which now governs the important appointments. So, also, even the Medical Society of the city and county has long been under the same government, by reason of the apathy of its membership, who abandon the *annual* meetings, which often require weeks to obtain the required quorum of thirteen, who then parcel the offices among themselves.

These Kappa Lambdas claim the right by prescription to *represent the profession* on all important public occasions, especially if fees are in prospect; as seen in the medical councils convened in times of epidemics, and in the recent Parish Will case, when so many of them made a nice operation by medical opinions, liberally paid for, however incongruous and irrelevant in the courts of law. And with this *ex-officio* presumption, their leaders tamper with the laymen who appoint medical officers to posts of honor or emolument in hospitals and other remedial institutions, securing the preference to their clique at the expense of others who are " outsiders."

Hence it must be obvious, that our *young physicians*, who have too much conscience to enter into any *secret* conspiracy, or who not being the favored sons of Kappa Lambdas, or otherwise chosen into the conclave, find themselves the greatest sufferers by the existence of this greedy monopoly and exclusive power, acting as it does clandestinely and irresponsibly, itself being invisible. In short, it is an *imperium in imperio*, a combination of professional men *in* the profession, ignoring and proscribing all *outsiders*, irrespective of learning, science, skill or moral worth, these all being insignificant compared with membership in their exclusive and secret club.

Our young medical men, fresh from the colleges where Kappa Lambda professors have received their money, and declared them their *equals* on their graduation, if ardent and ambitious for distinction, find themselves under the ban in New York if they attempt to take position here. They feel keenly their disappointment in their honest efforts to gain the humblest places in our public medical charities; and not until after repeated defeat, by some invisible power behind the throne, do they discover the mysterious cause, by learning that their successful rivals were indebted to this secret society, overriding all their claims on the score of merit. The alternative left them is to sacrifice their independence by courting the favor of the Kappa Lambdas, or retire from the unequal contest with a power working wholly in the dark. The best of our young brethren, preferring principle to policy, retreat rather than yield their manhood. Many such have left the city, and others have left the profession forever; while still others have foolishly descended into quackery, seeking to find " honor among thieves."

This deplorable picture of the mischiefs of this *secret medical society* would be incomplete, unless allusion were made to the interests of the public, not less than the profession, which are jeoparded and outraged

thereby. One of their chief sources of emolument and self-aggrandizement is found in their monopolizing and multiplying consultations
with each other exclusively. A list of the club is handed to the
patient or his family, with the assurance that " these are the *most respectable* physicians in New York!" and a readiness is expressed to meet
either of *these!* but all outsiders are objected to, until it is discovered
that resistance is vain. A reluctant consent is then given to meet the
gentleman insisted on by the patient, and he is expected to consider
himself complimented by the opportunity; for though these exclusives
seek to be called in consultation by outsiders, it is a favor they never
willingly reciprocate, but only submit to the necessity, when the alternative is the loss of the fees and the patient.

It need scarcely be urged, that a consultation among a Mutual
Admiration Society must be a farce, being called and held rather for
the benefit of each other, than for that of the patient. When the
latter is to be served, as in a case of life and death, the purpose of a
consultation should be, to give the patient the advantage of the independent opinion of the best man in point of skill and experience; and
its purpose should never be to serve the consulting physician, because
belonging to the same club. In the latter case, the treatment of the
patient would most likely be unchanged by the consulting physician
out of regard to his *chum*, to whom he was indebted for being called,
and from whom he desires similar favors. The patient has therefore
a touching interest in these trading consultations of far more importance than their expense.

The danger to the purse of a patient under such circumstances is,
that unnecessary consultations will be called and multiplied by the
members of a secret club, pledged to help each other, and to *know*
nobody else if they can help it; and the only escape from such imposition on the part of the patient and his friends, is by calling in consultation some outsider, who, in defiance of the club, has a position
and reputation entitling him to such confidence. Moreover, a consultation may thus be had, in which the welfare of the patient will be
paramount, and in a critical case this ought to be secured at the sacrifice of every other consideration.

That there are among the Kappa Lambdas men who are above and
beyond any of the professional or moral delinquencies chargeable
against others, is unquestionable; nor would these be guilty of the trading arts, ascribed, and not without just cause, to the Kappa Lambdas, and from which as a secret society they cannot escape, whatever

disclaimer individual members may make. Their meetings are said to be social dinners, at which medical scandal is the condiment, even in the presence of the invited guests, who are those regarded in league with them, or prospectively chosen to add to their number, if they stand the probation. The dinner over, and the wines imbibed, the guests are excluded, and the secret session commences in a private room, where plans are concocted in the dark for their mutual advantage, and their aggressions upon outsiders are arranged. And so long as this secret club exists among us, our profession must be degraded, retaliations will be engendered, and the combination of medical men *se defendendo* against this dark conclave of familiar spirits, will continue, as now, to divide and degenerate the fraternity.

We are not surprised that the public press has at length begun to assail the profession for tolerating such a conspiracy, however much we may deprecate the public exposure of the humiliating facts, which are now sent out to the four winds by the recent publicity of what has so long been endured in secret. For these Kappa Lambdas not only smuggled a representative into the National Medical Congress for 1858, but they betrayed themselves at the recent election in the N. Y. Academy of Medicine, which they only carried by a *single vote*, after caucussing for weeks, and circulating tickets marked with *a dot** against the names of their clan who were to be voted for, and bargaining with certain weak brethren to withdraw from the canvass, with or without a *quid pro quo* in the future

The very existence of this secret society is high treason against our Code of Ethics; and by the Constitution, its members, as such, are excluded from the American Medical Association, which requires delegates to be sent by " regularly organized medical associations in *good standing !* and which have adopted our *Code of Ethics !*" This code justly protects the regular members of the profession from being fastidiously deprived of their rights in consultation, and secures the entire *equality* of all regularly licensed or graduated physicians, in all their rights and privileges; and hence the Kappa Lambdas have not adopted a code which would annihilate their secret society. Hence they never dared to send a delegate until last year, and his name is on the record by inadvertence, else he and they had been excluded by acclamation. Let the trick be tried at Louisville, and may we be there to see.

---

* A delegation of the tribe is reported as a feature in the late mongrel Quarantine Convention, but they did not turn up at Louisville.

25

MEDICAL POLITICS, BELLEVUE HOSPITAL, ETC.

Our advices from Albany, announced last month, turn out to have been again premature and erroneous, for our neighbor, Dr. Gurdon Buck, failed to reach the position he sought so ardently, and one of his competitors, every way his inferior, Dr. A. N. Gunn, has succeeded in grasping the prize, and has been appointed *Health Officer;* so that politics is again in the ascendant over the public health and safety, and the spoils are divided among the party. Under the same auspices, Dr. Jerome, a country doctor, from somewhere out West, of whom we hear favorably, is made Resident Physician of the Marine Hospital, a post demanding a species of qualification for detecting and treating pestilential disease, which he must now learn, or perform his duty by a hired proxy, as the Health Officer will do, taking care of the fees for himself and the party, by whom they will both be taxed. *Where?* either the Quarantine or Marine Hospital is to be located, has not yet transpired, for the Staten Islanders have expelled both from their shores—Long Island has excluded them by law—and New Jersey will tolerate neither on any part of her coast. But they may as well be in the moon, for all the practical benefit resulting from the present system of Quarantine to our commerce, or to the public health. The incumbents, however, are sure of their salaries and fees, which are the " main chance."

The Legislature have just closed their session, and the Sanitary bill, new Charter bill, &c., have all been defeated by a corrupt lobby of partisan politicians, who disagreed as to the division of the spoils. The ignorant and mischievous organization of our Board of Health and kindred departments, will therefore continue without any medical element, and be, as heretofore, a curse to the city, and a disgrace to the civilization of the nineteenth century.

The pending revolution in the Medical Board of Bellevue Hospital, thanks to the Medical Governor, Dr. Bruninghausen, has begun to ripen, and promises to overcome the resistance of the would-be-monopolists, whose treachery in reaching their own positions is now likely to meet its reward. By concealing the existence of a vacancy in their Board, lest the Governors might exercise their prerogative by appointing some one, *not* of their clique, they have kept Dr. Parker as the *locum tenens* of Dr. Lidell, until the ruse was discovered by another vacancy having been made by Dr. Smith's open resignation. To fill the latter seven select names were sent to the Governors, when Dr. Bruninghausen inquired after the other vacancy, till now undiscovered. Whereupon *four* other vacancies were created by adding to the Medical Board *two* physicians and *two* surgeons; and there being thus *six* vacancies, the Board of Governors have very properly filled them all, as follows, viz.:

Surgeons.—Drs. Alexander B. Mott, Charles Th. Meier, J. W. S. Gouley, W. H. Church.

Physicians.—Drs. J. W. Green, A. C. Loomis.

We trust that these new elements being introduced into the Medical Board will have a salutary effect uppon its organization, which sadly needs reform; and we have an abiding faith, now that there is a medical man among the Governors, which we have so long urged, that the expenses for *drugs, medicines, &c.*, will not reach the extravagant figure of $8,000 ! in one year, as in 1858. See Report.

Dr. Bruninghausen is an able and highly intelligent physician, and cannot fail to win golden opinions, if he continue the work of reform he has commenced, and in which he has been thus far sustained by his colleagues.

The new appointees, chosen from so many competitors, are indebted to the Board of Governors, and not to the old Medical Board, for their places, as some of them have reason to know. They are all qualified men, and will sustain themselves in their new positions, whether judged by comparison or otherwise.

It will not escape observation, that for the first time in the history of our medical institutions, six appointments have been made, without a single Káppa Lambda among them, and in defiance of their combined opposition. Is not the inference authorized, that this conspiracy has reached its *dénouément*, and that the Governors have had enough of the dictation of that sect in the old Board ?

Some threats have been volunteered that there would be resignations among the latter, but there need be no apprehensions on that score, even if forty should be added instead of four. So long as this hospital and its inmates are left without a medical head in a Resident Physician, who shall be a salutary check on the irresponsible members of the Board, and protect the inmates from experimental treatment and unsurgical operations, and at the same time preserve the tax-payers from the wasteful extravagance of expenditures for rum and medicines, the old Board will not be driven from the plunder. But placing the hospital under a medical head, will be the signal for the old rats to quit.

Statistics of Medical Colleges for the Session 1858-9.

We insert the following statistical table, which includes all the schools we have heard from. It is necessarily incomplete, but we have kept the table standing, and add the reports from other colleges which have reached us before our May number. Information from every school in the country is respectfully solicited, that we may state the aggregate in the next number of the GAZETTE. If any errors occur, we shall be thankful for corrections from any quarter.

	Students.	Graduates.
Jefferson Medical College	570	256
University of Nashville	436	103
University of Pennsylvania	409	144
University of New York	350	128
University of Louisiana	335	98
College of Physicians and Surgeons, (N. Y.)	180	39
Medical College of Georgia, (Augusta,)	165	58
Pennsylvania Medical College	109	33
University of Michigan	143	——
New Orleans School of Medicine	140	36
Harvard University	139	30
St. Louis Medical College	185	40
Philadelphia School of Medicine	75	18
New York Medical College	107	25
University of Buffalo	67	13
University of Vermont	80	20
Shelby Medical College	53	11
Dartmouth Medical College	——	9
Albany Medical College	——	48
Medical School of Maine	50	——
Missouri Medical College	——	23
Rush Medical College	——	31
Cleveland Medical College	69	19
Atlanta Medical College	136	39
Ohio Medical College	139	33
Starling Medical College	——	——
Ogelthorpe Medical College	50	13
Savannah Medical College	34	8
Memphis Medical College	——	——
University of South Carolina	195	——
Medical College of Virginia	70	20

University of Virginia	107	—
University of Maryland	—	—
Yale Medical College	—	—
Castleton Medical College	51	—
Berkshire Medical School	—	—
University of Iowa	—	—
University of Louisville	—	35
Kentucky School of Medicine	103	28
Transylvania University	18	6

DR. CLOSE, OF PORT CHESTER, N. Y.,

Is a venerable and reputable physician, and desires to be heard in reply to Dr. Platt, on the subject of Veratrum Viride, by a brief article, which we insert in this number.   His son, Mr. Geo. C. Close, of Brooklyn, is a respectable and educated apothecary, and very much regrets the reference to him which Dr. Mead, of Albany, has made, who will share his regret when he learns that the allusion to him and his store was without his knowledge or consent, though found in his father's letter, which all parties admit authorized Dr. Mead's inference. Mr. Close is opposed to "advertising" his tinctures in any form, but conducts a legitimate business, in which he deserves success.

DR. JOHN BELL'S

Inaugural Oration before the Philadelphia County Medical Society occupies a larger space in this number than we are wont to give to one article.   With those who read it throughout, however, we shall need no apology for its length; or if we did, it will be found in its intrinsic excellence and merit, for in matter and manner it is worthy of its veteran author, who is known to be one of the best scholars and writers in the profession.   We marvel that it was not printed by the Society which was honored by its delivery, and this lack of service we have here endeavored to supply.

NEW YORK STATE LUNATIC ASYLUM.

This greatest of our State charities, located near Utica, N. Y., have transmitted their annual report to the Legislature, a document highly creditable to the managers and superintending physician, Dr. Gray, who, with his subordinates, are fulfilling their mission to its hundreds of inmates in a manner entitling them to the gratitude of the State.

DELAY OF OUR MAY NUMBER.

This issue of the GAZETTE has been delayed in view of the meeting of the American Medical Association, and its precursor, the Convention of Medical Teachers, from which conjoint assemblage much had been expected. But the chairman of the special committee of last year, Dr. J. R Wood, nor, as appears, either of his colleagues, thought it worth while to attend the Convention they had prayed for, nor did any of the leading spirits, in invoking this "conference of medical teachers," take interest enough in the concerns of medical education to come up to Louisville at all. The absence of all such, and the seemingly concerted declinature of so large a majority of the larger and older schools to attend the meeting they had themselves called, would indicate that but little is to be expected from the colleges of the country in the way of "Reform," that oft repeated, and much abused battle-cry, by which certain of the brethren are wont to ventilate; unless the profession at large shall take the initiative, and lead on the needed work. But when the profession refer it to the teachers, and the teachers refer it back to the profession, and neither has the courage to move, who is to set the ball in motion? Two "Committees of Conference," one from this Teachers' Convention, all "professors," and another from the Association, from which all professors are excluded, are now charged with the whole responsibility of reform until June, 1860; when, if they "report" anything *practical or practicable*, the work may commence, which it has not yet. The late "Convention of Teachers" is regarded by all parties as a failure; but "blessed are we who expect nothing, for verily we shall not be disappointed."

Annual Meeting of the American Medical Association at Louisville, Kentucky, May, 1859.

The Convention of the *Medical Professors* of the country, called by the American Medical Association to meet at Louisville, Ky., one day in advance of their own annual meeting, met and adjourned on May 2d, having done nothing, for reasons which will be obvious when we name the colleges *not represented at all!* which are the following, viz.:

Universities of New York, Pennsylvania, Maryland, Virginia, Louisiana, Buffalo, Nashville, Jefferson Medical College, Yale College, &c., &c., neither of whom have sent here even a single delegate.

Still, however, delegates appeared from twenty of the schools, chiefly of the South and West, viz.: Charleston, S. C.; Augusta, Ogelthorpe, and Atlanta, Geo.; St. Louis and Missouri; Kentucky and Louisville; Shelby and Memphis, of Tenn.; Michigan University; Cincinnati, O., and Cleveland, O.; Lind and Rush, of Illinois; University of Iowa; Richmond, Va.; Harvard, of Boston, and Dartmouth, of N. H. Prof. Crosby, of N. H., presided, and Prof. Blackman, of Ohio, acted as Secretary. The absence of representation from so many of the older and larger schools prevented any definite action, and hence an adjournment until next year, after providing for a committee of five professors to confer with the Association through a similar committee to be asked for, and report at next annual meeting.

This morning, May 3d, the American Medical Association met at Mozart Hall. The President, Dr. H. Lindsley, of Washington, D. C., took the chair, with Drs. Sutton, Crosby, and Edwards, Vice-Presidents; Drs. Semmes and Bemis, Secretaries, and Dr. Wistar, Treasurer, in their places. The usual proceedings were had, inaugural address delivered, &c., when Dr. Reese, of New York, chairman of the Committee on Nominations, reported the following officers for the year, viz.:

. *President.*—Dr. Henry Miller, of Louisville.

Vice-Presidents.—Dr. Tripler, U. S. A., Dr. Askew, of Del., Dr. L. A. Smith, of N. J., Dr. C. West, of Indiana.

Secretaries.—Dr. Bemis, of Ky., and Dr. E. Ives, of New Haven, Ct.

Treasurer.—Dr. Caspar Wistar, of Philadelphia.

All of whom were elected by acclamation.

The reading of papers was in order, discussions, &c., which occupied the time until Wednesday inclusive. The special and standing committees were appointed, and the time and place of the next annual meeting fixed at *New Haven, Ct.*, on the first Tuesday in June, 1860, the constitution being altered to allow this change of time.

The following names constitute the Standing and Special Committees, as reported from the *Nominating Committee*, consisting of one delegate from each State represented, and of which *Dr. D. Meredith Reese, of New York,* was elected Chairman, and *Dr. W. Brodie, of Michigan,* Secretary, viz.:

New Haven, Ct., was selected as the place for the next annual meeting, and the time fixed for the *first Tuesday in June,* 1860. Dr. Eli Ives was appointed Secretary, to be associated with Dr. Bemis, who holds over.

Committee of Arrangements.—Drs. Charles Hooker, Chairman,

Stephen G. Hubbard and Benjamin Silliman, Jr., with power to add to their numbers.

Committee on Prize Essays.—Drs. Worthington Hooker, Chairman, Jonathan Knight and P. A. Jewett, of Connecticut; Dr. C. C. Shattuck, of Mass.; and Dr. Usher Parsons, of R. I.

Committee on Publication.—Dr. F. G. Smith, Chairman, Dr. C. Wistar, Dr. Hollingsworth and Dr. Hartshorne, of Philadelphia; Dr. Askew, of Delaware; Dr. Bemis, of Ky.; and Dr. Ives, of Conn.   .

Committee on Medical Literature.—Dr. Henry Campbell, of Georgia, Chairman; Dr. D. F. Wright, of Tenn.; Dr. O. W. Holmes, of Boston; Dr. S. G. Armor, of Ohio; and Dr. W. H. Byford, of Ill.   •

Committee on Medical Education.—Dr. D. Meredith Reese, of New York, Chairman; Dr. W. K. Bowling, of Tenn.; Dr. Chas. Fishbach, of Indiana; Dr. John Bell, of Philadelphia; and Dr. Z. Pitcher, of Michigan.

Special Committee of Conference with the Committee appointed by the Teachers' Convention, and to report in May, 1860, selected by the President, Dr. Miller, viz.:—Dr. Thomas W. Blatchford, of New York, Chairman; Dr. Francis Condie, of Penn.; Dr. Bozeman, of Ala.; Dr. Brodie, of Mich.; and Dr. Sneed, of Kentucky.

Special Committees.   . •

On Morbus Coxarius and the Surgical Pathology of Articular Inflammation.—Dr. Lewis A. Sayre, of New York.   :

On the Surgical Treatment of Strictures of the Urethra.—Dr. James Bryan, of Philadelphia.

On Drainage and Sewerage of large Cities; their influence on public health.—Drs. A. J. Semmes, C. Boyle, and G. M. Dove.   `

Dr. Reese, from the Nominating Committee, in his final report, named several other special committees. But for these and other particulars our readers are referred to the full report of proceedings, which will appear in our June number, but for which we have no room at present.

Among the most important changes resolved on at this meeting was that introduced by Professor Lindsley, of Tennessee, and which was adopted, by dividing the Association at every annual session into sections, and to which the reading and publication of all the scientific and professional reports of special committees are to be referred. See our June number for official report.

THE QUARANTINE AND SANITARY CONVENTION

Has recently held another gathering in this city, still more prolific of words, resolutions, speeches, &c., than any former one, and especially as some of the medical profession have ventilated their eloquence on important topics, exposing their ignorance and inconsis'encies in the presence of municipal officers, who practically understand more on the subjects of consultation than these pretended medical experts. Opinions have been given in public worth less than the paper on which they are written; and this by medical men who never saw a case of yellow fever in their lives, and who would flee the city with their families to-morrow for personal safety, if any alarm or panic should be gotten up by popular rumor. And yet, such men have gravely voted their opinions about the personal communicability of the disease, and the danger of *fomites!* the Latinity of which is all Greek to them. The senior and foremost among them, not long since, publicly declared his belief that cholera was so contagious that the walls of the houses containing cases would reproduce it years afterwards, as they were *fomites* through winter and summer! He even doubts now, as do many of his sage compeers, whether *persons* may not prove *fomites!* for yellow fever, as their clothes undoubtedly are, in his opinion, but they hesitate to say so. The knowledge of most of these men is derived from books, but they are superficial readers, else they would have withheld their crude opinions on subjects on which they blunder so discreditably, that no municipal body of intelligent civilians will confide the interests of commerce, and the lives of a million of people, to any Quarantine they may devise, in their presumptuous folly. We shall have more to say next month. The Reports from Drs. Clark, Bell, and others, are able, and these will redeem the body from contempt

Another Weekly Journal.

The Medical and Literary Weekly has been issued by Drs. Taliaferro and Thomas, at Atlanta, Geo., in newspaper form, at $2 per annum. The editors give evidence that it will be a spirited and sprightly sheet.

LETTER FROM BRUNSWICK, MAINE.

The MAINE Medical School here has about the usual number, probably a few more than last year, when they had just fifty. We are expecting to have a new building in a year or two, as there is now before the Maine Legislature a bill for a grant of a township for that purpose. If we get it through, we shall at once commence the new building. In haste, very truly yours, B.

CONTENTS.

RECEIPTS for 1859—Continued.

Drs. Perkins, Elliott, Meier, Bernacki, Blackman, A. Moore, S. M. Elliott, O. White,
J. B. Flint, Close, Cary Burnett, Bennett, Lindsley, Scraggs, Norris, Guernsey, Pacetty.

AMERICAN

MEDICAL GAZETTE.

| Vol. X. | JUNE, 1859. | No. 6. |

ORIGINAL DEPARTMENT.

Twelfth Annual Meeting of the
AMERICAN MEDICAL ASSOCIATION.

LOUISVILLE, *May* 3, 1859.

The Association met at eleven o'clock, A. M., in Mozart Hall, the President, Dr. Harvey Lindsly, of the District of Columbia, in the chair, supported by Drs W. L Sutton, of Kentucky, Thomas O. Edwards, of Iowa, Josiah Crosby, of Massachusetts, and W. C. Warren, of North Carolina, as Vice-Presidents, with Drs. Alexander J. Semmes, of the District of Columbia, and S. M. Bemiss, of Kentucky. acting as Secretaries. Dr. Caspar Wister, of Pennsylvania, Treasurer, was also in attendance.

The President announced the Rev. Mr. Robinson, of Louisville, who opened the proceedings with prayer.

Dr. Robert J. Breckinridge, chairman of the Committee of Arrangements, then welcomed the delegates to the city.

Prof. Joshua B. Flint, of Louisville, accompanied by Drs. Sutton, Chipley, Spilman, and Snead, then came forward and addressed the President as follows:

Mr. President—At a late annual meeting of the " State Medical Society of Kentucky," the following resolution was unanimously adopted, and the gentlemen before you, all ex-Presidents of the Society, constituted a committee charged with carrying it into effect:

"*Resolved*, That J. B. Flint, with such associates as he may select, be a committee to wait upon the American Medical Association, so soon as it shall have opened its session in Louisville, and in behalf

26

of this Society bid it welcome to the medical jurisdiction of Kentucky, assure it of the cordial interest of the profession of the State in the objects and purposes of its institution, and of the readiness of this Society to co-operate in all its endeavors to promote the honor and usefulness of our common calling."

In regard to the assurances of welcome, Mr. President, so far as they apply to yourself and your associates as individual guests of your Kentucky brethren, those gentlemen would hardly pardon me for adding a word to the general terms of the resolution. Already, if I mistake not, there are demonstrations of the spirit of hospitality, which render any assurances on that subject worse than superfluous.

But I am happy to assure you, Mr. President, that the Association over which you preside, in its corporate capacity, with its well-known purposes and ends, will find an equally cordial reception in the generous community which it has now honored with its presence. The people of Kentucky, sir, are generally prepared to appreciate as it deserves every enterprise of a public-spirited or philanthropic character which presents itself to their notice, and I think I may say especially disposed to befriend the cause of Medical Education. They have certainly done somewhat not a little to their credit in evidence of their intelligent interest in Medical Science and the best means of its advancement. Through the munificence of the State, in one case, and of this liberal city in the other. two medical libraries have been procured in Kentucky, each of which is superior to any and all the public collections of medical books that can be found in most of the other States of the Union. Not more than two of our sister States, so far as I can learn, can be compared with us in this interesting particular.

One of these libraries, belonging to the Medical Department of the University of Louisville, at its best estate, numbering 4,000 volumes, you will doubtless visit during your sojourn among us; and, although much defaced and mutilated by the conflagration which layed that institution in ruins two years ago, you will still find it to be a large and choice collection—adequate to the requisitions of medical research, and presenting satisfactorily the course of medical literature from the time of Hippocrates to the present day. •

The other library to which I refer belongs to the Medical Department of Transylvania University, and contains 8,000 volumes. I hope that not a few of the members of the Association, before leaving Kentucky, will find their way into that also, in the course of a visit to the beautiful inland city in which it is located—a city distinguished throughout the land for the general intelligence and refinement of its population, as well as for the eminent public men who have signalized it as their home; but to medical men, not only of our own, but of foreign countries, especially memorable as the residence of the great lithotomist of our day, and surgical patriarch of the West—Benjamin W. Dudley.

Such benefactions as these to the means of medical study attest, as I have already intimated, so enlightened an interest in the improvement of our profession, as to guarantee not only a welcome to the Association which represents it, but efficient co-operation in its endeavors on the part of the profession and people of Kentucky.

May your present session, Mr. President, be an agreeable one to the members of the Association, and prove eminently beneficial to the interests of American medicine.

The Secretary, Dr. Bemiss, then called the roll of members of the Association, and the following gentlemen were in attendance:

District of Columbia.—Harvey Lindsly, Cornelius Boyle, Alex. J. Semmes.

Virginia.—L. S. Joynes, P. C. Spencer, A. S. Payne.

Georgia.—Henry F. Campbell, Joseph Jones, W. H. Doughty, J. T. Banks, A. G. Thomas, John W. Jones, J. G. Westmoreland.

Louisiana.—S. O. Scruggs, R. A. New.

Maryland.—G. W. Lawrence.

South Carolina.—Henry R. Frost, H. W. Gibbs, John F. Gaston, W. H Huger, Francis J. Miles.

Pennsylvania.—Caspar Wister, Robert K. Smith, James Bryan, W. B. Atkinson, Frank Riesor, Wm. Hunt, John Shrack, D. D. Clarke.

Rhode Island.—James H. Eldridge.

Ohio.—Thomas W. Gordon, A. H. Baker, W. W. Dawson, Thos. M. Taggart, H. E. Foote, John C. Beck, C. G. Comegys, S. P. Hunt, James Graham, B. F. Richardson, T. J. Mullen, J. B. Smith, Rob. Thompson, Charles S. Tripler, Stephen Bonner, John A Murphy, E. P. Tyffe, Daniel Tilden, J. Helmick, George Fries, A. E. Heighnay, Joseph Clements, J. G. Rodgers, H. G. Carey, Wm. Mount, C. McDermott, R. L. Rea, W. H. Lamnie, B. S. Brown, G. A. Doherty, J. C. Devise, G. C. E. Weber.

New York.—Lewis A. Sayre, Thomas W. Blatchford, David Meredith Reese, J. Carey Selden, A. L. Saunders, Douglass Ely, David L. Rogers.

Tennessee.—John H. Callender, J. C. Newnan, James M. Kellar, H. R. Robards, J. S. White, W. K. Bowling, E. B. Haskins, F. Rice, J. B. Lindsly, T. L. Maddin, D. F. Wright, W. C. Cavanaugh, R. C. Foster, E. D. Wheeler, B. W. Arant, W. D. Haggard, Paul F. Eve.

Michigan.—Moses Gunn, Z. Pitcher, Wm. Brodie, John Bennet.

Delaware.—H F. Askew.

New Jersey.—Landon A. Smith, E. Fithian, Joseph Fithian, Alex. N. Dougherty, Abraham Coles.

New Hampshire.—Dixi Crosby

Kentucky.—J. W. Singleton, N. B. Anderson, H. K. Pusey, Churchill J. Blackburn, W. H. Miller, R. C. Hewitt, John L. Dismiskes, J. B. Flint, John Hardin, W. A. Turner, M. Goldsmith, Llewellyn Powell, G. W. Bayless, L. P. Yandell, David Cummins, B. M. Wible, A. B. Cooke, D. W. Yandell, D. D. Thomson, R. J. Breckinridge, S. M. Bemiss, John B. Book, Henry Miller, T. P. Satterwhite, G. W. Ronald, Lewis Rogers, J. Hopson, J. Q. A. Foster, L. Russell, Hugh L. Givins, O. H. Spilman, H. D. Stirman, N. B. Marshall, E. D. Force, T. S. Bell, R. P. Letcher, A. Callaway, E. D. Weatherford, J. D. Landrum, D. J. O'Reilly, Samuel Reid, John H. Polm, W. S. Chipley, W. D. Holt, W. E. Gilpin, A. E. Steuart, Wm. Hayes, Thos. Marshall, W. L. Sutton, C. P. Mattingly, Stanton F. Bryan, J. W. Bush, H. M. Skillman, L. Buckner Todd, W. R. Evans, W. C. Snead, W. B. Caldwell, W. H. Gardner.

Alabama.—George D. Norris, J. B. Coons, W. P. Reese, A. J. Reese.

North Carolina.—Edward Warren.

Missouri.—Montrose A. Pullen, J. M. Allen, John H. Watters, Joseph N. McDowell, Stephen Ritchie, M. L. Linton, J. R. Washington, Chas. A. Pope, W. M. McPheeters.

Wisconsin.—C. B. Chapman.

Iowa.—D. L. McGugin, Thos. O. Edwards, Daniel Meeker.

Indiana.—Charles Fishback, B. S. Woodworth, W. R. Winton, Calvin West, Isaac Capelberry, J. N. Green, R. D. Maury, Geo. Sutton, Isaac Mendenhall, M. H. Hardin, L. D. Personett, A. B. Butler, R. E. Haughton, D. W. Taylor, S. S. Boyd, J. H. Brower, A. McPhecters, J. Langes, Joel Pennington, L. H. Kennedy, J Joel Wright, H. G. Sexton, Joseph Somers, John Moffit, D. Morgan, H. P. Ayres, Wm. Dickey, D. H. Jessup, Joseph H. D. Rogers, Benj. Newland, John Sloan, T. R. Austin, R. R. Town, A. Clapp, F. W. Beard, Wm.

Reeder, D. M. Jones, Chas. Bowman, R. S. Shield, Jno. M. Kitchen, S. Davis, Geo. W. New, J. H. Woodburn, S. M. Linton, C. Brown, A. G. Boynton, F. M. Mothershead, T. Bullard, W. A. Clapp.

Massachusetts.—Pierson F. Kendall, G. Shattuck, Benj. F. Heywood, Sol. D. Townsend, Josiah Crosby, J. B. Upham, Enos Hoyt.

Illinois.—J. W. Fruer, Daniel Brainard, N. S. Davis, R. N. Isham, J. H. Hollister, H. A. Johnson, D. W. Young, O. Goodbrake, H. Noble, J. M. Steele, A. H. Ince, J. N. Graham, J. B. Curtis.

The President then appointed the following gentlemen a committee on voluntary essays: Drs. L. P. Yandell of Kentucky, Bryan of Philadelphia, and Comegys of Ohio.

Dr. R. J. Breckinridge, from the Committee of Arrangements, announced the hours of business from 9 A. M. to 1 P. M. and 3, P. M., until such hour as the Convention should adjourn upon resolution, which arrangement was adopted.

Dr. Harvey Lindsly, the President of the Association, then read his retiring address, which was listened to with marked attention, and was an eloquent tribute to the dignity of the medical profession and the importance of its improvements.

After he had concluded, Dr. L. A. Smith, of New Jersey, moved that the thanks of the Association be tendered to the President for his able and eloquent address, and it was ordered to be placed in the hands of the appropriate committee for publication, among the proceedings of the meeting.

Dr. Caspar Wister, chairman of the Committee on Publication, read the annual report, and on motion of Dr. Sayre, of New York, the following resolutions appended to it were unanimously adopted:

" *Resolved,* That hereafter every paper intended for publication in the Transactions must not only be placed in the hands of the Committee of Publication by 1st June, but it must also be so prepared as to require no material alteration or addition at the hands of the author.

" *Resolved,* That authors of papers be required to return their proofs within two weeks after their reception, otherwise they will be passed over and omitted from the volume."

Adjourned until 3 o'clock, P. M.

AFTERNOON SESSION.

Dr. W. L. Sutton, one of the Vice-Presidents, took the chair, in the absence of the President.

Dr. D. Meredith Reese, of New York, chairman of the Committee on Nominations, reported the following officers for the ensuing year:

President.—Henry Miller, of Kentucky.

Vice-Presidents.—H. F. Askew, Delaware; Chas. S. Tripler, U. S. Army; L. A. Smith, New Jersey; Calvin West, Indiana.

Treasurer.—Caspar Wister, Pennsylvania.

Secretary.—S. M. Bemiss, Kentucky.

Dr. Sayre moved the adoption of the report, which was unanimously agreed to.

Dr. Brainard, of Illinois, moved the appointment of a committee to conduct the newly-appointed officers to their respective chairs. The Acting President selected Drs. Brainard, of Illinois, Mattingly, of Kentucky, Sutton, of Indiana, McDowell, of Missouri, and R. J. Breckinridge, of Kentucky, and they accordingly performed the duties assigned to them.

The newly-elected President, on taking the chair, addressed the Convention in substance as follows:

Gentlemen of the American Medical Association—I am wholly at a loss to command language to express the deep sense of obligation put upon me by calling me to the Presidency of your Association. It is an honor any man may well be proud of; and although I admit in all sincerity that you might without difficulty have selected an individual more worthy the position, I may be allowed to say you could not have conferred it upon one who would prize it more highly or cherish it longer with the most grateful recollection. I do esteem it the greatest honor ever conferred upon me by the profession that I love, and to which I have devoted a long life; nay, more—it is the greatest honor that could be conferred upon any man by the medical or any other profession in this or any other country; for any decoration of honor or any mark of approbation conferred by a crowned head I should regard as a bauble in comparison. Who are you, gentlemen, when rightly considered? You are the rightful representatives of the great American Medical Profession—an army forty thousand strong, and a body of men, no matter what captious criticism may say in disparaging comparison with the European branch of the profession, in my humble judgment, far superior to the same number of medical men to be found in any quarter of the globe. Although, as a body, you may not be so learned, so critically and nicely framed in all the minutiæ of the profession, yet for strength, integrity, and precision in all the great principles guiding to a successful combat with disease, this body is equal, if not superior, to that of any kingdom of Continental Europe.

To be called to the Presidency of such a body of men, is, in my sober judgment, the greatest compliment that could be conferred on mortal man, provided that man is a devotee of medicine, who has given his whole mind, soul, heart, and strength individually to the profession, and has that high regard for it which will not suffer any less noble pursuit to interfere with the daily though laborious duties of the profession.

Coming so recently from a sick-bed, and still enfeebled in health, I beg to be excused from further remarks, and desire you to accept this brief and imperfect acknowledgment of the distinguished honor conferred upon me, instead of what, under other circumstances, I might be disposed to say.

The President, after this graceful address, sat down amid much applause, when Dr. R. J. Breckinridge moved that the thanks of the Association be tendered to the retiring officers for the faithful and assiduous manner in which they have conducted the business committed to their charge, which was unanimously adopted.

A long and discursive debate then ensued on the admission of members by invitation. The plan of organization permits practitioners of respectable standing from sections of the United States not otherwise represented at the meeting, to receive appointment by invitation of the meeting after an introduction from any of the members present, or any absent permanent members, to hold connection with the Association until the close of the annual session at which they are received, and to be entitled to participate in all its affairs as in the case of delegates. The point of difficulty seemed to be, whether the invitations should be extended by the Committee of Arrangements or by open vote of the Association. It was finally settled by referring all the applicants' names to the Committees of Arrangements and Credentials.

Dr. J. B. Lindsly, of Tennessee, offered the following:

" *Resolved*, That a committee of three be appointed by the chair to inquire into and report upon the propriety of dividing the Association into sections, for the purpose of performing such parts of its scientific labors as may relate to particular branches of medicine and surgery."

Dr. Brodie moved its reference to the Nominating Committee.

Dr. Brainard explained at some length the object of the resolution of inquiry, and urged its adoption, as the means of giving more effect and usefulness to the proceedings of the Association, the reports of which had heretofore gone out unmatured in consequence of the want of concentrated action.

A motion by Dr. Sayre to lay the motion on the table was negatived, and the motion of Dr. Lindsly was then adopted.

Dr. Davis moved that no person be permitted to speak more than twice on the same subject, or more than ten minutes at one time, except by consent of the Association, which was adopted.

The Standing Committee on Prize Essays was called on for their report, but without a response. This was also the case with the Committee on Medical Education. The Committee on Medical Literature had no report to present.

A letter from Dr. J. G. F. Holston, of Ohio, chairman of the Special Committee on the Microscope, was read, reporting progress, and begging a continuance for more extended investigation, which was referred to the Committee on Nominations.

A letter from Dr. Stephen Smith, of New York, from the Special Committee on Medical Jurisprudence, had the same reference.

The Special Committee on Quarantine was not ready to report.

Dr. Mattingly, of Kentucky, from the Special Committee on Diseases and Mortality of Boarding Schools, asked a continuance until next year, in order to obtain further information requisite to the full investigation of the important subject   This was referred to the Committee on Nominations.

The Special Committee on Surgical Operations for the Relief of Defective Vision, on Milk Sickness, and on the Blood Corpuscle, had the same reference.

A report from the Committee on Medical Ethics, signed by Dr. John Watson, of New York, was read, laid on the table, and made the special order for to-morrow, at 12 o'clock, M. This is an important subject, and will probably give rise to much debate to-day.

Continuances were asked by the Committees on the Pons Varolii, Medulla Oblongata, and Spinal Marrow—their Pathology and Therapeutics; on American Medical Necrology; on the Hygienic Relations of Air, Food, and Water, the Natural and Artificial Causes of their Impurity, and the best Methods by which they can be made most effectually to contribute to the Public Health; on the Effect of the Virus of Rattlesnakes, &c., when introduced into the System of the Mammalia; on the Climate of the Pacific Coast, and its Modifying Influences upon Inflammatory Action and Diseases generally; on the Constitutional Origin of Local Diseases, and the Local Origin of Constitutional Diseases; on the Physiological Effects of the Hydro Carbons; on Epilepsy; on the Causes of the Impulse of the Heart, and the Agencies which influence it in Health and Disease; and on the best Substitute for Cinchona, and its Preparations, in the Treatment of Intermittent Fever, &c.; all of which were referred to the Committee on Nominations.

The Special Committee on Government Meteorological Reports made a report, written by Dr. R. H. Coolidge, of the U. S. Army, but read by Dr. Paul F. Eve, of Tennessee, which was referred to the Committee on Publication.

The committee, appointed in May, 1857, on Criminal Abortion, submitted a report, written by Dr. Storer, of Boston, which was read by Dr. Blatchford, of New York, and referred to the Committee on Publication. The following resolutions appended to this report were unanimously adopted:

" *Resolved,* That while physicians have long been united in condemning the act of producing abortion at every period of gestation, except as necessary for preserving the life of either mother or child, it has become the duty of this Association, in view of the prevalence and increasing frequency of the crime, publicly to enter an earnest and solemn protest against such unwarrantable destruction of human life.

" *Resolved,* That in pursuance of the grand and noble calling we profess—the saving of human lives—and of the sacred responsibilities thereby devolving upon us, the Association present this subject to the attention of the several Legislative Assemblies of the Union, with the prayer that the laws by which the crime of procuring abortion is attempted to be controlled may be revised, and that such other action may be taken in the premises as they, in their wisdom, may deem necessary.

" *Resolved,* That the Association request the zealous co-operation of the various State Medical Societies in pressing the subject upon the Legislatures of their respective States, and that the President and Secretaries of the Association are hereby authorized to carry out by memorial these resolutions.

The Convention then adjourned till to-morrow morning at 9 o'clock.

SECOND DAY.

WEDNESDAY, *May 4th*, 1859.

The President, Dr. Miller, called the Association to order at 9 o'clock.

Dr. D. Meredith Reese, chairman of the Committee on Nominations, called attention to the fact that the committee could not act definitely until the place for next year's meeting should be designated. He stated also, that the Medical State Society of Connecticut had requested that an amendment to the Constitution, proposed two years since, should be taken from the table, relative to the time of meeting.

It was moved by Dr. Blatchford, and seconded by Dr. Sayre, that the amendment to the third article of the Constitution be taken up, which proposes to add after the words "first Tuesday in May," the words " or first Tuesday in June;" and after the words " shall be determined," the words " with the time of meeting."

The amendment was adopted by a constitutional vote.

Dr. D. M. Reese also stated that the Connecticut brethren had extended a kindly invitation to the Association to hold its next meeting at New Haven, through Dr. C. Hooker; which invitation was referred to the Committee on Nominations.

Dr. Reese also called attention to the necessity of some radical change in the mode of appointing committees to prepare treatises on scientific subjects to be reported at the annual meetings. It had been seen that, on yesterday, a large majority of the committees made no reports, and did not even see proper to send in any communication explanatory of delay. The difficulty heretofore has originated in the mode of selection adopted by the Nominating Committee. It has been customary for gentlemen to hand in their names and the proposed subjects on slips of paper, and the committee, without further investigation, have so published in the annual reports. Thus it has happened that appointments have been most injudiciously made, and gentlemen, to whom a special duty has been assigned, have been found to know less of that than any other subject. He therefore hoped that no committee of last year would be reappointed or continued from which no report had been had, and no communication received.

On motion, the Nominating Committee was unanimously instructed to act upon the suggestions of the chairman, who also stated that there should be some definite expression of disapprobation as to the course of those gentlemen who had volunteered essays, and had their names reported in the newspapers and spread over the land, and then paid no further attention to the matter.

Dr. Flint, from the Committee on Prize Essays, begged leave to report that they received four dissertations in time for a careful and thorough examination, and two others, quite voluminous, only two days before the meeting of the Association. The latter we have felt constrained to exclude altogether from the competition of the present year, on account of the absolute impossibility of reading them with a critical purpose and effect. The others have been carefully examined by all the surviving members of the committee—one estimable associate, Dr. Evans, having been called from all his earthly labors before the active duties of the committee began.

More than one of the four essays we examined exhibited much labor, and a commendable scholarship in their preparation—are voluminous, and in some respects very meritorious papers; but, in the unanimous judgment of the committee, neither of them possesses the degree and species of merit which should entitle its author to the Association prize.

The committee beg leave futhermore to report, that in their opinion, and as the suggestion of their own recent experience, the Association should determine in more precise and formal manner than has yet been done, the terms and conditions of competition and of success in the contest for prizes, for the government alike of contestants and the committee of adjudication, and that a committee be now appointed to consider and report upon the subject.

Dr. J. B. Lindsly, chairman of the committee appointed to inquire into the propriety of dividing the Association into sections, for the better performance of its work in considering the various branches of medicine and surgery, recommended the adoption of such a plan, as being indispensably necessary to making this body a working scientific association. They do not deem it necessary to enter into any argument in favor of this plan, it being the one already universally adopted by similar bodies. They would simply recommend, for the present, a division into the following sections, as being most suitable to facilitate the transaction of business, viz.:

1. Anatomy and Physiology.
2. Chemistry and Materia Medica.
3. Practical Medicine and Obstetrics.
4. Surgery.

The committee do not propose that this subdivision of labor shall in any manner interfere with the regular business of the Association as now conducted; but only that after having assembled each day in general session, each section shall meet separately for the purpose of hearing and discussing papers on such subjects as properly belong to them, and they therefore recommend that the Committee of Arrangements for the ensuing year be requested to provide suitable accommodations for the services of these sections, and that each of said sections shall be authorized to make such arrangements as may be required for the proper transaction of its business.

This report was considered and adopted, after a very able speech in its support by Dr. Davis.

Dr. J. W. Singleton, of Ky., moved the suspension of the rules for the introduction of the following:

"*Resolved*, That in the death of Dr. A. Evans, of Kentucky, the Association has lost one of its most manly and efficient members, and society a friend and benefactor."

The resolution was unanimously adopted.

Dr. W. L. Sutton, under the resolution appointing a committee on registration of births, marriages, &c., proposed a plan of general action, an abstract of which he read on motion of Dr. Gibbs, of S. C., and on motion of Dr. L. P. Yandell, the subject was referred to a committee, to report during the present session.

Drs. Sutton, Lindsly, W. R. Gibbs, Bryan, Pitcher, and Shattuck were appointed such committee.

Dr. Blatchford stated that he had received from Dr. Willard, Secretary of the New York State Medical Society, fifty volumes of their Transactions for 1859, for distribution to the medical press, the medical colleges, and all medical societies of the South, and sent with a request for an interchange of civilities. Gentlemen present can be supplied by application to Dr. Bemiss; and if the number sent be not sufficient for the supply, they will be cheerfully forwarded to any gentleman by application to the Secretary, Dr. S. D. Willard, Albany, N. Y., the postage being included in the application, which is twenty-two cents.

A voluminous report from Dr. Thomas Logan, of California, on Medical Topography and Epidemics, was received, and referred to the Committee on Publication.

The chairman of the Committee on Voluntary Essays stated that he had received a paper on a case of extra-uterine fœtation from Dr. Enos Hoyt, of Transylvania, Mass., and another on a case of accidental poisoning by strychnine from Dr. Douglas Bly, of Rochester, N. Y. He also presented a very voluminous paper entitled " Observations on some of the Changes of the Solids and Fluids in Malarial Fever, by Joseph Jones, Professor of Medical Chemistry, in the Medical College of Georgia, at Augusta." By request, Prof. Jones gave a verbal abstract of his paper and an exposition of his theory, and on motion of D. W. Yandell the communication was referred to the Committee on Publication

Dr. D. W. Yandell announced that the following railroad companies had agreed to pass delegates to this Convention over their roads at half price: Pittsburg, Fort Wayne, and Chicago; Pennsylvania Central; Jeffersonville; New Albany and Salem; Louisville and Nashville, and Cleveland and Pittsburg.

On motion, a vote of thanks was tendered to these companies for their liberality.

Dr. J. B. Flint offered the following resolution:

"*Whereas*, Our brethren of Great Britain are engaged in erecting a monument to the memory of John Hunter, whose invaluable services in behalf of Physiology and Surgery are recognized and honored, as well on this side of the Atlantic as in Europe; and whereas, this Association, as the representatives of American Medicine, would rejoice in some suitable manner to participate in so grateful a testimonial of gratitude and respect: Therefore,

"*Resolved*, That a committee of three be appointed to consider in what manner this participation can best be effected, so as to be acceptable to our British brethren, and consistent with our means and opportunities of action, with instructions to report at the next annual meeting."

The resolution was adopted, and Drs. Flint, Bowditch, and Shattuck appointed as the committee.

Dr. Harvey Lindsly offered the following:

"*Whereas*, Parliamentary rules of order are numerous, complicated, sometimes obscure, and often inapplicable to such a body as the American Medical Association; and whereas, from the nature of the pursuits of medical men, they cannot be familiar with these rules: Therefore,

"*Resolved*, That a select committee of three members be appointed to prepare a system of rules for the government of this Association, as few in number, as concise and as perspicuous as possible, to be reported at the next annual meeting."

This resolution was adopted, and Drs. Lindsly, Comegys, and Blatchford appointed as the committee.

The paper of Dr. Bly, on Accidental Poisoning by Strychnine, was read by its author; and, as individual cases are not reported in the Transactions of the Association, thanks were returned for the communication, with a request that it be published in some medical journal.

An invitation from Grand Master Morris, of the Masons, was received, urging medical brethren to attend the Masonic Convention now in session in this city.

The Nominating Committee made the following report:

The next annual meeting to take place at New Haven, on the first Tuesday of June, 1860. Dr. Eli Ives is elected Junior Secretary.

Committee of Arrangements—Drs. Chas. Hooker, Stephen G. Hubbard, and Benjamin Silliman, Jr., with power to add to their numbers.

Committee on Prize Essays—Drs. Worthington Hooker, Conn.; G. C. Shattuck, Mass.; Usher Parsons, R. I.; P. A. Jewett, Conn., and John Knight, Conn.

Committee on Publication—Drs. F. G. Smith, Philadelphia, Pa.; Wister, do ; Bemiss, Louisville, Ky ; Ives, New Haven, Conn.; Hollingsworth, Philadelphia, Pa., and Askew, Wilmington, Del.

Committee on Medical Literature—Drs. Henry Campbell, Ga.; D.
F. Wright, Tenn.; G. Wendell Holmes, Mass.; S. C. Armor, Ohio,
and W. H. Byford, Ill.

Committee on Medical Education—Drs. D. M. Reese, N. Y.; W. R.
Bowling, Tenn.; Chas. Fishback, Ind.; John Bell, Penn.; Z. Pitcher,
Mich.

The following Special Committees were appointed:

On Morbus Coxarius, and Surgical Pathology of Articular Inflammation—Dr. Lewis A. Sayre, of New York.

On the Surgical Treatment of Strictures of the Urethra—Dr. James
Bryan, of Philadelphia.

On Drainage and Sewerage of Large Cities, their Influence on Public Health—Drs. A. J. Semmes, D. C., Chairman; Cornelius Boyle,
and G. M. Dove.

On Puerperal Tetanus, its Statistics, Pathology, and Treatment—
Dr. D. L. McGugin, of Keokuk, Iowa.

On Hospital Epidemics—Dr. R. K Smith, of Philadelphia.

On Puerperal Fever—Dr. S. N. Green, of Stilesville, Ind.

On Anæmia and Chlorosis—Dr. H. P. Ayres, of Fort Wayne, Ind.

On Veratrum Viride—Dr. James B. McCaw, of Richmond, Va.

On Alcohol—Its Therapeutical Effects—Dr. J. R. W. Dunbar, of
Baltimore, Md.

On Meteorology—Dr. J. G. Westmoreland, Atlanta, Ga.

On Milk Sickness—Dr. Robert Thompson, Columbus, Ohio.

On Manifestations of Disease of Nerve Centres—Dr. C. B. Chapman,
Wisconsin.

On the Medical Topography of Iowa—Dr. T. O. Edwards, Iowa.

On Microscopic Observations on Cancer Cells—Dr. Geo. D. Norris,
New Market, Ala.

On the Philosophy of Practical Medicine—Dr. James Graham, Cincinnati, Ohio.

*On some of the Peculiarities of the North Pacific, and their Relations
to Climate*—Dr. Wm. H. Doughty, Ga.

The following Special Committees were continued or altered:

On Microscope—John C. Dalton, Jr., N. Y.; David Hutchinson,
Ind.; A. R. Stout, Cal.; Calvin Ellis, Mass.; Christopher Johnson,
Maryland.

On Diseases and Mortality of Boarding Schools—Dr. C. Mattingly,
Ky., and Dixi Crosby, N. H.

On the Various Surgical Operations for the Relief of Defective Vision—Drs. M. A. Pallen, Mo.; T. J. Cogley, Ind., and W. Hunt, Penn.

On the Blood Corpuscle—Dr. A. Sager, Michigan.

On American Medical Necrology—Dr. C. C. Cox, Maryland.

*On the Hygienic Relations of Air, Food, and Water, the natural and
artificial causes of their impurity, and the best methods by which they can
be made most effectually to contribute to the public health*—Dr. C. C. Cox,
Maryland.

On the Effect of Virus of Rattlesnakes, &c., when introduced into the System of Mammalia—Dr. A. S. Payne, Virginia.

On the Climate of the Pacific Coast, and its modifying Influences upon Inflammatory Action and Diseases generally—Dr. O. Harvey, California.

On the Constitutional Origin of Local Diseases and the Local Origin of Constitutional Diseases—Drs. W. H. McKee, North Carolina, and C. F. Heywood, New York.

On motion of Dr. Brodie, Dr. A. J. Semmes was requested to serve as Secretary *pro tem.* during the remainder of the session.

The Association took up the special order, being the report on Medical Ethics, to which had been referred the action of the Dubuque Medical Society, which, after debate, was laid over until 12 o'clock to-morrow.

On motion of Dr. H. F. Campbell, a section of meteorology, medical topography, and epidemic diseases, and of medical jurisprudence and hygiene, was added to those already adopted by this Association.

Amendments to the Constitution of the Association were then taken up, and a provision was acted upon, that no individual who shall be under sentence of expulsion or suspension from any State or local medical society, of which he may have been a member, shall be received as a delegate to this body, or be allowed any of the privileges of a member, until he shall have been relieved from said sentence by such State or local society. This amendment to the Constitution was adopted.

The next amendment, lying over from last year, was the proposition of Dr. Kyle, of Ohio:

That the Constitution of the Association be so amended as to prohibit the admission as a delegate, or the recognition as a member, of any person who is not a graduate of some respectable medical college.

This amendment was rejected, but, on the question of reconsideration, a long and animated debate ensued, which called forth all the oratorical abilities and much of the personal feelings of the delegates. Without arriving at a vote, the Association adjourned for dinner.

The following gentlemen have been admitted to the Association as members by invitation:

Indiana.—B. C. Bowan, N. D. Field, John S. Rowe, R. Curran, D. Wiley, J. A. Windle, A. V. Talbot, J. W. Davis.

Ohio.—W. C. Hall, N. B. Davis.

Tennessee.—J. M. Brannoch.

Kentucky.—W. N. Gaither, S. B. Field, W. S. Cain, J. A. Hodge, S. B. Merrifield, Joshua Gore, H. M. Berkeley.

Missouri.—J. M. Allen.
Alabama.—Drs. Bozeman and Turney.
New Hampshire.—David Kay.
United States Army.—Charles S Tripler.

AFTERNOON SESSION.

Upon the reassembling of the Association, the discussion was renewed on the motion to reconsider the vote by which the amendment
to the Constitution was negatived, prohibiting the admission as a delegate or the recognition as a member of any person who is not a graduate of some respectable medical college.

Dr. Kincaid moved a further amendment to insert the word "hereafter" after " prohibiting."

Dr. Askew, of Del., one of the Vice-Presidents, in the chair, ruled
the amendment out of order at the present stage, or until the Association decide upon the question of reconsideration.

After a long discussion, Dr. Davis, of Ind., moved to lay the motion to reconsider on the table, which was carried, 97 yeas, nays not
counted; so the amendment stands registered.

The next proposed amendment to the Constitution was that suggested by the New Jersey Medical Society, asking for such changes
as would establish a Board of Censors in every judicial district of the
Supreme Court, who should examine and grant diplomas to all proper
members of the Association.

This was temporarily laid on the table, for Dr. Crosby to offer a report of the Medical Teachers' Convention, which met on Monday last.
He strongly recommended a committee from this body to confer with
the Teachers' Committee, and felt great confidence that something
beneficial to medical education would be the effect of such conference.

Dr. Comegys moved the appointment of a committee of five to confer with the committee of Medical Teachers and report at the next
annual meeting, provided that no medical teacher be selected on the
part of this Association.

This again gave rise to an excited debate, clearly showing that there
was a great deal of bad feeling between the professors and the laymen
of our profession. Prof. McDowell, of Missouri, was extremely happy
in some of his hits, and kept his auditors in a roar of laughter. He
acknowledged that Philadelphia and New York had the advantage
of location; the railroads took students there as they did the horses
and cattle of the West, and sometimes its asses.

(To be concluded in the July number.)

SELECTIONS.

ON THE SPECULUM VAGINÆ.

By John P. Mettauer, M.D., LL.D., of Virginia.

The employment of this instrument, of late years, in the exploration and treatment of uterine affections, has become almost as common as the stethoscope and percussion in the diseases of the thoracic organs. Even inexperienced practitioners, who have barely laid aside the swathings of their pupilage, presume to employ it, and speak authoritatively of the mode of applying it, as well as of the diseases demanding its use. They seem to regard the operation as a thing of little importance, as far as female delicacy is concerned, and to believe that poor woman should submit to it, even if a disease of the uterus is only suspected to exist, that might possibly render the speculum necessary hereafter.

Every enlightened and humane physician will concede that a necessity will sometimes arise for the employment of the speculum, as well as other modes of exploration, repulsive to female delicacy. In such cases a sacrifice of delicacy becomes a duty, and sensible women unhesitatingly submit to its wise and sacred behests.

The writer has undertaken this communication for the purpose of showing that the speculum, in the investigation and treatment of uterine diseases, has been needlessly employed, and its value, as a means of diagnosis, greatly abused. That the instrument is entirely unnecessary in a large majority of uterine diseases, the writer's experience abundantly testifies. His experience with the speculum, too, has long since satisfied him that the evidence furnished by it is often unsatisfactory, and not to be relied on; nay, in some instances, it is actually deceptive, by reason of the changes caused in the state of the os and cervix uteri, by the pressure of the instrument on them. It has frequently been the case, in the hands of the writer, that the pressure of the speculum has so changed the color and presenting surface of those parts, as actually to defeat the objects of the examination; and such will often be the case in engorgement of the uterus, and when there is malposition of it from retro or antiversion. Generally, in determining as to the existence or non-existence of induration, engorgement, the deviations of position, internal ulceration, and, very frequently, of ulceration of the os itself, no matter how carefully and skillfully used, it affords little if any information of a reliable and use-

27

· · ful nature. Even when the three or four bladed instrument is employed, the operation and results will be obnoxious to these objections in a great degree, and they are the only reliable forms of vagino-uterine speculums in displaying the parts to be examined, and are also more readily and easily introduced; yet, little difficulty will be encountered in the use of any of the speculums now in use, even with a mere novice, who has carefully studied and learned the form, course, and depth of the vagina, the highly wrought and fanciful account of such difficulties, published in the *Monthly Stethoscope and Medical Reporter*, No. 2, vol. 2, for 1857, to the contrary notwithstanding.

It is not pretended that the speculum is useless, or absolutely unnecessary in vaginal and uterine diseases. Far otherwise—as the writer has employed it in those diseases in some instances with the best results. It is to the officious and indiscriminate employment of it that he objects, and to the exclusion and neglect of the more reliable and delicate mode of examination by the " toucher."

The speculum has not found general favor in France, although much employed in that country. At the head of its opponents there, the name of the distinguished Velpeau stands conspicuous; and it is matter of gratulation to the writer to find his views supported by such high authority; yet he had entertained those views and carried them out in practice years before he was aware that Velpeau had expressed similar opinions and objections.

It is probable that the physicians of this country and France more generally and indiscriminately employ the speculum than any others in the civilized world; and it is probable also that the taste for using it is due, in a degree, if not wholly, to the cliniques, as well as to the hospital practice connected with the medical schools of those countries, where female delicacy and exposure are regarded with little concern, as the subjects of the use of the speculum are derived from the most degraded classes of society, with whom modesty is only known by name. In many instances, the writer has met with women laboring under organic diseases of the uterus, who declared to him that they would sooner take their chance to live or die with the disease, than submit to the use of the speculum; and all are more or less opposed to it, even those who finally submit to its employment. Really, it is not to be wondered at, that a modest, delicate woman should feel unwilling to submit her person to such a revolting exposure; and the writer candidly owns that he has never yet applied the speculum, or even examined by the toucher, without being more or less abashed and disconcerted, by reason of the exposure the operation necessarily imposes on females. Even the ordinary modes of investigation by question and answer often greatly shock a modest female, and in a degree, in some instances, embarrass the diagnosis of her diseases.

When organic disease of the uterus exists, and the rational symptoms fail in furnishing the requisite amount of information necessary to form a satisfactory diagnosis, nearly every intelligent woman will consent to a physical examination, if made sensible of the necessity for it, especially if the proposition to do so is delicately presented; and such being the case, it is the duty of the physician, as far as is consistent with safety, to save his female patients all needless shock of feeling from delicate questions or personal exposure.

Entertaining such views of this delicate subject, the writer some ten years since directed his attention to the investigation of organic diseases of the uterus, guided by the toucher, chiefly; and after repeated trials, affording ample experience, he unhesitatingly states that the information it furnishes is far more reliable and satisfactory than that derived from any form of speculum, in determining as to the existence and nature of such diseases. In numerous instances, during the time above stated, he has tested the correctness of his diagnosis in uterine diseases guided by the taxis. Most of the examples presented ulceration of the os, but in many cases the cervix was also implicated more or less extensively. Ten of them exhibited the os patulus, exceeding in size a Spanish dollar, and deeply ulcerated, the cervix indurated considerably beyond the interior boundary of the corresponding border of the ulcer, and the general health greatly impaired.

After carefully examining into the condition of the os and cervix uteri by the toucher, he was enabled to detect ulceration with great certainty, as well as induration, engorgement, and all of the deviations of position.

An ulcerated os uteri presents to the experienced touch the same feel as an ulcer on the exterior of the body; and an accompanying induration of the surrounding parts is a very common attendant of such ulceration, as it is also of many external ulcers. Induration of the cervix, however, is decidedly more apt to accompany intra-cervical ulceration; and as it is uniformly met with in such ulceration of the cervix, clearly ascertained to exist, as well as frequently in ulceration of the os likewise, it may safely be inferred that it represents ulceration in all those cases in which the cervix is inaccessible to the touch, when indurated, without ulceration of the os.

In deciding as to the existence of induration of the os or cervix uteri, the speculum is absolutely useless. Even in ulceration, the information it imparts is unsatisfactory and unreliable. In engorgement and inflammation, it furnishes no information that is not derivable from the toucher, elucidative of those conditions, and is far more offensive to the feelings of a delicate woman than the investigation by the taxis.

The discharge, said to be characteristic of, and peculiar to ulceration of the os and cervix, is not by any means constant in appearance, nor does it furnish conclusive evidence in all cases that ulceration does exist when met with. If present, and just issuing from the os uteri, either in its semifluid or ropy condition, the speculum, if then applied, would only prove that the morbid secretion unequivocally proceeded from the os uteri. The discharge of this diseased product externally, however, affords as satisfactory evidence of the existence of ulceration of the os uteri, as if actually seen escaping from the uterine cavity, because its characters are sufficiently marked to remove all doubt of its identity.

Although furnishing pretty satisfactory evidence of the existence of organic diseases of the uterus, of itself, the revelations of the toucher should invariably be taken in connection with the other symptoms usually met with in such diseases, in forming a diagnosis. The ulcerated os and cervix, when accessible to the touch; the induration; the peculiar discharge; pelvic and dorsal pains; inability to stand' long at a time; frequently, abdominal pains; disodered digestion; nervousness; depression of spirits, and the peculiar desponding expression of countenance termed "facies uterine," when taken together, leave little room to doubt as to the existence of ulceration of the os and cervix uteri.

The speculum will be demanded in those cases in which the os uteri cannot be reached by the finger, as then no other reliable plan could be adopted for exploring and treating such examples. Fortunately, these latter instances are rarely to be met with, as the writer has only witnessed two out of over a hundred cases treated by him in ten years. It will also be required in scirrhus uteri, when the indurated cervix is to be excised; and when adhesions between the os or cervix and vagina exist. And it will be indispensable in cauterizing the uterus with the incandescent iron, and in leeching or scarifying the organ.

For the purpose of cauterizing the os and cervix, the writer employs the nitrate of silver, and the acid nitrate of mercury, conveyed to the parts, concealed by a canula directed by the index finger of the right hand; and the operation should be repeated once in three or four days, or after longer intervals, if the previous operation is followed by prolonged bleeding, until the cure is perfected. The nitrate of silver is best adapted to the mild or slight examples of ulceration; while the acid nitrate of mercury should be used when the ulcers are deep and extensive, and especially if the cervix is decidedly implicated. It is best, however, to begin the treatment with the nitrate of silver; and if amelioration seems tardy, then to employ the acid nitrate of mercury in alternation with the caustic silver.

The position most convenient to the operator for examination, as well as for the application of remedies, is on the left side, with the thighs flexed on the trunk, and the legs on the thighs. The person should invariably be covered, and the nates placed near the border of a bed. In this posture, the parts can generally be reached and examined with the index finger of the right hand with entire convenience; and it is also the best for the application of the speculum, as well as the cauterizing agents employed through it.

The first trials, in the use of the caustic, upon the plan advocated in this paper, will, in all probability, be attended with some difficulty; but gentle efforts, repeated again and again deliberately, will soon impart the requisite dexterity of manipulation to insure success; and, after learning how to apply the remedy, the ease with which it can be done will astonish both patient and physician.

A crayon formed of the nitrate of silver, or the stick itself, may be used, applied as already intimated; and, for the application of the acid nitrate of mercury, a short, full camel's hair brush, or mop, saturated with the undiluted solution, answers best. The canula should be fully ten inches in length, of proper calibre to contain the crayon, or mop, and open at both ends, so as to allow the handle of the crayon to project sufficiently beyond the free, or outer extremity, so as to be held and wielded by the operator's left hand; and it may be formed of silver or glass; the latter material the writer employs, and decidedly prefers.

To guard against vaginal irritation, from accidental diffusion of either of the caustics over its surface, after being applied to the uterus, a weak solution of common salt should invariably be injected into the vagina immediately after any cauterization—using for the purpose a female glass syringe—taking care at the same time that this saline solution is effectually applied to the upper portion of the passage immediately around the cervix uteri. After this the vagina may be abluted daily with simple water or mucilaginous infusions, such as slippery-elm or flaxseed teas, applied tepid or cool, as may be preferred by females. The saline wash may also be used tepid or cool, according to the fancy of different patients.

The bowels should be kept in a soluble, easy condition, using for the purpose, when necessary, mild aperients, especially gentle aloetic preparations. When induration of the cervix exists, and if the habit is anæmic, the iodide of iron will be proper. If anæmia, without induration, is present, and more especially should there be nervous debility, and marked depression of spirits, frequently tending to deep despondency, the phosphate of iron will be indicated. It will sometimes be necessary to resort to vegetable tonics in these cases; and in many instances nothing answers better than good porter. The cold infusion of wild cherry bark (prun. virgin.)will very often supersede all other vegetable tonics; and the cases most likely to be benefited by it are those attended with undue nervousness, as well as debility. When the liver is torpid, and the bowels refuse to respond to the action of aperients, the nitro-muriatic acid mixture will be found signally beneficial. The diet should invariably be simple, and moderately nutritious.

It will greatly promote recovery, to require patients to remain in bed, or in a recumbent posture, during treatment; and for months after recovery, every species of traveling will be hurtful. The utmost care should be taken to guard patients against exposure to variable temperature. Catarrhal disturbances invariably aggravate uterine diseases of every kind, and in none do they prove more hurtful than in ulceration and induration of the os and cervix.—*Va. Medical Journal.*

LONGEVITY.

[The two following papers on Longevity are selected from the last number of the *New Orleans Medical and Surgical Journal*, and cannot fail to interest our readers.—ED. GAZ.]

"Can the limits of human life be extended? This is the question propounded by a celebrated professor of chemistry in a memoir presented to the Academy of Sciences: 'upon the causes of old age and senile death.' This chemist is M. Ed. Robin. He believes human life may be prolonged, and, courageous in this opinion, seeks for rational means to arrive at his conclusion. He will seek a long time still, says the reader. Such is our opinion, and, no doubt, M. Robin's, who, waiting further developments, furnishes us matters of interest on this topic.

"Living beings may be compared to furnaces, always kindled; life exists only in a state of combustion; but the combustion which occurs in our bodies, like that which takes place in our chimneys, leaves a residue, a detritus, ashes. This detritus, which is always accumulating, is, according to M. Robin, the prinicpal cause of old age and senile death.

"Food, whatever may be its nature, whether vegetable or animal, liquid or solid, is charged with mineral matters which are left in different parts of the organism by the process of combustion. At first, these serve for nutrition; but when the bones are all consolidated they continue to flow into the system, and then incrust and mineralize different parts of the mechanism.

"The manner in which mineralization causes old age in man is clearly pointed out: on the one hand, ossification of the cartilages of the sternum, greater rigidity of the posterior ligaments of the ribs, cause the respiration to become slower and slower, limit its extent, and finally render it altogether diaphragmatic; on the other, ossification of the vessels and their valves, diminution of the calibre of the arteries, obliteration of the capillaries, reduction of their number, and enlargement of the pulmonary cells, render the circulation more and more difficult, and diminish the respiratory surface.

"The air coming in less close contact with the blood does not so well aërate it; this liquid, therefore, becomes of a deeper color, engorges the venous system, as in asphyxia; and experiments upon the quantity of carbonic acid exhaled, upon animal temperature, upon the passage of certain elements of the blood in the urine, do not permit us to doubt that, beginning with a certain age, a combustion gradually less abundant takes place.

"As the combustion and heat diminish, so do the electrcity and nervous fluid; therefore, sensibility and contractility are lessened, motion and the general activity decrease; enfeebled by all these causes, the nervous action contributes in its turn to diminish the combustion, and ...... all the world knows the result of this.

"By force of such arguments, which have some good in them, M. Robin hopes to prove that it is easy to retard old age, and death in a large number of animals, by abating the phenomena of slow combustion

" In consequence, he proposes to institute three series of experiments upon animals whose lives are of short duration. One class will be fed upon those aliments which contain the smallest proportion of mineral matters of an incrusting nature; another upon food entirely deprived of these matters by appropriate dissolvents, and the last upon ordinary food; but with it is to be administered, beginning with a certain age, lactic acid, which has incontestably the power of dissolving mineral matters, and would appear to be sufficient to dissolve, during life, those which have been already deposited in the organism.

" If it be demanded what we think of the subject which M. Robin has chosen for his researches, we would reply that we highly approve them, and encourage the author to persevere. We well know what will be said: Paracelsus ! Van Helmont ! etc. But names, whether good or bad, have but little weight with us; and, for approving the researches of M. Robin, which are connected with one of those beliefs the most generally and deeply felt by humanity, which, in our opinion, would alone justify them, we have another reason still, or a principle, which we may reduce to the following formula: *Every quality which appears to be an exception in a species, indicates a new rule, to which this species may be subjected.*

" Applying this principle to the present subject, we say, there are macrobites or centenarians in the human species; then macrobie is compatible with the human organization, and since it exists, its cause may be determined. Now, to posess a knowledge of the cause is to be master of the effect; and that which has heretofore been the exception, may become the rule.

" The long life of the patriarchs provokes a smile. But in times less distant from our own, facts may be found which are but little more credible, and which cannot be disputed. It may gratify our readers to cite some of these facts:

" Ponce Lepage died in 1760, in the Duchy of Luxemburg, at the age of 121 years; a short time before his death he cultivated his field, and made excursions on foot of six or seven leagues. Eleanor Spicer died in Virginia, in 1763, aged 121 years. All her senses were perfect at the time of her death. Madame Barnet died in Charleston in 1820, aged 123 years. She recalled perfectly events which had occurred a century before. Grandez died in Languedoc, aged 126 years. He was a journeyman goldsmith, and was in the habit of working till ten or twelve days before his death. The Englishman John Newell died in 1761, at the age of 127 years, in the full enjoyment of reason. Another Englishman, John Bayles, a sheep-seller, died in 1706, aged 130 years. During the last years of his life he drove his flocks of sheep to the neighboring markets. Margaret Lawler, English, died in 1739, aged 135 years. A few days before her death she walked some three or four miles and returned home the same day. Joseph Barn, a negro, died in Jamaica in 1808, aged 140 years. A few days before he was in the habit of walking four miles. Polotiman, a surgeon in Lorraine, died in 1825, at the age of 140 years. The day before his death he operated upon a cancer with much dexterity. Thomas Parr died in London in 1635, at the age of 152 years. Until he was 130 years old he engaged freely in all 'the labors of a farmer, and even threshed his wheat.

"Obst, a village woman of Silesia, died in 1825, aged 155 years. She had labored in the field the evening before her death. Joseph Surrington, a Norwegian, died in 1797, aged 160 years. He preserved to the last his reason and his senses. John Bowin, born in the Bannat of Tameswar, died in 1740, aged 172 years. Peter Zortan, a countryman of the preceding, died in 1724, aged 185 years.

"If the life of these extraordinary beings be examined, it will be found very difficult to determine the causes of their longevity; the privilege which they enjoyed appears to have been compatible with every mode of living. For instance, Annibal Camoux, who died when 121 years, and who figures in one of Horace Vernet's paintings, drank much wine, and lived upon the coarsest food; so also the surgeon Polotiman never passed a day without being intoxicated; the peasant woman, Obst, who died at the age of 155, drank ordinarily two tumblerfuls of brandy daily. [At a recent meeting of the Detroit Historical Society, it was stated that a French resident of that city died a few years since at the age of 116 years, during 104 of which he never drew a sober breath.—ED.] From such examples it might be concluded that drunkenness gave one a lease for a long life.

"But on the other hand, Eleanor Spicer, who lived to her 121st year, never drank spirituous liquor; Grandez, who died at 126 years, never drank wine; John Effingham, who died at the age of 144 years, knew liquor only by sight. In addition to this contrast, here are some facts through which it is difficult to see clearly: Dennis Guignard, who died at the age of 123 years, dwelt in a cavern dug in sandy stone; Drahakemberg, who died in his 146th year, had been captured by Corsairs, and endured for fifteen years all the hardships of a cruel captivity; Jean Lafitte, who died at the age of 136 years, had contracted from early youth the habit of bathing two or three times a week, and preserved this habit to the end of his life; Jean Causeur, who died aged 146 years, lived chiefly on milk food (*laitage;*) Jean d'Outrego, who died at 146, lived upon Turkey wheat and cabbage; Thomas Parr, who died aged 152 years and 9 months, fared all his life upon bread, old cheese, milk, whey, and table-beer; and in conclusion, Peter Zortan, who died at 185 years of age, lived solely upon vegetables.

"All of this is sufficiently contradictory, nor is it easy to deduce from these facts rules for a regimen proper to produce macrobie; so that it is not here that it is necessary to seek for them. The knowledge afforded by these facts is sufficiently precious without demanding more from them; like all exceptions to natural laws, they furnish us with a revelation. By proving to us that human life may be prolonged far beyond its ordinary limits, they invite us to researches, which, in their absence, would not have been thought of, except to reject at once the idea of them. It is now left to us to discover the causes, and to conquer the means to obtain the result. This research does not appear to us a matter of indifference; and if, in order to enjoy longevity, it is sufficient to subject one's self to a regimen of lactic acid, we would willingly submit to it.

"If it were true that the art of greatly increasing the duration of human life was accessible to us, we could only applaud the contrast of future longevity, with the brevity of existence in the past. However short the life of our fathers, it sufficed for them to sow an ample harvest of sorrows; and however long may be the lives of our sons, or ourselves, it will not suffice to exhaust the noble pleasures which the remunerating future holds in reserve for good and honest men."

Dr. Legrand remarks upon the above: "So let it be, say we; and we have only to add, that Harvey has left us some curious details in regard to Thomas Parr, whose autopsy he made. He was married at 120 years, and at 130 he was summoned before the House of Commons for a misdemeanor. Harvey is said to have been an eye-witness to a coition successfully accomplished by Thomas Parr, at 140 years of age. One is not a great anatomist without being possessed by the demon of curiosity!"—[Translated from *L'Union Médicale.*]

In the "Curiosities of Medical Experience" it is stated that "Henry Jenkins lived to 169, and we have on record the case of a negress aged 175. The Hungarian family of John Rovin were remarkable for their longevity: the father lived to 172, the wife to 164; they had been married 142 years, and their youngest child was 115; and such was the influence of habit and filial affection, that this *child* was treated with all the severity of paternal rigidity, and did not dare to act without his *papa's* and *mamma's* permission."

To these might be added a number of reliable cases who lived more than 150 years, and some to 180. We will mention only three of the most recent: Marie Prion died in 1838, aged 158 years. A Polish peasant died in 1834, aged 188 years; and about ten years since, Madelon, a negress and a native of Louisiana, died at Pass Christian, Mississippi, who had seen her century and a half. Her daughter and grandson, living at that time, had reached a very old age; and Madelon is reported not only to have recovered the sight which she had lost, but to have been blessed with a third set of masticators.

These instances of modern longevity suffice to prove that in this respect, at least, mankind is not retrograding. The oldest of the biblical patriarchs did not surpass them. Abraham attained but 175 years, and his son Isaac only 180.

As to ancient Methuselah and the balance of the antediluvians, it is supposed, for good reasons, that their years were estimated by our seasons, and should consequently be divided by four. However, in non-medical works are recorded many cases of persons who lived two, three, and even more than four centuries; but, once trusting ourselves to these, we find such records vastly eclipsed by the equally reliable case of the Wandering Jew, who was *actually seen* by various parties some 600 years ago, and is thought by some credulous individuals to be still engaged in those peregrinations which he has so industriously prosecuted for the last 1800 years and more!

Dr. B. Dowler, in his researches upon the vital statistics of New Orleans, found in the African Cemetery that there was one centenarian in every fifty interments selected at random, which gives a proportion thousands of times higher than is recorded of any other race, or in any other part of the world.

[Although these enumerations (here alluded to by my friend and editorial associate, Dr. Chaillé,) were made at random, they were all taken from *monumental inscriptions*, and may virtually (without on my part intending it) have the *numerical effect of selection, if, as is probable, the ratio of monumental inscriptions be less for infants and young persons than for the adult and the aged class.*—B. DOWLER.]

There are various sources of error which might render these selections at random unreliable as a true indication of the ratio of centenarians to the total mortality; still there is no doubt that among the natives of Louisiana and our Gulf shore, there is to be found a larger proportionate number of persons who have passed their hundredth year, than in other parts of the United States or in Europe. The official statistics of the deaths in New Orleans for the past three and a half years give us sixteen centenarians, which is one in less than nineteen hundred of all the deaths. If from this calculation the yellow fever deaths be excluded, as they should be, (since these are among our unacclimated strangers,) the proportion would amount to one in less than fourteen hundred. In either case the ratio is far more favorable than is afforded by any European statistics.

The United States census for the decade ending with the year 1850 equally proves how favorable our Southern climate is to longevity, the number of centenarians being vastly greater, in proportion to the population, in the Southern than in the Northern States, and this holds true whether in reference to the black or white race, the slaves or freemen. In no States is the proportion of centenarians so large as in Texas and Louisiana.

The learned physiologist, M. Flourens, has written an interesting work on "Human Longevity." He concludes that the normal duration of man's life is one hundred years, and fortifies this conclusion by researches in comparative anatomy and physiology. He states that the duration of life, in mammalia at least, is proportionate to the duration of growth; the duration of growth to that of gestation, and the duration of gestation to the height. The larger the animal, the longer the gestation, etc. Buffon and other naturalists, as far back as Aristotle, have asserted that there was a fixed ratio between the duration of life and that of growth; but M. Flourens claims to have discovered the certain sign that marks the term of growth, which is the union of the bones with their epiphyses, after which the animal necessarily ceases to grow.

He finds in all animals which he has subjected to his observations and investigations, that the duration of their lives is five times that of their growth. For instance, the union of the bones with their epiphyses (i. e., the term of growth) occurs in the camel at 8 years, and this animal lives about 40 years; in the horse at 5 years, and this animal lives about 25 years; in the ox at 4 years, and this animal lives about 20 years; in the lion at 4 years, and this animal lives about 20 years; in the dog at 2 years, and this animal lives about 10 years; in the cat at 1½ years, and this animal lives about 8 years. From these and many similar examples, he concludes that, since in man the union of the bones with their epiphyses is effected at 20 years of age, the normal duration of his life must be 100 years.

We may conclude this paper, which, perhaps, is more curious than instructive, with the following quotation from Flourens: "Just as the duration of growth, multiplied a certain number of times, say five times, gives the ordinary duration of life, so does this ordinary duration, multiplied a certain number of times, say twice, give the extreme duration. A first century of ordinary life, and almost a second century, half a century (at least) of extraordinary life, is then the prospect science holds out to man." We leave it for those who love it more than the undersigned, to say, Amen!

CHAILLÉ.

Observations on Longevity, with Cases.

SUPPLEMENTARY TO THE PRECEDING ARTICLE:

By B. DOWLER, M.D.

The maximum estimate of the world's population among the best statisticians is 1,200,000,000 souls; of this number sixty-one die every minute. And although a considerable number die of accidents, an overwhelming majority perish by diseases, which the future progress of medicine may possibly, for the most part, prevent or cure, until the natural decadency of old age

"Shall end this strange, eventful history."

It is but sixty-three years since Jenner vaccinnated the first child. Before his discovery, according to some of the best statistical writers, one-thirteenth of the human race died of small-pox. Here is a remedial measure of easy application, which, if rigidly enforced, eliminates the most fatal of all exanthematous fevers from the bills of mortality, and consequently enhances the mean duration of life, while it affords presumptive proof that similar means of prevention or cure are within the category of possibility in relation to other maladies. If a preventive or cure should be discovered for consumption, one-fifth of the human race would be transferred to the account of longevity, or, at least, to that of an increased expectation of life.

Hygiene and morality—both eminently practicable, but generally not practiced by erring humanity—are to a great extent adequate to the task of eliminating many of the causes of premature death. Thus, intemperance, war, murder, syphilis, and many similar causes of the

short duration of life, would be extinguished by observing the merely
negative rule of virtue found in the first reading lesson of the old school
primer, namely, " *My son, do no ill.*" Inaugurate morality, hygiene,
the physical comforts; let physic and surgery advance as they have
already advanced during the present half century, and each revolving
century will add, perhaps, an improvement in the human constitution,
with an increased mean duration of life, and probably an increasing
number of extreme cases of longevity. Every day's occurrences confirm the Sacred Record that many " do not live out half their days,"
simply because they are not temperate, just, virtuous, and provident.
A degraded moral status conjoined to the physical evils of extreme
poverty and bad hygienic conditions, with a reckless neglect of the
incipient stages of disease, are the great abbreviators of human hopes
and life, and not solely the decrees of the Eternal.

The learned Dr. Sherlock, who lived two centuries ago, in his work
on Death, in reference to the question of the assumed absolute and
unconditioned determination of each person's life, says: " This is that
famous question which Beverovicius, a learned physician, was so much
concerned to have solved, and consulted so many learned men about;
as supposing it would be a great injury to his profession did men believe that the time of their death was so absolutely determined, that
they could neither die sooner nor live longer than that fatal period,
whether they took the advice and prescriptions of physicians or not.
But this was a vain fear; for there are some speculations which men
never live by, how vehemently soever they contend for them: a skep-
tic who pretends there is nothing certain, and will dispute with you
as long as you please about it, yet will not venture his own arguments
so far as to leap into fire or water, nor stand before the mouth of a
loaded cannon when you give fire to it. Yet these men will eat and
drink, to preserve themselves in health, and take physic when they
are sick."(140-1.)

During the historic period, outside of the longevity recorded in the
Sacred Writings, it is probable that the average or mean duration of
life has increased, owing to the progress of medical knowledge and the
increase of the physical comforts throughout the civilized world. Authentic examples of great longevity seem to have been also greatly
multiplied.

Pliny the Elder, nearly contemporaneous with the beginning of our
era, in his vast work of fact and fiction, (*Historia Naturalis,*) gives the
most remarkable examples of longevity among the ancients. He
mentions some instances of longevity taken exclusively from the re-

gion between the Apennines and the Po, as found on the record of the census instituted by Vespasian, and within these narrow limits he enumerates fifty-four persons who had reached the age of 100 years, fourteen of 111, twenty of 125, forty of 130, forty of 135, thirty of 140. In the single town of Valciatium, near Placentia, he mentions six of 110, four of 120, one of 150 years."—(*New Am. Cyc.*: New York, 1858.)

Before proceeding to make a few remarks on longevity, it is intended to give an enumeration of cases from 120 years upward, having excluded such as Dr. Chaillé has already given, nearly all of which, however, had been previously noted in my list. Imperfect as the latter is, I am not aware that any one so extended has hitherto been published. I have excluded cases recorded by authorities, when contradicted by other authorities. The authorities which are relied on in this catalogue are not generally named, because such citations would occupy much more space than the facts themselves. Owing to my limited leisure, I may have omitted to copy not a few cases which I have on record, but not easily found on this occasion.

DIED, AGED 120: *Death of a Venerable Servant.*—Sarah Mallory, a colored woman belonging to the estate of the late Capt. Gilbert, died at Norfolk on the 22d of March, 1859. She is said to have been born in 1740, and was therefore in the 120th year of her age. The *Day Book* says: " Her youngest child attended her funeral, as the last of the family. His back is bent, and his locks frosted o'er with the snows of eighty-seven winters. She remembered many of the exciting scenes which were enacted during the Revolution, and the surrender of Cornwallis at Yorktown was but as yesterday to her. At that time she was forty-one years of age, and her youngest child nine years old." Héléne Massy, free woman of color, at Mr. James Papplye's plantation, July 30, 1849. (*N. O. Delta.*) Mary Goodsall, negress, at Spanish Town, Jamaica (December, 1830); Mrs. Mary Inness, Mount Grace, Jamaica (December, 20, 1820); William Marshall (1792); Flora Gale,——; Dominick Joyes (1765); Moneula, negress (1780); Mrs. Moore (1765); John Mackay (1766); Sir Fleetwood Sheppard (1768); John Ryder,——; Mrs. Adams,——; John Chump (1769); Mrs. Sands (1770); Patrick Blewet——; Richard Gilshenan (1771); Barbara Wilson (1772); Sieur de la Haye (1774); H. d'Arcary de Beaucovoy (1778).

LIVING AT 120: *"Old People.*—The natives of Louisiana are remarkable for the extraordinary instances of longevity which they afford.

During the past six months we have noticed the death of several old persons who had exceeded the age of 100 years. We, the other day, saw a negro woman in Conti street, 109 years of age, who lives with her daughter, 82 years old. Her eyesight, hearing, and health are tolerably good. A more extraordinary case of longevity is that of an old French lady living at No. 140 Marigny street. Incredible as it may seem, she is said to have attained the age of 120 years, and the story seems to be true, for there are old people alive now who remember her a very old woman in their youth. Of course she is extremely infirm, and the cold weather of the present winter has affected her health so much that her demise is daily expected. This climate is undoubtedly one of the most favorable to longevity in the world."— (*N. O. Bee*, Feb. 6th, 1856.)

DIED, AGED 121: C. Lane, of Campbell County, Virginia (1821); Elizabeth Hilton (1760); Francis Bons (1769); Mrs. Gray (1770); William Farr, ——; Owen Tudor (1771); Margaret McKay, ——; John Whalley (1772); Henrietta Long (1788).

AGED 122: "*Death of the Oldest Man in Pennsylvania.*—Timothy Sweeny, aged 122 years, died in Fairview Township, Butler County, on the 27th ult. Mr. Sweeny was born in the year 1737, in Curahan, Parish of Ardfert, County of Kerry, Ireland, and emigrated to this country in 1837, being then 100 years old. He was never known to have had an hour's sickness, having the full use of his faculties to the last, with a delicacy of hearing and quickness of perception that was really miraculous for one who had journeyed so far beyond the allotted bounds of earthly existence. His last day on earth was spent, as usual, at the genial fireside of his daughter, Mrs. Nolan, surrounded by affectionate grandchildren; and nothing occurred to warn them that in the sleep of the night the patriarch was to sink silently and at once into the deep slumber of the grave."—(*Pittsburg Post*, March, 1859.) Margaret Annesley (1752); Catharine Giles (1758); Mrs. Carman (1771); Andrew Brizin Debra (1774); Mrs. Neale (1785); Archibald Cameron (1791).

AGED 123: Martha Preston (1769); Jean Arragus (1779); Matthew Taite (1792).

AGED 124: Thomas Wishart (1760); Catharine Brebner (1762); Andrew Vidal (1774); Abraham Vanverts (1774); Thomas Bright (1708); Elizabeth Stewart (1725); Andrew Bueno (1753); Robert Parr (1757).

AGED 125: John Dance, Virginia; —— Rice, ——; John Tice (1774); Mr. Gernon (1780); Mr. Frome (1785.)

AGED 126: Robert Montgomery (1670); John Bales (1706).

The journals of 1844 contained the following statement: Mr. John Hightower, of Marengo County, Alabama, died in August, 1844, aged 126 years; was a soldier of the Revolution; was in Braddock's defeat, and was wounded in that battle. His age can be established by an authentic family record.

A negress living in Virginia, aged 126: A correspondent of the *Richmond Enquirer*, writing from Powhatan, December 30, 1854, says:

"There is a negro woman in Powhatan, now living in my immediate neighborhood, whom I have talked with, who was born the year after George II. ascended the throne of England, and four years before the birth of George Washington! She is now 126 years old, and was, of course, very near half a century old at the time our Declaration of Independence was proclaimed, the 4th of July, 1776.

" I state this upon information that I believe to be true, and the appearance of her person serves to confirm it. Her memory seems to furnish her an indelible record of all the events, great and small, of her long life, when aroused from the state of drowsy forgetfulness that frequently betides her. When I saw her she was wide awake and full of chat. She had remarkably fine eyes, and, I was told, could thread a needle and sew nearly as well as she ever could.

" She said she had been the mother of sixteen children, all of whom died of old age, and that there was precisely one year and one day between their births, respectively; that she had never been sick, never had a physician to see her, and never took a single dose of physic in her life. She talked cheerfully and fluently, and quoted many passages of Scripture readily and appropriately.

" Whenever she touched upon religion, her mind seemed to become absorbed at once; and the (to me) unexpected fluency and beauty of her language indicated ' the gift' that we sometimes hear of. Though no doctor, I was prompted by curiosity to feel her pulse, to see if it beat like other people's. I found it quite regular and strong. I inquired if she had never lost her eyesight. She said, ' No, never, nor appetite either.' "

AGED 127: Davie Grant (1658); Mrs. Bampton (1758); William Hughes (1769); Madame Girodolle (1772); Daniel Mullecry (1775); Martha Jackson (1776); John Newell (1761).

AGED 128: John Jacob, of Mount Jura, ——; Mary Yates (1776); Edglebert Hoff (1755); Mary John, —— ; Mr. Fleming (1771); Abraham Strodtham (1772).

28

AGED 129: Thomas King (1768); Joseph Gale (1769); John Gough (1771).

AGED 130: Donald Cameron (1759); John De la Somet (1766); George King; John Taylor (1767); William Beaty (1774); John Watson (1778); Robert Macbride (1780); William Ellis; Satira, negress, Antigua (Feb. 17, 1823); Tom, belonging to Mrs. Bacon, South Carolina (1829); Lucretia Stewart, Jamaica (1817); Margaret Darby, negress, Fellowship Hall, Jamaica (April 6, 1821,) retained her faculties to the last. •

AGED 131: Elizabeth Taylor (1764); Peter Gardner (1775).

AGED 132: Jeremy Gilbert, Northamptonshire.   .

AGED 133: Elizabeth Merchant (1761); Mrs. Keith (1772).

AGED 134: Francis Ange (1767); John Brookey (1777); Jane Catharine Lopez, negress, Kingston, Jamaica (1808).

AGED 135: Jane Harrison (1714).

AGED 136: James Sheile (1759); Catharine Noon (1768); Margaret Foster (1761); John Mouat (1776).

AGED 137: John Richardson (1772); —— Robertson (1793); H. Francisco, Whitehall, near New York (1820).

AGED 138: William Sharpley (1757); Joan McDonogh (1768); Mrs. Clum (1772). LIVING CASE: —— Fairbrother, of Lancashire, was still living (1771).

AGED 139: Thomas Dobson (1766); Mary Cameron (1785).

AGED 140: A negro woman died on the 4th of July, 1858, at Kenner, aged 140 years. She was born in Guinea, Africa, and retained her faculties until within a short period of her death. She belonged to Minor Kenner. William Leland (1732); James Sands (1770); Rebecca, negress, Falmouth, Jamaica, her age having been correctly traced from the deeds of her owners; Abraham Paiba, Charleston, South Carolina.

AGED 142: Swarling, a monk (973). About fifteen years ago, (1844,) the following case was reported and credited as true: Late papers from the Island of Jamaica announced the death, at Spanish Town, of a black man named John Crawford Ricketts, at the extraordinary age of one hundred and forty-two years; and what may be considered as very unusual, he was in good health till within about two weeks of his death.

AGED 143: Charles McFindley (1773). Baron Humboldt mentions, that while he was in Lima, an Indian, Halario Pari, died at the age of 143.   •

AGED 145: Evan Williams (1782); Countess of Desmond.

AGED 146: Thomas Winslow (1766); Joseph, negro, of the estate of Morice Hall, Jamaica (1821); Anne Wignell (1812).

AGED 147: Solomon Nibel, in Laurens District, South Carolina.

AGED 148: William Mead (1652).

AGED 150: Francis Confit (1768); Marcus Aponius, Ramino, Italy; Marc Albuno, Ethiopia; Catherine Heath, Jamaica (Sept. 3, 1831), never had a child, retained her faculties to the last.

AGED 151: Mrs. Judith Crawford, of Spanish Town, Jamaica (Nov. 21, 1829).

AGED 152: John Bowels (1656); Henry West, of Upton, Gloucestershire.

AGED 154: Thomas Damme (1648).

AGED 160: Robert Lynch, a negro, the property of Sir H. East, at St. Andrews, Jamaica (Dec. 5, 1830).

AGED 164: Mrs. Margaret Moser, Montgomery County, Pennsylvania (in 1854), aged 164 years, four months and seventeen days. —(*Baltimore Sun.*)

AGED 175: Louisa Truxo, negress of Tucomea, South America (1780).

AGED 180: At Frederictown, United States, a mulatto (1797).

Longevity of certain Animals.—Mr. Wilson relates from Hufeland's *Art of Prolonging Life*, that a gentleman from London, a few years ago, received from the Cape of Good Hope a falcon that had been caught with a golden collar, on which was inscribed in English, AN. 1610. It had been at liberty 182 years.

M. Buffon says that Count Maurepas had in a moat of his a carp known to be 150 years old. Gesner says that a pike was caught in Suabia, in 1497, having an inscription dated in 1230, showing that its age, at the least, was 267 years. The Rev. Mr. Kirby, in his *Bridgewater Treatise* (372), says: "A pike was taken in 1754, at Kaiserslautern, which had a ring fastened to the gill-covers, from which it appears to have been put into a pond of that castle by the order of Frederic II., in 1487, a period of 267 years."

In the fourth volume of Buffon's Natural History, the late Mr. Audubon, of Louisiana, is quoted as saying, that in company with Mr. Augustin Bourgeat, he killed an alligator seventeen feet long: "It was apparently *centuries old;* many of its teeth measured three inches; we took some of them for powder charges."

On Thursday, the 23d of July, 1858, while Mr. Joseph Hartman, of Bedminster, was in his meadow, with the mowers, he found a large land tortoise, upon the bottom of whose shell there was the following inscription in legible characters, viz.: A. E. F., 1736, which would make it at this time 122 years old.—(*Doyleston (Pa.) Democrat.*)

The *Leicester* (England) *Mercury* (1854) has the following statement:

" A GOOSE NINETY-THREE YEARS OLD.—Mr. Fverett, farmer of Kirby Lodge, near Rockingham, has a goose which he vouches to be at least ninety-three years old. It has been on his farm full fifty years, and passed the former part of its life on the farm adjoining. It is a large, fine fowl, with a head and neck as white as snow, and has lately hatched a brood of goslings from its own eggs. Mr. E. has a book stating its age and history, which he can authenticate."

But it is time to pass from this digression to the starting-point, human longevity.

A few examples of long life, yet not reaching 120, relating chiefly to the South, will be subjoined:

" *Longevity.*—Instances of extreme old age are perhaps more frequent in this city than in any other city on the continent. Every week or so we hear of the demise of some ancient individual whose years run up to the neighborhood of a century, and occasionally of one who has made a commencement on his second century. Yesterday a free woman of color, named Suzanne Blandine, died at her residence, No. 8 Greatmen street, at the age of 105. She was a native of St. Domingo. As she died suddenly and unexpectedly, the coroner was sent for, but the decision of the jury of inquest was that she had died of old age."—(*N. O. Picayune*, Feb. 21, 1856.)

" *Longevity.*—We learn, on unexceptionable authority, that Victorie Simon Mercier, a colored woman, who died yesterday in a house on Royal street, between Conti and St. Louis streets, had reached the patriarchal age of 111 years. She was the eldest sister of the wet nurse of the father of Dr. Mercier—fourteen years older. She remained active and sensible to the last. On Friday last she walked a distance of three squares."—(*N. O. Picayune*, Oct. 3, 1855.)

In the parish of St. James, December, 1846, a negro died at the age of 110.

In his History of South Carolina,(1808,) Dr. Ramsay mentions that during the eleven preceding years, one person had died in that State, aged 100; two at 103; one at 104; one at 105; one at 108; one at 109; one at 112; one at 114. He further mentions that two were then living in the same State, at the age of 111; three at 102; one at 104; one at 107; two at 110. (ii. 418, *et seq.*) He says: " Mr. Neighbors died aged 114—his wife 109. The latter, at the age of 105, broke her thigh in three places, which healed very kindly."

Dr. H. Howard, in his History of North Carolina, (ii. 288--9, A. D., 1812,) says: "Mrs. M'Allister died in 1798, in the town of Fayetteville, N. C., aged 112. Living in the same village: Mrs. Tommie, at the age of 106; Mrs. Cruise, 105; James Mears, 106; Ab. Grimes, 104; Duncan Campbell, 108; while others were living at the age of 106, 103, 100, etc. In 1794, William Taylor, aged 114, and William Howard, aged 108, were living in North Carolina."

Benjamin Bushe, born in Massachusetts, died at Greensborough, Vermont, March 21, 1845, aged 115.—(*Nat. Intel.*)

M. Ferry, who, at the age of 82, wrote the article *Vieillesse*, in the *Dict. de la Conver.*, thinks that couriers, particularly in Chili, oftenest attain great longevity. The speed demanded of these runners or couriers requires great muscular exertion, with consequent exposure, which more recent statistical observers consider, though contrary to former opinion, unfavorable to health and longevity.

The effect of occupation and exposure upon health and longevity has been recently stated in the following summary: "It has oftentimes been asserted that those exposed to severe labor in the open atmosphere were the least subject to sickness. This has been proven a fallacy by Mr. Finlaison, Actuary of the National Debt Office, in London. Of persons engaged at heavy labor in out-door exposure, the percentage of sickness in the year is 28.05. Of those engaged at heavy labor in-doors, such as blacksmiths, etc., the percentage of sickness is 26.64—not much difference, to be sure; but of those engaged at light occupations in-doors and out, the percentage of sickness is only 20.80, 21.58. For every three cases of sickness in those engaged at light labor, there are four cases among those whose lot is heavy labor. The mortality, however, is greatest among those engaged in light toil, and in-door labor is less favorable to longevity than laboring in the open atmosphere

"It is established clearly, however, Mr. Finlaison says, that the quantum of sickness annually falling to the lot of man is in direct proportion to the demands of his muscular power. How true this makes the assertion: every inventor who abridges labor and relieves man from the drudgery of severe toil, is a benefactor of his race. There were many who looked upon labor-saving machnies as great

evils, because they have supplanted the manual toil of many opera-
tives. A more enlightened spirit is now abroad; for all experience
proves that labor-saving machines do not destroy the occupations of
men, but merely change them. Man is relieved from drudgery by the
iron sinews of the machine, and his own are left to move more lightly
and free in pursuing avocations demanding less physical, but more
mental and noble exertion."

Upon this subject Sir Henry Holland asks and ingeniously answers
the following questions: " To what extent the bodily powers may be
preserved, by maintaining their assiduous exercise—whether, to take a
single instance, the muscular organs may be kept longer in vigor by
exertion to the full extent of ability at each successive period of life?
or whether the powers, whatever they be, which minister to their actions, are longer and better sustained by comparative repose? Taking
life, not as a definite, exhaustible quantity of an unknown influence,
but as expressing a common result of the actions of many parts differently constructed and endowed, we are furnished with what comes
nearest a satisfactory answer: Whatever habits sustain the greatest
number of organs or functions in a healthy state (having regard also
to the relative importance of these functions) may be considered as
most conducive to length of life. The positive fatigue of any organ
from its exercise must be deemed an excess—of little import, it may
be, in single instances; certainly injurious by frequent or habitual
repetition. All exercise of a natural function within this limit may
be viewed, without material risk of error, as salutary in itself, and
maintaining the integrity of the organ concerned longer than the
opposite of inertness and disease. The same rule may be applied
without error to the mental functions. Disuse is not preservation.
We have reason to believe that the integrity of these faculties is best
and longest sustained by habitual exercise, within those bounds which
are reached without fatigue at each successive period of life."—
(*Notes*, 254–5.)

Experience, however, often makes sad havoc of the finest theoretical definitions—an example of which I may here relate, though it
does not coincide with Dr. Holland's explanation—an example, the
truth of which will sufficiently excuse its egotism. I confess—all are
willing to confess that which is far from disgracing themselves in the
estimation of others—I confess to great intemperance in the use of the
eyes. In early life parental authority and the withholding of lamps
and candles were insufficient to prevent my prolonged night-reading.

I substituted the light of ignited wood, when denied other means of
illumination. I have read scores of volumes in the open sunlight, on
horseback, when traveling to visit the sick, etc., and have practiced
reading, writing, and proof-reading at night to a vast, if not a profitable extent, not only seeing well all the while, but with an increasing
vision, which of late amounts to microscopic power of a low order,
without any disadvantage except a very slight degree of short-
sightedness.

The effect of climate upon the mean and the extreme duration of
life has not been ascertained by reliable statistical data. Some writers claim, in this behalf, superiority for the rigid climate of Scandi-
navia; others for the eternal summer of the South, which, according
to them, is the paradise especially of the aged.

The winter season of cold climates appears to be peculiarly dangerous to the aged, often causing senile catarrh, apoplexy, palsy, typhoid
pneumonia, etc. Hence, on theoretical grounds it might be assumed,
in the existing deficiency of exact statistical data necessary for either
a reliable comparison or a contrariwise probability, that, inasmuch as
the calorifacient power of the old is impaired, a warm climate, other
things being equal, must be more favorable to senile life than a variable, cold one.

" Men who have passed the meridian of life in England suffer less
from heat than younger persons; and, indeed, life might often be prolonged by removing from a cold to a warmer climate at the period
when the power of producing animal heat becomes more feeble."—
(*Med.-Chir. Rev.*, July, 1844.)

" In climates very warm, and at the same time very dry, the human species enjoy a longevity perhaps greater than what we observe
in the temperate zones. Europeans who transport themselves at an
age somewhat advanced into the equatorial part of the Spanish colo-
nies, attain there, for the most part, a great and happy old age."—
(*Humboldt: New Spain; Anno* 1803.)

" In those wild regions [Upper Oronoco] we are involuntarily reminded of the assertion of Linnæus, that the country of palm-trees
is [was] the first abode of our species, and that man is essentially
palmivorous: ' *Homo habitat intra tropicos, vescitur palmis, lotophagus:
hospitatur extra tropocos sub novercante Cerere carnivorus.*' "—(*Syst.
Nat.*, i. 24. *Humboldt: Narrative*, v. 208.)

Mr. Lewes, in his recent Life of Goethe, says: " Old age is a relative term. Goethe at seventy was younger than many men at fifty;

and at eighty-two he wrote a scientific review of the great discussion between Cuvier and Geoffroy St. Hilaire, on Philosophic Zoology, a review which few men in their prime could write. But there are physiologists who deny that seventy is old age. M. Flourens, for example, maintains that from fifty-five to seventy man is at his most virile period; and M. Reveillé Parise, in his work, *La Vieillesse*, declares that between fifty-five and seventy-five, and sometimes beyond, the mind acquires an extension, a consistence and a solidity truly re markable—'*C'est véritablement l'homme ayant atteint toute la hauteur de ses facultés.*' * * * Sophocles is said to have written his mas terpiece at eighty. The reflective powers often retain their capacity, and· by increase of material seem to *increase* it," etc. To multiply authorities on this subject would be too severe a trial of the patience of Young America. Youth of that class, unfortunately no myth, would, like a prodigal heir, make no manner of objection if the old would make a little more haste, so as to leave their places, honors, and estates to the rising generation. There is, blessed be Bichât! a very different class of young men. Young in years, but old in labors, researches, and discoveries. Professor J. Aikin Meigs, who adorns what he touches, has, in his late eloquent and truthful address to the juvenile graduates of the Pennsylvania College, enumerated many medical writers and discoverers, who, in early life, sounded the utmost depths yet reached in science. It is true, as Professor Meigs declares, "that young men are the apostles of new truths the world over." Rising above the dense, dark stratum of ancient dogmatism, like the mountain peaks, they are the first to receive and reflect the light of advancing knowledge.

Medical Convention for Revising the Pharmacopœia of the United States.

The Medical Convention for revising the Pharmacopœia, which met at Washington, in May, 1830, provided for assembling a conven tion for the same purpose, in the year 1860, by the following reso lutions:

" 1. The President of this Convention shall, on the first day of May, 1859, issue a notice requesting the several incorporated State Medi cal Societies, the incorporated Medical Colleges, the incorporated Colleges of Physicians and Surgeons, and the incorporated Colleges of Pharmacy, throughout the United States, to elect a number of dele gates, not exceeding three, to attend a general convention to be held at Washington on the first Wednesday in May, 1860.

"2. The several incorporated bodies thus addressed shall also be requested by the President to submit the Pharmacopœia to a careful revision, and to transmit the result of their labors, through their delegates, or through any other channel, to the next Convention.

"3. The several medical and pharmaceutical bodies shall be further requested to transmit to the President of this Convention the names and residences of their respective delegates, as soon as they shall have been appointed, a list of whom shall be published, under his authority, for the information of the medical public, in the newspapers and medical journals, in the month of March, 1860."

In accordance with the above resolutions, the President hereby requests the several bodies mentioned to appoint delegates, not exceeding three in number, to represent them in a convention for revising the Pharmacopœia of the United States, to meet at Washington on the first Wednesday in May, 1860; and would also call the attention of these bodies to the second and third resolutions, and request compliance with the suggestions therein contained.—*Med. News.*

PUNCH ON HOMŒOPATHY.

Mr. Punch is accustomed to receive letters and treatises, imploring him not to call homœopathy fudge, and some of them attempting to assign reasons why he should not. In all these communications, the medical opponents of homœopathy are called "allopathists." "Allopathist" as contradistinguished from "homœopathist" of course means a person who treats diseases with other medicines than those which produce similar diseases, that is, who endeavors to cure unlike with unlike, instead of endeavoring to cure like with like. Who are the allopathists? Mr. Punch has an extensive medical acquaintance, but he does not know any. No intelligent medical practitioner attempts to cure diseases in general with specific medicines of any kind. There are very few such medicines known to the medical profession. The principle on which diseases, for the most part, are treated by rational and scientific physicians and surgeons is that of removing impediments to the natural process of recovery; or that of assisting the curative efforts of nature, not necessarily, and not always, by causing people to swallow drugs. When drugs are given by such practitioners, they are generally given with a view to their indirect influence on disorders. For instance, the combination popularly known as the "black and blue reviver," which directly affects internal parts of the trunk, may be "exhibited" for the relief of a headache, or for the removal of an inflammation of the great-toe.

Professor Holloway is perhaps an allopathist; however, he does not tell us on what principle his pills and ointment cure all diseases. The various doctors who advertise their patent medicines in the quacks' corners of newspapers of the baser sort, may be allopathists also; and likewise the medical profession possibly contains a few fools or impostors who are so describable. But the few specifics used in the ordinary practice of physic may absolutely even act on the homœopathic principle, that "like cures like;" thus differing from homœopathic doses only in not being infinitesimal, and, Mr. Punch supposes, in being efficacious.

In none of the communications about homœopathy received by Mr. Punch is there anything like scientific proof that infinitesimal globules produce any other than infinitesimal effects. Cases of alleged cures, subsequent to the swallowing of these globules, prove nothing, until they amount to enormous numbers. Professor Holloway, and Messrs. Du Barry & Co., adduce plenty of such proofs; perhaps not fictitious. Mere swallowing and cure can be connected as cause and effect only by immense clouds of cases in which the cure is almost the invariable sequence of the swallowing. It does not signify whether the thing swallowed is a great bolus or a pill of the size of a pin's head, containing an invisible dose.

Quinine is acknowledged, on the strength of a vast accumulation of evidence, as a remedy for ague. It cures ague in one grain, two grain, three grain doses. Will quinine, or anything else, in infinitesimal doses, cure ague as obviously in an equal number out of a vast multitude of cases? Will an infinitesimal quantity of sulphur exert any curative influence on that cutaneous affection which delicacy expresses by the euphuism of the Caledonian violin?

Mr. Punch's homœopathic friends seem to forget that statements of facts which are contradictory to common sense and received science, require rigid proof. None of them propose any method by which the active properties of an infinitesimal globule can be demonstrated. Neither homœopathists, nor mesmerists, nor spiritualists, either offer or accept the test of any *experimentum crucis*; and when Mr. Punch asks for it, they answer by abuse, and the comparison of themselves to Galileo, and those who laugh at them at the inquisition.—*Med. News.*

An Act to incorporate the Medical Society of the State of North Carolina, and for the establishment of a Medical Board of Examiners.

Sec. 1. *Be it enacted by the General Assembly of the State of North Carolina, and it is hereby enacted by the authority of the same,* That the association of regularly graduated doctors, calling themselves "The State Medical Society," be and they are hereby declared to be a body politic and corporate, to be known and distinguished by the name and style of "The Medical Society of the State of North Carolina;" and by that name and style shall have perpetual succession, and a common seal; that they, or a majority of them and their successors, shall be able and capable of in law to take, demand, receive and possess, money, goods and chattels, land and tenements, and apply the same to the use and for the advancement of the purposes and objects of the said society; that the said Medical Society, or a majority of them and their successors, shall be able and capable in law of suing and being sued, pleading and being impleaded; that they shall be authorized to make all by-laws, rules and regulations, necessary and proper for their own government and for carrying out the purposes contemplated in this act, and for the promotion of medical science and the elevation of the medical profession in this State, not inconsistent with the constitution and laws of North Carolina.

Sec. 2. *Be it further enacted,* That from and after the 15th day of April, 1859, no person shall practice medicine, surgery, or any of the branches thereof, or in any case prescribe for the cure of diseases, for fee or reward, unless he or they shall have been first licensed so to do in the manner hereinafter described. *Provided,* that no person who shall practice in violation of this act shall be deemed guilty of a misdemeanor.

Sec. 3. *Be it further enacted,* That in order to the proper regulation of the practice of medicine and surgery in the State of North Carolina, there shall be established a board of regularly graduated physicians, to be known by the name and title of "The Board of Medical Examiners of the State of North Carolina."

Sec. 4. *Be it further enacted,* That the Board of Medical Examiners of the State of North Carolina shall consist of seven regularly graduated physicians.

Sec. 5. *Be it further enacted,* That it shall be the duty of the said Board to examine all applicants for license to practice medicine and surgery, or any of the branches thereof, in the State of North Carolina, on the following branches of medical science, viz.: Anatomy,

Physiology, Surgery, Pathology, Medical Hygiene, Chemistry, Pharmacy, Materia Medica, Therapeutics, Obstetrics, and the Practice of Medicine; and if on such examination he or they be found competent, to grant to such applicant or applicants a license or diploma authorizing him or them to practice medicine and surgery, or any of the branches thereof, in the State of North Carolina. *Provided*, that five members of the Board shall constitute a quorum, and that four of those present shall be agreed as to the qualifications of the applicant.

Sec. 6. *Be it further enacted*, That the said Board shall be at liberty to examine for and grant license to practice medicine or surgery, or any of the branches thereof, in this State [to or any of the branches thereof in this State] to any person so applying, [who shall give any person so applying,] who shall give satisfactory evidence to the Board that he is 21 years of age, and of good moral character; such applicants if found competent shall have granted to them the license before mentioned, signed by the Board of Medical Examiners or a majority thereof, and if found incompetent they shall be rejected.

Sec. 7. *Be it further enacted*, That to prevent delay and inconvenience, two members of the Board of Medical Examiners may grant a temporary license to applicants therefor, and make report thereof to the next regular meeting of the Board, for confirmation, provided that such temporary license shall not continue in force longer than the next regular meeting of the Board, and that such temporary license shall in no case be granted after the applicant has been refused a license by the Board of Medical Examiners.

Sec. 8. *Be it further enacted*, That it shall be the duty of the Medical Society of the State of North Carolina to furnish to the General Assembly of the State of North Carolina, by their [Society] Secretary, a list of   members of that Society, from which list the General Assembly shall elect seven to constitute the Board of Medical Examiners before mentioned, to continue in office for the term of six years from the date of their election. *Provided*, that whenever any member of this Board shall cease to be a member of "The Medical Society of the State of North Carolina," either by resignation or expulsion, his office of Medical Examiner shall be thereby vacated.

Sec. 9 *Be it further enacted*, That the members of the State Medical Society shall have power to select the Board of Medical Examiners, except when the Legislature chooses to exercise this right.

Sec. 10. *Be it further enacted*, That the Board of Medical Examiners thus appointed shall assemble in the city of Raleigh and Morganton, alternately, on the first Monday in May in every year, and shall remain in session from day to day, until all applicants who may present themselves for examination within the first ten days after their meeting shall have been examined and disposed of.

Sec. 11. *Be it further enacted*, That the Board of Medical Examiners shall be and they are hereby authorized to elect all such officers and to frame all such by-laws as may be necessary to carry this law into effect, and in the event of any vacancy by death, resignation or otherwise, of any member of said Board, the Board, or a quorum thereof, shall be and they are hereby empowered to fill all vacancies.

Sec. 12. *Be it further enacted*, That the Board of Examiners shall keep a regular record of its proceedings in a book kept for that purpose, which shall always be open for inspection, and shall cause to be entered on a book kept for this purpose the names of each applicant for license, and the name of each applicant licensed to practice medicine and surgery, and the time of granting the same, together with the names of the members of the Board present, and shall publish the names of those licensed in two of the newspapers published in the city of Raleigh within thirty days after the granting of the same.

Sec. 13. *Be it further enacted*, That the said Board shall have power to demand of each and every applicant thus licensed, the sum of ten dollars before issuing a license or diploma, and the sum of five dollars for each temporary license, to be paid to the Secretary of the Board.

Sec. 14. *Be it further enacted*, That the members of the said Board shall receive as a compensation for their services four dollars each per day during the time of their session in the city of Raleigh, and in addition thereto, their traveling expenses to and from the city of Raleigh, to be paid by the Secretary of the Board, out of any moneys in his hands, upon the certificate of the President of the Board of Examiners.

Sec. 15. *Be it further enacted*, That any person who shall practice medicine or surgery in this State, without having first applied for and obtained license from the said Board of Examiners, as provided for by this act, shall not be entitled to sue for or recover before any magistrate or court in this State any medical bill for services rendered in the practice of medicine or surgery, or any of the branches thereof.

Sec. 16. *Be it further enacted*, That the said Board shall have the power to rescind any license granted by them, when upon satisfactory proof it shall appear that any physician thus licensed has been guilty of grossly immoral conduct.

Sec. 17. *Be it further. enacted*, That the Secretary of the Board of Medical Examiners shall give bond with good security to the President of the Board, for the safe keeping and proper payment of all moneys that may come into his hands under the provisions of this act.

Sec. 18. *Be it further enacted*, That the provisions of this act shall not apply to any person or persons now engaged in the practice of medicine or surgery in this State, but shall be construed as applying to those only who may hereafter propose to commence the practice of the same in the State of North Carolina.

Sec. 19. *Be it further enacted*, That this act shall be in force on and after the 15th day of April, 1859, and shall be considered a public act.

On the Comparative Influence of the Male and Female Parent upon the Progeny.

By J. B. Thomson, L.R.C.S., Edinburgh,

Resident Surgeon, General Prison, Perth.

The following cases appear to me illustrative of a very curious and not unimportant chapter of anthropology, viz.: "The comparative influence of the male and female of the human family upon their progeny"—a subject upon which very crude and indefinite notions are held, not only by the public, but by the members of our profession. It is a settled point with many, that it is foolish to search after any laws regulating the transmission of particular textures, features, and constitutions from either parent to the offspring. These philosophers are satisfied with the unsatisfactory views of the poetical Lucretius:

> " Fit quoque, ut interdum similes existere avorum
> Possint, et referant proavoram sæpe figuras,
> Inde Venus varias produit sorte figuras
> Marjorumque refert voltus xocesque, comas-que."

While it is admitted that we can found little upon mere supposed general, physical, or psychical resemblances, I think the method of inquiry followed in this paper is a correct one, and that a number of individual instances of the transmission of abnormal peculiarities from parent to progeny being accumulated and balanced, will lead to a safe and scientific induction.

Mercatus, in his work, "De Morbis Hereditariis," says truly, that the parents, grand-parents and great-grand parents transmit quality, character, form and structure, proportion and disproportion, or any preternatural condition of a single member or organ, part or parts. Of this statement there can be no doubt. We may go further, and affirm that, where we find such irregularities and defects plainly appearing in one parent, and reappearing in any of the offspring, such irregularities or defects are due to the influence of that parent. The order of causation is not to be questioned. And, further, when striking abnormal conditions, physical or mental, are transmitted in families, the statistics of such should form data upon which to found a proof whether and in what proportion the influence of the male or of the female predominates. Beginning with physical peculiarities of the external structure, transmitted from parents to their progeny, let us examine "the transmission of skin peculiarities."

CASE I.—*Hereditary transmission of webbed fingers.*—A. M., Alva, has had a family of nine children, five sons and four daughters. He himself and his four daughters are webbed betwixt the middle and ring fingers, or close-fingered, as their mother calls it, *i. e.*, the skin stretches across and unites these fingers together. None of the sons have this peculiarity. A. M.'s grandfather had the same; also his mother and two sons and one daughter; his uncle, two daughters and one son having all the fingers of both fingers webbed together. A. M.'s daughter has one daughter webbed between the middle and ring finger of both hands.

CASE II.—*Hereditary transmission of webbed fingers and toes.*—(This case, from a recent number of the *Lancet*, is so similar to the former, that I make no apology for transferring it to this paper, for the sake of illustrating my argument.) W. S. has three fingers united throughout by skin, viz., the middle, the ring, and the little fingers of both hands. His mother has the same, but W. S. is the only one of seven children so malformed. Her uncle (her father's brother) had the same, and her paternal grandfather had the three smaller toes on each foot similarly united.

CASE III.—*Hereditary transmission of extra fingers and toes partially webbed.*—J. B., Menstrie, has a daughter with six toes on each foot, the little toe and its neighbor being well webbed; also two little fingers on each hand partially adherent by skin. J. B.'s great grandfather had the left hand also partially webbed. No other member of this family can be traced to have had any abnormal physical conformation.

CASE IV.—*Supernumerary toes and fingers webbed.*—J. R., Tillicoultry, has the following peculiarities in his family, viz.: One girl webbed between the little toe and its neighbor; one son with two little fingers on each hand, and two little toes on each foot. No hereditary trace of these peculiarities can admit the account of the mother as the true cause. She says, that when she carried this boy in utero, she met with an accident which split her little finger in two, so that it always afterwards looked like two fingers.

From the small number of cases now set forh, it would be unsafe to draw any strong proofs, lest we should be placed in the category of the philosopher in R·sselas, who was always coming to conclusions without anything being concluded. But, although we admit that such a small number of cases is not proof positive, we must allow that they point to the following deductions, viz.:

1. That the male parent has a principal share in the transmission of hereditary skin peculiarities to the offspring.

In Case I., we have a grandfather, a father and an uncle sending down an abnormal condition directly through the belonged to all those descendants who inherit this skin peculiarity. On the other hand, we have a grandmother and granddaughter transmi:ting the same directly to their children

In Case II., the paternal grandfather, and in Case III., the great-grandfather, was the origial progenitor, to whom the physical malformations were traced back. Leaving out No. IV., where the origin is very doubtful, we have the following proportional cases, in which the immediate influence of the female parents:

CASE I.—Transmitted immediately by Male,	10—Female,	4
II. " " "	3 "	1
III. " " "	2 "	0
	15	5

But these cases point to another interesting deduction:

2. That the skin peculiarity in all these cases, where it could be traced back, had its origin in a male progenitor. In No. 1, it came in with a grandfather, and in No. 3, with a great-grandfather. A curious question here arises: Did the influence of the originator of this malformation extend itself through several generations who bore his peculiar characteristic? Is it true, as Dr. Harvey has recently asserted, that the male is the real producer of the species? Is it true that the influence of the male, in certain instances, extends beyond the first impregnation?

The consideration of these cases, which show the influence of the male to be greater than that of the female parent in the transmission of skin peculiarities, led me to look at the history of certain skin diseases which are hereditary, and the following instances occurred to my recollection:

Case of the porcupine family.—The original porcupine man, Edward Lambert, had six children and two grandsons with the same singular skin as himself, resembling, it is said, an innumerable company of warts of a dark-brown color, and a cylindrical figure, rising to an inch in height. In this case, the disease originating in a male, continued to all the family of six, and descended to the grandchildren.

Leprosy, too, seems to be chiefly derivable from the male parent. In Dr. Simpson's curious inquiries into the history of leprosy, we find quoted from the old Burgh Records of Glasgow, (1589,) "Robert Bogell, son to Patrick Bogle," both lepers in that city.

The modern experience of this malady in Norway, where it has so unaccountably increased of late years, has led to serious inquiry how it is to be prevented. Leprosy, or the spedalkshad, is held by Drs. Boeck and Danielson to be purely hereditary; and so strong is the opinion of the male being the chief propagator, that the proposal has not only been laid before the Storthing or Norwegian Parliament to prohibit the marriage of a leper, but it has been a topic of public and professional discussion how far it would be just to deprive the male infants of leprous parents of the power of propagation. Ligature of the vasa deferentia, we learn, has been seriously contemplated as a national measure.

The analogy of the lower animals confirms these views of the paramount influence of the male in transmitting generally the character of the skin to the progeny. The spawn of the salmon being impregnated with the male trout, the skin and the spots upon it showed the characters of the trout, and *vice versâ*, the salmon being the male. With birds, generally, the outer textures follow the male parents. With quadrupeds, the same rule holds. An intelligent and experienced sheep farmer informs me that it is the practice to cross the blackfaced sheep on the Ochils with the Leicester ram. The Ochil ewes are blackfaced, and have horns. The Leicester ram is not blackfaced, and has no horns. The breed follow the Leicester ram, whitefaced, and in the proportion of about 85 per cent. have no horns. A few years ago, on the estate of Alva, there was a black ram with five horns, two on either side, and one in the centre. The breed by the common white ewe took the abnormal character of this ram, with a few exceptions. We know also that the products of the male ass by the mare, and of the stallion by

29

the she-ass, can be distinguished by the skin having the distinctive characteristics of the sire.

Numerous examples of this law must be well known to cattle-dealers; and this subject is admirably treated by Mr. Orton, of Sutherland, in his ingenious papers "On the Physiology of Breeding."

We may safely, I think, conclude from the facts before us:

1. That in the lower animals, and in man also, the influence of the male is greater than that of the female parent in the transmission of the skin texture to the progeny.

2. That the exceptional cases (probably more in man than in the lower animals) lead us to look for some primary or secondary law presiding over the physiology of generation.

I intend to continue this inquiry as to the influence of the male on the other textures and organs of the body, in a series of cases and notes. —*Montreal Med. Chron.*

COMMUNICATIONS.

OUR PHILADELPHIA CORRESPONDENT.

No. 12.

Army and Navy Boards—Medical Schools and Professors— Disease and Death.

> " Life's but a walking shadow: a poor player,
> That struts and frets his hour upon the stage,
> And then is heard no more. It is a tale
> Told by an idiot, full of sound and fury,
> Signifying nothing.'   SHAKSPEARE.

DEAR GAZETTE—The Spring is upon us, the toils of the Winter campaign are over, and professor and pupil are reflecting on the past, and laying plans for the future. The Navy Board of Medical Examiners is still in session. The number of applicants, we learn, is unusually large. The requisitions of the Board are said to be very strict; so much so, that many of the candidates are frightened from the lists before the day of trial. Among the requisitions is one which we think is unusual, viz.: the candidate is required to sign a paper stating that, on his honor as a man, he is not aware of any hereditary disease affecting his family. This cuts off all young men liable to phthisis, or supposed to be liable to phthisis from hereditary causes. Almost any physical defect is made a sufficient cause for rejection. You will recollect, perhaps, that the veterinary surgeons make a distinction between simple physical defects (wind-galls, for instance,) and more serious matters affecting the health or usefulness of the animal. The latter are considered sufficient cause for pronouncing the animal unsound; while the former are so numerous and trivial, as not to be esteemed worthy of notice. A similar distinction, probably, would not be out of place in the selection of surgeons for the army and navy. One condition we would consider absolutely essential. Young men should *not* be addicted to the use of intoxicating drinks as a beverage. A good moral character is as necessary in the army or navy to a medical practitioner, as it is in civil life.

We hear that a number of the assistant surgeons of five years' standing are being dropped from the service, for neglecting their professional studies; this is technically denominated *bilging*. Dr. Ruschenberger seems determined to attain not only grade and position in the navy for the profession, but to bring the profession up to a proportionately high standard of acquirements. Some of the young men complain sadly of what they esteem arbitrary measures, and charge him with prejudice and unfairness. Whether this be true we know not; but his efforts appear to us to be well calculated to elevate the professional standard in the navy. If our observations are correct, there are a great many young men, applying for admission to both the army and navy, whose habits and qualifications, or want of qualifications, prevent them from succeeding in civil life, who, through political, social, or family influence, hope to establish themselves at the public charge.

In our last, we spoke of an effort which was being made in the Legislature of our State to sweep out of existence the political, medical, and social corruptions existing in the Board of Health and Guardains of the Poor, by having these bodies appointed by the Councils and the Courts, instead of being elected by the pot-house politicians. This has been done with an unusual amount of unanimity and public approbation. Henceforth the Medical Board of the celebrated Blockley will be under the control of a body of intelligent and respectable men. There is a rumor afloat that the present chief of this institution will be subjected to a censorial investigation in the County Medical Society, in reference to a series of alleged immoral, if not criminal, practices, degrading to the character of the profession, and to the membership of the above-named Society; the moral character of its members being a subject to which it pays annually increasing attention.

Madame Rumor now also speaks of the disorganization of one of our medical schools. The late resignation of the Professor of Practice in the Pennsylvania College has been followed, it is said, by symptoms of an *émeute* in the rest of the faculty. The truth is, GAZETTE, as I have said before, there is plenty of room here for a new medical institution! which, by meeting some of the just demands of the profession of the day, by increasing the medical requirements of the student, giving prominence to clinical and other practical branches, and prolonging and multiplying the courses of instruction, would, with a well-constituted faculty, in time, secure a success unprecedented in our city. There is, in fact, a general belief in the necessity of some such alleviation in the curricula of medical instruction; and Dr. Davis, of Chicago, is but embodying, in his attempted organization of a school, some of the ideas of the day.

Since writing the above, we learn that the Faculty of the Pennsylvania College has retired in a body, and that the gentlemen of the Philadelphia College have possession of the charter, hoping, in this way, to combine the patronage of the two schools. This, however, will be impossible. The Alumni of the Philadelphia College, which number several hundreds, will, of course, desire to see the name of their *alma mater* perpetuated. The resignation of Dr. Pepper from the Pennsylvania Hospital has been followed by that of Dr. G. B. Wood from the same institution, and a member of the late Faculty of the Pennsylvania College has been elected to fill his place — Dr. Francis G. Smith, who is a *gentleman* and a scholar—titles which are rather rare among the noisy cliques of our profession. The appointment is in every way a good one. Dr. Wood has also resigned from the University, the resignation to take place next spring. A respectable medical journal of our city, in speaking of Dr. Wood's retirement, says: "There are few men in this country who have served their profession as faithfully, honorably, and *disinterestedly*, as Dr. Wood." We agree with this sentiment in all but the last part. Dr. Wood has probably drawn more money *directly* from the pockets of the profession than any other medical man living; and has secured its highest honors, and worn them proudly. We know of little more which the profession can bestow upon Dr. Wood.

Our Philadelphia delegation to Louisville was, I learn, very small, and not at all composed of the more windy portion of the profession. The distance and the Sanitary Convention, doubtless, prevented some of the gentlemen from attending the American Medical Association.

When honors are both cheap and easily acquired, the aspirants for them increase in number.

The diseases of the season, this winter and spring, among us, are of a twofold character—bronchitic and typhoid. Bronchitic affections, including croup, pneumonia, pleurisies, &c., have been exceedingly prevalent. In addition to this, there has been in all diseases a typhoid tendency. Within fifty to one hundred miles of our city, there have been whole districts afflicted with typhoid fevers. There are many cases here now. The spring is cool, but forward, and to the diseases mentioned we may add a good many cases of eruptive fevers, measles, scarlet fever, &c.

Philadelphia is perhaps more actively engaged in medical instruction now, in all its departments, than it has ever been. More active talent is concentrated in it by far, more variety exists in that talent, and we predict that the next half century will make her the medical emporium of the civilized world. Books, journals, hospitals, orators, and societies here abound, and will abound; for our position is based on what Napoleon considered essential to the support of government itself—public opinion. We are not among those who think that man, in any of our professions, has degenerated. Our Rushes, Physicks, Dewees, Dorseys, Bartons, are well represented by men now living, who might be named, who sustain and push on the great car of science and progress as vigorously as did their ancestors. The truth is, the contest is so fierce for eminence in our profession now, that when a weak or incompetent physician becomes elected by an accident to a post which he cannot fill, it is he and the institution he represents which suffer, not the cause of science or the profession at large. Competition is more free every year, and a broad grin on the medical countenance of the initiated greets the dolt, and dogs his heels while in office. We want some new institutions, and the want being felt, will soon be supplied.

We are sorry to learn that our newly-adopted citizen, Professor Dickson, has met with a severe bereavement in the death of an amiable and intelligent daughter. Our thoughts involuntarily turn to those beautiful lines of Sir Walter Scott, in the "Lady of the Lake," where the old Douglass meets his affectionate daughter:

"If there's a tear so pure, so meek,
It would not stain an angel's cheek,
'Tis that which pious fathers shed
Upon a duteous daughter's head."

And we may add,

> "Ah! it is sad when one thus link'd departs!
> When Death, that mighty severer of true hearts,
> Sweeps through the halls so lately loud in mirth,
> And leaves pale Sorrow weeping by the hearth."
>   MRS. NORTON.

But my sheet is nearly full, and the time to post my epistle has arrived, so farewell.   Yours, &c.,   SENECA.

Letter from the Hon. Judge Meigs.

D. MEREDITH REESE, M.D.,   AMERICAN INSTITUTE, *April* 16, 1859.

Dear Sir—I have pleasure in showing to you *London Punch* of March 26th. On the last page see Mr. *Allopathic* Punch kicking the *Homœopathic ass!* The glorious cause of true science, in which you are so often called to contend with that delirium of our "*ism-atic*" folks, makes me lend my feeble applause on all occasions.

Long may you live to do much good!

I am, with the greatest esteem, your grateful servant,

H. MEIGS, *Recording Sec'y.*

Lilliputian Pills.—An intelligent correspondent entreats *Punch* to study Homœopathy. *Mr. Punch*, in return, implores his intelligent correspondent to study Anatomy, Physiology, and the nature of diseases. He will then see that the rule of healing disease by assisting nature, and removing impediments out of nature's way, is not theory, but ascertained science.

If brevity is the soul of wit, it is also the essence of argument—especially the argument of *Punch*, whose enlightened readers know almost everything, and are bored by discussions which teach them nothing.

No doubt a lady at the top of a house can smell a cigar smoked in the hall. More than that, a hound can smell the foot-print of a distant fox. But there is no proof that what immediately affects the sense of smell is ponderable matter at all. If it is, it requires nerves of special sense to perceive it, and thus proves the aphorism which *Mr. Punch* proposes to accompany "Like cures Like;" namely, "Infinitesimal Quantities produce Infinitesimal Effects."

Of course no quantity is, in strict language, infinitesimal; but the word is current. Say Peninfinitesimal, if you like, instead.

It is also very doubtful if the force or influence of contagion is ponderable substance. Suppose it to be so, what infinitesimal globule will produce an effect on the human body so remarkable as scarlet fever?

The circumstances affecting statistics must be stated to make them worth a thought. If a given number of inflammations had to be treated on the old plan of bleeding and drenching, and an equal number homœopathically, *Punch* has little doubt that the disadvantage, in point of recovery, would be greatly on the side of the former, and that this class would show a much superior mortality per cent. A certain number of such diseases will get well if let alone; will not get well if improperly interfered with. *Mr. Punch* believes that homœopathic cures correspond precisely to this number; their treatment, regimen apart, consisting in the administration of next to no medicine at all.

Will homœopathy set to a leg? Will it cure a broken arm? These questions may seem absurd; but it is as hard to conceive infinitesimal doses doing these things, as it is to conceive them producing any material effect on the human frame.

Will homœopathic globules make a dry skin perspire; cause a torpid liver to pour out bile, or any inactive gland whatever to secrete; or compel to work any lazy scavenger organs, whose office it is to cast rubbish out of the system? If not, they will not effect the conditions on which the cure of diseases depends, and without which all who know anything of the matter know that it is impossible.

EDITOR'S TABLE.

Annual Meeting of the American Medical Association at Louisville, Kentucky, May 3d, 1859.

Of this medical anniversary, as it was our privilege to be present, we take occasion to say, that although the attendance from the North and East was comparatively small, yet there were present over 300 delegates, representing 25 States. The business of the session was conducted to its close with harmony and dispatch, and of the measures adopted our readers may judge by the detailed report in this number of the GAZETTE.

The reception of the Association by the profession and citizens of Louisville far transcended our expectations, though our Nashville experience prepared us for a high estimate of Western hospitality. The entertainments for every evening were numerous and elegant; and in every instance many of the fairest daughters of Kentucky were present to greet and welcome the strangers with their smiles. The gaiety and refinements of Louisville society were exemplified at these splendid *soirées*, given in the mansions and spacious palaces occupied as residences by the physicians not only, but by many of the private families of this prosperous and wealthy city. It would be invidious to particularize, when all were equally characterized by genuine Southern generosity and magnificence, while the reception given to all, and by all, at each of these crowded assemblies, was cheerful, cordial, and affectionate. We saw nothing in the way of excess or intemperance betrayed by any member of the body, or either of the guests, although everywhere there was a bountiful prodigality and profusion of the choicest luxuries and the most costly viands, from which the far-famed Kentucky Bourbon and other vinous and alcoholic combinations were not excluded. Possibly the presence of so many medical men, and the example which each is required by his profession to exhibit, may have imposed the duty of moderation on all. If any forgot what was due to our liberal hosts, and to the gorgeous array of beauty, adorned as it was with Oriental richness and splendor, we can only affirm that the trespass escaped our eye. We saw nothing to regret, but everything to admire, in our extemporaneous introduction to the *élite* of Louisville society.

Among those who spontaneously invited and welcomed us to their beautiful residences, and to whom the Convention were indebted for princely entertainments, we venture to name the Hon. James Guthrie, the eminent Louisville patriot and statesman, whom we all delighted to honor. Mrs. Ward most cordially invited the Association to a *matinée*, given in her spacious and beautiful residence, at noon, on the close of our meeting on Thursday, which was attended by the entire body; and on the evening of that day a citizen's reception was given at the Masonic Temple, which, in splendor and richness of entertainment, is said to have been seldom surpassed.

Among the objects of interest in and about Louisville, which are varied and instructive, none attracted more attention than the inspection of Dupont's Artesian Well, which has been bored in the heart of the city, to the depth of 2,080 feet; and whence perennially issues a flow of water to the extent of 330,000 gallons in twenty-four hours, or 229 gallons per minute, and rising by its own pressure 170 feet above the surface. The bore of this well is 5 inches in diameter for 76 feet, and below this it is reduced to 3 inches.

The water is found to be highly mineral and medicinal, abounding in saline ingredients and sulphureted hydrogen, analogous to that of the Blue Lick Spring in taste and properties. The proprietor has issued a pamphlet, by Professor J. Lawrence Smith, of the University of Louisville, conveying every needed information. A colored gentleman, yclept *Doctor Sanders!* is ever on the spot, to detail the wonderful healing virtues of the waters, on which he discourses eloquently, in a style so unique and grandiloquent, that we obtained the promise that we should be furnished with a verbatim report, and a daguerreotype of the black doctor of Louisville, whose genius transcends that of a regiment like the black doctor now flourishing in Paris. We hope soon to receive the manuscript.

At the termination of the labors and enjoyments of the Association, the members scattered to their homes. Some of us *viâ* Lexington, to visit the grave and monument of Henry Clay; others to the Mammoth Cave, *en route* for a Southern tour; but all hastening homeward, where, we trust, all have arrived in safety.

P. S.—It is due to the Pennsylvania Central Railroad to say that the delegates were furnished with excursion tickets from Philadelphia to Pittsburg at half fare, by a prearrangement made through Dr. Caspar Wistar. The conductors on all the other routes from Pittsburg to Louisville professed to be without instructions, and ignored the arrangement which had been definitely agreed to at their respective head-quarters, the public announcement of which gave credit to the companies for a generosity which they did not merit. The line from Cincinnati to Columbus have since refunded the fare, by politely inclosing it to our Treasurer, for three of us who had paid it under protest. But the full fare to Pittsburg was exacted by the Steubenville line. Let our Western brethren, coming East next year, remember the Pennsylvania Central, which merits their patronage for honorably fulfilling its engagements, and is moreover one of the best and most delightful roads in the country.

MEDICAL EDUCATION.

We trust that none of our readers will fail to examine the "Act of the Legislature of North Carolina," which has just been passed and is already in force, providing for an independent Medical Board of Examiners, without whose license, "*no person shall practice medicine, surgery, or any of the branches thereof; or, in any case, prescribe for the cure of diseases, for fee or reward, within the limits of the State.*"

This glorious old State, which has thus become the pioneer in the "Reform" so much needed in Medical Education, is without a single Medical College, and to this fact is doubtless due the harmony with which the profession there have united in procuring the passage of this law. A wise Legislature have thus afforded to the citizens of that State the same protection from unqualified physicians which our Federal Government has provided for the soldiers and sailors of our army and navy; the only protection possible against the flood of incompetent and dangerous men who are annually graduated by our schools and colleges, and, by virtue of their degree, licensed to practice " *in toto mundo.*" Always excepting our army and navy, where a Medical Board of Examiners rejects them by scores, every succeeding year, though fresh from the colleges, with their diplomas certified in Latin and the mystic M.D. affixed to their names.

In following this example, and erecting this barrier at the very threshold of the profession, North Carolina has equalized all the colleges of the country, by requiring all their graduates to appear before their own State Board of Examiners; and fixing the value of diplomas from any school as mere literary testimonials, but *no license to practice.*

She has done more by this act to advance " *Southern* Medical Education," as it has been called, than has been effected by all the sectional appeals ever made through their journals. And should her example be followed by all the sister States of our confederacy, all the reforms so clamorously insisted upon will be secured as by a *coup-de-main*, and the profession may have peace on this vexed question, and the people will have security.

If some of the overgrown colleges should suffer loss by this equalization of the worth of their diplomas, their loss will be gain to other and smaller schools, and both the profession and the public be largely benefited. The separation of the teaching from the licensing power, which we have so long and so often urged, is fast becoming the settled judgment of the profession, and in which many of the eminent teachers of the country fully concur.

The law of North Carolina, just passed, may be defective and require amendment for its practical working, but it must be regarded by all as "Progress in the right direction."

CITY INSPECTOR.

This officer, who, by the charter, is the executive head of the Department of Health in this great city, and whose bureaus include the statistical and sanitary inspection; registration of births, marriages, and deaths; cleansing of the streets; the removal of nuisances; the care of the markets, &c., &c , has heretofore been filled by a politician, chosen without reference to his qualifications, for the important duties devolving on him, but solely for the purpose of dividing the spoils of public plunder with the dominant party, the lucky incumbent being expected to reserve the lion's share for himself. This office was once only held by a physician, Dr. John H. Griscom, for two years, but he failed to be re-elected, and has been a standing candidate ever since, but without success.

The term of the present *hold-over* incumbent expired at the close of the year 1858, his salary being $5,000 per annum, and the *annual* patronage of the office being some $70,000 for salaried offices at his disposal, besides the contracts for street-cleaning and sundry other perquisites, said to be *productive*, on a large scale, to the chief officer of the department. In anticipation of the vacancy on the 1st of January last, when the nomination of a successor devolved on the Mayor, by and with the advice and consent of the Board of Aldermen, a meeting of the profession was called last fall with the view of securing the appointment of some medical man to this medical office, Dr. Griscom and Dr. McNulty being at that time prominent candidates. The action of this meeting was duly chronicled in the GAZETTE at the time, and the object earnestly commended. But though the Mayor then favored the appointment of a medical man, yet unfortunately he was led by Kappa Lambda officiousness to fall into the hands of bad advisers, Dr. John Watson & Co. being allowed in consultation. Hence, on the 1st of January, Dr. S. C. Foster received the nomination of the Mayor. On this name being sent to the Board of Aldermen, it was referred to a special committee to inquire who and what he was, and on the legitimate ground that he was unknown to the Board; and the Mayor, on inquiry, admitting that he was equally unknown to *him*, the nomination having been made under the influences we have indicated. It soon became apparent, however, and has since been avowed, that Dr. F. was of the wrong stripe of politics, and the delay in reporting on his case betrayed the settled purpose to allow the incumbent to *hold over*, by retaining the new nomination under advisement, and thus preventing the Mayor from offering a substitute by another nomination. Whereupon Dr. F's name was withdrawn by his consent, and the name of Mr. Purdy, the wheel-horse of the Democracy, was sent in.

The Aldermen, however, refused to relinquish their vantage-ground, and have ever since rejected or returned all the Mayor's repeated nominations, and the incumbent has still retained possession of the office. But on attempting to compel the Mayor, by *mandamus*, to pay his salary, and thus recognize his continuance in office, the Supreme Court have blocked the game, by a denial of the writ prayed for, and adjudging the office of the City Inspector vacant since **January 1st, 1859.** Whereupon the Mayor has taken forcible possession of the office, and ejected the hold-over incumbent, in which course he is not sustained by the Aldermen, who are disposed to await the decision of a higher tribunal, to which the case is to be taken up. The end is not yet, nor can it be certainly foreseen.

During the pendency of this controversy, great efforts have been made to invoke the aid of the Legislature to abolish the office of City Inspector, and organize the department anew. The Sanitary Association have done good service in this work, and might have succeeded but for the same counsels which misled the Mayor, and the persistent effort to include in the proposed reform in the Board of Health the name of the President of the Academy of Medicine, and other obnoxious individuals. The Legislature refused any alliance of the State with private corporations, in so important a matter as constituting the Board of Health of this great city, and we honor their judgment. Hence, nothing has been done at Albany to relieve the city from the incubus of this City Inspector controversy.

Meanwhile, the summer is upon us, our streets filthy beyond comparison with any other city in the land, and we have now no City Inspector, even to record our mortality, should a wasting epidemic overtake us. The responsibility rests upon the Mayor and Aldermen, who jointly, as we think, are to blame. If the Mayor would even now nominate some reputable medical man, known to himself and the Board of Aldermen, as qualified for the professional and executive duties of the office, without regard to politics, he would either be confirmed, or some better reasons than those heretofore given would have to be alleged for non-concurrence. Among those on his slate, he will find the names of John H. Griscom, J. McNulty, Elisha Harris, and W. W. Sanger, from which brief list any stripe of politics may be propitiated, and either of them would make a better officer than either of the rejected nominees. Let him *advise* with the recusant Aldermen and try again, before the alarmists shall get up a panic in relation to the public health, which, by the blessing of Providence, was never better than now.

QUARANTINE AND SANITARY CONVENTION.

The critical notice of this body and its doings, which we promised, is in preparation by a friend, who only waits for the official proceedings before completing it. We only hint that if it is too long, it will not be read. What is needed is simply and only an exposure of the doctrine of " fomites," as endorsed by the Convention, as identical with the old and exploded superstition of " contagion," *tout la même chose* under another name. Dr. Hosack himself, the prince of contagionists, would be content, if he were living, with the doctrines of this Convention in relation to yellow fever. So also all the stupidity, abuses, cruelties, and extortions of our present rotten borough system of Quarantine, will be perpetuated, if the " fomites" nonsense is not shown up to the public authorities in its true light, notwithstanding all the explaining and expounding, modifications and qualifications, of Drs. Stevens, Watson & Co.

A peddler's pack or sailor's jacket may raise a panic, and blast our commerce, and scatter our citizens, if either should be suspected as " fomites," and a single case of sporadic fever should be ascribed to either.

Let the people be enlightened, and taught that for the generation of the atmospheric source of yellow fever either at Havana, New Orleans, or New York, a temperature of 90° of F. is necessary, and must be continuous for weeks; and that yellow fever under such circumstances may be manufactured anywhere, and will become epidemic if filth and putrefying vegetation, and crowded apartments, and foul air abound, as in a dirty city.

Let it be proclaimed, that neither cotton, hides, nor bilge-water, in ships arriving from yellow fever ports, ever did or ever can be the fomites, or media of importation, but that the cause of yellow fever resides in the air, and in the air alone. The *atmosphere* from a yellow fever port may be shut up in the holds of a vessel, may develop the disease in the passengers and crew, and when the hatches are removed at Quarantine or at the wharves of a city, if permitted to enter, the poisoned air may infect all who breathe it. If in a hot climate, it may spread into the surrounding air, and if this be foul and reeking with filth, may be wafted by the winds for a greater or less distance, the air being the source of infection in every case.

Let it be publicly known that personal contagion of yellow fever, or any other fever except small-pox, is a fable, the very error of the moon; and if the sick be removed from the air which infected them into a healthy atmosphere, it is a physical impossibility that the sick, fomites and all, can communicate the disease to the well. Hence those Quarantine laws, which detain the well on board an infected vessel an hour, are based on superstition and cruelty. Nor can the detention of the vessel, longer than for the purpose of cleansing, purification, ventilation, &c., be justified, all the fomites in the case being contained in the air of the vessel. So that the ruinous abominations of Quarantine laws and the impositions of its officers should be regarded as the relics of barbarism, and the system be henceforth conformed to the spirit and science of the age.

NEW YORK SANITARY ASSOCIATION.

A public meeting of this body was recently held in the 14th Street Medical College, when, after a lecture by Dr. Griscom on "Light in its Sanitary Relations," and a Report made by P. M. Wetmore, Esq., on behalf of a committee, explaining the causes of the failure of the sanitary bills before the late Legislature, the following timely and excellent address was delivered by the Hon. Erastus Brooks, which we copy with much pleasure:

To the Scientific and Professional Men of this Assembly:

MR. PRESIDENT—I do not expect to say anything novel or new. As a citizen of New York, in common with yourselves, I feel a deep interest in the welfare of the people of the metropolis; and regarding, under Providence, the health of the people as a primary source of all human happiness, I have not felt at liberty to decline the invitation of your Committee of Arrangements briefly to address this meeting. I know that a vast amount of disease exists here; and I believe, by human agencies, that a great deal of it can be alleviated. The exposure of the evil, I hope, will lead to some immediate remedy; and if in no other way, upon the principle of the old and familiar proverb, that an ounce of prevention is worth a pound of cure. I do not know, as an unpretending observer of the medical art—ignorant, I confess, alike of medical compounds and of all suitable prescriptions for specific diseases—what the most proper remedy for any bodily disease in the world may be. Nor have I that confidence in the medical art itself, which amounts to a conviction that there are any remedies yet discovered which, unaided by the patient himself, can result even in an approximation to perfect cure. Still less have I confidence in any of the discoveries and inventions which have their origin in quackery or empiricism.

I see before me a world of natural beauty, the grand creation of the beneficent Architect of the universe. It is clothed in robes of light by day, and covered with a mantle of darkness by night. It has all the appropriate elements of the perfect excellence of its great Author: the sun, moon, and stars for light and warmth; the green earth—plain, valley, and hill-side—for the double purpose of a place of rest, and for producing all that can contribute to human life and comfort; sparkling waters from unfailing fountains to quench the thirst; the choicest fruits and sweetest flowers to gratify the senses; seas and oceans for commerce and intercourse; and, to crown all, as the last, best, greatest work of the Deity, the creation of man, in the image of God, and with a mission to him amounting to a command to replenish the earth and subdue it—to have dominion over the beasts of the field, the fish of the sea, the fowls of the air, and over every living thing that moveth upon the earth, including every herb and tree yielding seed. No wonder that, when God saw everything that he had made, that he pronounced it very good.

The application I wish to make is this: That to mar all these beauties of creation and all these objects of a wonderful life by those having a divine origin and destined to immortality, betrays not only a want of gratitude and an absence of the commonest wisdom, but it naturally creates a feeling of the deepest humiliation. In this sense, sir, as a question of moral duty, and in the light of palpable facts, let us survey some of the objects of interest immediately around us.

During the week past our city was filled with neighbors and strangers, discussing with an intensity of feeling our obligations towards the idolatrous people of the Old World, towards the Indians of the Far West, the negroes of Africa, the slaves of the Southern States, and all those varied questions of practical or abstract interest which, on one side or the other, arouse the passions or sympathies of all those who become partisans or friends of every question of public interest. As charity begins at home, and as repentance, too, should begin there also, I am right glad, sir, that an hour or two of this evening is to be devoted to our personal duty in reference to the official and personal crimes, vices, and negligences of our own city and households. Here is a field for the broadest theoretical philanthropy, and room enough for the truest practical benevolence. Here, too, in laying bare the evils from which we suffer, I would adopt the motto of one or all of you who believe in the medical art—*saucio sanare*—and only wound to heal. If anywhere on earth there is missionary ground where, in the spirit of Spenser's Ideal, one may engage himself, mind and heart, in

" Making a sunshine in a shady place,"

—it is right here.   You have had too much occasion to see and know this, in making and observing your legislators.   Your Senate Chambers and Halls of Assembly need cleansing as much as the stables of the classic Augea, and I hope, sir, both for this work and in the severe toil of purifying the foul places of our own city, this Sanitary Committee, now in session, may have all the courage, strength, and success of old Hercules himself.   I have recently been a visitor to some of the tenant houses of the city, where I have beheld scenes of wretchedness and degradation almost beyond comprehension.   One may indeed, if he will, like the good Howard in our midst, dive into the depths of dungeons, plunge into something as bad, if not worse than the infection of hospitals, and in more than a thousand places survey the mansions of sorrow, misery, depression, and contempt. Florence Nightingale, Elizabeth Fry, or our countrywoman, Dorothy Dix, could easily here enter upon a voyage of discovery and a circumnavigation of charity.   We have for an example, in the 8th Ward of this city, what is called the "Rotten Row," where 250 families and 1,250 persons are crowded into a space of about 180 by 50 feet, with, in one case, six people in one room, making common cause with the hens and pigs.   It is as bad, or worse, in some of the other wards and tenant houses of New York.   There is one house in Oliver Street, 16 feet by 30, with three floors and an attic—three rooms to each of the first and second floors, and ten rooms in all—in which have been crowded no less than fourteen families, with no entrance but an alley, and the yard literally reeking with filth.   I have visited a worse house in Cherry Street, where 120 families, or 500 persons, have been crowded upon two lots of ground, in a house five stories above the basement, and 150 feet deep.   Such filth, wretchedness, and suffering as one may see in these dens, miscalled human habitations, are almost beyond comprehension.   I asked myself two questions when within these dark, damp dungeons.   First, are the builders of these charnel houses human beings?   And second, how long can their occupants survive such loathsome degradation?   Every brick and particle of mortar seems to cry from the ground, like the blood of Abel for the murder of his brother, against this daily sacrifice of life upon the altar of human avarice.   Their owners or lessees may go forth clothed in purple and fine linen, and fare sumptuously every day; but the blood which crimsons their own cheeks, and flows, like the wine of life, in rich currents through their own veins, is but the spoil of the sick and the bruised, the languid and poverty-stricken Lazaruses who lie sick and dying at their gates, begging for the crumbs that fall from the master's table. Their love of gain is like the poisonous asp at the mother's breast, and every touch a leech sucking out the life-blood from those whom God formed and fashioned in the image of his own immortality.

I call attention to the fact that the deaths in this city for the last forty-six years have increased in a ratio vastly beyond the increase of population, and that, comparing London with New York, the mortality in the former city, to make the two cities equal, might be even thirty-six thousand deaths a year more then they are. The number of the dying here indeed is frightful, especially among the children; and were it not for our institutions of charity, our lying-in asylums, insane, reform, and orphan schools, our child's nursery and hospital, and kindred associations, public and private, for saving the souls and bodies of destitute adults and children, it would be vastly more than it is. And I rejoice to add, Mr. President, that under the auspices of a noble woman, whose genius and enthusiasm are not more remarkable than her large heart and cheerful, constant labors for the poor, an Infants' Home, a true foundling hospital, is to become a reality in our midst, and that before the rude blasts of winter can again lay the icy hand of death upon our neglected little ones, shelter, home, food, and raiment, and what is better, loving hands to enfold them, will be found for the multitudes who now die of neglect. Till when, may God temper the wind to his shorn lambs. Again, Mr. President, many of the cellar population of this strange city live in deep, damp cells, six feet, and more, under ground, exposed during every rain to the peltings of the pitiless storm. I am told by one of your association that this class of our population is not less than 25,000, which is not one-tenth of the number crowded into the tenant houses of this city.

The bodily ailments generated in these pestilential places are the very worst which flesh is heir to. The touch of disease becomes almost at once the hand of death, and if the victims escape for the day, the month or year, the seeds of disease are sown in a broken constitution, which hurries them to premature graves. The atmospheric diseases in the crowded portions of a city like this are legion; and how can it be otherwise, when there are 20 or 30 families in a house? One of your reports shows that in the Sixth Ward of this city, with all the

30

great improvements of the last twenty years, the deaths are one in 23, or in the First Ward one in 21.96; or, in contrast with the Fifteenth Ward, as one in 55, or one in 69.

Living in a free Republic, with a free Press, free Schools, and all the appliances of a high order of Intelligence, we are very far from where we ought to be in the attainment of practical knowledge upon our sanitary condition. I fear, sir, that among what are called the favored classes we are in this respect behind some of the governments of the Old World, which in other respects are more distinguished for their despotisms than for anything else. Some of the most despotic nationalities in the world make the amplest provisions for the health and physical comforts of the people. There are gardens and music, picture galleries and holidays, where the poorest subject of the King has as free an ingress as the Prince of the Realm. · How well did that singular man, Peter the Great, understand how to begin and advance an Empire which in the space of a few generations has become the third in Europe! It was in the Public garden of Peterhoff, and in the wide airy streets of the Capital, that the germs of civilization were planted. And, sir, I cannot but honor the present head of the French nation for the physical revolutions he has been working out in that centre of all European attraction, the City of Paris. Whatever there obstructs desired improvement, be it the Palace of the Prince, the highway of the King, costly edifices or majestic warehouses, yields to the determination to secure air and room for the thousands who throng that crowded capital. I cannot but wish the Emperor success in all this; and I hope I may, at this hour, be pardoned for saying also, that I wish him the most immediate and abundant success in every effort he is making to secure liberty and independence for the long oppressed people of Italy, to whose liberation he is pledged.

I honor this city, too, for its munificence in making provision for a Public Park, worthy not only of this great metropolis of the New World, but worthy of an Empire. I never, in public life, voted more cheerfully for a public improvement than for this one; and if it shall be wisely administered, we shall all soon forget the costs and the taxes, great as they are, in the large returns of public health and honest employment, which is the best possible interest that can be given for an investment in the cause of intelligent humanity.

Men of New York, in closing my desultory remarks, may I not say that you owe to the city of your birth or adoption the choice of rulers, who shall teach those around them, and much more in their own example than in precept, that—

> " The quality of mercy is not strained,
> But droppeth, as the rain from Heaven,
> Upon the place beneath."

And, rulers of New York—you who are the chosen chiefs of the City—its Mayor and Commonalty—its Governors and Board of Health—its Police and Heads of Departments—look well to your own accountability and reputation. Every man in office is to his constituents, his conscience, and his country, responsible before Heaven for the manner in which he administers his public trust. If life and health are sacrificed by a neglect of duty—come that neglect from what is done or what is left undone—the wrong act lies at your door. The law of the land makes the taking of life by violence an offence punishable with death. The divine law requires personal accountability in the discharge of every personal and delegated duty, while that Golden Rule founded upon that Higher Law that has the sanction of peace on earth and good-will to men, commands us to do unto others as we would they should do unto us. What, indeed, would become of this city of ours, if there were not a big hole at the top of it, to let down a little of God's daylight, and, with it, some little of the sweet air of Heaven ? I would, then, invoke from rulers and people, landlords and tenants, tax-payers and non-tax-payers, a deeper interest than has hitherto been manifested in the health of the City. The latter is the happiness of the body, just as virtue is the happiness of the mind. I call, therefore, upon the charitable and humane—those who live in dwellings of their own—those who build and buy houses—those who sell and those who hire—those who have children of their own, and those who, having none, yet wish well to those young plants, which, in their tender years, are as delicate as the frailest flowers of summer, before the rude winter's blast—to have mercy upon those exposed to disease and death in their very midst. God has made for all the full light of the Sun and the free air of Heaven, and I have shown from the Book of the highest wisdom that power and dominion over all upon the face of the earth rests with the last object of His creation—MAN himself. Upon us, then, inhabitants of this great and exposed City, belongs a double share of responsibility. Let us assume it like men, and in this, the spring-time of the year, with summer heats and summer diseases at hand, acquit ourselves as becomes a moral and just people.

MEDICAL NEWS AND HOSPITAL GAZETTE.

Our contemporary of the above journal would be wiser to "let strife alone before it is meddled with," else he may possibly burn his own fingers by his flippant fling at the N. Y. Academy of Medicine, and its' action in the late onslaught upon Dr. Horace Green. He writes under a grievous misapprehension of the facts, or he is open to the charge of misrepresenting them, by his comments on Dr. Mott's letter. Why did he not publish both sides of the mooted question, including Dr. M's own qualifications of that letter, amounting to a retraction? His readers would then have learned that there is no conflict here between the "friends of the *swabbing* practice" and Dr. Mott, who uses the sponge probang and "swabbing" himself in his public and private practice, as does Dr. B., and every other surgeon in N. O. Such criticism can only provoke a smile, nor is his the style to do good with, as he must be aware.

OUR YOUNG SURGEONS,

Who are laudably ambitious for distinction and practice in these days, are wont to find their "Jordan a hard road to travel." Dr. Ayres, of Brooklyn, has had this experience. He lately devised and executed an autoplastic operation for congenital exstrophy of the bladder and its accompanying deformities in a female, who had been suffered to grow up to mature years under the observation of older surgeons, no one of whom had the courage or patience to attempt the relief of her hideous and loathsome deformity. Dr. Ayres's operation turned out to be a success, and his treatment has given his patient a new lease of life, leaving only a trivial disability, which to her is an unspeakable blessing. We reported the case in the GAZETTE, and, as in duty bound, commended him as he deserved.

Had he gone into the newspapers with it, as other and older surgeons do with other and even minor operations, taking care that his own hand was not visible, he would have been assailed for extra professional advertising, by the very men whose advertisements of their own names, as nominally connected with hospitals, are repeated *ad nauseam.* Or had his operation possessed neither novelty nor merit, he would have escaped the carping of envy, for nobody cares to attack mediocrity. But he chose to report his case to the profession in a legitimate way, thus to encourage others to undertake the relief of similar cases, instead of abandoning them as utterly beyond all surgery, as is most generally done.

For this he has been anonymously assailed in the *Boston Medical and Surgical Journal*, whose editors must allow us to say, that they might be better employed than allowing their correspondent to detract from the merits of a young surgeon, whose name accompanies his report, without the responsibility of the criticism being assumed by the signature of the writer.

NEW YORK CITY LUNATIC ASYLUM.

The report of the Resident Physician, Dr. Ranney, shows the crowded state of this pauper institution, there being an excess of 200 patients beyond the capacity of the present buildings, which, only affording adequate accommodation for 450 inmates, have been crowded the year round with over 600, the present number being 655!! The mortality of the year has been 95, much less than might be anticipated in view of the discomforts of so closely-packed rooms, and so greatly disadvantageous to the medical and moral treatment required by the suffering inmates.

This hospital is too large, and had far better be substituted with two smaller ones, than to increase the buildings as proposed. No superintendent, with his corps of assistants, can do justice to 650 insane persons, whose needs are vastly greater than any other class of patients. Moreover, as Dr. Ranney shows, if only the pauper lunatics, rightfully chargeable to the city, were received, the present buildings are sufficiently ample for the present. The suggestions of the report on this topic deserve the attention of the Governors.

NEW YORK ACADEMY OF MEDICINE.

The last meeting was taken up with a discussion on an attempt to exclude all *patented* articles from the notice of the Academy hereafter, which was unsuccessful, of course, while one of its own members has just *patented* a ventilating apparatus, which is to be brought before the Academy.

Dr. Harris then commenced the reading of a paper on the personal contagiousness of yellow fever, &c., attempting to vindicate the vote passed at the Quarantine Convention, "*fomites!*" and all. It was not completed, however, and it will be time enough to criticise it hereafter.

Dr. Corson then rose to a question of privilege, and complained that he had been misapprehended and misrepresented in relation to his course with the publication of the paper lately read by him before the Academy. Although in type, it had not been technically published or circulated until he had the consent of the Council, which the President could testify; and he had since obtained the consent of the Academy. He therefore claimed to have acted honorably throughout. If the GAZETTE's report of a former meeting was understood to imply censure in this regard, let it stand corrected. *Fiat justitia, ruat cœlum.*

UNIVERSITY OF THE CITY OF NEW YORK.

The announcement of this, the leading medical school of our city, will be found in this number of the GAZETTE; and by the statistical table published in our last No. it appears that, numerically, it stands the *fourth* school in the United States in matriculants, and the *third* in the country in its graduates. We observe that its regular course of lectures, at the next session, will continue *four months and a half,* and that five cliniques are held by the Faculty every week. No change has been made in the Faculty this year. See our advertising columns for details.

UNIVERSITY OF THE PACIFIC.

MEDICAL DEPARTMENT AT SAN FRANCISCO.

In our last number we inserted a paper from Professor E. S. Cooper, who has distinguished himself as a surgeon by many brilliant and successful operations. We are now in the receipt of the announcement of the new medical college at San Francisco, which opens in May, with a full Faculty, and continues eighteen weeks. The fees are $180 for a full course, $5 for matriculation, and $50 for graduation. The Faculty include Doctors Morison, Rowell, Cole, Cooper, Carman, and Barstow.

PRIZE MEDAL.

Dr. Jacob Harsen, of this city, has lately invested $2,500 in founding a prize medal for the highest attainments on the part of the students in Clinical Medicine at the *New York Hospital.* Those who excel in any *other* hospital, whatever be their merits by comparison, are excluded from competition for this prize.

Will not some benefactor remember the students at Bellevue and the State Emigrants' Hospitals, both of which have more clinical students, and are larger institutions?

UNIVERSITY OF BUFFALO

This medical school, whose Faculty will compare favorably with that of any college in the country, makes its announcement in the present number of the GAZETTE. We learn that three hospitals are accessible to students, where clinical opportunities are afforded by Professors Hamilton, White, and Rochester, of whose capabilities as teachers it were superfluous to speak. The enlarged class of last year is ominous of greater prosperity in the future. See advertisement.

UNIVERSITY OF NASHVILLE

In referring our readers to the standing advertisement of this medical school, we cannot forbear congratulating the Faculty that their class of last year places them the *second* in the list of American colleges, the Jefferson school at Philadelphia being alone in the numerical advance. Such prosperity is unprecedented.

THE KAPPA LAMBDAS.

A letter from *Dr. John H. Griscom* is published in the inaugural address of Dr. Brinsmade, President of the State Society, last year, in which Dr. G. says:

" *Kappa Lambda of Hippocrates* has 24! members; average attendance 12!; meets monthly at the dwellings of the members; objects—general *improvement* in medical science!" Pro-di-gi-ous!

MISCELLANEOUS ITEMS.

Dr. James L. Phelps, as appears by the printed record, was the delegate from the Kappa Lambdas, in 1856, to the American Medical Association, at Detroit. Our correspondent is in error, therefore, when he states that *Dr. John G. Adams* was the *only* delegate ever sent. It is safe to predict that they will never send another.

Drs. John H. Griscom, Alexander H. Stevens, John Watson, and *E. L. Beadle** are supposed to have represented the Kappa Lambdas, in the late Quarantine and Sanitary Convention, for they clearly took the lead, all the other medical men seeming to follow in their wake; and it would seem they "went it *blind!*" else they could not have so stultified themselves by voting as they did on the "*fomites*" resolution, in which all parties have written themselves down ———; unless, forsooth, they claim to have meant to be understood in a Pickwickian sense.

---

* This gentleman only having the *honor* of delegation.

Professorial Changes, &c.—Dr. Geo. B. Wood has resigned his chair in the University of Pa., to take effect in the spring, so that he will lecture through the next session.

Dr. Alfred Stille having resigned his chair in the Pennsylvania Medical College, the Faculty of that school have disbanded. The *Philadelphia College of Medicine* have thereupon organized under the Gettysburg charter, relinquished by the former College, and will be the third medical school in Philadelphia.

We hear rumors of several other changes in the medical schools of Philadelphia, occasioned by the advanced age and failing health of several of the professors, and which cannot be long delayed. These changes will make openings both in the Jefferson and University Schools, which will be eagerly sought as the best positions in the country.

In the New York Medical College the chairs of Anatomy and Obstetrics have been vacated by the resignation of Profs. Childs and Barker. We have not heard who are to succeed them.

In the College of Physicians and Surgeons, of New York, we learn that Dr. Geo. T. Elliott has been appointed *adjunct* Professor of Obstetrics, and Dr. Thos. M. Markoe, *adjunct* Professor of Surgery. The announcement that Professor Gilman had resigned his chair was *another* blunder of the " Press," copied, as usual, by the complaisant "Reporter." The object of these appointments was to prevent these gentlemen going into the N. Y. Medical College.

Dr. Francis G. Smith has been appointed Physician to the Pennsylvania Hospital, in place of Dr. Geo. B. Wood, resigned.

Profs. Hun and Dean have resigned their chairs in the Albany Medical College, and Drs. Townsend and Quackenbush will supply their lack of service. The course will begin in September of this year, and the spring course is henceforth abandoned.

A new Medical College is about to be opened at Mobile, Ala. Dr. Nott takes the chair of Surgery, and has sailed for Europe to select museum and apparatus.

The Medical Classes in Philadelphia last winter reached the number of 1,163!

Dr. Burge's Apparatus for fractured thigh is becoming popular among surgeons in private practice. The price, it will be seen, is *forty dollars.*

The Bugeaud Toni Nutritive Wine is in great request among patients suffering from malarial and periodic fevers. It is composed of pure Malaga wine, Peruvian bark, and Cacoa, and is grateful to the palate of dyspeptics, who find it highly useful as a tonic; and it is also prized by convalescents, as preferable to any other form of cordial. See advertisement.

The senior *Dr. Marsh,* whose new radical cure truss is announced on our cover, has just returned from a professional visit to San Francisco, &c., in California. His instrument has the warm approval of

Dr. E. S. Cooper, the eminent surgeon of the golden State, and Dr. M. has found his visit available in enhancing the reputation of his truss, and in extending in that new State his own high character in mechanical surgery, by introducing his various appliances for the cure of defects and deformities, to which good work he has devoted so many years of his life. He thinks that the necessity of the new operations for the radical cure of reducible hernia may to a great extent be superseded by the surgical adaptation of his truss, which he can modify to suit any case.

Dr. David Sands, of A. B. & D. Sands, the proprietors of McMunn's Elixir of Opium, has returned from his European tour, undertaken for the benefit of his health, which has been much improved by the voyage. He found that the value of the Elixir of Opium is recognized by the profession abroad, as well as at home. We are daily witnessing its utility in public and private practice, the testimony of which by the profession is ever accumulating.

Transactions of the Medical Society of the State of New York, for 1859.—This volume is received, and will be found to be quite equal to any of its predecessors in the variety and practical character of its contents. Many of the papers it contains evince very great ability and originality. The address of the retiring President is admirable. Copies may be obtained by addressing Dr. Sylvester D. Willard, Secretary, at Albany, N. Y.

Sailed for Europe.—We see among the passengers by the Persia, the names of Dr. Chipley, of Lexington, Ky., and Dr. E. D. Fenner, of New Orleans. Several of our New York physicians have taken passage in the Arago, which sails as we go to press.

CONTENTS.

UNIVERSITY OF NEW YORK.
MEDICAL DEPARTMENT.
SESSION, 1859-60.

The Session for 1859-60 will begin on Monday, October 17, and will be continued until the 1st of March.

Faculty of Medicine.

Rev. Isaac Ferris, D.D., LL.D., Chancellor of the University.

Valentine Mott, M.D., LL.D., Emeritus Professor of Surgery and Surgical Anatomy, and ex-President of the Faculty.

Martyn Paine, M.D., LL.D., Professor of Materia Medica and Therapeutics.

Gunning S. Bedford, M.D., Professor of Obstetrics, the Diseases of Women and Children, and Clinical Midwifery.

John W. Draper, M.D., LL.D., Professor of Chemistry and Physiology, President of the Faculty.

Alfred C. Post, M.D., Professor of the Principles and Operations of Surgery, with Surgical and Pathological Anatomy.

William H. Van Buren, M.D., Professor of General and Descriptive Anatomy.

John T. Metcalfe, M.D., Professor of the Institutes and Practice of Medicine.

J. W. S. Gouley, M.D., Demonstrator of Anatomy.

J. H. Hinton, M.D., Prosector to the Professor of Surgery.

Alexander B. Mott, M.D., Prosector to the Emeritus Professor of Surgery.

Besides Daily Lectures on the foregoing subjects, there will be five Cliniques weekly, on *Medicine, Surgery, and Obstetrics.*

The Dissecting-room, which is refitted and abundantly lighted with gas, is open from 8 o'clock, A. M., till 10 o'clock. P. M.

Fees for a full course of Lectures, $105. Matriculation fee, $5. Graduation fee, $30. Demonstrator's fee, $5.

UNIVERSITY OF BUFFALO.

Medical Department.—The Annual Course of Lectures in this Institution commences on the FIRST WEDNESDAY IN NOVEMBER, and continues sixteen weeks. The Dissecting-rooms will be opened on the first Wednesday in October.

Clinical Lectures at the Buffalo Hospital throughout the entire term, by Professors Hamilton and Rochester.

FACULTY.

James P White, M.D., Professor of Obstetrics and Diseases of Women and Children.

Frank H. Hamilton, M.D., Professor of the Principles and Practice of Surgery and Clinical Surgery.

George Hadley, M.D., Professor of Chemistry and Pharmacy.

Thomas F. Rochester, M.D., Professor of Principles and Practice of Medicine.

Edward M. Moore, M.D., Professor of Surgical Anatomy and Surgical Pathology.

Theophilus Mack, M.D., Lecturer on Materia Medica.

Sandford Eastman, M.D., Professor of Anatomy.

Austin Flint, Jr., M.D., Professor of Physiology and Microscopy.

Benj H. Lemon, M.D., Demonstrator of Anatomy.

Fees—including Matriculation and Hospital Tickets, $75. Demonstrator's Ticket, $5. Graduation Fee, $20

The Dean is authorized to issue a perpetual ticket, on payment of one hundred dollars.

Students who have attended a full course of Lectures in this or any other institution, will be received on payment of $50. The fee from those who have attended two courses elsewhere is $25

For further information or circulars, address,

THOMAS F. ROCHESTER,

Buffalo, 1859.   **Dean of the Faculty.**

AMERICAN

MEDICAL GAZETTE.

| Vol. X. | JULY, 1859. | No. 7. |

ORIGINAL DEPARTMENT.

Twelfth Annual Meeting of the
AMERICAN MEDICAL ASSOCIATION.

(CONTINUED FROM THE JUNE NUMBER.)

Dr. T. M. Blatchford, of New York, offered as a subtitute the following preamble and resolution:

"*Whereas*, Of all the subjects which can engage our attention in our associate capacity, that of Medical Education is paramount; and *Whereas*, harmony of action is essential to success in establishing definite qualifications entitling to admission in our ranks; and *Whereas*, nothing can be gained by hasty action in a matter so vital to our very existence, as a permanent Medical Institution: Therefore,

"*Resolved*, That further action be suspended for the present upon the subject of the resolutions offered at the last meeting of the Association by the chairman of the Special Committee on Medical Education, and that a committee, consisting of S. W. Butler, of Pennsylvania, L. A. Smith, of New Jersey, Dixi Crosby, of New Hampshire, C. A. Pope, of Mo., and T. Buckler, of Maryland, shall be appointed to confer with the committee appointed at the meeting of Medical Teachers, to report some plan for action at the next meeting of the Association."

This amendment was lost, and the original resolution adopted.

The resolutions from the New Jersey Medical Society were then taken from the table and referred to the Committee of Conference.

Dr. Davis offered a resolution instructing the same committee to confer with the State Medical Societies for the purpose of procuring more decisive and uniform action throughout the profession in carrying into effect the standard of preliminary education adopted by this Association, at its organization in 1847. This was carried.

Dr. Gibbs, from the committee to examine into a plan of uniform registration of births, marriages, and deaths, offered the following report:

They have given the same a careful consideration, and they unanimously recommend that the report be adopted, and referred to the Committee on Publication.

They also recommend that the same committee be continued, with instructions to add to the report, in time for publication in the ensuing volume of Transactions, a form of registration law which may be likely to answer the requirements of the several States.

Dr. Sayre, of New York, offered the following:

" *Whereas*, The medical profession at large have an interest in the character and qualifications of those who are to be admitted as their associates in the profession: Therefore,

"*Resolved*, That each State Medical Society be requested to appoint annually two delegates for each college in that State, whose duty it shall be to attend the examinations of all candidates for graduation; and that the colleges be requested to permit such delegates to participate in the examination, and vote on the qualifications of all such candidates."

This was, on motion, referred to the Committee of Conference.

The paper of Dr. Jones, presented at the morning session, was taken from the Committee on Publication and referred to the Committee on Prize Essays.

Dr. Eve moved to record the name of Dr. Benj. W. Dudley, as a permanent member, which was adopted by a unanimous vote, the delegates all rising to their feet in token of respect.

Adjourned till to-morrow morning, at 9 o'clock.

THIRD DAY.

THURSDAY, *May* 5, 1859.

The President called the Association to order at nine o'clock, and the reading of the minutes of yesterday was dispensed with.

The first business in order was an amendment to the Constitution, laid over from last year, and proposed by Dr. T. L. Mason, of New York, to insert in the first line of the second paragraph of Article II., after the words "shall receive the appointment from," the words "any medical society permanently organized in accordance with the laws regulating the practice of physic and surgery in the State in which they are situated, and consisting of physicians and surgeons regularly authorized to practice their profession." Also, to add to the sixth paragraph of the same article the words " but each permanent member of the first class designated in this plan of organization shall be entitled to a seat in this Association, on his presenting to this body a certificate of his good standing, signed by the Secretary of the society to which he may belong at the time of each annual meeting of this body."

Dr. Lyndon A. Smith, of New Jersey, said amendments to the Constitution should be adopted with care; and though, perhaps, that now proposed might be desirable, still, as Dr. Mason, who had proposed it, was not present to explain his views, he moved that the subject be laid over until next year. This suggestion was adopted.

Another constitutional amendment, proposed by Dr. Henry Hartshorne, of Pennsylvania, and laid over from last year under the rules, provides to add to Article II. the words: " No one expelled from this Association shall at any time thereafter be received as a delegate or member, unless by a three-fourths vote of the members present at the meeting to which he is sent, or at which he is proposed."

This amendment was adopted.

Another amendment, proposed by J. Berrien Lindsly, of Tennessee, was called up, to omit in Article II. the words " medical colleges, hospitals, lunatic asylums, and other permanently organized medical institutions in good standing in the United States;" and also to omit the words: " The faculty of every regularly constituted medical college or chartered school of medicine shall have the privilege of sending two delegates. The professional staff of every chartered or municipal hospital containing a hundred inmates or more shall have the privilege of sending two delegates; and every other permanently organized medical institution of good standing shall have the privilege of sending one delegate."

This was laid on the table until the next annual meeting.

An invitation was received from Mons. Groux, requesting the delegates to meet him at the hall of the University at noon to-day, to witness experiments on his congenital fissure of the sternum, which was deferred until four o'clock this afternoon, as the Association had previously accepted the hospitality of Mr. and Mrs. Robert J. Ward at the former hour.

Dr. Singleton offered a series of resolutions from "Young Physic," deprecating the introduction of schisms, and reflecting on the harmony of the Association; which, after a vigorous speech from Dr. McDowell, was unanimously laid on the table, with a request that it should not appear on the minutes. Dr. Davis regarded the evidences of harmony and good feeling exhibited here this year as greater and more cheering than on any previous occasion, and deprecated any insinuation that unkindly sentiments existed.

Dr. McDermott submitted the following resolutions:

"*Whereas*, A vast proportion of the disease and misery that afflict our race is caused by the excessive use of intoxicating liquors; and whereas, in the opinion of this Association, the evils of intoxication can be most effectually remedied by the establishment of Inebriate Asylums, wherein the victims of intemperance may be subjected to such restraints and treatment as shall effect a thorough reformation of their habits: Therefore, ,

"*Resolved*, That this Association recommend the establishment of inebriate asylums in the various States of the Union.

"*Resolved*, That the State and County Medical Societies, and all members of the medical profession, be requested to unite in diffusing among the people a better knowledge and appreciation of the beneficent purposes and important benefits that would be conferred upon society by the establishment of such asylums throughout the various sections of the country."

This resolution was referred to the mover, as a Special Committee, with a request that he would report thereon at the next meeting of the Association.

Dr. Shattuck offered the following, which was adopted:

"*Resolved*, That the committee appointed in May, 1857, on Criminal Abortion, be requested to continue their labors, and especially to take all measures necessary to carry into effect the resolutions reported by them on the first day of the meeting."

Dr. Yandell, from the Committee on Voluntary Essays, made a further report that a communication had been received from Dr. Langer, of Iowa, on Subcutaneous Injections as Remedials, which, on motion, the author read.

The essay was referred to the writer as a special committee, with the request that he would report further at the next annual meeting of the Association, and continue his investigations.

Invitatious to visit the Insane Asylum and the Library and Museum of Transylvania University were received.

The President appointed as the Committee of Conference, to meet the committee from the Teachers' Convention, the following gentlemen: Drs. Blatchford, Troy, N. Y.; Condie, Philadelphia, Pa.; Bozeman, Montgomery, Ala.; Brodie, Detroit, Michigan; and Sneed, Frankfort, Ky.

Dr. D. Meredith Reese, from the Nominating Committee, made the following final report:

Special Committees continued.

On Quarantine.—Drs. D. D. Clark, Penn.; Snow, R. I.; Jewell, Penn.; Fenner, La.; and Houck, Md.

On Medical Ethics.—Drs. Schuck, Penn.; Murphy, Ohio; Linton, Mo.; Powell, Ga.; Eve, Tenn.

On Tracheotomy in Membranous Croup.—Dr. A. V. Dougherty, N. J.

On Mercurial Fumigation in Syphilis.—Dr. D. W. Yandell, Louisville, Ky.

On the Improvements in the Science and Art of Surgery, made during the last Half Century.—Dr. Jos. McDowell, St. Louis, Mo.

On the Cause and Increase of Crime, and its Mode of Punishment.—Dr. W. C. Sneed, Frankfort, Ky.

On the Education of Imbecile and Idiotic Children.—Dr. H. P. Ayres, Fort Wayne, Ind.

On the Uses and Abuses of the Speculum Uteri.—Dr. C. H. Spillman, of Kentucky.

On the Topography of Vermont.—Dr. Perkins, of Vermont.

On the Pons Varolii, &c.—Dr. S. B. Richardson, of Kentucky, and Dr. Fishback, of Indiana.

On the Physiological Effects of the Hydro-Carbons.—Dr. F. W. White, of Illinois.

On the Effect of the Perineal Operations for Urinary Calculi upon Procreation in the Male.—Dr. J. S. White, of Tennessee.

The paper from Dr. Ellis, of Massachusetts, on the subject, " Does the microscope enable us to make a positive diagnosis of cancer, and what, if any, are the sources of error?" was referred to the Special Committee on the Microscope, of which Dr. Dalton is chairman.

On motion, the report was adopted as a whole.

Honorary resolutions were passed to the memory of the following members of the Association, deceased: Dr. W. W. Boling, of Alabama; Dr. Thomas D. Mütter, of Penn.; Dr. P. C. Gaillard, of S. C.; Dr. Jabez G. Goble, of New Jersey; Dr. John K. Mitchell, of Tenn.

Dr. R. K. Smith, of Philadelphia, submitted the following:

" *Resolved,* That the death of Dr. John K. Mitchell, one of the members of this Association, has been to this body a loss keenly felt by every man who knew him. His eminence as a teacher, his varied acquirements in every department of learning, and his generous social qualities in every relation, endeared him to every member of the profession who had the pleasure of his personal acquaintance.

"*Resolved*, That the family be notified of the action of this Association."

Other more formal resolutions were offered, and feeling eulogies pronounced.

Dr. Sayre offered the following, which were adopted by acclamation:

"*Resolved*, That the thanks of the American Medical Association are eminently due and are hereby presented to the citizens of Louisville, Ky., for the princely hospitality publicly and privately extended to the members of this body during its present session.

"*Resolved*, That to the Committee of Arrangements and the profession of Louisville, generally, our thanks are due for their kind and assiduous attention to the Association, and for the hearty welcome with which they have greeted our convention in their flourishing city."

After the transaction of some other unimportant routine business,

On motion of Dr. Davis, the Association adjourned, to meet at New Haven, on the first Tuesday in June, 1860.

The registration book during the day announced the names of Drs. D. G. Thomas, of New York; William S. Cain, of Kentucky, and Peter Allen, R. K. McMeans, and W. R. Kable, of Ohio—making 305 members in attendance during the session of the Association.

CONVENTION OF MEDICAL TEACHERS.

MORNING SESSION.—At a meeting of the last National Medical Convention, held in Washington City, it was *Resolved*, That there should be a National Convention of the Teachers from the Medical Colleges in the United States, and that they should meet in the city of Louisville, Ky., the day before the meeting of the National Medical Convention. In accordance with this resolution, they met on Monday morning, May 2, 1859, at Mozart Hall.

After prayer by Rev. J. H. Heywood, Dr. Dixi Crosby, Professor of Surgery in Dartmouth College, N. H., was called to the chair, and Dr. George C. Blackman, of Ohio, appointed Secretary.

Dr. Crosby returned his thanks to the Convention in a neat and appropriate speech.

Dr. D. F. Wright offered the following resolution:

"*Resolved*, That all members of the Faculties of Medical Colleges, now present, shall be considered members of this Convention; but that when more than one from the same College is present, but one of them shall cast the vote of that institution."

A substitute was offered by Dr. Baker, of Ohio, that a committee of three, on credentials, be appointed by the chair. This substitute for the original resolution was then carried, and the chair appointed the following gentlemen to serve on that committee: Dr. Shattuck, from Massachusetts, Dr. Haskins, from Tennessee, and Dr. Baker, from Ohio.

The Convention then adjourned for thirty minutes, to allow the Committee on Credentials time to report. At the expiration of the time, the committee reported the following colleges as represented, with the gentlemen as delegates:

Dartmouth College, N. H.—Prof. Dixi Crosby. *Shelby Medical College, Tenn.*—Profs. E. B. Haskins and D. F. Wright. *Missouri Medical College.*—Prof. J. H. McDowell. *St. Louis Medical College.*—Prof. N. L. Linton. *Medical College of South Carolina.*—Prof. H. R. Frost. *Medical College of Georgia, Augusta.*—Prof. H. F. Campbell. *Medical Department of the University of Michigan.*—Prof. Moses Gunn. *University of Louisville, Medical Department.*—L. P. Yandell and L. Powell. *Cincinnati College of Medicine and Surgery.*—Prof. H. Baker. *Jefferson Medical College, Philadelphia.*—Profs. Robly Dunglison and Franklin Bache. *Lind University of Chicago.*—Prof. N. S. Davis. *Oglethorpe Medical College, Georgia.*—Prof. A. G. Thomas. *Medical College of Ohio.*—Prof. Geo. C. Blackman. *Kentucky School of Medicine*—Profs. M. Goldsmith and Geo. W. Bayless. *Iowa University.*—Prof. McGugin. *Medical College of Memphis.*—Prof. H. R. Robards. *Medical College of Virginia, Richmond.*—Profs. B. R. Welford and L. S. Joynes. *Atlanta Medical College, Georgia.*—Profs. J. G. Westmoreland and John W. Jones. *Medical Faculty of Harvard University at Boston.*—Prof. Geo. C. Shattuck. *Rush Medical College, Chicago, Ill.*—Profs. Daniel Brainard and Joseph W. Freer. *Western Reserve Medical College, Cleveland, Ohio.*—Prof. G. C. C. Weber.

On motion, the report was received, and the committee allowed to report further the names of delegates during the day.

The next business in order was the election of officers for the permanent organization of the Convention.

On motion, the officers of the preliminary meeting were declared elected.

Prof. Crosby, in taking his seat as President, said the Convention had derived one advantage from the re-election of the present officers, as they were spared being inflicted with additional speeches of thanks. He concluded by saying that, unless changed by the Convention, he had the authority to make rules for conducting business. He therefore ruled that no member shall speak longer than ten minutes, nor more than twice on the same subject.

A motion was offered by Dr. D F. Wright, of Tenn., allowing all persons present from the different Medical Colleges to sit as members of this Convention. This was amended by Dr. Davis, of Chicago, by adding that no college should be allowed more than one vote on any proposition. This was carried.

Dr. Davis, of Ills., offered a resolution authorizing the appointment of a committee of five, as a Business Committee. This being carried, the President appointed the following gentlemen: Drs. Davis, of Ills., Gunn, of Michigan, Frost, of S. C., Shattuck, of Mass., and Yandell, of Louisville, Ky.

The Convention then adjourned for thirty minutes, to allow the committee time to prepare business.

At the expiration of the time, the committee reported six resolutions, which were accepted from the committee, and were, on motion, brought up in order. The following are the resolutions:

" *Resolved*, That this Convention recognize the great advantages to be derived from the action of the American Medical Association in prescribing the terms and conditions on which medical degrees shall be conferred and licenses to practice medicine shall be granted, and that any expression of opinion as to methods or periods of instruction from the American Medical Association should be received with deference and respect, and that all pains should be taken to enforce any rules or regulations recommended by that body.

"*Resolved*, That this Convention earnestly recommends the American Medical Association to adopt such measures as will secure the efficient practical enforcement of the standard of the preliminary education, adopted at its organization in May, 1847, and that the Medical Colleges will cheerfully receive and record the certificates alluded to in said standard, whenever the profession generally, and the preceptors, will see that students are properly supplied with them.

"*Resolved*, That no Medical College should allow any term of practice to be a substitute for one course of lectures in the requisitions for graduation.

"*Resolved*, That hospital clinical instruction constitutes a necessary part of medical education, and that every candidate for the degree of Doctor of Medicine should be required to have attended such instruction regularly for a period of not less than *five months*, during the last year of his period of pupilage.

"*Resolved*, That every Medical College should rigidly enforce the rule requiring three full years of medical study before graduation, and that the diploma of no Medical College shall be recognized which is known to violate this rule."

The first resolution created some degree of excitement, and provoked considerable debate, when the Convention adjourned until three o'clock.

AFTERNOON SESSION.—The debate still continued on the first resolution, as reported in the forenoon. Dr. Bayless, who had the floor at the time of adjournment, offered the following amendments: to substitute, in the fourth line, the word "recommended" for "prescribe," and all after the words "deference and respect" be stricken out.

The debate on this resolution still continued warm, most of the gentlemen participating, when Dr. Joynes offered the following as a substitute:

"*Whereas*, It appears that a large portion of the Medical Colleges of the United States are unrepresented in this Convention; that no changes in the present system of education can be effected unless adopted by the schools generally:

"*Resolved*, That it is inexpedient at this time to take any action upon the propositions contained in the report presented by the Special Committee on Medical Education at the last meeting of the American Medical Association.

"*Resolved*, That with the view of obtaining a more general union in counsel and action upon this important subject, this Convention do now adjourn, to meet again on the day preceding the next annual meeting of the Medical Association, and at the place which may be agreed upon for such meeting, and that the several Medical Colleges in the United States be requested to appoint each a delegate to such adjourned meeting of this Convention."

An amendment was offered by Dr. Wright, by adding another resolution to the effect that a committee be appointed to examine the different propositions offered. The vote of the Colleges being called on this resolution, the vote stood ten for the substitute and nine against.

The following gentlemen were appointed by the chair to serve on that committee: Dr. L. P. Yandell, of Louisville; Dr. G. Shattuck, of Massachusetts; Dr. G. C. Blackman, of Ohio; H. F. Campbell, of Georgia; Dr. M. Gunn, of Michigan.

The meeting was then adjourned.

The Connection of the Nervous Centres of Animal and Organic Life, with the Results of Vivisection.

By John O'Reilly, M.D.,

Licentiate and Fellow of the Royal College of Surgeons in Ireland; Resident Fellow of the New York Academy of Medicine.

My presence being casually requested, in the middle of November last, to take a part in a discussion relative to the anatomy and physiology of the placenta, it so happened, on that occasion, that I was induced to advance original views in the course of the debate on the matter which took place.

In order to sustain the position I assumed, relative to the nervous connection between the mother and fœtus, it became necessary to study the action of the nervous systems of animal and organic life. I state these particulars for the purpose of showing I had not directed my attention to these important subjects previously, and as an apology for the abrupt manner in which the papers were written.

To promulgate new doctrine with a view of overthrowing the old, unless founded on unquestionable facts, must, to a great extent, be deemed a heresy.

No person entertains a higher opinion of the labors of Prochaska, Bichat, Richerand, Sir Charles Bell, Payne, Hall, Müller, Brown-Séquard, Bernard, Grainger, Todd, and Dalton, than I do. I trust, therefore, I will not be considered as detracting from the reputation of these distinguished physiologists, when I assert they have failed to fully or truly expound the relationship existing between the nervous systems of animal and organic life.

It will be recollected, that I asserted that the lenticular ganglion acted under the control of the Pineal gland, or ganglion, through reflex action through the brain, and the *exceedingly* small filament of the third nerve communicating with it; and that the contraction and dilatations of the iris were thus regulated, as well as the adjustment of the muscles of the eyeball, supplied by the third pair of nerves; that the par vagum acted under the influence of the central ganglion; that tetanic spasm of the muscles was produced by irritation of the organic ganglia; that coma was induced by compression of the central ganglion.

In a conversation I recently had with my esteemed friend, Dr. Busteed, Professor of Anatomy and Physiology at the New Veterinary College, who is not only a capital anatomist, but an excellent operating surgeon, and one to whom I am greatly indebted for kindly volunteering to test my theory by vivisection, I stated my conviction, that the carotid plexus governed the circulation of the blood, and prevented the brain from being broken up, or deluged with blood, when attacked with inflammation, as well as protected the lives of persons indulging to a fearful and amazing extent in the imbibition of intoxicating drinks.

As it may be deemed superfluous to make further allusions to the statement made in my former paper, I beg to refer to the essay itself.

In order to afford facility to others to make experiments for their own satisfaction, I will state the mode of proceeding: The best animal that can be selected is a sheep; none other can be kept sufficiently quiet. The instruments required consist of a hand-saw, chisel, dissecting-knife, forceps, and retractors; sponges, water, ligatures, and plugs of paper about a quarter of an inch in thickness should be in readiness. The sheep, being placed on a firm table, should be held by assistants. The scalp is now to be freely removed, together with the muscles attached to the cranium. A coffin-shaped piece of the skull is next to be taken away, about four inches long and three in width; the narrow extremity should terminate at a line drawn transversely about one inch and a half above the superciliary ridges, whilst the posterior should extend about one inch beyond the occipital protuberance. This being accomplished, the dura mater is next to be dissected off by dividing it on each side of the falx, separating it from its attachment to the crista galli; here some hæmorrhage will take place from the longitudinal sinuses; but it need not be apprehended. The membrane being reflected back, the tentorium cerebelli is next to be detached. In doing this, the lateral sinuses will be opened, rendered manifest by a gush of venous blood, which, if not restrained, will soon render further dissection useless; several sheep were prematurely killed by this accident; the top of the finger should be pressed against the part until a plug of paper is pushed into the sinus, which will prevent further trouble from this source. Having now exposed the cerebrum and cerebellum, the posterior lobes of the cerebrum should be separated from the cerebellum. In doing this, there will be some hæmorrhage, which may be restrained by the application of ligatures. Having reached the fissure of Bichat, the posterior border of the corpus callosum, together with that portion of the fornix incorporated with it, must be divided in the mesial line from before backward, and held asunder by retractors. The velum interpositum is now exposed; it must be divided in the same direction. Hæmorrhage to some extent will be the result, which may be arrested by the application of cold water. The venæ Galleni, which carry blood from the plexus choroides to the straight sinus, are inclosed in a duplicature, divided from the velum interpositum, and cannot escape being derived. The tubercula quadragemina are now brought into view. A small pale, yellowish-red body will be seen anteriorly resting against the nates, connected to the optic thalami at the sides, and placed just above the iter a tertio ad quartum ventriculum; this is the Pineal gland or ganglion. It will be perceived in the latter part of the dissection described, which is very difficult to perform, in consequence of the oozing of blood, that every time the point of the knife goes into the neighborhood of the gland, the sheep plunges.

The gland being now open to observation, you gently seize its body with the forceps, extending the points towards, or nearly as far as its attachment to the thalami. Oscillations of the iris will be at once the effect. Move the gland more freely, and the pupil will contract to a very small diameter in an instant. Still further press the gland, and make traction, and the eyeball will move rapidly in all directions.

Here let me anticipate a question that may be asked, namely: How do you know but the fourth nerve, which goes to the superior oblique muscle, and the sixth, which is distributed to the external rectus, is not engaged in these movements of the eyeball?

My answer is, it would be all nonsense to suppose so, inasmuch as the fourth nerve arises by three filaments from the valve of Vieussens, and the sixth from the superior extremities of the pyramidal bodies, and are several leagues distant, figuratively speaking, from the Pineal gland, and have no connection with the lenticular ganglion.

Make more firm pressure and traction, and the sheep will vomit and be thrown into a tetanic spasm; the neck will be curved, the legs thrust violently forward, every muscle in the body will appear to be engaged, and you will hear the by-standers exclaim, "You have killed the sheep!" The forceps being now relaxed, the sheep will shortly recover, and you can go through the same process. Sometimes, instead of the vomiting, the sheep will bleat most pitifully, and then be thrown into the tetanic spasm. Press the gland down towards its attachment, and you will observe the pupil to dilate.

Another way may be taken to expose the gland, which consists in separating the hemispheres of the cerebrum, slicing off the lobes on a level with the corpus callosum; in doing which it is probable a small opening may be made into the lateral ventricles, which will be soon known to have taken place by the sheep commencing to snore, in consequence of the blood passing into the ventricles and compressing the gland. The corpus callosum is next to be reflected back. The anterior pillars of the fornix are next to be detached and thrown back as far as possible, which is rather difficult, in consequence of its connection posteriorly with the corpus callosum.

The clot of blood being removed, the gland will present itself, and the sheep will breathe naturally. The brain may be cut in all directions and freely removed, without apparently producing the slightest effect on the sheep. It may be pressed on with same indications. Not a single vessel will be observed to give blood *per saltum*, notwithstanding the deepness of the incisions; and the animal suffers no pain so long as the gland, or the part of the brain the gland is attached to, is not interfered with.

Having now described the operations as performed by Dr. Busteed, I will proceed to state the result of the experiments:

First Sheep.—After exposing the brain, Dr. Busteed passed in a very fine needle, with a view of piercing the gland; the sheep was instantly attacked with violent convulsions, which continued until the butcher cut the sheep's throat. The brain was now removed, and the needle was found to have passed through the peduncle of the gland.

Second Sheep.—After exposing the gland, compression produced dilatation of the pupil and tetanic spasm, when the sheep's throat was cut.

Third Sheep.—Hæmorrhage rendered the operation unsatisfactory.

Fourth and fifth Sheep.—Contraction, dilatation, rolling of the eyeballs, and tetanic spasms.

Sixth Sheep.—Similar results, together with vomiting, on the gland being drawn from its attachment, which was instantly followed by tetanic spasm and death of the sheep.

Seventh and eighth Sheep.—Contraction and dilatation of pupil; rolling of the eyeballs. Pressure with traction caused the sheep to bleat most pitifully, as if suffering extreme torture, followed by tetanic spasms. In these two cases the experiment was performed in the manner secondly described, and the sheep were observed to commence snoring. After the hemispheres of the brain were removed in both cases, the bodies of the lateral ventricles were slightly opened, allowing the blood to flow in. On removing the fornix and the clot of blood, the sheep breathed naturally. Supposing the seventh sheep had died in the tetanic spasm, the butcher cut off the head, when the body of the sheep plunged violently, and life was not extinct for about three minutes.

Ninth Sheep.—Contraction and dilatation of pupil, rolling of the eyeballs, tetanic spasms, and death. Here let me observe, the bleating of the sheep was caused by the irritation propagated through the recurrent branch of the par vagum, to the organic nerves in the larynx, derived from the superior cervical ganglion. .

' I will now endeavor to demonstrate that the great Sir Charles Bell did not thoroughly understand the use of the spinal nerves. I will quote Sir Charles's remarks. He says: "On laying bare the roots of the spinal nerves, I found that I could cut across the posterior fasciculus of nerves, which took its origin from the posterior portion of the spinal marrow, without convulsing the muscles of the back; but that on touching the anterior fasciculus with the point of the knife, the muscles of the back were immediately convulsed."

Here let me remark, the anterior and posterior roots of the spinal nerves, as Mr. Grainger has beautifully shown, receive filaments from the pre-vertebral ganglia, and consequently the anterior roots of the spinal nerves could not be irritated without touching the filaments of the ganglia, thus showing the fallacy of the experiment.

The spinal nerves are messengers, instituted to carry instructions relative to sensation and motion, from the nervous centre of animal life to the nerves of organic life, situated at remote parts of the body.

If all the muscles in the body can be thrown into spasmodic action by irritating one ganglion in the brain, it follows, as a consequence, that the spinal nerves are not actually required for that purpose.

Comparative anatomy shows that the spinal nerves are not essentially required for the movement of the muscles. The invertebrata have no spinal chord or spinal nerves; yet the snail slowly winds his way with his domicile on his back, and if he happen to be decapitated during his perambulations, he is not much discomfited, but will soon reappear with a new head. The little busy ant moves with astonishing rapidity and enjoys good visual organs, thus showing the perfection of its nervous system. I cannot help remarking, it would take an admirable anatomist to prepare the retina of the ant for demonstration; as well as a powerful microscope to bring into view the foramen of Sœmmering. I am induced to make these remarks to show persons, who will not believe anything unless revealed by the microscope, that nerves exist where they are not able to discover them.

Dr. Hall states the real objects of his researches as follows:

First.—To separate the reflex actions from any movements resulting from sensation and volition.

Secondly.—To trace these actions to an acknowledged source, or principle of action in the animal economy—the vis nervosa of Haller acting according to newly-discovered laws.

Thirdly.—To limit these actions to the true spinal marrow, with its appropriate incident and reflex nerves, exclusively of the cerebral and ganglionic systems.

Fourthly.—To apply the principle of action involved in these facts to physiology, viz.: to the physiology of all the acts of exclusion, of ingestion, of retention, and of expulsion in the animal frame.

Fifthly.—To trace this principle of action in its relation to pathology, viz.: to the pathology of the entire class of spasmodic diseases. And,

Sixthly.—To show its relation to therapeutics, especially to the action of certain remedial, and certain deleterious physical agents

Finally.—To these objects, taken together as a whole, or as a system, that I prefer my claim, and I do not pretend that an occasional remark may not have been incidentally made by some previous writer bearing upon some one or other of them.

It does not come within my province to discuss whether Prochaska, Payne, Hall, or Campbell is entitled to the honor of the discovery alluded to by Marshall Hall; but I affirm, inasmuch as spasm of the muscles can be induced by irritating the Pineal gland, or central ganglion, that the discovery, no matter who claims it, is shaken to its very foundation, and thrown completely in the background, inasmuch as a large mountain, called the Pons Varolii, separates the Pineal gland from the medulla oblongata. It is not, therefore, necessary to prove that Marshall Hall arrived at false deductions, having drawn them from false premises.

Dr. Brown-Séquard has shown that certain parts of the body are susceptible of producing epileptic attacks on being irritated; and has demonstrated the fact by tickling a monkey under the angle of the eye, and thus inducing epilepsy. Here let me remark, that monkeys are prone to very vicious habits, and are continually practicing masturbation—thus rendering their organic nervous system in the highest degree excitable, and prone to epileptic seizures. Every person knows that tickling the soles of the feet will produce convulsive attacks; and if continued, will end in death. The phenomena just enumerated are considered the result of reflex action, and excitation of excito-motor, or incidental nerves.

It is a certain fact that the application of belladonna to the eyelids causes dilatation of the pupil; it is equally true that the iris is furnished exclusively with nerves from the lenticular ganglion.   How can the matter be accounted for by the explanation of either Brown-Séquard or Marshall Hall?   I would answer, it cannot.   What occurs is this—the belladonna exercises a sedative action on the organic nerves in the skin, which inosculate with the nasal branch of the fifth pair; and is conveyed by the latter to the brain central ganglion, and by reflex action from the ganglion to the brain, fifth nerve, ophthalmic division of the fifth, nasal branch of the latter, and lenticular ganglion by its communicating branch, and thence to the ciliary nerves that go to the iris.   This is a most beautiful illustration of reflex action according to my theory, and solves a difficulty that I believe no man has satisfactorily done before.

When a young lady is spoken to about her lover, she instantly blushes.   How is this to be accounted for?   The mind communicates with the central ganglion, the latter by reflex action through the brain and facial nerve to the organic nerves in the face, with which its branches inosculate.   This may be said to be a fanciful theory; but does not the stomach blush during the process of digestion?   Is it not supplied by branches from the solar plexus which inosculate with the branches of the par vagum?   Here I must state, it appears from the experiments of Bernard, as well as the examples just given, that the blood becomes oxygenized whenever the animal and organic nerves are acting in conjunction, and confirms the doctrine I advanced on a former occasion, that the fœtal blood was arterialized by nervous influence in the placental lobule.   Marshall Hall gives us an example of reflex action: the grasping of the ovary by the fimbriated extremity of the Fallopian tube during impregnation.   The fœtus of the kangaroo, after leaving the uterus, becomes attached to the nipple of the dam. The infant, after being born, seizes the nipple of the mother in its mouth. Are not these examples analogous to the one pointed out by Marshall Hall?   I think they are, and at the same time think it would be a very difficult thing to demonstrate nerves passing from the lips of the fœtus to the true spinal marrow of the dam in the one case, or the lips of the infant to the mother in the other.   How can these things be explained?   The answer is—by vital action.   What is vital action? It is an intelligent power, inherent in and emanating from the organic nervous system.   It is the breath of life, which, when blown out, terminates man's earthly career, and leaves him an inanimate mass—such as he was when God made him out of the slime of the earth. It is what is generally known as instinct. How can this be proved? By recollecting the part the lenticular ganglion plays in the regulation of the movements of the iris, and the otic in the tensor tympani muscle, as I have already described in my former paper.

I am satisfied many persons will deem me very presumptuous for controverting the opinions of Marshall Hall; but my aim being truth, I am regardless of criticism. "*Magna est veritas et prevalebit.*"

I think I have sufficiently elucidated my theory to enable any person to understand the pathology of catalepsy, chorea, paralysis agitans, spasm of the glottis, convulsions from dentition, spasmodic asthma, sea-sickness, and other diseases too numerous to specify.

When persons are exposed to the vapors of certain gases they are said to die of apnœa, from $a = non$, $\pi\nu\epsilon\omega = spiro$; which translated means, in popular language, "shortness of breath," or asphyxia, from $a = non$, $\sigma\phi\upsilon\xi\eta = pulsus$, which may be literally translated, the stroke of death. What causes death under such circumstances? The blood becomes charged with carbonic acid, and acts as a poison on the organic ganglia, which are thus rendered powerless in their function of causing the muscles to contract; hence it is the heart immediately ceases to pulsate, and the consequent death of the individual.

The mode in which arsenic, tartar-emetic, tobacco, and other poisons destroy life, is by their destructive influence on the organic nervous system.

As some may suppose I am stating things not called for in an article of this kind, I will conclude by observing, the experiments detailed were performed by Dr. Busteed in presence of Dr. Gallagher, Mr. Roderigal, myself, and several other persons. I have further to remark, that I will leave it to others to decide whether I have made a discovery or not, with respect to the anatomy and physiology of the placenta, or the connection of the nervous centres of animal and organic life.

If I have appropriated the offspring of any other man's brain to myself, I candidly acknowledge I have done so in blissful ignorance of the name of the author; and will make a suitable acknowledgment on being apprised of the name of the individual, and where his work is to be found.

If my former communications commanded no attention, I attribute it to my not being known as a teacher, or being connected either with a college, a hospital, or any other public institution. I do not feel

32

surprised, being thus circumstanced, that many should think I could
have no knowledge of the subjects I attempted to elucidate. Everybody knows a professor is looked upon as being something extraordinary, and that it may be said of him—

> " Ard still they gazed, and still the wonder grew,
>   That one small head should carry all he knew !"

230 FOURTH STREET, WASHINGTON SQUARE,
      June, 1859.

NOTE.—The following extract, taken from the third volume of the
Cyclopædia of Anatomy and Physiology: Article, Nervous Centres,
by R. B. Todd, is worthy of attentive perusal, as showing the *important connections* of the ganglion, as well as the opinion entertained of
its use by Des Cartes, who, it is almost unnecessary to state, considered the gland the seat of the soul, without being able to demonstrate
the fact, or show any connection between *it* and the other ganglia.
And here let me state, that this latter observation I believe to be true
of every writer since Des Cartes wrote his work; and that my discovery consists in showing the Pineal gland is the chief ganglion, and that
it is connected with all the other ganglia, and presides over them.

" PINEAL GLAND.—We may here conveniently notice the position
and connection of the *Pineal gland*. This body, rendered famous by
the vague theory of Des Cartes, who viewed it as the chief source of
nervous power, is placed just behind the third ventricle, resting in a
superficial groove, which passes along the median line between the corpora quadrigemina. It is heart-shaped, and of a gray color. Its apex
is directed backward and downward, and its base forward and upward. A process of the deep layer of the velum interpositum envel-
ops it, and serves to retain it in its place. From each angle of its
base there passes off a *band* of *white matter*, which adheres to the inner
surface of each optic thalamus. These processes serve to connect the
Pineal body to the optic thalami. They are called *the peduncles of the
Pineal gland*, also *habenæ*. In general they are *two* in number, one for
each optic thalamus. They may be traced forward as far as the *anterior pillars* of the *fornix*. Posteriorly these processes are connected
along the *median line* by *some white fibres* which adhere to *the base* of
the *Pineal gland*, as well as to the *posterior commissure* beneath, and
which seem *to form part* of the *system* of *fibres* belonging to that commissure. *A pair* of *small bands* sometimes pass off from these fibres,
along the optic thalami, parallel to the peduncles above *described*."

SELECTIONS.

Medical Society of the State of Michigan.
President's Address,

By J. A. ALLEN, M.D., of Kalamazoo.

Gentlemen of the State Medical Society—Much has been accomplished by the Medical Profession within a few years past. It is, perhaps, safe to say that within the last quarter of a century it has been revolutionized. Old things have passed away, and all things have become new. Not that twenty-five years ago the profession were all wrong, or even in the greater part. Truth twenty-five years ago was as true as now, and will be unchangeable in all time to come. But truth is Janus-faced, and wears quite opposite appearances to different beholders. The pair of eyes which look out upon it have quite as much to do with its import, as the thing itself. And thus we repeat, the profession, entertaining and receiving similar truths, has been revolutionized within a moderate term of years. The "Pilate-question," what is Truth, has been differently solved, and, as we are happy to believe, more in accordance with the great plan which it is the true mission of the scholar, whatever his sphere of investigation, to unfold.

Under the leadings of this revolution, medicine has emerged from the domain of occult arts, has thrown off the trappings and paraphernalia of an ignoble mysticism, has forborne to claim special privileges not conceded to all other arts and sciences, has substituted the *savan* for the seventh son of a seventh son, the calm, philosophic student for the loud-voiced quack, and now treads the straight highway of all knowledge, unallured by the by-ways of dishonest assumption, untempted by the shallow successes which ever befall the shallow pretender, who still rises highest in vulgar estimation, as the bubble glows brightest at the very point of utter collapse. It is a noticeable fact, that there is now less apparent effort on the part of the profession to convince the world that it ought to be respected, than there was even ten or five years ago, simply because the profession has become *intrinsically more respectable.* Legislatures are no longer besieged by anxious petitioners for legal barriers to be thrown up against medical Philistines or Galileans. So far as respectability is concerned, and competency to wage successful internecine warfare with all the hordes of quackdom, though baptized with whatsoever German or Anglo-Greek patronymics, the profession as a body feels amply prepared to take care of itself.

At the present moment, there is not a phase of spurious medical practice, whatever its pet denomination, be it Thomsonism, Homœopathy, Hydropathy, Indian or self-styled Eclectic, but " has touched the full meridian of its glory, and hastes now to its setting."

And their decline is traceable not to the furious onslaughts made upon them by indignant disciples of the true God of Medicine, but from the inherent seeds of decay derived by hereditary transmission from their Egyptian prototypes, who wrought divers wonders by their enchantments, but whose rods were finally devoured by that of Aaron.

It is worth remembering that it was not the noise of the rams' horns which caused the walls of Jericho to crumble into ruin, although it is very likely the blowers thought they were entitled to lasting credit for their extraordinary exertions.

It is Truth which gives vitality, and power, and victory, and immortality. Our endless clamoring about it half the time does little more than to throw suspicion that we do not half believe in it ourselves.

For a moment let us glance at what has been done by the medical fraternity within a period which our own recollection comprehends.

Anatomy, which a few years ago was scarcely more than a dry catalogue of names and localities of parts of greater or less magnitude, subservient mainly to the mechanical uses of the surgeon, has expanded to the proportions of a philosophic science, necessitating the possession of the entire organic creation as its stupendous lexicon. In fact, human anatomy, without combination of comparative anatomy, compares in interest, importance and instruction, about as the Cadmian alphabet does to the works of Milton or Shakspeare. The one scarcely reaches higher upon the mental faculties than memory, their lowest servitor; the other calls upon the highest powers of the understanding and reason. Physiology was but little known, and even in the best appointed medical colleges was dismissed with a few discursive remarks, and those mainly upon the laws of optics, acoustics and mechanics, but it has now merged in itself Histology, with all its intricate and manifold manifestations among all things, whether animate or inanimate, upon which the law of change is written. It has followed close in the wake of every organic motion, whether sensible or insensible, and diligently sought the *how* and the *wherefore*. It has simplified and harmonized apparently complex and contradictory phenomena, bringing them out from under the sway of occult demoniac vital forces, and arranging them with other orderly phenomena of the physical universe. It has assiduously separated the explicable from the temporarily inexplicable; and even with reference to the latter, dares to investigate *how* results are brought about, though it may not as yet determine satisfactorily *why*.

As its latest and crowning triumph, it has pointed out clearly and unmistakably the simple, but exquisitely beautiful, mechanism by which the different parts of the living body are reciprocally affected by their respective changes; nay, more, undaunted by the traditional mystery which shrouded " the silver shining cords," it has unraveled their web, and now treads the before-time labyrinth as fearlessly as Theseus, by the aid of the clue of Ariadne, trod the one of antiquity. There is now no more of mystery about the mode of action of the nervous system, than there is about the telegraph or steam-engine.

We need not hesitate to assert that Chemistry and the other sciences collateral to medicine, such as Microscopy and Natural History, owe their present proud position more to the investigations and studies of medical men, than to those of any or all other classes.

Meantime, the practical branches, including the diagnosis and treatment of external and internal diseases, bringing to bear upon them all forces capable of modifying the whole body or its parts, whether by the mild influences of air and moisture, food, exercise and sleep, or the potential agency of direct medication, or the still more striking (because presented fully to the eye even of the inexpert) achievements of the surgeon, have kept even step with the progress of the abstract and more or less recondite sciences.

Statistics and details are before the world to prove what we assert, and we challenge contradiction.

The per centage of cures or relief, by means of medical and surgical appliances at the present time, so remarkably exceeds that of former years, that even a proportion of our own profession half incline to the belief that either diseases or the constitution of men have changed for the better. Brief departure into the line of the old methods, or more satisfactorily still, neglect of any, or reliance upon inert treatment, however, will soon demonstrate, to the thinking man, the error of this idea.

The average duration of human life, thus wonderfully increased, is now recognized as a new element in the calculations and reasonings of the political economist and the statesman. It is to some persons a surprising fact that this increase in the duration of human life, owing entirely to the improved methods and resources of our profession, would be sufficient of itself to keep up the ratio of our national increase, and consequent diffusion over the now uncultivated territories of our domain, were the immense foreign emigration now pouring in upon us utterly to cease. Truly this is something which should command the attention of all who desire the prosperity of our common country.

It was not, therefore, mere favoritism or special legislation for the benefit, personally, of a particular class, which determined the establishment of our own State Medical College, with all its ample facilities for acquiring a knowledge of the noble art and Godlike science of medicine. It is not for merely personal objects that this organization takes upon itself its responsibilities, and proposes to itself its manifold duties. This association was not organized, nor does it continue its labors, that Drs. A, B, and C may be elevated to notoriety, or that sundry sordid objects may be accomplished. It has a wider scope—a profounder design. It looks to triumphs upon a grander scale over disease and death, the common enemies of the race. It looks to large additions to the term of human years, to sounder bodies, and consequently sounder minds, among the whole people, and concurrently with these the growth and enrichment of the State. It seeks to preserve as long as possible the "old men for counsel and the young men for war."

Medical men, in common with all scientific investigators, recognize at the present time more than ever before, that inquiries with reference to physical laws, in order to give results of any noteworthy magnitude, must take a wider and more comprehensive range than can be attempted by any single, although it be a master mind. The time has gone by when it is believed by any considerable number that, to use Lord Bacon's expressive simile, the great truths of nature can be wrought out from one's own cogitations, as the spider weaves its web from its own entrails. As the real laws which govern the apparently eccentric phenomena of nature, such as the winds, the hurricanes, the fall of rains, explosion of meteors, earthquakes, &c., can only be determined by widely-extended observations, girdling and investing the entire planet, thus do we believe that disturbances of Plato's microcosm, which occur apparently so disorderly as to justify the old mythologies attributing them to the wrath of offended deities, are nevertheless under the orderly control of laws, discoverable by continuous observations over all the continents, and islands, and seas.

Nequaquan nos homines sumus, sed partes hominis: exomnibus aliquid fieri potest, idque non magnum—ex singulis fere nihil. Thus wrote Sca liger long since, and the centuries cannot contradict it. The greatest of minds accomplishes "almost nothing" single-handed, but by union *something* can be done. Indeed, we are scarcely men unless we unite our efforts to those of others—we are but disjointed fragments. There remains much to be done, and your speaker would scarcely do justice to the position he occupies through your unmerited kindness, did he not venture a few suggestions, which occur to him as appropriate.

The order of remark is scarcely material, and circumstances compel me to be somewhat rambling and discursive. The profession should combine to secure periodical and complete reports of the three principal epochs in every person's history, viz.: birth, marriage, and death. Without this clue, there can be no rational comparison of the relative salubrity of different districts of country, nor any accurate data upon which to found one of the most important problems of political economy, namely: given a certain population in a particular district, how long before it will be doubled or reduced to a moiety? a question involving the very highest interests of the commonwealth.

A registration of births and deaths, combined with periodical reports from the various *entrepôts* of immigration, would furnish a reliable, constant census. I need not here speak of its advantages in a merely civil point of view—inheritances and the like; but, considered only in a professional light, it would tend to the elucidation of a vast number of unexpected truths.

The causes of death ought in every case to be recorded. I am aware that many have ridiculed this feature, because reports of this kind are frequently made by uneducated professional or non-professional persons, and hence are often erroneous. But this difficulty is of very little comparative importance. The mathematicians are in possession of adroit methods of calculating the elements of error, so as to approximate an absolutely correct result—and this is a process easily initiated in the case before us—the elements of error are apparent. Such a registration would give a good idea of the prevalence of particular diseases in particular districts, and would ensue in discovery of the causes of their choice of locality; in other words, the general law of their fixation or movements would be eliminated. The "essential relation" would eventually be ferreted out, and not improbably the local scourge be banished, or rendered comparatively innocuous.

In order to this result, the State Geologist should give us an accurate acquaintance with the physical characteristics of all parts of our peninsulas. All the appliances of art and science to ascertain the meteorological peculiarities would speedily be brought into requisition; and, as Lieut. Maury would have us follow up the track of the winds, and vapors, and storms, laden with thermometers, barometers, thygrometers, *et id genus omne,* so would the medical profession follow up the trail of disease. Systematic, comprehensive action is what is needed. If the medical profession throughout the United States were organized as are their brethren in the army and navy, and every case treated, whether resulting in recovery or death, duly reported to some central bureau, there to be subjected to analysis and scientific examination, under all the light which modern science is capable of throwing upon them, we do not doubt that within five or ten years medicine would take such a prodigious stride in advance, that the undertakers throughout the land would stand aghast, fearing lest, like Othello, they may find their "occupation gone."

But this cannot be done, and we need not delay upon it. But registration as the duty of civil officials is feasible, and we ought earnestly to urge it upon those we have chosen to make and unmake our laws.

As citizens of the State, we believe such a registration would show Michigan to stand in the very front rank for salubrity and longevity. We all know that the great tide of emigration has gone by us for a few years past, mainly from the impression assiduously propagated by interested parties, that this State is less healthy than some of her compeers at the West.

This error a faithful registration would speedily dispel, and the augmented population and wealth which would then throng upon us to improve our matchless resources, our soil of unsurpassable fertility, and inexhaustible store of mineral and forest riches, would quickly repay thousand-fold the trivial expense involved.

Incidental to this subject, permit me to say a few words with reference to epidemics. We need a careful chronicle of their visits and peculiarities from every part of the State. Isolated reports are comparatively valueless.

What Dr. So-and-So saw, or thought he saw; what wonder-working charms he carried in his dilapidated saddle-bags; how many he cured or dismissed to the Superior or nether regions, although facts very interesting to Dr. So-and-So and his committee of old ladies, are, in a scientific point of view, hardly worth the paper on which he communicates them to the popular medical or secular paper, according as he believes or *dis*believes in the code of ethics.

It will not do, in this age of the world, to frame opinions or shape practice upon any such cobweb fancies as these. Some, or all of us, have learned, to our cost, that it is not princes only to whom we should not confide our faith.

For be assured, that as certainly as the solid earth sustains our mortal bodies, so certainly are we fashioned and vitalized, kept in orderly health or racked by disorderly disease, alike by the controlling power of harmoniously operating laws, which it is our province and mission to disclose. Some years since, in connection with two distinguished medical gentlemen, I had the honor of serving upon a committee of the National Medical Association, whose duty it was to report upon the epidemics of a large section of the Northwest. Accordingly, we issued a vast number of circulars in the usual form, calling upon the profession to contribute reports to the committee, promising ample public acknowledgments for all favors received. What was the result? In reply to something over six hundred circulars, addressed by myself alone—at least two hundred of which contained a special request, *in writing*, that the person receiving it should reply in particulars—there were exactly *six* epistles of greater or less latitude or longitude received. Less than one per cent.

I need scarcely say that the thing was an entire failure. But it has been paralleled again and again, and will find successors every time the experiment is tried.

The difficulty and the remedy are alike obvious. That large class of practitioners who are in active and successful business have, or think they have, little or no time for writing out their observations and experience. To be worth anything, such reports should be full and explicit, clear and methodical. He whose duty it becomes to collate them, ought not to be obliged to stumble and wade continually, but be permitted to launch boldly upon a clear sea. To accomplish this object, then, let us have another sort of circulars issued, with definite printed interrogatories, with blank spaces for replies. The questions should be carefully digested, as few as possible, and admitting replies brief and succinct. It would be scarcely more trouble for a physician, however extensive his practice, to fill out and return one of these methodical reports, than to make out the papers in a single policy of life insurance. We should thus in a short space of time have material for analysis and study, which could not fail to

throw a flood of light upon the nature, and, consequently, the prophylaxis and treatment of epidemics.

Such blanks might be furnished by this or other local medical societies, and each of its members be required to report them to the society
as often as deemed expedient. Here is something tangible and practicable, and I beg leave respectfully to submit to your honorable body
whether it be not best at this meeting to take the initiative in the
matter. The blanks once filled up, should be referred to a competent
bureau, or committee, whose duty it should be to collate all the facts
presented, carefully abstaining from interlarding with vain speculations or vicious theories, which may be permitted to infest their own
minds, but not allowed to vitiate the sources of knowledge.

Whether the chemists are right in creating and renewing body and
spirit by the retort, the spirit-lamp and test-tube; or whether Prof.
Paine be engaged in a laudable undertaking in moving the world
back five hundred years, and attempting to galvanize into needless
resurrection the fossil theories and fanciful dreams of olden times, are
questions which ought not to find a place in reports of the kind contemplated. Let us sow our inquiries broadcast over the peninsula;
then shall there be returned to us plentiful harvests of truth and
knowledge.

It need scarcely be observed, that a similar method may be adopted
in procuring information in every department of medical inquiry. To
obtain general replies, we must make the facilities for answering less
a tax upon the time and labor of our overworked brethren, than the
discourtesy of not answering would be upon their proverbial sensibili-
ties. A thousand will answer yes or no, where one would sit down
and write an elaborate essay.

Facts standing isolated are little better than fictions. Systems
based upon them are more deleterious to human advancement than
even those of Stahl and Paine, which rest upon no foundation save
the figments of seething brains. The latter are but unreal, and
therefore harmless, visions; while the former, having something of the
substance of truth in them, are prolific of mischievous results.

It does not, as some have seemed to suppose, require the highest
order of intellect to secure the largest proportion of " the clear and
warrantable body of truth." It does not require even any very superior talent of memory—that worst abused, because least understood,
of all our faculties. There are those who would overawe our imagin-
ations by stupendous display of this mechanical faculty. Their minds

reflect back upon us the images that strike their surface, *absorbing none*, as the pool or the creek returns the rays from overhanging or passing objects. If they write books, words and phrases plentifully abound, but wide and comprehensive thought, far-reaching investigations and profound reflections, are absent. The truth is, " *order is* Heaven's first law," " in fact as well as in verse," and a heterogeneous conglomerate, " dry rubbish shot here," though it fill whole encyclopædias, is as far from true knowledge as midnight from noon. Hence we must have systems, classifications, tabulations, and exact and comprehensive methods.

Without these, we can do nothing worth our while. Traditional experiences; authors, new or old, " with margins crammed with citations " of other authors, be they new or old; even the scattered and flickering rays of our own farthing candles, however assiduously trimmed, will do but little to illumine the thick darkness which ever surrounds us. We must bring each our little store to the common centre, so that the hillock shall become a mountain, the water-drops flow together into rivers and seas, and the farthing candles become a pillar of fire in our van.

At the present time it has become more indispensable than ever before that the physician should be thoroughly educated—educated not only in the special branches directly subservient to general practice, but in that wider sense which involves a more or less intimate acquaintance with all the departments of general science and literature. We can thoroughly understand no single branch of study, unless we ascend to the level of all sciences.

Especially in medicine, where the range of inquiry is so expanded and various that no man can extend the boundaries of knowledge in any direction, but what the medical man will be directly profited by its occupancy.

The subject of medical education has therefore very appropriately attracted much of the attention of the profession. To maintain the invincibility even of the " Old Guard," great care must be taken with the recruits. Practically, it would be desirable that no young man should be encouraged to enter upon the study of medicine until his mind has been matured, his perceptions vivified, and all his faculties developed and disciplined by an enlarged and liberal scope of preliminary studies. It is indisputable that a great number enter upon this study too little matured by years, and *less* qualified by previous instruction. This arises from the notion that the art, and a sufficient quantity of the science for practice, can be gained without that exact and generous education which other learned professions require. And this, to a certain extent, is true. A certain readiness in concocting pills and horrible mixtures, and a certain fluency in the use of elongated technicalities, is readily acquired, and the neophyte may easily convince a confiding community that he is amply qualified for the high duties of warding off or relieving disease. The daily bread is thus procured with facility, and, alas! too often, both physician and patients believe that this is enough—that this is all.

But not this, is our idea of the true physician. It is perhaps impossible at once to raise the standard to its proper height, but it is incumbent upon this Society, in its own sphere of action, to aid and assist those whom the State have especially intrusted with medical teaching, in an effort to come up at least to the standard which the Regents of the University seemed disposed to fix. We know the difficulties that surround this subject practically at the Medical College, and know that it is not a step to be hastily taken; but we honestly believe that it would be far better for the profession and the State, could a high grade of preliminary attainment be insisted upon before matriculation.

It is but an act of simple justice to say that none are more anxious to establish this rule than the learned gentlemen of the Medical Faculty at Ann Arbor. They recognize its importance, but as practical men they also know that its enforcement would ruin their institution, as it would any other of the kind from Maine to Louisiana. The course adopted, requiring respectable academical attainments prior to actual graduation, is so far a good one, but it has this disadvantage— it does not reach all those who ultimately go out from the institution as practitioners. A large proportion of the students at Ann Arbor never finally graduate; they go abroad with the prestige of having attended medical lectures at the State University; the community suppose their graduation a matter of course, and hence the Medical College shares alike in the honors or discredit which may attend their future career. We of the State Medical Society ought to do our part to put an end to the difficulty at once, by sustaining such a public opinion as will justify the Faculty in coming up to the desirable requirement, even though it materially diminish the number in attendance upon the lecture-rooms of the Medical Department of the University.

Beyond this, we ought not to receive into our offices as private students those not thus qualified—this will strike at the root of the matter.

The profession is already full, too full, even of those having tolerable acquirements. It is an easy achievement to don the M.D. The art of medicine is, in some respects, like the art of music—there are hosts of *fiddlers*, few thorough artists. The popular ear is easier tickled by a "plantation melody" than by the divine strains of some grand oratorio. And thus, practically, so far as mere popularity is concerned, and success in securing many calls and plentiful dollars, it is about as well to know little as to know much about the real pith and marrow of the science; in fact, a liberal degree of ignorance is more likely to give that noisy boldness or oracular self-sufficiency, which especially attract the applause of the multitude.

But this kind of success, according to my understanding of the matter, is not what this Society seeks to promote. We seek to increase the grand total of knowledge; to advance the interests of society at large, by informing the minds of those to whom the public health is committed. The task is a public one, and panders to no private success or failures. Among the means to be employed there is scarcely any which offers higher opportunities for discovery and improvement than close, exact, comprehensive—in fine, *educated* observation at the bedside of patients. It is here where the master-spirit is recognized by those capable of appreciating him. Others may glitter upon the printed page, or attract admiring crowds to the display of their wisdom upon the street corners or lounging-places of the town, but the leading spirit of the *clinique* is their sovereign and our sovereign. The galloping mode of medical instruction, which poverty of students, with the commingled poverty and rivalry of the colleges, have introduced, must be superseded by better methods. We hesitate not to assert, both from personal observation and the concurrent testimony of men best qualified to judge, that the prevailing mode of teaching in medical colleges is vicious and defective in the extreme. It takes students years to unlearn the radical errors which they have received, even from instructors of the highest rank in the lecture-room. And this, perhaps, not so much from the fault of the lecturer, as from the nature of the subject. It is about as difficult to convey to a student by oral instruction any definite ideas of particular diseases, as it is to explain colors to a blind man or sounds to the deaf. It cannot be done. And yet the task is attempted, year after year, with most solemn persistency, and ludicrous results. The lecturing Sisy-

phus rolls the stone almost up to the sight of his disciple, but before
the disciple can grasp it, away it rolls to the bottom of the declivity,
whilst the pupil sits in nebulous gloom far up the amphitheatre, obliv-
iously waiting his turn at the stone he has never yet seen.

The long lecture term, with its immeasurable expenditure of breath
and brains, is but the lengthened shadow of the clinic. It is the clinic
only which is the truly substantial part—the lecture ought to be but
an incident of darkness not yet dispelled. Perhaps it is still urged,
as the daguerreotypists, that useful class of our fellow-citizens, urge
upon their handbills: "Secure the shadow ere the substance flies!"
Happy is it if the lecturer's descriptions approximate their objects as
closely as the daguerreotype, with its moveless surface, approaches
the human form divine, with all its wealth of curiously wrought
mechanism, and living soul within. The like is not seen in any other
branch of science. In this science of medicine, where minute, absolutely indescribable differences utterly reverse all appliances, the student is sent upon a sea he has never sailed, upon decks he never trod
before, to lands he never saw, to races whose language he knows not,
with a cargo whose value he is ignorant of, to be blamed or applauded
for subsequent failure or success.

The lecture should, so far as possible, be upon the case then and
there presented. In this lies the only safety of physician and patient,
and medical colleges should be estimated accordingly as they afford
this true method of teaching. We grant that lectures could not be as
discursive, perhaps not as eloquent, but more truth would be imparted,
and imparted in such a way as not to involve error as its consequence.
The careful study of a single case is worth more to a medical student
than the memory of most medical volumes; for in that single case will
be found wrapped all the great problems of the science and the art.
Power to solve these will bestow power to solve others. What to
observe, and how to observe, and then what is the meaning of these
indications? These are the great questions, and the student who faithfully seeks solution of these will succeed.

But not to enlarge, it will be seen that we believe the present time
is competent to afford a better mode of teaching than prevailed a
quarter of a century since. And this we believe to be possible by
elevating the clinic to the highest place in the schedule.

Locate your college upon and around the clinic, if you would have
it rest upon any other than a sandy foundation. Upon that rock you
may build as high, and spread as wide as inclination and finances will

permit; but if anything must go, spare the clinic and amputate the rest.

But as now constituted, the most of the colleges are playing Hamlet, with the part of the melancholy and philosophic prince excised and left out, and a poor play they make of it. Practically, according to these views, our own medical college ought to be planted upon a large and constant clinic. If that is not to be found where it is now located, let the influence of this Society, and of the profession generally, be brought to bear in its removal to where it may be found. The hospitals and asylums should be thrown open to the student, and all the appliances which progress has brought to light should be brought to aid in his advancement.

The State has wisely done what it would have been simply a disgrace not to have done—founded an Asylum for the deaf and dumb in the city of Flint, and an Asylum for the insane at Kalamazoo. The Asylum at Flint is already prosperously operating, and it is sincerely believed that the present Legislature will provide the means to put the institution at Kalamazoo in successful operation

I am not personally familiar with the workings of the Flint Asylum, but with reference to the one commenced at Kalamazoo I can speak from actual observation. The profession may rest assured that the delay which has attended its construction has been unavoidable. Not a dollar has been wasted, excepting by the accidental conflagration of the central or receiving building. The plan and details of the structure are such as must receive general commendation from those having at heart the welfare of the unfortunate insane.

If the building were this day completed in every part projected, every room would be demanded by patients. In my opinion, both humanity and the honor of the State require that this institution should be put in a state of completion in all its parts and appurtenances, so soon as material and labor can accomplish it. This done, and the superintendency of the highly accomplished and skillful gentleman whom the Trustees have been so fortunate as to secure, will place the Michigan Insane Asylum upon a footing which cannot fail to show results as yet unsurpassed by any institution in this or any other country.

But besides the two classes of patients thus provided for, there is another, which almost equally demands the interest of the profession, and the public care. This class is scattered throughout every part of the State, many of them in the county poor houses, but mostly in the families of persons of scanty means, not yet thrown upon the public bounty, but gradually and surely approaching that finale. Disease and infirmity render them helpless, and poverty prevents them from availing themselves of the means of recovery. Some, it is true, have the care, if such it may be called, which may be extended to them in the county houses; but this Society knows, the profession knows, and the public ought to know, that this is seldom or never of the kind which will afford relief.

The medical skill employed by the several counties is rarely of a high order. The medical attendance is usually sold at auction to the lowest bidder, and hence is most likely to fall into the hands of those whose time and acquirements are of the lowest grade of valuation. But waiving this defect, the surroundings are not conducive to recovery. Experience demonstrates this, and we need scarcely to allude to it. The philanthropist must admit at once that something ought to be done for that unhappy class who are not only poor, but sick and imprisoned in the county houses. In addition to these, a large number who have some means, but not enough to afford the best facilities for cure, require a place where they may be surrounded with everything that the present stage of enlightenment in medical practice affords for relief or cure, and yet upon such moderate terms as to be within their compass.

There are also a large number of transient persons who, when taken sick or injured by accidents, usually fall a prey to boarding-house keepers until their money has disappeared, and then too often die from absolute neglect.

For all these the State Hospital would afford a welcome retreat, and it is not hazardous to say the general cost of their support would be very materially lessened. Aid which now must be constant and permanent, would thus become but temporarily necessary.

By rendering this hospital subservient to the clinical department of the State Medical College, the patients would, while helpless themselves, be made to contribute to the general welfare, proving that "there is a soul of goodness even in things evil," and "from the nettle, danger, can be plucked the flower, safety." This is not hypothesis or visionary: I do not even suggest an experiment; it is a thing already demonstrated. Thus the State Medical College could at once take rank with institutions of the very highest order. The counties and towns would find their large poor rates very materially lessened. A large amount of suffering would be prevented, and cures, otherwise hopeless, be achieved.

For these and other reasons which might be adduced, I venture to commend this subject to your mature consideration, hoping that eventually ways and means may be found to bring about the object so much to be desired. Our duty, as medical men, is by no means restricted to the doling out of pills, or the amputation of offending members. There is a higher sphere than this. It becomes us to consider all things which influence in any manner the perfection of body and mind, and that not only in the narrow individual sense, but also as affecting the interests of communities, of nations, of the world.

It will be seen that I have briefly contemplated several very important subjects. Each of them require notice, and each of them might require longer consideration than possible at this time to give them altogether.

We cannot accomplish everything at once, but we can make a beginning. *Possunt, quia posse videntur*—all things are possible to him who earnestly attempts.

This association, now comprehending in its actual working membership but a limited number of the profession in the State, may readily be converted into one which shall embrace every scientific physician within our borders.

Of these but comparatively few may attend upon our annual meetings, but each will be represented by his contributions. Our various committees will not then be obliged to rely upon their individual resources, but will command the services of every one who honors or wishes well to the profession.

The interests which are involved, and the public character of the objects sought, will require that its transactions have a large and general circulation, beyond what the means to be raised by voluntary contribution or assessment shall reach. And here an honorable example is afforded us—the great State of New York, appreciating the importance of the information thus to be gained and diffused, requires its State Medical Society to report its proceedings to the Legislature, and thus from them it is spread before the people. Most surely there is nothing which more concerns a State than its sanitary condition. A healthy country will attract inhabitants; and, besides this, the inhabitants are ever desirous of knowing what will conduce to the better physical condition of the men, women, and children, as well as the cattle, sheep, and horses. The State promotes agriculture by liberally

33

appropriating moneys to the maintenance of agricultural fairs and the like. It will surely not refuse to advance the great public object that we have in view, by aiding us in diffusing the information which this Society is willing, voluntarily and gratuitously, to collect. The facts collected together, which might be reported under the sanction of the Society, might, perhaps, then be referred to the bureau of the Super-intendent of Public Instruction—a department of the government which already recognizes the importance of other things than com-merce, trade, and the raising of grains. But in whatever way it be done, it will not only strengthen the bonds of this Society, but must inevitably contribute to the higher development of the State in actual material prosperity. It is a matter eminently worthy of your reflec-tion, and it is to be hoped may be carried into effect during the pres-ent meeting.

I am happy to believe, and in that belief to congratulate the Socie-ty, that there is a growing spirit of harmony among the members of the profession; the fraternal feeling which should spring from similar pursuits in life, correspondence of interests and objects of study, has been gradually spreading, so that we hear less and less, year by year, of the dissensions that have been so often charged upon us, as almost characteristic of the profession. Time and reflection have cooled some old asperities, which once agitated the Æsculapian craft. There is engendered a larger spirit of forbearance towards independ-ent thought, and a more catholic toleration of every honest effort in the right direction. Not that any of the manifold varieties of "exclu sive systems" and charlatan practices are looked upon with less disfa-vor by high-minded, scientific, and philosophic practitioners, but be-cause we recognize that medicine is yet comparatively in its embryo condition, and that large liberality must be indulged to those who honestly labor to develop it to maturer proportions. In current phrase, the medical world is not yet finished, painted and ready to be fenced in. As was said in olden time, if one of the brethren do really cast out devils, he need not be blamed because he follow not with us. Dictation now will not be borne by independent medical men. That time has gone by. Truth is neither old nor young, and its possessor is rich indeed, whether his years be a score and a half, or three scores and a half. It is not houses or lands; it is neither years, nor even honors; it is neither form nor deportment which causes one man to differ essentially from his fellow. The real diversity exists in that amount of "the clear and warrantable body of truth" which they respectively possess.

The "code of ethics" cannot prevent innate vulgarity and ignorance from being manifested; it cannot prevent true worth and knowledge from shining with a clear and steady light. In this there is wealth of encouragement to the medical scholars, and to all scholars. True greatness of mind is manifested in rising above mistaken views, even when these are pinned upon the garments of old and venerated doctrines.

During the past year, death has removed several of our number; and here I cannot forbear to refer to one who was particularly zealous and efficient in sustaining this organization—Dr. Lucius G. Robinson, of Detroit—a gentleman of education and refinement, with a mind well stored with scientific principles, ready in expression, whether orally or by writing. Beyond these, his amiable disposition and fine friendly feeling endeared him to all who knew him intimately, and commanded the respect and esteem of those who were less fortunate in this regard. He has passed from our midst in the very flower of his years, just as the profession throughout the Northwest had become familiar with his name, through the *Medical Journal* he founded, and also ably conducted. His seat is vacant here, but his memory will be retained in our hearts as the successful practitioner, the earnest lover of his profession, the firm, fast friend, and Christian gentleman. Dr. Leland, of Detroit, also, has been unexpectedly called from this earthly sphere of action. Of a retiring and unassuming deportment, he was not widely known beyond the immediate circle of his family and field of practice. But wherever known, whether in this Society, of which he was a member, or in the round of his practice, he was highly esteemed and highly appreciated. We may well honor his memory by perpetuating it upon our records, whilst we pay the tribute mourning for his untimely decease.

Gentlemen of the Society, it is in your hands to decide whether this association shall maintain a vigorous and profitable existence, or drag out a feeble continuance to a speedy dissolution.

In my opinion, the former can be secured by enlarging the sphere of action; aspiring to be general and comprehensive, rather than to be local and fragmentary.

The material to work upon is abundant, and it requires but concentration and fixed purpose to place the Michigan State Medical Society upon a par with the most distinguished institution of the kind of this or any other country. I see around me gentlemen with clear heads, well-disciplined minds, acute perceptions, and large attainments. Let us have these laid under severe contribution, that those of us who are favored with less of each may be benefited in the result.

For the honor conferred on me by election to this honorable position, accept my sincerest thanks. From the Profession of the State I have, with but few exceptions, ever received kindlier words and acts than my abilities or services would ever warrant; and I can only tender in return my gratitude, and the pledge never to discontinue effort to render the whole science of medicine more worthy of popular esteem, because based on clearer, more comprehensive, more exact and immutable truths.

[From the Montreal Medical Chronicle.]

THE "DEAD ALIVE."

By R. B. NASON, Esq., M.R.C.S.

Sir—An article, "The Dead Alive," in your January number, demands of me a veritable statement of the case alluded to. The subject of the inquiry is still living, and some time past has afforded me scope for observation.

I have only been waiting for a termination of the case, either in convalescence or death, to enable me to give to the profession, through your valuable columns, a full and truthful history of this rare and curious case, replete with interest. The exaggerated statement which has gone the round of the press has produced such great curiosity in this immediate neighborhood, that I have been applied to by many parties, professional and non-professional, to be permitted to see the case, the parents of the patient having refused admittance to all strangers.

The case having extended over a long period, and fearing a detailed account might occupy too much of your valuable space, I have condensed the matter as much as possible; but should the profession consider the case worthy of a more enlarged history, I will gladly at some future period meet their wishes, as far as my rough notes, aided by my memory, will supply it.

In August, 1858, I was requested to visit Miss Amelia Hinks, aged twelve years and nine months, daughter of a harness-maker, and residing with her parents in Bridge Street, Nuneaton. She was supposed to be suffering from pulmonary consumption. I found her much emaciated, and complaining of headache; great lassitude; loss of appetite; short cough; secretions morbid; catamenia not appeared. I prescribed an alterative, to be taken at night, and a ferruginous tonic three times a day; a generous, though mild, nutritious diet, which she continued some time with benefit. I could not detect any chest disease. She then went into the neighborhood of Leanington, for change, to visit some friends, and after a short stay became much worse. Her parents, being apprised of her state, fetched her home as soon as possible. On her arrival I was requested to see her. I found her very attenuated, and complaining of great debility, headache, and loss of appetite; tongue clean; bowels confined. From this time she began to refuse food and medicine, and friends wished her not to be disturbed for anything, and daily and hourly anticipated her death. She was watched night after night, in anticipation of that event happening, and on the 18th of October, about half past three A. M., she apparently died. She is said to have groaned heavily, waved her hand, (which was a promised sign for her mother to know that the hour for her departure was come,) turned her head a little to the light, dropped her jaw, and *died*. In about half an hour after her supposed departure she was washed, and attired in clean linen; the jaw was tied by a white kerchief; penny-pieces laid over the eyes; her hands, semi-clenched, placed by her side; and her feet tied together by a piece of tape. She was then carried into another room, laid on a sofa, and covered by a sheet; appeared stiff and cold; two large books were placed on her feet, and I have no doubt she was considered to be a sweet corpse.

About 9 A. M. the grandfather of the supposed dead went into the death-chamber to give a last kiss to his grandchild, when he fancied he saw a convulsive movement of the eyelid, he having raised one of the coins. He communicated this fact to the parents and mourning friends, but they ridiculed the old man's statement, and said the movement of the eyelids was owing to the nerves working after death. Their theory, however, did not satisfy the experienced man of eighty years, and he could not reconcile himself to her death. As soon as I reached home, after having been out in the country all night, I was requested to see the child, to satisfy the old man that she was really dead. About half past ten A. M. I called; and immediately on my entrance into the chamber I perceived a tremulous condition of the eyelids, such as we frequently see in hysterical patients. The penny-pieces had been removed by the grandfather. I placed a stethoscope over the region of the heart, and found that organ performing its

functions perfectly, and with tolerable force. I then felt for a radial .
pulse, which was easily detected, beating feebly, about 75 per minute.
The legs and arms were stiff and cold; the capillary circulation gone.
I carefully watched the chest, which heaved quickly, but almost im-
perceptibly; and immediately unbandaged the maiden, and informed
her mourning parents that she was not dead.   Imagine their conster-
nation!   The passing-bell had rung, the shutters were closed, the undertaker was on his way to measure her for her coffin, and other
necessary preparations being made for interment.   I ordered friction
to the rigid limbs, moderately warm flannel to be applied, and other
restoratives; and in about two hours she spoke, and requested to be
taken to her mother's room, having been in the winding-sheet seven
hours. She told her friends that she heard all they said, and knew
they were laying her out; and that she heard the passing-bell ring, but
could not speak. She passed a very large quantity of limpid urine,
and refused food.

    At four P. M. the following day she groaned heavily, bid the by-stand-
ers farewell, and relapsed into the same cataleptic state, and remained so six hours and fourteen minutes. I saw her in that state, and
tried to raise her; she fell, listlessly regardless of position or danger;
and in whatever form the body was placed, it remained. She took no
food between the attacks, but asked for water to wet her lips; and
requested that nothing more in the shape of food might be given her,
for she did not wish to eat nor drink again until she did so in heaven.
For a whole week she took nothing, but lay perfectly quiet, with her
eyelids firmly closed and her teeth in apposition. At the expiration
of that time I told the parents of the patient that I considered it their
duty to insist upon food being taken. She was coaxed and threatened, but all in vain. She would not answer any question put to her,
and whatever food was forcibly put into her mouth she ejected. I
then, by means of a gag and an elastic tube, fed her with beef-tea,
arrowroot, and other nutritious food. At this time she commenced
moaning, and continued night and day, never ceasing for ten days.

    After this painful state of things, her friends thought she must sink
from exhaustion; but she did not appear to have sufficient power to
stir; in whatever position she was placed, she remained, until changed
by some attendants.

    Her mother now drew my attention to the absence of kidney secre-
tion, and assured me that for many days she had not voided urine.
As there were more utensils in the room than the one set apart for her

special use, I desired all to be removed but one, taking care that no other person made use of it. Ten days elapsed, but still no urine was discovered. I then told her mother that it was impossible—perfectly inconsistent with life; and asked if there were any closet or secret place in the room to which she had access. There was one, but it was filled with dirty linen. I asked permission to search it, when I found most of the linen saturated with urine. She had watched the opportunity of her friends' absence, and gone quietly into this closet and relieved her bladder.

At two A. M. one morning, whilst her parents were sleeping, she got out of bed, set fire to various articles in the room, and made her escape into the street in her night-dress, crying, " Murder !" The fire was, fortunately, extinguished, through the great presence of mind of the father, though at considerable cost, his hands being badly burned. She now began swearing most blasphemously, and continued to do so without intermission for sixty hours, after which she became exhausted, and relapsed into a state much resembling her former condition, in which state she has continued to the present time. Her eyelids firmly closed, her teeth set fast, and muscles rigid. Her bowels are moved about once a week, and she passes urine daily into the bed; not, I believe, from any want of power of the sphincter. For the last month there has been great difficulty in feeding her by the mouth. The determination she evinced to resist food was extremely annoying; but I felt inclined to be as determined as she, and from that time have fed her three times a day by the rectum, giving her about half a pint of strong beef-tea and wine, alternately with the same quantity of new milk, arrowroot, eggs, &c. After the first lavements, and when I was prepared to operate the second time, she raised her hand to her mouth, and repeated the movement two or three times, evidently wishing to convey the impression that she preferred food to be administered in a more agreeable manner; but I found, on trying to give her food by the mouth, that she was obstinate as ever. I therefore persisted in administering food by the rectum. I ordered a certain number of biscuits to be placed on a chair near the head of the bed; the next morning they numbered one less. In the evening I requested the number might be made up, and three had vanished. We found unmistakable evidence that she had eaten them.

. Dec. 4th.—Her friends beginning to despair of her, and feeling anxious to know what physical strength remained, as also whether she had the will to eat and power to masticate, I devised a scheme which,

if carried out properly, would not only prove to her friends that she
could open her eyes and mouth too if she thought she was unobserved,
but in a great measure aid me in my diagnosis, and give me a hint as
to my future treatment.   I said in an audible tone, in the presence of
the patient, that I insisted on the father and mother sleeping in another apartment; for she by her conduct was destroying their health.
She should be locked in the room by herself all night.   Having said
so, we arranged that the father should be secreted in a closet in the
chamber, with the door sufficiently open to allow him to watch her
movements through the night.   At one A. M. she raised herself up-
right in bed, opened her eyes, looked all around the room, turned
down the bedclothes, and got out of bed as nimbly as ever, and walked directly to a quantity of food, which had purposely been laid for
her.   She turned it over, tasted, and finally took a good supply into
bed, quietly drawing the bed-clothes over her.

8th.—It is five weeks to-day since she spoke to any one.   Her eyelids have been closed the whole of the time, and her mouth, too, excepting when forcibly opened; the pulse has varied very little, between
70 and 80.   Her body appears much better nourished.

Having now given a description of the case to the present time, it
remains for me to give my opinion as to the nature of this mysterious
case.   Considering that her mother has been at times hysterical, and
that there has been sufficient evidence of the early development of the
generative organs in most of the female members of the family, coupled
with most of the prominent features of the case before us, and from
many trifling, though important, incidents, which from defective
memory I have omitted, I am inclined to consider it one of hysteria
of an aggravated character, complicated probably with a morbid condition of the brain.   I entertain hopes that, provided I can sufficiently
nourish the body until the uterine organs are more fully developed, my
patient may continue to be " *The Dead Alive!*"

I am, sir, your obedient servant,

RICHARD BIRD NASON, M.R.C.S., L.S.A.

BRIDGE STREET, NUNEATON, *December 14th*, 1858.

NAVY MEDICAL BOARD.

The Board of Naval Medical Examiners, consisting of Surgeons W.
S. W. Ruschenberger, L. B. Hunter, J. D. Miller, and Passed Assist-

ant Surgeon George H. Howell, adjourned *sine die*, May 23d, 1859. Assistant Surgeons Thos. J. Turner, (appointed in 1853,) R. P. Daniel, William G. Hay, and William T. Hord, (appointed in 1854,) were found qualified for promotion.

Of the competitors before the Board for the ten vacancies which will probably occur, in the course of the year, in the grade of assistant surgeon, the following have been selected:

1. William Bradley, Pa.; 2. Edward F. Corson, Pa.; 3. David Kendleberger, Ohio; 4. Joseph D. Grafton, Arkansas; 5. Robert L. Weber, Pa.; 6. Robert J. Freeman, Va.; 7. William E. Taylor, Va.; 9. James McMaster, Pa.; 10. James W. Herty, Ga.

The five first named have been already appointed, and it is probable the others will receive commissions in the Medical Corps of the Navy prior to the meeting of another Board.

It is supposed that the increased activity of the naval service, in connection with the comparatively small number of medical officers, a large proportion of whom, from age and physical disability, are incapable of active duty, will induce the next Congress to authorize a considerable augmentation of the medical corps. Should this conjecture prove to be correct, it is probable that from forty to fifty assistant surgeons will be required to fill new appointments in the course of the year 1860. Those young members of the profession who are desirous to obtain admission into the Naval Medical Corps should begin now to prepare for the competition which will be open in the course of the next spring.—*Med. News.*

AMERICAN MEDICAL LITERATURE.

We have never felt any sympathy with those who desired to prematurely force forward the Medical Literature of this country by a sort of hot-house process, believing that a natural healthy growth was inevitable, which would make up for any slowness of maturation by its excellence and permanency. We observe with much pleasure the evidences of progress in this direction which are daily multiplying, and it affords us gratification to chronicle each new step in advance. When Prof. Dalton, of New York, recently issued a systematic work on Human Physiology, we felt assured that it would at once take its position among the most advanced expositions of the science that our language afforded. We are therefore pleased to find the following tribute to its merits, which we extract from the April number of the *Westmin-*

ster Review—well deserved praise, which, as we have reason to know, emanates from one of the most distinguished physiologists of Great Britain.

"In striking contrast with the six ponderous tomes of which the Cyclopædia consists, (one of its five volumes being so bulky that a division of it is indispensable for use,) is a compendious treatise that has recently issued from the American press, by a rising young physiologist, who had previously gained · considerable distinction by his original investigations. His ideas of the science are based less upon the systems which have been commonly accredited, than upon the investigations which have marked its progress during a recent epoch; so that instead of interweaving the latter with the former, after the fashion of the most systematic writers and teachers, modifying the older doctrines in so far as may be necessary to make them accordant with later researches, he has taken, as it were, an altogether new point of departure, and has set himself to consider on what plan and with what materials the fabric might be best built up, if it were now to be erected *de novo*. There is, we think, considerable advantage to science in the occasional advent of fresh minds which do not allow themselves to be fettered by its traditions, but determine to prove and examine everything for themselves. Unfortunately, some of these seem to differ from their predecessors for the mere sake of establishing a claim to originality, or of gratifying their own love of antagonism and faultfinding. This, however, is not a fault which can be laid to Dr. Dalton's charge. His object has been, not to invalidate the researches of others, but to establish and corroborate them by original investigation, so as to present to the world a compact and reliable summary of the principal verities of physiological science that shall be in accordance with the most advanced knowledge of the time; and we are happy in being able to recommend his treatise as admirably fulfilling this intention. We may differ from him in his estimate of the value of particular facts, and in the conclusions he deduces from them; but the work is highly creditable to his judgment and industry, and is not surpassed by any with which we are acquainted as a concise summary of human physiology, giving due prominence to those points which have the most intimate bearing on medical practice. We must not omit to mention that the illustrations are nearly all original, and are of high merit; and that the whole getting-up of the book does great credit to the American press."—*Med. News.*

MEDICAL DEPARTMENT OF THE ARMY.

The Army Medical Board, which recently convened in this city, have recommended the following gentlemen for appointment in the Medical Staff of the Army:

No. 1. George Suckley, M.D., New York.

No. 2. Dewitt C. Peters, M.D., New York.

No. 3. Charles H. Alden, M.D., Pennsylvania.

Assistant Surgeons, Alexander B. Hasson and Jonathan Letherman, were examined by the Board, and found qualified for promotion. —*Med. News.*

Verdict for Professional Services of Six Hundred Dollars.

We are indebted to a facetious correspondent for the following interesting details. Read them *after dinner;* they will repay the perusal:

The injustice of juries as regards professional ligitation is a common experience of physicians throughout the country. Verdicts in their favor are exceedingly rare, and hardly ever obtained without mutilation of legitimate professional fees, to an extent which scarcely leaves a balance for the payment of law expenses.

There is obviously no alternative but to suffer the imposition of dishonesty, rather than to embark with more time and money in a dubious and vexatious lawsuit. Sometimes the provocations are, however, too strong to be borne; and an injured physician, despite of all warning precedents, and odds against a favorable termination, may resort to this *ultima ratio creditorium.*

Such appears to have been the case with Dr. Andrews, of East Brooklyn, who brought an action against Fagan, for the recovery of professional fees amounting to $600.

The defendant resides with two younger brothers at East Brooklyn. They are lords of the same shanty and manor of ten acres, which latter they work to good advantage. By penury, abstinence, (except in the matter of whiskey,) persevering exertions, fat contracts, etc., they have accumulated a tolerable competency, which yearly increases by cautious and profitable investments. So far, so well for Mr. Fagan.

To pass away the monotony of their domestic life, they had occasionally a social drink, and on reaching the proper pitch, the festivities were wound up with a general pitch-into-one-another all round, when *claret* was tapped without stint or ceremony. On one of these occasions the younger Paddy indulged in the pleasant diversion of dissecting the senior Fagan, in a manner so effectual, that it made him tremble for the precious lives of himself and brother. After a profound family deliberation, it was resolved to invite the attendance of Dr. Andrews, for the purpose of patching up the dilapidation.

The Doctor, promptly arriving at the scene of action, found Paddy the elder in a rather precarious situation—punctured like a sieve, and the family claret so freely shed as almost to take the blush out of the patient's red hair! Misther Fagan was then sewed up and done for, and his dissolved integrity united as well as the accommodations of the shanty—

> ("As nate a mud cabin as ever was seen;
>   And considering it was but to keep
>   Poultry and pigs in,
>   I'm sure it was always most illigant clane.")—

and his imposing position on a bundle of straw would permit. But one of the wounds had entered the fundamental basis of existence by perforating not only his "abominable" cavity, but also the small intestine, allowing the free escape of Paddy Fagan's spirit! The alarmed (but now disarmed) brothers, dimly realizing the danger of having their bachelors' hall thus broken up "sine die," (i. e., even without the dying of the elder one,) enjoined the Doctor to spare no pains or plasters, and they would come down handsomely for that same "in liberal spirit," and might the Lord bless him!

The Doctor,

> "Taught by that Power that pities him,
>   Began to pity them,"

and, *item*—he saved poor Paudeen's life!

His task was laborious, requiring more than ordinary skill, tact, and circumspection, besides much time and devotion.

Dr. Andrews, during his term of attendance on the patient, could not escape the importunities of the disconsolate kinsmen, who thus took up the balance of his time.

In all, he had made some seventy visits, lasting from thirty minutes to five hours. Among them were twelve night calls, particularly requested by the patient and his kids.

When Fagan found himself in boots again, he handed over to the Doctor one hundred dollars in gold, imagining this sum to be a handsome remuneration, and the latter accepted the proffered amount as payment " on account," tendering subsequently a bill for the balance, $500. This demand Mr. Fagan considered " outrageous," without further considering the Doctor—hence the action.

Drs. Daniel Ayres, Louis Bauer, and George Cochrane. of Brooklyn, being put on the stand by the plaintiff, with a view to a valuation of the professional services of Dr. Andrews, testified as follows: That the charges for professional attendance rested on three points, viz.:

1. The *amount* of professional services;
2. The *quality* of professional services; and,
3. The *responsibility* to be incurred while in charge of the case.

In applying these principles to the case of Fagan, they had no hesitation in stating that as to No. 1, the services of Dr. Andrews were very laborious: the visits numerous, and of long duration—some of them during the night—and that they could not be classified under the head of ordinary visits in country practice at 50 cents each. As to No. 2, they further considered that the case had required more than ordinary skill and tact in its management; that in both, the Doctor had exceeded all reasonable expectation, for which the highest encomium was due to him. And as to No. 3, that Fagan's case being one of public notoriety, had placed upon the Doctor extraordinary responsibility, which should not be undervalued. For the failure in such cases, more especially in small townships, reflects most seriously upon the attendant's professional qualifications, the public being neither capable nor inclined to appreciate the difficulties of the injuries.

A few failures of this description would have the effect of depriving the physician of an otherwise well-merited professional reputation and practice. They considered, therefore, the charge of $600 every way reasonable, and in keeping with professional usage.

The defence, though admitting the amount, the skill and responsibility of the services, tried to establish a lower scale of prices. It maintained that a *cadaver*, a carcass, (which Walker defines as the decayed parts of a *thing* without completion or *ornament*, which latter qualification his most ardent admirers even had not the face to claim for him,)—the cadaver, it maintained, commanded no more than its regular market price, say $15; that Fagan had been a corpse, half dissected by fraternal exuberance, and was therefore decreased in value, estimating such value at not exceeding the sum of five dollars bankable currency—(the current figure, by-the-by, for "stock" generally sought after by fishmongers and orangemen;) and that a fee of $100 was more than the Doctor could have reasonably demanded.

The jury, composed of very intelligent citizens, (and always considered so by the party in whose favor they find,) thought differently, however, of the *value* of Fagan, (if *not* of his *worth*,) and after brief deliberation, returned a verdict in favor of the plaintiff for the full amount, with costs.

This termination was as unexpected as it is exceptional; and I thought it might benefit the profession by being put on medical record.—*Med. and Surg. Reporter.*   BROOKLYN.

[From the N. O. Medical News.]

Dr. E. D. Fenner's Treatment of Yellow Fever.

Our colleague and friend, Dr. E. D. Fenner, left for Europe on the 14th inst. He will visit all the principal hospitals of England, Ireland, Scotland, and the Continent, as far as time and opportunity will allow, and we have no doubt he will return to us in the fall both physically and mentally prepared to surround with increased interest and usefulness the Chair of Theory and Practice, in the new school, which he has for three years so ably and faithfully filled. Dr. Fenner is one of the working medical men of the South, and what gives inestimable value to his labors is the fact, undenied and undeniable, that he promulgates only those doctrines which he conscientiously believes to be *true.* We anticipate for our pages this summer interesting contributions from his pen, giving the result of his observations abroad.

On board the steamer which bore him hence it will be seen that his mind still dwelt on home and its medical interests, and he has furnished us the following letter, which will be appreciated by all who know him:

Veratrum Viride and Chlorine in Yellow Fever.—MY DEAR COLLEAGUE: As some practitioner may desire to try the new treatment for yellow fever which I brought to the notice of the profession in the October and November numbers of our Journal last year, I have concluded, before quitting the country, to leave you some plain directions for carrying out the same.

I repeat what has been said before, that I think we have in the veratrum viride and chlorine mixture medicines which are fairly entitled to be *considered remedies for yellow fever.* They will at least fulfill the following indications, viz.: *completely control febrile excitement, and keep up the secretions of the liver, kidneys, and skin.* Now these are not *all* the indications that are presented in yellow fever, but they certainly are the principal ones, and those to which our remedies are chiefly directed. If the febrile excitement be very moderate, the V. V. will hardly be called for.

My directions, in brief, are as follows:

At the commencement of the attack order a hot mustard foot-bath and. evacuate the bowels with a mild cathartic, such as castor oil, citrate of magnesia or Seidlitz powders. If the stomach be irritable, with bilious vomiting and a coated tongue, give a gentle emetic of ipecac. or salt and mustard.

After this, if the fever be high, give five drops of the V. V. in a little water every four hours till the pulse be brought down to seventy, when the V. V. will be stopped, or the interval between the doses prolonged so as to keep the pulse at seventy. At the same time begin with the chlorine mixture, and give two table-spoonsful every four hours —thus, V. V. at 2, chlorine at 6; V. V. at 8, chlorine at 10, etc. If the fever be moderate from the first, the V. V. may be dispensed with, and the chlorine alone relied on and given more frequently, say every second hour. These doses are for adults. Children, even sucking infants, bear the chlorine well, but the V. V. should be very cautiously given to them.

The repetition of foot-baths, sinapisms, spongings, enemata, etc., must be left to the judgment of the practitioner. I have no doubt that quinine in some way would be a valuable adjunct to these remedies, but I will not direct it at present.

The following is the chlorine mixture:

R.—Acid. Hydrochloric,

    Aqua Distillata *aa.* ℥ii. Mix, and add

    Potass. Chlorat. ʒii.

Let this be labeled, and kept on hand. For use prescribe as follows:

R.—Chlorine Mixture ʒii.

    Aqua Distillat. oj.   m.

S. Give two table-spoonsful every two or four hours, *(pro re nata.)*

For drink I like orange-leaf tea, lemonade, barley-water. *Covering* —generally one blanket. Do not rise up in bed after the first day until fairly convalescent.

With these two remedies as my main dependence, in twenty-five cases of the bad epidemic last year I lost only two: one a pregnant lady, who was delivered at the critical stage of the fever; the other a very delicate lady, with no recuperative energy.

Dr. W. E. Kennedy told me he treated fifteen cases with these remedies, and lost but one.

Dr. C. Beard treated eight cases, and lost none.

Dr. S. Choppin treated eight cases, and lost one

Other physicians told me they had tried these remedies with happy effects. I hope others will try them, if yellow fever should again appear in any of our cities or villages.

In my trip to Europe, my attention will be directed mainly to Medical Institutions and the prominent medical men of the day, of all which I shall endeavor to write you from time to time, as occasion may allow. I go in search of knowledge for the benefit of our students and those who will intrust them with their lives in coming time. Hoping to return with renovated energy, and to meet both you and a host of them at the opening of our lectures in November next, I remain, dear B.,

Yours, faithfully,   E. D. FENNER.

ON BOARD STEAMER R. J. WARD, MISSISSIPPI RIVER, *May* 16, 1859.

[From the N. O. Medical News.]

CALOMEL VERSUS CONSTIPATION.

[Heroic Practice—Calomel in Ounce Doses!—600 Grains of Calomel and 40 of Opium in Nine Hours!]

By T. J. HEARD, M.D., of Galveston, Texas.

Messrs. Editors—The following case is not without interest, and I present it to your readers on its own merits:

Mr. B , aged about 35 years—of bilio-lymphatic temperament—eat a great quantity of cheese and crackers about the 1st of May, 1858. From this excess a severe attack of flatulent colic, associated with gastric irritability and obstinate constipation, resulted. My partner, Dr. P., was called to him, and treated him in the most approved manner for five days. I was absent from town (Washington, Texas) at the time, and Dr. P. sent for me in consultation; not that he could reasonably expect any material aid from me, I being much younger than himself, but in order to be sure that all should be done for the patient. I called with him to see B., and a more miserable object I have never beheld. The Dr. had given everything that promised benefit, including croton oil by the mouth, and tobacco by the rectum. The poor fellow was cold, and shivering from the intensity of the pain in his abdomen; tympanitis was as great as it could be, apparently; the pulse was a mere thread, and very frequent; the voice was sepulchral; thirst was intense; he had not slept during his illness, and his stomach rejected everything put into it.

We applied a mustard poultice over the whole abdomen, and left, to call again in six hours. At 8, P. M., we returned; he was in about the same condition; the abdominal pain had been so great that he did not feel the mustard, although it had produced a terrible blister. We requested Mr. A., at whose house the patient was staying, to have a coffin made that night, as there was hardly a doubt that he would die before morning, and the abdomen was so much distended that we anticipated its bursting soon after death. There seemed scarcely a doubt that the poor fellow was laboring under intussusception, and that the case was altogether hopeless.

Next morning, about 10 o'clock, I was passing the house on my way to the country, and I called to ask when poor B. died, and, to my utter astonishment, found him in about the same condition as that in which we left him. He immediately commenced imploring me to kill him—saying he knew he could not live; that his coffin had been made for him, and he was ready and willing to go; that he desired an end put to his suffering. I had, in my vest pocket, an ounce of calomel, which I made him swallow, only allowing water enough to wash it down. At 1, P. M., I called, and found that B. had slept about an hour, had taken some buttermilk, and had vomited but once. I reported this to Dr. P., at 2, P. M. He said the apparent improvement was not from the effect of the calomel, but was owing to loss of vitality in the invaginated intestine. At 4, P. M., I saw B. again. He had taken more buttermilk, and had slept some. I ordered for him 300 grains of calomel, and 20 grains of opium, to be divided into two powders—to be taken at intervals of three hours. At 8, P. M., both powders had been taken, and the patient was in about the same condition as at 4, P. M. We left two more powders as above. At 6, A. M., of the succeeding day, I called to ask for B. On opening the door, behold, the bed was empty! I called for some one to tell me when poor B. died, when, from an adjoining room, the patient (a poor half-witted fellow) cried out, "What in the h—l do you want?" I asked, "Is that you, B.?" "Yes—it is nobody else." I asked, "What are you doing there?" He replied, "What in the h—l do you suppose I would be doing, after all that calo-

34

mel?" B. was purged for one week, was not ptyalized, and was afterwards in better health than he had been for years.

The reader must determine whether the result ensuing on the administration of the calomel was coincident, or a genuine illustration of cause and effect. I give the facts as they occurred.

[As in all cases wherein great quantities and great variety of medicines are administered, it must be difficult to decide the question raised by this case. Of two things we feel well assured, however, viz.: that these heroic doses of calomel rarely, if ever, do any harm; and that opium, to be given with benefit in intensely painful cases, must be given in heroic doses, or it is useless. We have, ourself, had a severe case of neuralgia in which not less than eight grains of the best pulverized opium, at one dose, and repeated in two hours, would produce relief; and within a year we have administered, with our own hand, four-grain doses of sulphate of morphine, every six hours, for two days, to a case of idiopathic tetanus in an adult negro, with only the effect of producing gentle sleep. A less quantity of the remedy was utterly useless. We have long been satisfied that many patients suffer for the want of opiates and the kindred remedies in sufficient quantity, while the practitioner stands by with his judgment trammeled by the knowledge he has acquired of doses from the books or the lecture-rooms.—D. W. B.]

[*What will Dr. Bigelow say?*—D. M. B.]

PUERPERAL CONVULSIONS.

By FRANCIS H. RAMSBOTHAM, M.D.,

Obstetric Physician to the London Hospital, etc.

On Monday, February 7, 1859, at 5 P. M., I was sent for by Mr. Pryce, of Walworth, to Mrs. G., Beresford Street, aged twenty-eight, a stout, plethoric woman, pregnant for the first time, between six and seven months. She had complained, for six days before the attack, of drowsiness, confusion of ideas, with slight pain in the head, stertorous breathing, and puffy hands and face. She had never been the subject of hysteric or epileptic fits. In the afternoon of Sunday she experienced a severe attack of vomiting and purging, and at 9, P. M., was seized with a violent convulsion. The fits recurred very frequently— the people about her said every ten minutes—through the night and during Monday. She remained perfectly insensible the whole time, her breathing heavy and stertorous. On my arrival, however, there had been an intermission of nearly an hour free from fits, and she had just swallowed two or three tea-spoonsful of tea for the first time since the beginning of the seizure. Nevertheless, she was still quite unconscious, with widely-dilated pupils, acting sluggishly to the stimulus of light. The uterus occasionally became hard, and there seemed to be a disposition for the commencement of premature labor. She had been bled twice during the night, losing about thirty ounces of blood at the two operations; and in the day had been cupped on the back of the neck, and twelve leeches had been applied to her temples. The hair had been cut off, ice was applied to the head, and a turpentine enema had been administered, which had brought away a large quantity of foetid stools. I had some difficulty in reaching the os uteri with my finger, for it was very high, and inclined more than usually backward. It was dilated to the sixpence, just admitting the end of the finger, and the membranes were felt tense. Before withdrawing my hand I ruptured the membranes, and gave exit to a considerable discharge of liquor amnii; I then felt a limb, but could not make out which. Her size was greatly diminished. She had no more fits while I stayed in the house. I recommended that as long as she remained unconscious three grains of calomel should be placed on her tongue every two hours, in the hope of its passing into the stomach; and that another turpentine enema should be injected. There were only two more fits after I left; labor-pains supervened, and she was delivered at 2, A. M., (Tuesday;) the knees presenting. Her consciousness gradually returned soon after delivery; though headache continued. On Saturday, the 12th, Mr. Pryce wrote to me, that he had seen her that morning sitting up, after a refreshing sleep of five hours; that she still complained of her head, and felt relief from the cold application. The cochia after delivery were very scanty; she took ten grains of calomel, and for two days the sphincters performed their duty imperfectly. It is remarkable that she has no recollection whatever of anything that occurred for six days before the attack appeared, although she was following her ordinary occupation all the time; and except for the headache and drowsiness seemed as usual. No albumen could be detected in the urine. She is now convalescent.

Holding the opinion, as I do, that an attack of puerperal convulsions is merely a modification of cerebral apoplexy, I consider that this young woman's life was saved by the prompt and decisive bleeding.—*Med. Times and Gazette.*

Pardonable Secrecy.

A Secret Ward.—"In one part of the establishment at Wurzburg, there is a suite of six or eight apartments, which is called the *Geheime Abtheilung*, or secret department. This feature distinguishes many of the German lying-in hospitals, and it enables the victims of seduction and illicit love to conceal their shame from the open gaze of the world. Here, the young lady, who has 'loved not wisely, but too well,' may retire from society before her disgrace becomes apparent, her friends believing meanwhile, in some pleasing fiction, that she has gone on a tour to visit England, or to enjoy the gaieties of Paris. Here she enters, seen by no human eye, save that of the hospital attendants, who are all trustworthy, and sworn to implicit secrecy; here she lives till her confinement is past—never called by her name, but merely designated by a number; and when the event is over, she again passes out into the world, and perhaps talks of the celebrities she has seen in Pall Mall or Rotten Row, or of the beauties of the Champs Elysées."—*Dr. Adam.*

Seasonable Conservatism in Obstetrics.

On the Indications for the Application of the Forceps.—Among the indications, those derived from the insufficiency of pains are the most frequently assigned, and the most liable to give rise to errors in practice. The head remains at the floor of the pelvis, the pains, though more or less strong, being insufficient in the individual case to expel it beyond the external genitals. The patience of the accoucheur becoming exhausted, (much sooner, indeed, than that of the woman,) he has resort to instruments in order to terminate the labor. That such a procedure, common as it is, cannot be justified, scarcely requires to be said.

Much more frequent in occurrence than these examples of actual insufficiency of pain (which the author has always found at this stage of labor, especially in primiparæ, a very rare circumstance) are the cases in which the head, in spite of strong pains, remains at the floor of the pelvis, and although pressed down by every contraction towards the mouth of the vagina, never distends the perineum. Well aware of the impropriety of too early or of useless operative interference, at the beginning of his practice, Dr. Speigelberg contented himself in these cases with temporizing and pain-increasing measures, too often, however, with the result of still having to employ the forceps at last, as it seldom happened that the pains alone proved sufficient. Under these circumstances, a large proportion of the children were still-born. Taught by this experience, he afterwards in such cases resorted to the forceps earlier, and was, as regards the children, much more fortunate. He was also exceedingly surprised at the ease with which the head, apparently so firmly fixed, was extracted. Traction was scarcely required at all, a suitable adjustment of the instrument and a few lateral pendulum-like movements commonly sufficing to effect the delivery. Sometimes all was completed with one hand, the other supporting the perineum. While in those cases in which the ergot had been used to effect the propulsion, retention of urine, erosions, and inflammation of the vagina or vulva were met with, no such occurrences followed the use of the forceps. The cause, which in these cases prevents good pains proving effective, and renders a forceps operation so easy of execution, is a purely mechanical one—arising from the too great flexure of the head upon the chest. The face is turned towards the coccyx, the vertex rests on the perineum, and the occiput lies under the symphisis at the mouth of the vagina. The uterus, acting upon the trunk of the child, forces the occiput by means of the vertebral column, deeper every pain, pressing the chin more forcibly towards the chest. For the birth of the child, however, it is necessary that the neck should be stretched out so as to raise the head from the chest. The contractions of the perineal muscles, especially the levator ani, which, as well as those of the abdomen, are in a state of voluntary or of reflex activity, force the cranium still further upward and backward, i. e., towards the chest. The pains, however, increased in severity, prove useless, and the operation of the forceps is easily explained. When the blades are passed in at the sides of the head in the direction of the prolongation of the axis of the outlet of the pelvis, they remove the chin from the chest, stretch out the neck, and terminate the delivery at once. The head had already been forced through the pelvis, and the forceps has only to conduct it over the perineum. They do not act by traction, but as a lever or instrument for bettering the position. They must be passed up slowly, or the perineum may be injured. What is here stated has been but little observed, and as far as Dr. Speigelberg is aware, Cazeaux is the only author who has clearly set it forth. If this excessive flexure of the head does not furnish the indication in nine out of ten forceps operations as stated by Cazeaux, at least it is the most frequent cause of their employment, and places this in the most favorable light. Just as the weakness of pains is a rare, so is this condition a frequent indication. Dr. Speigelberg hopes that this communication may not be interpreted into a recommendation to have recourse hastily or uselessly to operations. But he adds that some of the worst consequences result from abstaining from operations when solid indications for interference present themselves; and that skill in employing his instruments is of even less importance to the obstetrician than the power of detecting the cases which justify his resorting to them.—DR. SPEIGELBERG, *Monatschrift fur Geburtsk*, Band xi. pp. 124–126.

BENNET DOWLER.

An American physician and physiologist, was born in Ohio Co., Va., April 16, 1797. He was educated at the University of Maryland, where, in 1827, he received the degree of doctor of medicine. During the last 23 years he has practiced his profession in New Orleans, and since March, 1854, has been the editor of the *New Orleans Medical and Surgical Journal.* From an early period in his career experiments upon the human body, immediately or very soon after death, occupied a large share of his attention, and the results of his investigations, comprising some important discoveries with regard to contractility, calorification, capillary circulation, &c., were given to the world in a series of essays in 1843–'4. Since that time these and other original experiments have been extended, generalized, and analyzed by him. With one exception, he has found in the course of his experiments no fact invalidating the fundamental laws which he announced in his first publications relative to *post-mortem* contractility of the muscular system. He had prematurely assumed, early in his researches, in accordance with the prevailing theory, that the death rigidity, or *rigor mortis*, is antagonistic to, or incompatible with, the coexistence of muscular contraction; but he soon found instances which led him to maintain that the contractile function exists in all bodies immediately after death, although in some it is scarcely appreciable, while in others it is absent or feeble at first, but gradually increases. In all it is intermittent, and may be economized by proper management, or overtasked and exhausted, or even destroyed by a severe blow. He was consequently led to the conclusion that this force is inherent in the muscular tissue, and in every portion of it, being wholly independent of the brain, spinal cord, and nerves. During the last 18 years Dr. Dowler has shown by experiments on hundreds of human bodies

that the capillary circulation is often active for some minutes, and
even for hours, after the respiration and the action of the heart have
ceased, and occasionally after the removal of this organ; and that in
the same cadaver a high degree of calorification, together with active
capillary and chylous circulations, may continue simultaneously for
several hours. His researches on animal heat, in health, in disease,
and after death, which have from time to time been published in medical journals, have led to important discoveries, particularly with reference to *post-mortem* calorification, which his experiments have shown
will, after death from fever, cholera, or sun-stroke, &c., rise in some
cases much higher than its antecedent maximum during the progress
of the disease. From these experimental researches, as well as from
a rational interpretation of the respiratory action of the lungs, either in
their natural, diseased, obstructed, or disorganized conditions, Dr.
Dowler has been led to reject the long-received theory which ascribes
animal heat to the lungs, as the sole heating apparatus of the animal
economy. He maintains that the chemical history of respiration may
be interpreted either as a refrigeratory or heat equalizing process, and
that while the absorption of oxygen during respiration may generate
heat, on the other hand the parting of carbonic acid gas and aqueous
vaporization from the lungs, together with the incessant respiration
of the air, almost always much cooler than the body, must refrigerate
the animal economy; that for all that has been proved to the contrary, oxydation and deoxydation, repair and waste, composition and decomposition, inhalation and exhalation, are mutually compensating or
equiponderant in the regulation of animal heat; and that, while it
may be plausibly assumed that nearly the whole series of organs and
organic functions, especially those of nutrition, contribute directly or
indirectly to the origin and distribution of animal heat during life, *post-
mortem* calorification might to some extent be accounted for by assuming that respiration is not a heating, but a refrigeratory process,
which, ceasing with apparent death, ceases to liberate the free caloric
of the economy; whence the calorifacient function, not being in many
instances extinguished with the respiration, persists, and for a long time
accumulates faster than it can be radiated into the surrounding media.
He has not, however, been able to trace a necessary connection, ante-
cedence, or parallelism between *post-mortem* calorification and muscular
contractility, the development, degree, and duration of which may
or may not coincide. In March, 1845, Dr. Dowler commenced a series of experiments in comparative physiology on the great saurian or

alligator of Louisiana, which he regarded as much better for the purpose than any of the cold-blooded animals usually selected for vivisection.   From these experiments, which embrace a period of 10 years,
he has ascertained that after decapitation the head, and more especially the trunk, afford unequivocal evidences of possessing the faculties of sensation and volition for hours after a complete division of the
animal.   The headless trunk, deprived of all the senses but that of
touch, perceived, felt, willed, and acted with unerring intelligence in
removing or avoiding an irritant, such as an ignited match or bit of
paper; when even a simple touch or a positive irritant was applied
laterally, the body curved or receded in a contrary direction, while
the most convenient limb was also directed to the exact place where
the foreign body impinged, in order to remove it, if possible.   After
as well as before decapitation, after complete evisceration, and after
the subdivision of the spine and its cord in 2 or 3 places, each section
mutually and simultaneously perceived or felt in common the presence
or contact of a pain-producing agent.   In some instances Dr. Dowler
observed that the separated head could see a body, like the finger,
purposely directed close to the eye, as was shown by the violent opening of the mouth, as if to bite, and by the head jumping several feet
from the operating-table to the floor.   The vivisection of the spinal
cord satisfied him also that neither root of the spinal marrow is the
exclusive seat of sensation or of motion, and that motion as well as
sensory phenomena may be excited by irritation of either root; a result directly opposed to the celebrated theory of Sir Charles Bell on
the functions of these roots.   The vivisection of the inferior animals,
(hitherto the basis of experimental physiology,) as well as the pathological, anatomical, and experimental phenomena observed in man, has
therefore led Dr. Dowler to the following conclusions: that the functions and structures of the nervous system constitute a unity altogether
inconsistent with the anatomical assumption of 4 distinct and separate
sets of nerves, and a corresponding fourfold set of functions; that
there is no anatomical or other proof that one set of nerves transmits
impressions to, and a separate set from, a sensorial spot somewhere in
the brain,·nor that the nerves themselves are simple conductors and
wholly insensible; that the 2 separate sets of nerves usually assigned
to what is called the excito-motory action of the spinal cord are wholly hypothetical; that instead of 4 traveling impressions, there is but
one, the primary or sensiferous impression, which is simultaneously
cognized upon the periphery as well as in the centre, and not solely

by an unknown spot in the brain through the intermedium of a secondarily transmitted impression, being intuitively felt where it really is; and that sensuous cognition or sensation is immediate, intuitive, and not representative, nor the result of transmitted secondary impressions, but a directly felt relation, *ab initio*, between an object and a sentient subject, and not one between a mere secondary representation, idea, or transmitted impression of an object. The assiduous devotion of Dr. Dowler to researches connected with medical and physiological science has won for him a wide reputation as an experimenter, an anatomist, and a pathologist.—*New American Cyclopædia*.

BOOK NOTICES.

A TREATISE ON GONORRHŒA AND SYPHILIS. By Silas Durkee, M.D., Fellow of the Massachusetts Medical Society, &c. With 8 colored plates. Boston: John P. Jewett & Co. 1859.

The author of this work has furnished the profession with what has long been needed in this department, a plain, systematic, and practical book, in which, while he gives the literature of the subject all needed attention, including all the recent innovations and experimental experience of the syphilizationists and non-mercurialists of Europe, he treats the whole subject with an independence and originality which is refreshing in these days, when so many of the writers on kindred topics give us neither novelty nor merit.

We especially like the critical and discriminating spirit which characterizes every part of this work, and its freedom from any servile or sycophantic submission to what are called authorities. Dr. Durkee is a practical man, and his book is eminently utilitarian; his knowledge, acquired in the school of experience, being here freely communicated without reservation. It should be studied not merely by physicians and their pupils, but by all the quacks, whose ignorant and mercenary devices of imposture and extortion are here exploded, in contrast with the truth taught by rational science. And if the patients of the latter would read it, they might escape the fangs of these medical vultures, who prey upon their timidity and terrors.

A cursory examination is all we have yet had time to make of our copy, but we have read enough of its pages to predict that it will become a standard authority in this department, regarding it, as we do, superior to any of the works we have seen on the subject, whether foreign or domestic. It contains a number of plates, choicely colored from life, illustrating the ravages of constitutional syphilis upon the surface of the body, and these are free from the objectionable and disgusting obscenity which disfigures so many analogous works.

The author has honored himself by the dedication of his labors to his preceptor, Dr. Brinsmade, late President of the New York State Society, in terms of compliment which are well merited. We bespeak for the work a wide circulation, and predict its eminent popularity.

The typography, engravings, binding, &c., are worthy of the publishers, who have creditably performed their part, which is more than can be said of all the Boston trade.

A TREATISE ON BATHS; including Cold, Sea, Warm, Hot, Vapor, Gas, and Mud Baths; also on Hydropathy and Pulmonary Inhalation; with a description of Bathing in ancient and modern times. By John Bell, M.D. Second edition. Philadelphia: Lindsay & Blakiston. 1859.

This work is a complete Cyclopædia of Baths and Bathing, and exhausts the literature of the subject, which is one of growing interest. The author is so well known as a medical scholar, that it is sufficient to say that he has devoted very many years of his mature life to the investigation of Water as a preservative of health, and a remedy in disease. Nor can it be necessary to add that his book embodies more information on this topic than can be found in all the Hydropathic publications in existence. We renew the high commendation with which we heralded the first edition, as communicating that kind of knowledge which it is every man's duty to learn. It deserves a wide circulation.

ELEMENTS OF MEDICINE; a compendious View of Pathology and Therapeutics; or the History and Treatment of Diseases. By Samuel Henry Dickson, M.D., LL.D., &c. Philadelphia: Blanchard & Lea. 1859.

A second edition of this valuable work having become necessary, it has been subjected to a careful revision by the author, and now appears enlarged and improved. Professor Dickson's exalted reputation as a teacher and practitioner, acquired at the Universities of South Carolina and New York, has been rewarded and increased by his transfer to the Jefferson Medical College at Philadelphia, where he now occupies the chair of Professor of Practice in this, the largest medical school in America, a position which he adorns by his learning, his modesty, and his worth in all the relations of life. This elaborate work affords the proof of his profound scholarship, his ability as a writer, and his manly independence, for which we honor him, even when constrained to differ with him in some of his doctrinal teachings. In all that is practical, however, in this work, his experience, skill, and circumspection render him an authority worthy of the highest respect.

We should be glad to learn that this book was extensively read by the profession, for the science of medicine is so little studied in these degenerate days, and the tendency of the present age has such a proclivity to the cultivation of the mere art of healing, and this in specifics and specialties, that we fear its unpretending title will deter rather than attract readers. The "elements" on which all true science, all the principles of our divine art, are founded, seem at present to be undervalued, and without a revolution in the creed of the profession there is danger that the prestige of learning which formerly characterized medical men will be lost. Such books as this of Professor Dickson ought to revive the love of science, as the foundation of our art.

WOMAN, HER DISEASES AND REMEDIES. A series of Letters to his Class. By Charles D. Meigs, M.D., &c. Philadelphia: Blanchard & Lea. 1859.

This is the fourth edition, revised and enlarged, of the most popular and useful book which has ever appeared in this department of medical literature. If the venerated Professor of Obstetrics in the Jefferson College of Philadelphia had never rendered any other service to his profession and the public than the issue of this volume, he would have done enough to render his name and fame imperishable. But he has not ceased to labor on in his chosen field, having found time, amid his accumulated toils, to revise, enlarge, and essentially improve the work, of which this latest edition affords ample evidence. As we have taken occasion, on the appearance of each new issue of these letters, to commend the book for its originality and freshness, as well as the intrinsic excellence of its practical teachings, we can only repeat our estimate, regarding it as the best work on the subject of which it treats, alike for students and practitioners.

A DICTIONARY OF PRACTICAL MEDICINE; comprising General Pathology, the Nature and Treatment of Diseases, Morbid Structures. &c., &c. By James Copland, M.D., F.R.S., &c. Edited, with additions, by Charles A. Lee, M.D., &c. In 3 volumes, royal octavo. New York: Harper & Brothers. 1859.

This gigantic and standard work is at length completed, having been nearly twenty years in publication, having been issued serially and at long intervals, so that the reprint has been unavoidably delayed until now. Its intrinsic merits, however, will compensate for all this delay, which in fact has very considerably enhanced its value, the author and editor having been thus enabled to keep pace with the improving current literature of the profession, and introduce the latest novelties. The two volumes heretofore published are familiar to reading physicians, who will find in the third and final volume over 1,700 pages, completing the work, together with a copious index, table of classified contents, and the *prefaces*, or rather *post*-faces, of the author and editor. We shall notice the work hereafter.

TRANSACTIONS OF THE NEW JERSEY STATE MEDICAL SOCIETY.

This publication speaks well for our Jersey brethren. It contains a sound, discriminating address by the President, Dr. Coleman; a brief report from Sussex Co., by Dr. Ryerson; and a full and elaborate report from Essex Co., by Dr. Lehlbach, which includes a large number of cases, both medical and surgical, chiefly derived from Newark, N. J., where our science in all its departments is cultivated with ardor, and which may be regarded as the medical headquarters of the State. Very creditable operations in surgery are reported by Dr. G. Grant, of Newark, and Dr. A. N. Dougherty, of Newark; while Dr. B. L. Dodd, also of Newark, gives an obstetrical report of 100 cases, with practical comments; and statistical tables, &c., are furnished by Dr. Grant, the medical statistician of the State. Lithographic drawings, a map illustrating the topography of Orange, N. J., by Dr. S. Wickes, &c., add to the interest of this volume.

MALUM EGYPTIACUM—COLD PLAGUE, DYPHTHERIA, OR BLACK TONGUE. By Samuel A. Cartright, M.D., of New Orleans, La.

This pamphlet, from one of the most eminent physicians of the country, abounds in practical information vastly needed at this juncture. Of its author it may be justly said, " *Nihil tetegit, sed ornavit.*"

NEW YORK MONTHLY REVIEW OF MEDICAL AND SURGICAL SCIENCE, AND BUFFALO MEDICAL JOURNAL, for June, 1859.

The transfer of this Journal to New York, under its new title, is one of the results of the removal of Drs. Austin Flint, senior and junior, to this city, to the medical corps of which they will constitute a double acquisition, and we welcome both them and their Journal, and heartily wish them success.

ON THE FORMATION OF THE ARTIFICIAL ANUS. By C. Th. Meier, M.D., Surgeon to Bellevue Hospital.

This paper, which appears in the *Medical Monthly*, is now issued in pamphlet form. It was originally read before the N. Y. Medico-Chirurgical College, a new organization of physicians, surgeons, and Obstetricians of this city. Dr. J. O'Reilly, whose paper on Nervous Pathology appears in this number of the GAZETTE, is also one of the members.

EDITOR'S TABLE.

MEDICO-CHIRURGICAL COLLEGE OF NEW YORK.

Under this title a new Medical Association has recently been formed in this city, at the meeting of which on June 9th, we were present. As the minutes of the previous meeting were read, we obtained from the Secretary a copy; and deeming them of sufficient interest, we take pleasure in giving them place in the GAZETTE, and hope to report the proceedings of the new society monthly hereafter. Some forty or fifty of the working men of the profession have united in this movement. Papers are read, cases narrated, and pathological specimens are to be forthcoming, no less than eight of the latter being on the table, and commented on at length, at this late meeting, to be reported hereafter.

The College met May 26th. DR. ROBERT NELSON in the chair.

DR. MEIER read a paper on the Formation of an Artificial Anus; which is published in the AMERICAN MEDICAL MONTHLY.

DR. GARDNER said that the paper just read was extremely interesting to him for several reasons. He had witnessed several cases of this congenital difficulty, had reflected much upon the subject; and had listened, a few years ago, to quite a lengthened discussion upon the advisability of performing such an operation under any circumstances, save that when the occlusion was only by a simple membrane. At the Pathological Society of this city, where this discussion took place, there was a difference of opinion, but most of the surgeons inclined to the view that the operation was not warranted. This, it was said, was the opinion of Sir Benj. Brodie, and other of the English surgeons.

DR. GARDNER said, he had met with three cases of imperforate anus, the history of one of which would perhaps illustrate some of the views advanced in the paper read by Dr. Meier. He was called to see a child which had been operated upon by a trocar passed through the septum, between the *cul-de-sac* which existed at the normal site of the anus and the intestines, a distance of 1½ inch.

This wound made had partially healed, but he opened it again by passing a gum-elastic catheter, No. 8, injected tepid water, in this manner softened the fæcal matter, which passed out through the catheter. This operation he repeated daily for nearly two months, and after that he used graduated bougies, at regular intervals of one, two, three, or four weeks, thereby dilating the passage to a convenient calibre. The child is still alive, and is apparently well. It being a first child, there was the usual anxiety to preserve its life, notwithstanding this malformation, and to the excessive care and watchfulness of the mother may, in a great measure, be attributed the success of the manipulations resorted to. This case may show the result of a careful operation by means of a trocar in the perineal region, and the subsequent dilatation by artificial means. When the intestine is high up and has to be drawn down, Dr. G. thought the injury to the pelvic fascia would be necessarily so great as not to warrant the operation.

The other two cases he had seen, died; one was operated upon, the other not.

Dr. Dewees inquired if Dr. Meier had seen any case operated upon successfully in this manner.

Dr. Meier replied, that Amussat and Dr. Friedberg had both operated successfully; the cases he had mentioned in his paper. The case of Amussat was still alive in 1855, and was seen by Dr. Friedberg, who mentioned it in reporting his own case.

Dr. Dewees asked if there were any statistics as regards the relative frequency of this malformation in male and female infants.

Dr. Gardner remarked, that all the cases he had seen were male children. As regards the success of the operation, he believed that Dr. Batchelder and Dr. Sayre had both operated successfully through the perineum. Dr. B's case lived one year. He would inquire if in these cases there could be a re-formation of mucous membrane to line the artificial canal.

Dr. Budd asked Dr. Gardner if, in the case mentioned by him, the child had any control over the actions of the bowels, if there was anything which acted as a sphincter?

DR. GARDNER said, the great difficulty was to get a movement from the bowels; that there was more or less control over the bowels, but the great disposition now was to constipation.

DR. MEIER stated, in reply to Dr. Dewees, that he knew of no statistics upon the relative frequency of imperforate anus in the two sexes. Amussat, who has written a large volume upon the subject, makes no mention of this point. As regards this operation, simply as an operation, he thought there could be no objection to it. In Germany a surgeon would be blamed if he did not operate, and would render himself liable for damages. The operation through the perineum he preferred to all others, and the post-mortems performed by Amussat, upon the cases operated upon unsuccessfully by him in the groin or lumbar region, after a trial in the perineum, showed that if the perineal incision had been continued a little further, the lower extremity of the intestine would have been reached, and it might have been drawn down, the other organs being perfectly normal.

He thought the presence of muscular fibres in the perineal region would give an additional chance for the development of a natural means of retaining the fæces, which could not be if the operation was made in the lumbar or iliac regions.

DR. BRONSON said that the distance of the intestine from the perineum was not the longest on record, as Velpeau had recorded a case where it was ascertained to be three inches. The complication of the presumed passage between the intestine and the bladder was very important, as it had its bearing upon the chances of success in the operation. He had seen a case somewhat similar to the one reported, where the fæces were discharged through the urethra. An operation had been attempted, and it was said that gas had escaped through the wound, but no meconium. He had, in examining the patient, passed a probe up the wound in the perineum about ¾ of an inch, but could detect no entrance into the gut. He had not advised a repetition of the operation. The little patient continued to pass fæcal matter through the urethra. Whether the child was now living he did not know.

DR. CARNOCHAN was of the opinion that the surgeon should operate in all cases; for the attempt should be made to save life, however remote the chances might be.

DR. NELSON was of the same opinion; he thought an operation justifiable under any circumstances. In a legal point of view it is often very important, and is a surgical duty; not to operate is a dereliction of law. As to the pain, he esteems it of little importance, for he does not think there is much suffering in this respect in a young infant, whose nervous system has not been taught to suffer. As to the formation of mucous membrane, there was little necessity for it; a sort of pseudo-mucous membrane is produced in these cases, and often this occasioned the difficulty which arises in these cases, the same as in fistula in ano, which are lined with a membrane, if not mucous membrane, yet greatly resembling it. Dr. Nelson inquired if Dr. Meier thought there was any disposition towards a sphincter. Dr. Meier replied, that in one case, that of Dr. Friedberg, the action of the perineum was similar to the action of the sphincter, and after death the muscles of the perineum were found fairly developed.

DR. CARNOCHAN then presented two specimens of the calcaneus he had recently removed for disease of these bones instead of amputating, for which he had been consulted by the patients. In both instances they were discharging freely by a fistulous opening, and the health of the patients was greatly suffering.

There being nothing else before the Society, unfinished business was taken up, and the name by which the Society was hereafter to be known was discussed, and it was finally agreed that it should be called the N. Y. Medico-Chirurgical College.

DR. DEWEES was then elected Chairman for the next evening. Dr. Nelson, retiring from the chair, announced as the subject of discussion for the next evening, the Operation for the Exsection of the Os Calcis. After which the Society adjourned.

[For the MEDICAL GAZETTE.]

MAY 24th, 1859.

DEAR DOCTOR—I wish to call your attention to an advertisement in the London *Lancet*, republished in your city. It is an advertisement of the American Dispensatory, by John King, M.D., the eclectic partner of the detestable Cleveland. Is it proper for any medical journal to advertise the books of these quacks? Syme's Surgery, edited by Newton, another great eclectic quack, is set forth in the same advertisement, and care is taken to leave out the word *eclectics*, and the schools to which they belong, while Dr. Comegys, the translator of Renouard's History of Medicine, has his title and the name of the school (Medical College of Ohio) given in full. Now, if the publishers are to admit such advertisements, I, for one, will give them the benefit of a smaller number of subscribers in the West.

Will you, my dear sir, give your opinion on this matter in your Journal, and help those who are sorely tried with the *eclectics* in this city?

I am the more anxious that you should notice, as the influence and position of your Journal is felt all over the country; still more, the independence of the editorial department is so well known, that I am sure a few words from you will be of immense value.

A WESTERN READER.

[The foregoing communication is inserted because it reiterates a well-founded protest, which we and others have so often made against the American publishers of the London *Lancet*, and other foreign reprints, as well as certain medical journals, whose hunger for advertising pap tempts them thus to puff the most arrant quacks and their fraudulent plagiarisms. But this is only of a piece with certain New York medical book publishers, who not only sell the Eclectic and other quack books, but advertise largely and frequently in these quack journals, even announcing the eclectic forgeries in their catalogues! Cleveland, King, Newton, Sanders, *et id omne genus*, "steal their brooms *ready made!*" and can of course undersell their neighbors, who pay for their materials. Those publishers, instrument makers, or medical journalists, who either advertise in the Eclectic journals, or announce quack books of any kind, or insert their lying and brazen advertisements, should be ostracized by all true men, and all such should be put under the ban of the profession. So mote it be.—ED. GAZ.]

NEW YORK ACADEMY OF MEDICINE.

At the last meeting, Professor Smith opened the discussion on the Contagiousness of Yellow Fever, by reading an elaborate paper, condensing the testimony of the most eminent and trustworthy medical authorities, including that of the British, French, Spanish, and American physicians, all of which establish, beyond a reasonable doubt, that the old theory of contagion in yellow fever is now demonstrated to be utterly overthrown, and this by a multitude of incontrovertible facts which have been accumulating for half a century, and which perennial experience is everywhere corroborating; so that practical men nowhere countenance the idea of contagion in this disease.

Dr. Francis dissented from the paper, and made an earnest address.

We only wish that the equally baseless superstition of contagion in other epidemic and infectious diseases were as fully repudiated as in yellow fever, by Prof. Smith and every other medical teacher in the land. For, as American physicians were the first to explode this heresy of contagion in this fever, and compel all the medical world to abandon it; so should they be foremost in driving out of the profession the dogma of contagion in any fever but *small-pox*. The time is not distant when our profession shall see eye to eye on this subject, and the contagion of any other fever than variola will be annihilated, and only remembered as among the relics of ignorance and barbarism.

Dr. Stirling afterwards read a paper on Quarantine, and Dr. O'Reilly one on the Organic Nerves; which last was entirely original, and sustained by numerous vivisections. But it was kept back so late in the meeting, that very few remained to hear it. We opine that its merits will bespeak greater attention to it from foreign academicians than it received at home.

. Two original papers were received from Dr. B. Dowler, of New Orleans, but they were laid on the table, for lack of time.

UNIVERSITY OF LOUISVILLE.

The contemplated removal of Dr. L. P. Yandell to Memphis, Tennessee, has led to his resignation, which, from the kindly relations between him and his colleagues, is a source of mutual regret. It has, however, rendered it necessary to make some changes in the Faculty, amounting to a reorganization of this flourishing school. Medical Jurisprudence and Sanitary Science have been united into a distinct professorship, to which Professor S. M. Bemiss has been appointed. Pathological Anatomy and Clinical Medicine have been associated in like manner, and to this chair Dr. David W. Yandell has been elected; while Physiology has been divided among the other chairs in the school. We congratulate our brethren at Louisville on the judicious arrangement, and predict an increasing prosperity in the career of the University.

NOT A PHYSICIAN! BUT ONLY A HOMŒOPATH.

The Doctor King, recently hanged in Canada, and with a report of whose crime and punishment the public press is filled, was no doctor, but only a Homœopath; and as it is bad enough for our profession to bear the reproach of its own sins, we should not be confounded in the newspapers with those who do not legitimately belong to our fraternity, and whose fellowship we repudiate, though this is constantly

35

... ... reports of abortionism, forgery, poisoning and
... ... often ascribed to "doctors" in the published
... ... when it is notorious that the criminals are not physi-
... belong to the tribes of Homœopathy or other quackery,
... being purposely concealed, by the designation of
... in some cases, even calling them "physicians." Not
... all over the land, it was announced in capitals that a "re-
... physician had blown out his brains," when the parties who
... raised this calumny upon the profession knew that in this
... suicide had less claim to "respectability" than to medical
... and he, too, was a Homœopath. We remonstrated then,
... repeat our protest against the medical profession being treat-
... no other profession would tolerate. Shall the "members of the
... identified with every criminal pettifogger? Are the "clergy,"
... to be reproached by the publication of the crimes of every
Mormon elder, or spiritual trance preacher, by calling such impostors
... ministers of the Gospel," when they become suicides or murderers?
Or is it to be announced that an "editor" is in the "rogues' gallery,"
or "hanged," whenever some "penny-a liner" is punished by the law?
It is full time to "reform it altogether." Discriminate, if you please.

EXPENSIVE LUXURY.

One of the "weaklies," in a series of articles, is demonstrating that
our American medical colleges, for every 100 students, with 40 graduates, yield $4 ! to each professor ! for 6 months' labor ! And if
only 80 graduates and 90 students, then there is a *loss* to each professor of $11.14 ! These results are derived from figures, but are
after all only estimated, and on the average of all the schools. We
know some professors who would be grateful for the gain of even $4
per annum, and would pay largely if their annual loss were reduced
to only $11.14. And yet the ambition for professorships, even in such
schools, multiplies candidates for every vacancy, and they are raven-
ously sought, even by the very men who decry and depreciate the
schools. It is due to candor and truth, however, to add, that there
are medical colleges in the country which yield each professor an
annual income of from 3 to 6 thousand dollars, as the net proceeds
of each chair. This is the bright side of the picture, and ought to be
exhibited in contrast to the sombre view of the subject taken by our
weakly neighbors, the croakers.

THE FULL OF THE MOON.

In the N. Y. Academy of Medicine, among the circumstances in-fluencing the result of surgical operations, *the state of the moon!* was affirmed to be very important. One of the savans said that "opera-tions performed after the *moon* had attained its full, were more suc-cessful than those performed before it had done so." The chances of recovery after operations may be therefore calculated by the *Almanac*, to which surgeons and their patients should look. If some opera-tions we wot of were regulated by this *Lunarian* theory, they would be indefinitely postponed, for the patient would escape, by recovering without any operation. To account for the failure of many opera-tions is easy, when surgeons, so called, are "plenty as blackberries, and as *green* before they are ripe." To cover up unsurgical surgery under the lunary or astrological periods, is the "very error of the moon," better befitting the 16th century.

CONNECTICUT STATE MEDICAL SOCIETY.

This body has lately held its annual session, and we learn that the announcement that the next meeting of the American Medical Asso-ciation is to be held at New Haven in June next, was received with great satisfaction. Our brethren at New Haven will enter heartily into the work, notwithstanding the city will be crowded at the time by the session of the Legislature of the State. We anticipate one of the largest conventions of medical men ever held in this country, by reason of the attractions which gather about old Yale College and the city of elms. And we predict for the Association a hearty Yan-kee welcome.

DEATHS IN OUR RANKS.

Dr. Alexander Monro, known among anatomists as "Monro Tertius," his father and grandfather having preceded him in his pro-fessorship at Edinburgh, died April 10th of the present year.

Dr. Andrew Ranzi, Clinical Professor of Surgery at Florence, died recently, in that city.

Dr. Robert Mortimer Glover, of London, lately fell a victim to chloroform, during his experimental researches.

Dr. John Shelby, of Nashville, Tenn., is announced as recently de-ceased, æt. 74 years.

Dr. W. M. Boling, of Alabama, died lately in Montgomery.

COMMUNICATIONS.

OUR PHILADELPHIA CORRESPONDENT.

No. 13.

" This is the way physicians mend or end us,
  Secundum artem :—but although we sneer
In health—when sick, we call them to attend us,
  Without the least propensity to jeer."   BYRON.

  " The ingredients of health and long life are,
  Great temperance, open air,
  Easy labor, little care."   SIR PHILIP SIDNEY.

DEAR GAZETTE—You must not expect much news from our village
at this season of the year. In the first place, it is the most healthy
period of the year; in the second place, there is very little medical
teaching going on; and in the third place, the annual gatherings,
called conventions, are all over and gone. The last one we have had
here was that of the State Society.

This is the sixth time the Society has held its sessions in Philadelphia. The meeting was opened with prayer by an Episcopal minister,
and the delegates were welcomed to the city by a well-known reader
of Reports and Appeals, of our city, who said "the Convention were
the only legitimate representatives of the profession in the Key Stone
State." This of course excludes the " Northern Association," " Medico-Chirurgical College," " Phila. Medical Society," and the "College of
Physicians." The latter has been supposed to represent pretty much
all the dignity and science of the profession, not only of Philadelphia,
but of the United States; its President, we are told, some few years
since, preferring the presidential title to this institution as a card to
English society, to that of Professor of the University of Pennsylvania.

The President (a county member) delivered the usual Annual
Address, and an active member of the Philadelphia County Society
was elected President for the ensuing year, and the more important
offices were filled by other members of the Philadelphia delegation.

The next session will be held in Philadelphia; thus you see, if not a
Philadelphia Society, it is under the control of its medical men. The
number of counties represented have, heretofore, been less than half of
those of the State; a large proportion of the balance not having organized societies in them.

An attempt was made, by a party receding from the County Society, to have the old " Philadelphia Medical Society" represented in the Convention. This attempt failed—as all such have, and will. The matter of consultation with female practitioners and professors in Female Colleges was brought up, and, after considerable discussion, decided *against* such consultations. The objection made to the movement was, that it gave too much prominence to a set of quacks, who ought not to be noticed. .

Dr. Joseph Parrish introduced several of the feeble-minded children (idiots) from the institution under his charge, who gave an exhibition of their physical and mental improvement, which was received with much applause. We have visited said institution, and feel convinced that, through the physical, intellectual, and moral training of its inmates, much may be done towards bringing them up to a self-sustaining standard in the community; and this, by developing quite a number of their faculties. The "Institution for the Blind," which was visited by the Convention, bases its claims to public favor on the development chiefly of one faculty—that of music. In the latter case, less attention is necessary to the physical functions, there being little or no derangement of the health or strength of the patients; while in the former, the first great point to be attained is the proper development and balance of the physical structure, on which the intellectual and moral are to be built up.

This movement of Dr. Gugenbuhl will result in arresting the waste of humanity in one direction, and will save a large proportion of a very interesting part of the human species. Could it be preserved in other directions—infant mortality, intemperance, insanity, scrofula, wasting epidemics, wars, and the wear and tear of civilized society, &c.—we might hope for the ultimate elevation of humanity, prolongation of life, and the development of the higher virtues, in accordance with the wishes and aspirations of the philosopher and the philanthropist.

The Convention, after partaking of the hospitalities of some of our citizens, visiting some of the public institutions, electing its officers for the coming year, and attending to various other matters, adjourned at the end of the second day, to meet on the 2d Wednesday of June, 1860. This may interfere with the "National Association," at New Haven, Connecticut. The delegates next morning, Friday, June 10th, visited Atlantic City, bathed in the sea, dined in one of the hotels, and returned in the cars, at the expense of the profession of our city. Last year, it will be remembered, the excursion made was to the Lazaretto, which, by legerdemain peculiar to the Board of Health, was in part paid for by the city itself.

The weather in our city, thus far in June, has been a succession of very wet, very cool, and very hot days; producing thus early (nearly two months before the time) diarrhœas and dysenteries among the people; in other respects, the season is not a sickly one. Everything around the city betokens a full and abundant harvest, which the war, now raging in Europe, will probably make highly profitable to the farmer and the speculator. All kinds of fruit are, and probably will be, very plentiful; much greater attention being now paid than formerly to horticulture, in all its departments, as well as agriculture. Our strawberries this season are remarkably fine. It is true that the peach-orchards around Philadelphia are said to have died out, as well as many of the pear-trees, but a greater variety and abundance of the latter are cultivated at the North, while the quality and quantity of the former luscious fruit are much increased and improved by cultivators in Delaware, Maryland, Virginia, and other Southern States. Close attention to good sewerage, with the general cleanliness of the people, and the improvement of the times, make Philadelphia a remarkably healthy city. We are not cursed with the unnatural condensation of the population in confined and unhealthy localities, as is the case in some of our large cities; there is plenty of room and facility for the extension of the city, and almost every mechanic who earns from six to ten dollars a week can either rent or own his own house. Building Associations, which, it is known, have millions of money invested in them, especially among the Germans, facilitate very much the acquisition of a house by the persevering and industrious laboring man. The general observance of the Sabbath, which secures cleanliness, rest, and recreation, at least one day in seven, "for the ease of creation," tends at once to regulate the passions, secure the health, and improve the physical condition of the population of our Quaker city.

Just at present our people are crazy with the idea of constructing and using "Passenger City Railways." The comforts, facilities, and *bon marchè* of these conveyances, compared with the old lumbering and rickety omnibuses, increase the amount of travel enormously, which will no doubt result in some alteration in the character of our diseases. It is said the introduction of omnibuses into London increased the number of apoplexies and hæmorrhages by inducing people to ride who formerly walked. Another effect of the railroads (among us) is, the rapid extension of the city limits, preventing the aforesaid condensation of the people, and permitting all, both young and old, easy and daily access to the fresh air of the country.

Another matter which will add to our salubrity and morals is, the introduction of fountains and public city hydrants for the accommodation of the population in the great thoroughfares. The old city wells, whose waters have long since become useless by the impurity of the soil through which they pass, are to be reopened, hydrant pipes placed in them, to be kept cool for drinking purposes. This movement, though really inaugurated by the friends of Temperance in England, is here sustained by the community at large, and will no doubt, by the facility it will afford the thirsty wayfarer in obtaining, without money and without price, nature's beverage, result in great good to the cause of Temperance.

More attention still is necessary to the quality and quantity of water supplied to the city. Our "Fairmount Water Works," which, you will remember, succeeded those of Centre Square, though kept in full force, are not near sufficient to supply the wants of the city. Kensington and Spring Garden Water Works draw the water, one from the Delaware, the other from the Schuylkill River; and are said to afford a very impure and scanty supply of water. Some good-sized river (like the Croton in New York) should be turned *bodily* into our city, and such provisions made for the settling and purification of the water, as will secure at all times a fresh and healthy supply. This need of all large cities has ever required judgment and the expenditure of vast sums of money in supplying it, both in ancient and modern times. The aqueducts in and about Rome are among the most renowned monuments, which have stood for centuries, to the memories of Emperors, Popes, and wealthy citizens in the history of that great city.

An extensive plan and liberal outlay are necessary immediately in this direction, for the present and future wants of Philadelphia. Our rapidly increasing manufactories, as well as the general increase of the city, demand immediate attention to this subject. The burning of anthracite coal, different from the Western and other cities, where the bituminous is used, allows our atmosphere to remain comparatively pure, and free from those carbonaceous deposits which infect the air in other large cities.

Our moderate, provincial, or, if you like, Quaker habits, which, by curbing our desires, and restraining an inordinate ambition for the sudden acquisition of wealth, conduce, dear GAZETTE, (excuse the egotism,) to our health and longevity.

While the science and superior skill of our medical men not only protect us from the "coming disease" in the form of epidemics, but guard us in the hour of danger, when those physical afflictions are upon us, the medical profession of Philadelphia, high-toned, self-sacrificing, and second to no other in its practical application of the knowledge of the day, may be fairly put down as one of the blessings of the city, tending to increase the value of life, and the amount of health which we enjoy. Located as the city is, some sixty miles from the sea on the east, and an equal distance from the mountains on the west, we are not affected by the diseases produced by sea-air, or by those induced by the sharp winds of the mountains. A temperate latitude and location save us from the extremes of climate and locality; but I fear that I am referring too much to the real or supposed advantages of our city, and must curt my flying Pegasus, or perhaps subject myself to the charge of over self-laudation; this must be left to your own judgment, friend GAZETTE. In the mean time, our Medical Colleges remain in *statu quo;* their Deans are brushing up old announcements, or writing new ones. They are trying to "put their best foot foremost" in the coming contests for classes, men, and money. The few unsuccessful candidates of the past winter will probably pass through quietly, and obtain their diplomas in July. The belligerent leaders, who, during the present truce, are playing the amiable, the hospitable, and the courteous to each other, will soon begin to draw the lines of distinction between "your school and ours," and the autumnal breezes will waft in the raw material which is to form the armies of the allies.   Yours,   SENECA.

MISCELLANEOUS ITEMS.

Pure Blackberry Wine for Medicinal Use.—Mr. F. A. Rockwell, of Ridgefield, Conn., has turned his attention to the manufacture of a domestic wine from blackberry juice, adapted to medicinal purposes, in which the tonic and astringent properties which the fruit is known to possess, are fully preserved. This wine is pleasant to the taste, and will be readily taken by children, in many of whose bowel complaints it may be more useful than the drugs or nostrums generally used. It is to be placed on sale in the apothecary shops, so that physicians may prescribe it when they judge proper. The purity of this domestic wine, and that manufactured from grape-juice, is vouched for by most respectable testimony, and the proprietor is every way worthy of confidence. See advertisement.

New York Medical College.—Dr. E. R. Peaslee, of this city, has been appointed Professor of Obstetrics, &c., in the place of Dr. B. F. Barker, recently resigned.

Preparatory Medical Schools are multiplying, and Drs. Gaston and Talley have opened one at Columbia, S. C.

Amputation at the Hip-Joint, by J. Mason Warren, M.D., of Boston.—This entirely successful operation, rendered necessary by an osteo sarcomatous tumor of the femur, appears in a pamphlet, with a plate, depicting the formidable disease. We congratulate this distinguished surgeon on this achievement, which adds to his laurels.

Letter to each Delinquent Subscriber.

DEAR SIR:

Your bill for subscription to the *American Medical Gazette* remains unpaid, nor have I heard from you on the subject.

Please inform me in your reply whether you wish to continue your subscription.

An early answer will oblige yours, respectfully,

D. MEREDITH REESE,

NEW YORK, *July 1st*, 1859.   *Editor and Proprietor.*

Office of *Am. Med. Gazette*, 10 Union Square.

CONTENTS.

UNIVERSITY OF NEW YORK.
MEDICAL DEPARTMENT.
SESSION, 1859-60.

The Session for 1859–60 will begin on Monday, October 17, and will be continued until the 1st of March.

Faculty of Medicine.

REV. ISAAC FERRIS, D.D., LL.D., Chancellor of the University.

VALENTINE MOTT, M.D., LL.D.. Emeritus Professor of Surgery and Surgical Anatomy, and ex-President of the Faculty.

MARTYN PAINE, M.D., LL.D., Professor of Materia Medica and Therapeutics.

GUNNING S. BEDFORD, M.D., Professor of Obstetrics, the Diseases of Women and Children, and Clinical Midwifery.

JOHN W. DRAPER, M.D., LL.D., Professor of Chemistry and Physiology, President of the Faculty.

ALFRED C. POST, M.D., Professor of the Principles and Operations of Surgery, with Surgical and Pathological Anatomy.

WILLIAM H. VAN BUREN, M.D., Professor of General and Descriptive Anatomy.

JOHN T. METCALFE, M.D., Professor of the Institutes and Practice of Medicine.

J. W. S. GOULEY, M.D.. Demonstrator of Anatomy.

J. H. HINTON. M.D., Prosector to the Professor of Surgery.

ALEXANDER B. MOTT, M.D., Prosector to the Emeritus Professor of Surgery.

Besides Daily Lectures on the foregoing subjects, there will be five Cliniques weekly, on *Medicine, Surgery, and Obstetrics.*

The Dissecting-room, which is refitted and abundantly lighted with gas, is open from 8 o'clock. A. M , till 10 o'clock. P. M.

Fees for a full course of Lectures, $105. Matriculation fee, $5. Graduation fee, $30. Demonstrator's fee, $5.

UNIVERSITY OF BUFFALO.

Medical Department.—The Annual Course of Lectures in this Institution commences on the FIRST WEDNESDAY IN NOVEMBER, and continues sixteen weeks. The Dissecting-rooms will be opened on the first Wednesday in October.

Clinical Lectures at the Buffalo Hospital throughout the entire term, by Professors HAMILTON and ROCHESTER.

FACULTY.

JAMES P WHITE, M.D., Professor of Obstetrics and Diseases of Women and Children.

FRANK H HAMILTON, M.D., Professor of the Principles and Practice of Surgery and Clinical Surgery.

GEORGE HADLEY, M.D., Professor of Chemistry and Pharmacy.

THOMAS F. ROCHESTER, M.D., Professor of Principles and Practice of Medicine.

EDWARD M. MOORE, M.D., Professor of Surgical Anatomy and Surgical Pathology.

THEOPHILUS MACK, M.D., Lecturer on Materia Medica.

SANDFORD EASTMAN, M.D., Professor of Anatomy.

AUSTIN FLINT, JR , M.D., Professor of Physiology and Microscopy.

BENJ H. LEMON, M.D., Demonstrator of Anatomy.

Fees—including Matriculation and Hospital Tickets, $75. Demonstrator's Ticket, $5. Graduation Fee, $20

The Dean is authorized to issue a perpetual ticket, on payment of one hundred dollars.

Students who have attended a full course of Lectures in this or any other institution, will be received on payment of $50. The fee from those who have attended two courses elsewhere is $25.

For further information or circulars, address,

THOMAS F. ROCHESTER,

Dean of the Faculty.

ALBANY MEDICAL COLLEGE.

One Course of Lectures will be given at this Institution annually, commencing the *first* Tuesday of *September*, and continuing sixteen weeks. Degrees will be conferred at the close of the term, and also after the Summer Examination in June.

ALDEN MARCH, M. D., Professor of Surgery.
JAMES McNAUGHTON, M. D., Prof. of the Theory and Practice of Medicine.
JAMES H. ARMSBY, M. D., Professor of Anatomy
THOMAS HUN, M. D., Prof. of the Institutes of Medicine.

AMOS DEAN, Esq., Prof. of Med. Jurisprudence.
HOWARD TOWNSEND, M. D., Prof. of Materia Medica.
CHARLES H. PORTER, M.D., Prof. of Chemistry and Pharmacy.
J. V. P. QUACKENBUSH,M.D.,Prof. of Obstetrics.

Fees for the full course, $65. Matriculation fee, $5. Graduation fee, $20.

Material for dissection abundant, and furnished to students on the same terms as in New York and Philadelphia. Hospital Tickets free. Opportunities for Clinical instruction are believed to be equal to those afforded by any College in the country. Price of Board from $2,50 to $3,50 per week.

JOHN V. P. QUACKENBUSH, Registrar.

UNIVERSITY OF NASHVILLE.

Medical Department.—Session 1859-60.—The Seventh Annual Course of Lectures in this Institution will commence on Monday, the 2d of November next, and continue till the first of the ensuing March.

THOMAS R. JENNINGS, M. D., Professor of Anatomy.
J. BERRIEN LINDSLEY, M. D., Chemistry and Pharmacy.
C. K. WINSTON, M. D., Materia Medica and Medical Jurisprudence.
A. H . BUCHANAN, M. D., Surgical Anatomy and Physiology.

JOHN M. WATSON, M. D., Obstetrics and the Diseases of Women and Children.
PAUL F. EVE, M. D., Prof. of Prin. and Prac. of Surgery.
W. K. BOWLING, M. D., Institutes and Practice of Medicine.
WILLIAM T. BRIGGS, M. D., Adjunct Professor and Demonstrator of Anatomy.

The Anatomical rooms will be opened for students on the first Monday of October, (the 5th.)
A *Preliminary Course* of Lectures, free to all Students, will be given by the Professors, commencing also on the first Monday of October.
The Tennessee State Hospital, under the direction of the Faculty, is open to the Class free of charge.
A Clinique has been established, in connection with the University, at which operations are performed and cases prescribed for and lectured upon in the presence of the class.
Amount of Fees for Lectures is $105; Matriculation Fee, (paid once only,) $5; Practical Anatomy, $10; Graduation fee, $25.
Good boarding can be procured for $3 to $4 per week. For further information or Catalogue, apply to

PAUL F. EVE, M. D.,

NASHVILLE, TENN., July, 1859.   *Dean of the Faculty.*

CASTLETON MEDICAL COLLEGE.

There are two full Courses of Lectures annually in Castleton Medical College. The SPRING SESSION commencing on the last Thursday in February; the AUTUMNAL SESSION on the first Thursday in August. Each Course will continue four months. Degrees are conferred at the close of each term.

WM. P. SEYMOUR, M.D.,Prof. of Materia Medica and Therapeutics.
WILLIAM SWEETSER, M. D., Prof. of Theory and Practice of Medicine.
E. R. SANBORN, M. D., Prof. of Surgery.
WM. C. KITTRIDGE, A. M., Prof. of Med. Jurisp.

CORYDON LA FORD, M. D., Prof. of Anatomy.
P. D. BRADFORD,M.D.,Prof. of Phys. & Pathol.
GEORGE HADLEY, M. D., Prof. of Chemistry and Natural History.
ADRIAN T. WOODWARD, M. D., Prof. of Obstetrics.

FEES.—For Lectures, $50; for those who have attended two Courses at other Colleges, $10; Matriculation, $5; Graduation, $16; Board from $2.00 to $2.50 per week.

A. T. WOODWARD, M.D., Registrar.

CASTLETON, VT., Jan., 1859.

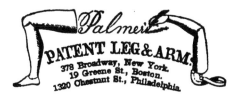

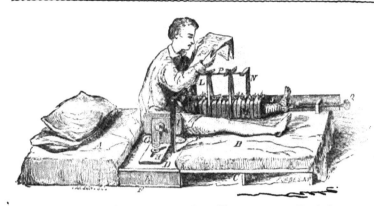

Burge's Apparatus for Fractured Thigh,

INVENTED BY

J. H. HOBART BURGE, M.D., of Brooklyn, N. Y.,

AND

WM. J. BURGE, M.D., of Taunton, Mass.,

has been thoroughly tested in actual practice, and has produced the most gratifying results. It is remarkably simple in its construction, easily applied, comfortable to the patient, adapted to fracture of either limb and to patients of any size. It is free from all the objections to which the ordinary straight splint is liable, and possesses other new features of great practical utility. By it the counter-extending pressure is confined to the nates and tuberosities of the ischia, and does not at all impinge upon the front of the groin, by which means one of the most frequent sources of annoyance and danger is obviated. No part of the body is confined except the injured limb and that to which it is immediately articulated, viz., the pelvis; thus the chest is left entirely unrestrained, and entire freedom of motion granted to the whole upper part of the body, which tends greatly to the comfort and health of the patient.

The pelvis is so secured as not to be liable to lateral motion or to sink in the bed.

Provision is also made for facility of defecation, thus insuring the greatest possible cleanliness, and preventing the necessity of disturbing the patient when his bowels are moved.

☞ Members of the profession may obtain this apparatus, complete in all its parts and nicely packed, by sending FORTY DOLLARS by mail or express to the address of

GEO. TIEMANN & CO.,

63 Chatham St., New York,

C. E. BORDEN,

Taunton, Mass., or

HIGBY & STEARNS,

· 162 Jefferson St., Detroit, Mich.

For further particulars see Transactions American Medical Association, Vol. X., and New York Journal of Medicine, May, 1857, and September, 1858.

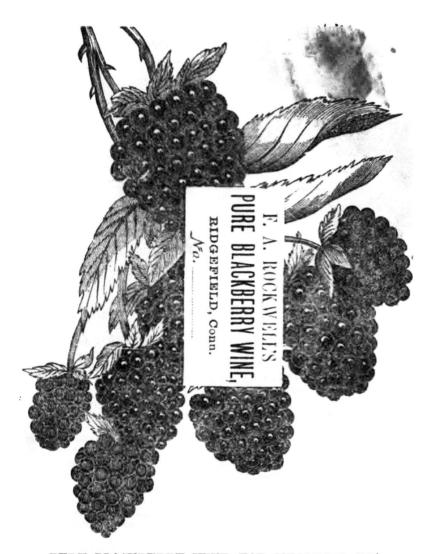

PURE BLACKBERRY WINE, FOR MEDICINAL USE.

Prices—Five Gallons and over, $2.50 per Gallon; $1 per Bottle; $10 per Dozen. Orders ? by the Case delivered in New York free of charge.

ALSO

PURE GRAPE WINE, FOR SACRAMENTAL AND MEDICINAL USE.

Prices—Five Gallons and over, $2 per Gallon; 75 cents per Bottle; $8 per dozen.

F. A. ROCKWELL, Ridgefield, Conn.

Agent in New York, E. GOODENOUGH, Bookseller, 122 Nassau St.

AMERICAN

MEDICAL GAZETTE.

| Vol. X. | AUGUST, 1859. | No. 8. |

ORIGINAL DEPARTMENT.

THE CONTAGIOUSNESS OF YELLOW FEVER!

BY THE EDITOR.

This is the question gravely proposed for discussion in the N. Y. Academy of Medicine, which, among its hundreds of members, scarcely includes a score who ever saw this fever, and still fewer who know anything practically of its epidemic nature or treatment. The information possessed by the mass of the brethren must be derived from books or teachers. All the older books, prior to this century, were written by contagionists; while nearly all the authorities, within the last 30 years, deny and repudiate the contagion of yellow fever, as has been shown in the able paper read in this discussion by Prof. Smith, and since corroborated by Dr. Harris. But the question is not considered settled, while there remain a few of the veterans of the olden time in our ranks, who adhere to the doctrine of contagion; and especially while any of the teachers in our schools, or any of our books of practice, continue to moot it, and hence this vexed question of controversy is still protracted.

It is in relation to our Quarantine system that this topic especially interests the profession and the public at this juncture, else it had never been brought here. If yellow fever be *contagious*, as is well argued, then it may be *imported;* and whether brought in ships by sea, or in railroads by land; whether it come by *persons* or *fomites*—if importation is possible, and it *is*, if it be contagious—then to prevent such importation is the highest duty of our Boards of Health, and would justify the most rigid Quarantine ever invented, at any sacri-

36

fice of money, trade, or commerce, and an impassable barrier should isolate our city from all intercommunication until all danger is past.

But if yellow fever is *not* contagious, then it is equally certain that it *cannot be imported*, either by land or water, neither by persons nor fomites; and hence all Quarantine, constructed on the contrary theory against this fever, is not only a needless expense, a wanton cruelty, a hideous outrage upon personal rights, but must of necessity prove a farce. To rely upon it for protection against a fever which may be of local origin, and hence overlook and neglect those sanitary measures, which, by removing the sources of the pestilence among ourselves, may allow the solar heat to generate yellow fever in our midst, is the very climax of folly. And yet this very absurdity is perennially perpetuated all over the land. Whether believing or rejecting contagion in yellow fever, medical men are everywhere found to countenance, uphold, and advise the persistence in all the superstitions which the contagious theory has engendered, from motives which we need not characterize. An enlightened Quarantine, against any *contagious* fever or malady, should be rigorously maintained, and hence the recent proposal to abolish all Quarantine finds no favor with practical men. But none is needed to prevent the importation of yellow fever, and for the reason that this fever is not, never was, and never will be, imported. And yet there are yellow fever ships, with passengers and crew who may or may not have sickened on the passage, but who if kept on board will sicken, but if sent on shore may escape. And in the event that any of them soon after develop yellow fever at our hotels, or with their friends, living in a healthy atmosphere, they cannot by possibility communicate the fever to anybody, for the reason that it is not contagious. But the Quarantine is still necessary, for such ships may be filled with infectious air, which, until they are cleansed and ventilated, may be sources of infection, poisoning all who inhale it.

The conflicting opinions which unhappily prevail, in and out of the profession, arise from the lack of discrimination between *contagion* and *infection*, not merely in these names, but in the things they respectively designate. And it seems to us that the profession owe it to themselves and the public, that such a body of medical men as constitute this Academy, should on so important a topic give no uncertain sound. Hence we should not only use terms which we understand ourselves, but which the public can interpret correctly, by requiring of us an intelligible definition adapted to the common mind.

In this brief paper, therefore, an attempt will be made both at definition and illustration, so that whatever may be thought of our opinions, all may perceive distinctly what we mean, without circumlocution or evasion.

Contagion, strictly speaking, is applied to diseases communicable by actual contact, or by equivalent proximity, to the sick by the well.

In this sense, the only contagious diseases are: 1st., syphilis; 2nd, gonorrhœa; 3rd, itch; 4th, erysipelas; 5th, hospital gangrene; 6th, the morbid poisons found in the dead bodies of animals, or in certain acrid vegetables; 7th, Egyptian ophthalmia, or other morbid secretions of animal bodies, as from certain mucous membranes, &c.; 8th, vaccina; and lastly, small-pox, which is the *only fever* thus communicable by contact.

Some of these require *im*mediate contact, others inoculation, by inserting the virus within reach of the absorbents, or upon the mucous membranes. Others propagate not only in these ways, but by *mediate* contact, morbid emanations being thrown off from the bodies of the sick and the dead, poisoning the air in close proximity, and thus communicating the disease to those who inhale it. The list given above is believed to contain all the maladies in this category.

Infection, though often used as a synonym of contagion, is now very generally distinguished from it wholly, and is applied to those diseases which do not require actual contact for propagation from the sick to the well, neither immediate nor mediate contact. This class originate in an atmospheric poison, a *materies morbi* in the air, the inhalation of which may produce the disease in the well, with or without a predisposition, by aerial contamination. This class are only communicable from the sick to the well in an unhealthy atmosphere, as in crowded and illy ventilated apartments, as in hospitals, jails, ships, or tenant houses, in which these diseases are found communicable from the sick to the well, who by such exposure become first predisposed, and then suffer an attack of precisely similar character. Or they may become endemic, i. e., the original atmospheric cause may contaminate more or less of the surrounding air, and infect all who inhale it, and such an endemic may develop an epidemic atmosphere of greater or less extent, and thus propagate itself.

Typhus, ship, jail, and hospital fever, cholera, dengue, yellow fever, remittents and intermittents, puerperal fever, scarlet-fever, measles, whooping-cough, mumps, influenza, diphtherite, &c., belong to this category, all of them *infectious* in an epidemic atmosphere, but none of them *contagious*, i. e., none of them communicable from the sick to the well in a healthy atmosphere. The sick being removed from the epidemic influence, and even dying ·in healthy districts, may be diligently nursed and attended without risk to the well, and this in all this class of maladies, for the reason that they are not contagious, nor communicable by contact.

Fomites, in the sense of the older writers, and in that of the recent resolution at the late Sanitary and Quarantine Convention, can only be predicated of contagion, and can have no possible application, either to yellow fever, or any other of the infectious or endemic diseases. Clothing and merchandise may carry a specific poison, as small-pox, and thus, as fomites, propagate this or any contagious malady. Hence the *importation* of this class of diseases it is the legitimate province of quarantine to prevent. But the importation of any article in foreign vessels, whether hides, wool, cotton, clothing, or provisions, cannot by possibility communicate the infectious or atmospheric epidemics, and hence they can never prove *fomites* of this class of maladies. But a vessel may bring infected air from an infected port, may infect passengers or crew on the voyage, or these escaping, may, on the hatches being opened at Quarantine, or at the wharves of a city, infect the surrounding air, which itself may become the " fomites," so to speak, of infection, to a greater or less extent, and a fatal endemic may thus be generated, if circumstances favor it by temperature and other agencies. Hence the cleansing, fumigation, ventilation, and whitewashing of such ships is the true business of quarantine officers, for disinfecting infected vessels, not from *contagion*, for there is none here; but from the infected air, which bears the poison of death in the form of an infectious atmosphere.

For the origination of yellow fever, and especially for its spread as an endemic, the heat of midsummer, 80 to 100° of F., must be continuous for weeks. If the humidity of the preceding spring have been great, and if the nights are cool, and malarious fevers are prevalent, these circumstances favor the development of yellow fever, and increase its extent and fatal malignancy. The combination of these circumstances is rarely witnessed in the Northern cities of our seaboard, but are frequent, or may recur annually, at New Orleans, Charleston, and other Southern ports, and in the W. I. Islands, as at Havana, &c. The fever is never prevalent anywhere without continuous heat, and ceases infallibly on the first autumnal frost. This ought to have precluded the idea of its being contagious, for the latter class are either unaffected by temperature, or, as with some of them, exclusively appear in cold weather. But this single fact no less conclusively points to the *local origin* of yellow fever, whenever and wherever it appears, and the sources of miasmatic exhalations, by heat, abound in those localities where yellow fever appears, and without an exception, intermittent, remittent, and other bilious, gastric, congestive, and inflammatory fevers are found to precede, accompany, and terminate with yellow fever epidemics. For, although at such periods all the concurrent maladies wear the livery and bear the type of the epidemic, yet the cases which, for the most part, are called yellow fever, are exceedingly various and unlike, presenting every phase of fever of the climate, modified by the malignancy of the prevailing yellow fever, though without many of its pathognomonic phenomena, and attended with much less fatality. During an epidemic, every variety of fever will be met with, admitted to be of malarious origin; and yet the malignant cases, differing only in the degree of intensity, congestive complications, and fatality; and hence called yellow fever, are most strangely and persistently ascribed by contagionists to some specific morbific cause, and their domestic origin denied, while the theory of importation is adopted.

It cannot be gainsayed, however, that by all history and all experience, all quarantine restrictions against yellow fever have been proved to be powerless in preventing its recurrence in those climates and under those conditions favorable to its origination. It annually reappears with the returning season, in many ports, into which the rigor of whose *cordon sanitaire* at Quarantine has rendered importation simply impossible. And that the sources and causes existing in the soil and climate of many tropical regions of the earth have often generated yellow fever, where no imagination could devise a suspicion of importation or foreign origin, is a conceded fact. Sporadic cases, indisputably characterized and authenticated, abound in the books, occurring in a single house, remote from all sources of contagion, sweeping off entire families; and where the local origin was proved by the attempts to remove the nuisances under the house, to which the disease was unerringly attributed; by which attempts every laborer perished by the same yellow fever which had destroyed the inmates. In like manner, after endemic visitations in many neighborhoods, the subsequent discovery and removal of the local causes have proved the local origin by totally preventing any recurrence, even when the circumstances were all favorable to its development. Just as certainly as the filling up of marshes or the draining of millponds have banished malarial fevers from neighborhoods which had been almost depopulated thereby, so also the yellow fever may be exiled from any locality, if the sources of its local origin are susceptible of removal. And it is only where the contingencies of climate and soil, heat and moisture, and the sources of miasmatic poison exist on so large a scale, and to such a vast extent as at Havana, New Orleans, &c., that sanitary science is powerless in suggesting a remedy. In such localities, Quarantines are worse than useless, for there is no importation in the case, the domestic origin of yellow fever resulting from a physical necessity, against which no restrictions can guard.

In multiplied instances the non-contagion of yellow fever has been proved beyond all successful contradiction by examples, in which the complete isolation of infected districts has been possible. And nowhere more demonstrably than in New York, during the epidemic of 1822, when the then Mayor first fenced up the infected streets, alleys, and houses, thus prohibiting all intercourse by land; and then employed boats on the river in removing all the remaining inhabitants from the infected district he had inclosed; and bringing both the sick and the well into the city, when it was proved that neither nurses, physicians, the public officers who stood at their posts, nor the grave-diggers who buried the dead, contracted the fever. So also in Baltimore, the section of Fells Point was thus isolated in 1819, and again in 1822, with precisely similar results. No single case of the fever occurred among the thousands thus removed, except the few who had been already infected, who sickened so soon that the origin of the disease was apparent. Thus the pestilence has been stayed in innumerable examples, when, if the fever had been contagious, or even contingently contagious, these precise measures would have depopulated the city and State; nor if contagion existed, could any part of the country communicating with New York, as in 1822, have escaped. It is a remarkable fact that these rational measures were dictated and carried out by men who, under the teaching of Dr. Hosack, were sturdy contagionists, showing that men may be muddled in their medical theories, and nevertheless sound in their practice. Such inconsistencies and self-contradictions inevitably characterize all the school of contagionists, as Dr. La Roche has abundantly shown in his great work on yellow fever, when commenting on Dr. Hosack, and especially upon Dr. Dickson, now of Philadelphia, whose recent edition of his book proves that while he theoretically clings to contagion, yet he disproves it by ignoring his theory, when he writes of the facts in practice testified by himself.

Let no one deceive himself into the belief that this is not a practical question, but a mere field of controversy. If yellow fever be *contagious*, it can be imported into New York by our daily and hourly arrivals, by sea or land, and our population may be decimated by its ravages in a single month; especially if *fomites* of any kind can carry this contagion. Every friend to the city and his race should become an alarmist; our force at Quarantine should be quadrupled, for yellow fever vessels are arriving daily. But if it be *not* contagious, contingently or otherwise, then peace and quiet may be proclaimed through all our borders, for we are in as much danger from leprosy or the plague; nor have we anything more to fear from the importation of yellow fever fomites, than if a cargo of broken legs were to reach Quarantine, we would have to apprehend that the legs of our citizens would be broken. The one is as "catching" as the other.

But there is a still graver practical mischief of this contagious theory, which affects our highest social relations and moral duties, and interests the public individually, involving not merely health, but life. In any city, visited by epidemic yellow fever, a belief in its contagion is the most fruitful source of its mortality, next to the equally baseless belief in its necessary fatality. The sick require for recovery the most tender and devoted attentions, from physicians, nurses, and relatives, which must be unceasing; but a belief in its contagion paralyzes effort, and excites fears which dry up the fountains of natural affection, and the sick are themselves prostrated by witnessing the terrors of all around. Personal safety often leads to flight, and the patients are too often neglected, if not deserted, for all that a man hath will he give for his life. Hence it comes to pass where contagious doctrines prevail, that the sufferers are left to the kind offices of strangers, the sick themselves often insisting upon the flight of their families and relatives, from despairing views inspired by contagion and its dangers. It is in such seasons that our profession, and their best assistants, female nurses, as at Norfolk, have to be summoned from abroad to minister to those from whom friends have fled, and whose removal from the infected district is impossible. Such martyrs are ever found to hasten at the call of duty, but they come from the ranks of the non-contagionists, to brave the infection at the peril of their lives.

It is hence that this subject derives its importance to the public, as well as our profession; and I have purposely, therefore, refrained from many salient points in the mooted controversy, which would have necessitated the citation of authorities, the detail of epidemics, and the multiplied theories which abound in the books on this subject of contagion, which has called forth more profitless controversy than any other in our literature. I have contented myself with this brief exposition of views, formed in the midst of yellow fever epidemics, with an ample field for observation, which, indeed, became my first experience in the profession, immediately after leaving the University. I have myself suffered a severe attack of this fever, by necessary exposure and toils in an infected district, where death seemed the rule, and escape the exception. It was my lot to witness scenes of pestilence never to be forgotten, and to mourn over the mischiefs of this theory of contagion, against which I was thus early an earnest protestant, as exemplified during the pestilence. I assisted in the measures then taken by the public authorities for mitigating the mischiefs of the epidemic, and in the sanitary measures to guard against its recurrence; and it was then that I was led to the high estimate I have ever since entertained of the paramount value of hygienic and sanitary measures, and medical police, and in this behalf have unceasingly labored ever since. It is thus that I have been led to take part in the present discussion. Of the relevance and worth of these thoughts the Academy will judge; of what is peculiar in my views upon contagion I am inclined to bide the ordeal of posterity, believing that the next generation of physicians will be disenthralled.

FOUR CASES OF RUPTURE OF THE UTERUS.

By AUG. K. GARDNER, M.D., Author of the Causes and Curative Treatment of Sterility, &c.

(Read before the New York Medico-Chirurgical College, June 23d, 1859.)

According to the statistics collected by Mr. Churchill, *rupture of the uterus*—the theme of this paper—occurs once in 1,331 cases. It is an acknowledged fact that it is not a consequence of prolonged labor, but on the contrary oftener occurs where the labor is speedy. It, therefore, is to be ascribed rather to an unnatural tenderness of the uterine tissues, which causes them to tear easily; to unusual violence of the uterine contractions, or to some impediment to the natural advance of the child, and the normal conclusion of the labor.

We are not compelled to go from home for our statistics, for our amiable friend, Dr. Trask, tells us that in 303 cases which he has collected, 16 were arm presentations, or one in about 16 cases; two breech cases, or one in 151 cases. As the proportional frequency of arm presentations is only one in 230 cases, and as breech cases occur once in 59 cases, the conclusion is that rupture of the uterus occurs oftenest in arm presentations, and very rarely in breech presentations.

But I do not intend to give the statistics or peculiarities of rupture of the uterus, for which I refer those interested to *Tyler Smith's Lectures on Obstetrics*, which I have recently edited, and will now proceed to give the report of those cases which have occurred to me in my professional walk in this city.

June 9, 1852, I was called to Mrs. Sweet, by Dr. Anderson, at 162 Wooster Street, in labor for several days. She had had two labors previously, one at seven months, and one died after a week's labor. She had been in severe labor, under the care of a midwife, since 1½ A. M. of the preceding day. At 9 A. M. Dr. Anderson first saw her, and found the cord prolapsing since 6 A. M., and without pulsation. When I saw her, at 3½ P. M., the os was not entirely dilated; as it was soft and yielding, and the pains slight, I advised secale canut. grs. x., every hour. The head presented, with the forehead to the right iliac anterior, which case is included in the category of the "forehead under the pubis."

At 10½ P. M., there being no change, I proceeded to perforate the cranium, an operation called for by the condition of the child and the length of the labor, yet delayed on account of undilated os uteri, and the fact that the head remained almost above the brim of the pelvis, scarcely entering the strait. The perforation was made with unusual difficulty, more than I have ever experienced up to the present time of writing this paper. This arose from the fact that the head was so high up, being almost out of reach, and there being great danger of wounding the promontory of the sacrum, which projected so much as to materially diminish the antero-posterior diameter. The tortuosity of the canal was so great as to make the danger of wounding the parietes or the undilated os very considerable, and only avoided by unusual time and care being devoted to this portion of the operation, and even then only at the expense of some severe injury to the hand which, within the vagina, guided the instrument. The head being finally opened, its contents broken up and evacuated, and its parietes collapsed, traction was vigorously made with the craniotomy forceps, and after the bulk was markedly lessened by the tearing away of the whole base of the skull, the head was brought down, making more than a half rotation in its descent. The shoulders were then delivered with great difficulty; one was towards the perineum, but returned at some distance in the strait. I passed a blunt hook into the axilla, and by strong effort delivered it; but when the arm was delivered it was under the pubis, thus effecting another half rotation in the same direction as the rotation when the head was extracted. The hook was again placed under the other axilla, like the former, towards the perineum, which was also delivered under the pubis. Vigorous efforts were necessary to deliver the abdomen, slightly tumefied, and again for the pelvis, which latter effected another rotation in the delivery. It should be noted that these rotations were all in the same direction. The placenta was soon removed, and the mother speedily and comfortably put to bed. The child was a male, weighing about 8 lbs.

August 4, 1853, I was again called to Mrs. Sweet by Dr. Anderson. She had been in labor since the 1st, the membranes rupturing at 4 p. m. The pains, however, were slight till the evening of the 3d, when she sent for Dr. Anderson at 10 p. m.; being out, did not see her till 10 a. m. the next day, when he immediately came for me. When I saw her, her appearance was very bad, having a hollow, ghastly look, clammy skin, which indicated some serious difficulty. She said that she had got along so poorly with doctors in previous labors, that she had determined to do without their assistance this time. I learned that her pains had been very strong all night, but about 6 a. m. they had suddenly almost entirely ceased, and that "she took a change" at the time. This intelligence made me suspect rupture of the uterus. On examination the abdomen was found very tender, but not tumefied. Placing her in position, a continuous flow of semi-putrescent and grumous fluid was noted. The head was discovered presenting, but so far distant, and apparently anterior to the pubis, that it could scarcely be felt by the ordinary surgical examination. On introducing my hand I discovered a flap, which at first was supposed to be an elongated neck of the uterus, but which was discovered to be the torn edge of the uterus. Being unable to move my hand freely, on account of the great narrowness of the antero-posterior diameter—so great as to press painfully, while making any attempt at rotating the head, upon my wrist—which is $2\frac{1}{4}$ inches in its long diameter, I withdrew it. On introducing the left hand, and passing within this "lip," I encountered the placenta, detached in its whole extent, and the occiput in the left iliac fossa; found one foot, and immediately brought it down; the other followed, and in a few moments the child was turned and delivered. The child was a female, of about 6 lbs., semi-putrid. The shoulders and head, much flattened, were delivered with some difficulty; placenta immediately followed, accompanied by firm uterine contractions.

On withdrawing my hand after the first introduction, the uterine contractions were so prompt as to eject a quantity of blood to the distance of two feet from the vulva. After the delivery the patient felt exceedingly prostrated; took some brandy and water with partial relief, and soon fell asleep. Pulse 148, and soft. She died the next morning, at 6 A. M.

Post-mortem made by Dr. Dalton. Abdomen somewhat tumefied, and resonant on percussion. On opening, slight peritonitis, and a small quantity of lymph on the peritoneal surface of the uterus, ovaries, and appendages. The uterus, &c., were removed, and on the anterior surface, immediately in relation to the pubis, a rent was discovered, filled with clots of blood, 6 inches in length, and almost severing the cervix from the body of the uterus.

On measuring the diameters of the pelvic strait, the antero-posterior was $2\frac{7}{8}$ inches, and the transverse $4\frac{1}{8}$. The specimen now exhibited was deposited by me in the museum of the N. Y. Medical College.

CASE II.

December 20th, 1853, was called at $10\frac{1}{2}$ A. M., by Dr. Daniel Adame, to Mrs. Reilly, 45 Harrison Street, in labor with her fifth child; her previous children being all dead-born and "cross-births" She was about 38 years old. Labor commenced at 4 A. M., and Dr. A. saw her immediately after. The os was fully dilated, and the pains regular and good, without any extravagant action. At about 8 A. M., the breech presenting sacrum to left, and the labor so far advanced that the female genitals of the child were visible, congested and dark, through the labia of the mother, and the doctor expected that in a few more pains she would be safely delivered. Suddenly, without any apparent reason, his attention was drawn to the more than usual retrocession of the child after the expulsive effort, and finally to the entire disappearance of the presenting portion, which had not receded after the last few pains. Vomiting now first commenced, and on the doctor passing his hand over the abdomen, he was surprised to find that the large soft uterine tumor had almost disappeared, and immediately under the abdominal parietes, which wer flaccid and yielding, was a hard tumor, evidently the head of the child, escaped into the peritoneal cavity, through a rent in the uterine walls.

On arrival, I found the head, as above described, in the region of the umbilicus, and agreed in the diagnosis of a ruptured uterus. At Dr. A's request, he first administering chloroform, I introduced my left hand, and easily finding one foot, brought it down, at the same time partially feeling the laceration near the pubis. Applying a blunt hook in the groin, the other leg was with some difficulty brought down, and by the same means each arm successively. The head, however, remained firmly fixed; and the cord showing that the child was dead, I punctured the head through the occipital bone, near the junction with the cervical vertebra, and diminishing its bulk, with the crotchet delivered the child. The placenta was lying detached, and nearly a quart of blood followed. The woman was then carefully bandaged, although her abdomen was tympanitic, and some brandy and morphia administered. This she soon vomited. She was at his time much prostrated, her pulse feeble, and at times almost imperceptible; the face looked badly, which it did when I entered. During the day and night following she took morphine freely, about ½ g every hour; also brandy, and occasionally inhaled a few drops of chloroform to mitigate any excessive pain. The next morning the abdomen was tympanitic; turpentine was applied to the abdomen with marked relief. In five minutes after its application she said that a flow was commencing, there having been none previously, which much mitigated her pain. At 4½, P. M., her pulse was 114, a not e

The rent was afterwards made out to be a longitudinal one, runn through the cervix and os uteri, and opening the walls of the ble How far it went into the body of the uterus was not fully deterr After various experiences, a year or more after, she was ope d upon in the Woman's Hospital, by Dr. Sims, and fully cured.

CASE III.

June 17, 1856, was called by Dr. Lewis Smith, at 10 A. M., to M W——, West 47th Street, who had had several children. She as taken ill the evening previously, and endeavored to get along with medical attendance, but finally sent for Dr. S., and he subsequently called Dr. Husted, who in vain attempted to turn. I saw her about noon. Dr. Smith found an arm and the cord presenting and the head within reach, and had brought down a foot. About an hour before I saw her, notwithstanding sh·had taken full doses of morphine, the pains continued very violent, and finally she felt something give way, and her pains then immediately ceased, and vomiting and collapse supervened. Dr. S. then succeeded in bringing down another foot, and when I saw her, the pelvis and lower extremities of a dead female child were delivered. The pulse of the mother was 146, the countenance haggard, and every indication present of there being severe local difficulty. With the blunt hook I delivered the arm, perforated head through the occiput, and finally delivered a large girl. In the afternoon she was permitted by the attendants to get out of bed, when hæmorrhage took place, and she died the next morning.. No autopsy was allowed, and the character of the lesion could only be surmised.

CASE IV.

May 26, 1858, I was called, at 3 A.M., to Mrs. Doyle, 72 Elm Street, by Dr. Simmons. She was in her seventh childbed—all previously without difficulty, but protracted. Labor had commenced at 12½ A. M., of the same day, when the membranes ruptured and a very large quantity of water escaped. The hand came down immediately, and when Dr. S. was called, he reports that there was no pulse at the wrist of the child, and the pains excessively violent. When I arrived he had given her laudanum, gtts. xxx., the right hand and arm was out of the vulva, the thumb to the pubis, and the position abdomino-anterior, with the head to the right. Dr. S administered chloroform, and I introduced the left hand, seized one foot, turned and delivered to the head, which sticking with the occiput under the pubis, and the fingers in the mouth; not sufficing to immediately extract it, at the same time using all justifiable force upon the body, I applied my tractor over the os frontis lying towards the sacrum, and speedily and easily delivered a fine male child, evidently some time dead, as there was no beating perceptible in the cord when the hand was introduced. The mother made a speedy getting up.

May 29*th*, 1859, I was again called by Dr. Simmons, to Mrs. Boyle, in her eighth labor. She had been kept awake during the night by premonitory pains, but Dr. Simmons was not called till 7 A. M. Os then undilated, and no presentation discovered. At 1 P. M., the membranes ruptured, and an immense quantity of water escaped. At the next pain the head and arm were thrust completely out of the vulva. The pains which ensued were very violent, and I was sent for, and arrived at 3 P. M., when I found her bathed in a cold sweat, pains persistent, but not violent; some vomiting. The abdomen tympanitic and tender to the touch. The right hand and arm were entirely protruded from the vagina, black and without movement. The thumb was towards the pubis, and the position was the back anterior, and the head on the left side of the mother. Chloroform was administered, and I then proceeded to introduce the left hand, easily effected, seized one foot, and withoutdifficulty turned, and brought down the other leg without any trouble. In introducing the hand into the uterus, the movements were somewhat restrained by what seemed to be the loose edge of the placenta, attached to the right side of the uterus and near the os, (as described by Dr. Barnes in his paper on "placenta prævia," and which position he gives as one of the causes of abnormal presentations.) A dark grumous fluid escaped along the arm in considerable quantities. The delivery was effected speedily and without force, except the head, which remaining in the strait— the cord having a scarcely perceptible pulsation—I did not think it justifiable to make any traction; and as it did not easily rotate with the finger in the mouth, I passed my vectis into the bottom of the sacrum over the forehead of the child, and without the least effort delivered. The child, a female, did not breathe. The placenta was detached, and immediately followed the child.

Immediately after the effect of the chloroform was passed away the patient complained of great pain in the abdomen, for which paregoric was administered and turpentine placed over the entire abdomen, which vesicated considerably, (and the blisters of which were subsequently filled with pus.)

No thought was given that there was any uterine lesion at this time, nor until the next morning, when I was sent for, with the statement that she had a vesico-vaginal fistula, as the water was flowing from her unrestrainedly.

Upon making an examination, it was discovered by passing a catheter that there was a rent in the vesico-vaginal septum, longitudinally with the vagina, and following this up it was found to run through the os and cervix uteri into the cavity of the uterus as far as the finger could pass.

The rupture of the uterus being thus determined, the Tinct. Opii was given as freely as was necessary to keep her quiet and free from pain; and the pulse, which was hard and firm at 140, was reduced somewhat in character and rapidity, and the profuse colliquative perspiration was checked. The subsequent day the tympanitis was relieved, and the dangerous condition apparently much diminished. The third day the pulse went up to 130, although taking Tinc. Opii. gtts. xxx. every hour. On taking gtts. of the Tinct. Verat. Virid., vomiting ensued, and by the next morning, when I saw her at 7 A. M., the pulse was 160, very flickering, and she died perfectly conscious and without pain at noon. No post-mortem permitted.

RESUME.

Of these four cases, one was a breech presentation, and three arm presentations; none of them primaperas; all of the children were females.

From the consideration of the case cured and the last case, both of which resemble one another in the character of the lesion and the causes of this injury, two thoughts are suggested. Do not the longitudinal ruptures occur more frequently than is supposed, oftener than those going around the cervix or in the fundus of the uterus? and secondly, are not ruptures of the uterus frequently overlooked, the same constitutional symptoms supervening after a difficult labor being considered to be the results of an unusual hæmorrhage, occurring, perhaps, from a detached placenta—to severe after-pains—or to puerperal fever, which has been developed with great virulence? I think that we should be more particular in making vaginal examinations after the placenta is delivered, in all those cases where intense fever and other constitutional symptoms come on with so much virulence and so immediately after the birth of the child.

NEW YORK, 141 E. 13th St.

AMERICAN INSTITUTE, *July* 2, 1859.

The July number of your MEDICAL GAZETTE, whose tone is ever bracing—*tonic*—shows the vanity of Hahnemann's nonsensical theory *heroically* in the case stated by T. J. Heard, M.D., of Galveston, Texas. The rescue from death by *an ounce of calomel* at one dose! a quantity which, divided homœopathically, say two billions of times, one part being a dose, would, if said one ounce had been administered in the same allopathic style as Dr. Heard's, form a mass of mercury of two billions of ounces—a weight which all the ships and vessels of the world could not carry!

If the homœopath doctor was kept for one month on like infinitesimal pills of bread, butter, meat, and drink, *he would be cured!*

How strange it is that experience should be so utterly lost upon us! From Hippocrates the *Rarey of old horse tamer*—should picked up facts for a hundred years himself to make out his aphorism—that millions of intelligent physicians have been gathering *experience* for ages in vain! As to doses of medicine, one may pun, and say "*experientia doseit.*" Your lines from Scaliger are wisdom. I turn them into plain English, as follows: "We are not men by any means! each is only a part of a man; something might be made out of all men—not great; but out of a single individual, next to nothing."

Julius Cæsar Scaliger, of Verona, was first a soldier, and in the battle of Ravenna, in 1512, lost his father and brother, and his mother died of grief. He was wealthy, became very learned, and lived until 1558.

Your reinforcement of the absolute necessity "of continuous observation" repels, like the electric negative pole, the modern *ism* in medicine. I feel compelled to consider these isms as *animalisms* instead of our true and only glory, *rationality.*

Long may you live to preserve that *priceless treasure of medical experience* for which you are the most able, fearless, and faithful *defender of the truth.* With great respect and esteem, I am yours always,

H. MEIGS, *Recording Sec'y of the Am. Institute.*

SELECTIONS.

Remarks on the Proceedings of the late Quarantine Convention, held at New York.

By B. DOWLER, M.D.

"NATIONAL QUARANTINE AND SANITARY CONVENTION, COLLEGE OF PHYSICIANS AND SURGEONS, New York, April 30, 1859.—On motion of P. M. Wetmore, amended by J. McNulty, M.D., it was ordered—That the Secretary be authorized to publish the record of the resolution of A. H. Stevens, M.D., and the vote thereon, as adopted at the preceding session of the Convention.

"*Resolved*, That in the absence of any evidence establishing the conclusion that yellow fever has ever been conveyed by one person to another, it is the opinion of this Convention that personal quarantine of cases of yellow fever may be safely abolished; *Provided*, That *fomites* of every kind be rigidly restricted."

This resolution, with its proviso, is the great result arrived at by the late Annual National Convention with an almost complete unanimity, the affirmative vote being eighty-five, the negative six only.

This adjudication has been hailed as definitive! Altogether satisfactory! A new foundation for sanitary legislation!

In no spirit of contradiction—with no wish to dissent from the opinions of the highly respectable National Convention—with no purpose to lessen the internal or external influence of the medical profession in the opinion of the public, by exposing its dissensions, a journalist may sink expediency in that of the well-being of society; he may be allowed to examine the dicta of an influential organization in matters which concern health, life, commerce, sanitary legislation and police. He may claim, until the contrary appears, the same honorable motives which govern those from whom he may reluctantly venture to differ in regard to unsettled questions of science, especially such as are supposed to be well or ill-adapted to promote health and prevent epidemics. Unawed and unbiased by great names and official proclamations, his duty requires neither silence nor acceptance contrary to his conscience and reason. The majority is not always right, nor the minority always wrong.

From the resolution with its proviso as above quoted, and from the debates of the Convention as already published, it appears that while this distinguished congress voted yellow fever to be non-contagious, goods or their fomites are voted to be contagious—" things, not persons, being the cause of the communicability of yellow fever."

Among the ninety-one votes cast on this memorable occasion, it is highly probable that not ten of the voters ever witnessed an epidemic of yellow fever, although some of the delegates professed to have read as high as three hundred volumes on this disease!

" *Prince Henry.* O, monstrous! but one half-penny worth of bread to this intolerable deal of sack! What there is else keep close; we'll read it at more advantage." " One half-penny worth" of logic will show that the proposition of the proviso stultifies and even virtually contradicts that of the resolution, as well as the fundamental ideas of nearly all that portion of mankind not members of the National Quarantine Convention.

> "Chief Justice Parker
> Made that darker,
> Which was dark enough before."

It is not intended on the present occasion to write a polemic for or against the contagiousness of yellow fever. Nor is it intended to attempt an exposition of the history, mystery, and expediency of quar-

antine in general.   A few remarks, however, upon the supreme result
of the late Quarantine Convention held at New York (which is one
of high import to the well-being of society, and deserves a closer
scrutiny than can now be given) may be allowable.

Yellow fever, it is said, originates from fomites; exclude fomites
and yellow fever is thereby excluded.   This truism is as evident as
that a part is less than the whole.   If Latin be more potent than the
mother tongue, here it is: "*Sublatâ causâ, tollitur effectus.*"   Fomites,
says the Convention, are in *things*, not in *persons*; therefore exclude
things, not persons, and yellow fever is thereby excluded.   This is
self-evident if the premises be true.   Eighty-five votes were, in this
case, wasteful and unnecessary, even though the members had neither
witnessed an epidemic yellow fever, nor read a book upon it.   Their
mothers would have told them so.   But what are fomites?   Definitions, typical examples, criteria, or some recognized standard must
be appealed to and universally admitted outside of the mad-house, else,
like the builders of the tower of Babel, no one will understand
the other.

" *Fomites.*   A term applied to substances which are supposed to
contain contagious effluvia; as woolen goods, feathers, cotton, etc."
Dr. Dunglison's Dictionary.

Fomites are not mere words. . Yet even in New Orleans, where the
ens epidemicum ought to be known, nothing is yet known but such hard
words.   The people, however, are in advance of the doctors in nomenclature, and withal more poetical; as they usually personify the great
unknown Ens by calling it YELLOW JACK, instead of *Fomites.*   Mother
wit against abstractions and hard words!

The popular mode of dealing with Yellow Jack among the unacclimated is, not by fumigation, but by running away to places where
his presence, for the time being, is not indicated by symptoms. ' As
they have not discovered fomites in things, they carry their things,
clothing, boxes and baggage, with them.   When the yellow fever declines, they return without fear to houses which sometimes had been
totally depopulated by death from this fever—houses shut up for
weeks after the last tenant had gone to the graveyard—houses from
which no one had attempted to remove the unknown fomites.   Thus
immediately after the subsidence of the great epidemic early in the
season of 1853, a vast number of persons returned to, or arrived at
New Orleans without having suffered from fomites in the things or
houses of the dead.

The Board of Health of New Orleans, in an official announcement, shows, for the month beginning with the 26th of November, 1853, that 6,707 passengers from foreign ports, chiefly immigrants, had arrived at our wharves in forty-seven sea-going vessels, by the river route. Now, if we add the number which had previously arrived, to the number which afterwards arrived from sea, the aggregate will scarcely fall below 10,000; while by other routes, chiefly by the river, the emigrants, absentees, and other unacclimated persons, as the steamboat population coming to the city, in September, October, November, and December, forty thousand more may be added, making fifty thousand—fifty thousand living experiments against contagion—fifty thousand exposures to fomites—the houses, goods, etc., of persons recently dead, including emanations from the few still sick, and yet, so far as the most careful observation could determine, the newcomers escaped all danger from yellow fever, although the weather was considered favorable for the extension of the disease. After the end of October, the deaths from this fever did not amount to thirty, although, as already stated, thousands of unacclimated persons were arriving, or soon after arrived, numbering about fifty thousand exposures to the assumed fomites of things. Medical history probably furnishes no example parallel with this in significance and extent.

Fomites exist, or they do not. If they are positive entities, what are they? whence are they? where are they? how many? In the name of fourscore and five witnesses, what are their sensible properties? Do they exist in all parts of space except such as are specially occupied by human bodies? Give their qualitative and quantitative analyses independently of the personality. Say, ye fourscore and five witnesses, who know and who vouch for these positive entities or fomites in *things*, which cotton, wool, and feathers, ought to sweep in a few weeks faster than and even against the winds over the continents of Asia, Africa, Europe and America, say, what are the characteristics of cholera fomites? influenza fomites? dengue fomites? typhus fomites? diphtheritic fomites? plague fomites? yellow fever fomites? Are all these in things, not in persons? Will they succumb to quarantine? or can they be "*restricted*" by it? Can fourscore and five restrict fomites without knowing them, without being able to point them out, as well the cotton and other *things* which they have actually entered and possessed?

The constituents of the Convention doubtlessly expected, as usual, that this assembly would explain the *ens epidemicum*, and point out the means of prevention—a feat never yet performed, so far as is known, in regard to a single epidemic. A short and plain route is open to such as admit that they are not born to solve the problems of the universe —namely, an honest confession of ignorance. To such as study the laws of Nature, without affecting to know the essential origin and connection of cause and effect, this confession is easy, because it is true. Newton, for example, investigated the laws of gravitation—the cause of gravitation was entirely beyond his gigantic grasp; indeed, he looked upon the cause as a perpetual volition of the Deity.

No one is bound to testify to what he does not know in order to please the public. If the cause of yellow fever does not originate in the human body, it does not follow that it must, as the only possible remaining alternative, originate in the air. The stars, the earth, metals, water, insects—in a word, everything known and unknown, may be a possible cause or antecedent, so long as nothing is positively known in the premises. No one can say that *things*, cotton, wool, feathers, cloths, lemons, etc., will not originate or carry the cause of yellow fever. All that can be said is, that this assumed origin and conveyance of fomites have not been proven by fourscore and five votes or otherwise.

So long, therefore, as the essential cause of yellow fever is unknown, no convention, least of all one not experimentally acquainted with yellow fever, can vote intelligently whether it originate in any one thing in the heaven above or in the earth beneath, without having carried out a twofold exhaustive process, namely, the synthesis and the analysis of all things in the universe; for, if one be left out, that may be the *causa vera*.

While, therefore, the personal contagiousness of yellow fever is scarcely probable in any well-accepted meaning of contagion, it is not a thing to be voted upon absolutely by yeas and nays. At least, those who vote against contagion, and yet know the dreadful fomites very well, as something very different from personal contagion, ought to sustain the *onus probandi* of their anomalous position. They ought, at least, to give some analogical evidence, derived from some indisputably contagious disease, as that of measles or small-pox, in order to show that yellow fever, itself perfectly innocuous *in persons*, will, nevertheless, communicate fomites to *things*, and thereby cause epidemics. The small-pox is communicated personally, and by things; by a direct contact, by a direct emanation, or by garments sent to a distance, or by the lymph or scab, as in inoculation, or by other less obvious means; always, however, more energetically by the near presence of the patient.

Admitting the very thing to be proven, namely, the contagiousness of the yellow fever thing, that is to say, its communicability by fomites contained in clothing, wool, cotton, etc., still the contradictory proposition, that the person affected with this disease cannot communicate it to another person otherwise than by means of goods, wares, merchandise, seems fundamentally contrary to the common-sense idea and all the known analogies of contagion. Yellow fever or yellow fever fomites (fomites, literally any thing that kindles or keeps the fire in) cannot exist without the subject in which it inheres. If there be any positive or sensible entity known as yellow fever fomites originating without the human body, it must be, according to the prevalent, yet *untenable* theory, an aerial infection, not an infection originating in articles of merchandise, as feathers, wool, cotton, mail matter, etc. If it be aerial, and exist independently of the yellow fever patient, no method has yet been devised for quarantining the wind. If the fomites originate with or come from the yellow fever patient, and be communicable by cotton and other merchandise, it must, *à fortiori*, be far more communicable by, with, and from the patient. If there be no fomites or harmful substance in or emanating from the patient, he can communicate none to his clothes, goods, chattels, wares, or merchandise. A contrary supposition is at war with facts, physics, and metaphysics. The fomites in goods, which pre-existed in the patient, must be, judging from analogy in the latter, of far greater intensity. Small-pox or measles may sometimes be transmitted by goods, but far more by the presence of patients suffering from that malady, as already mentioned. Perhaps a single person might communicate small-pox to the majority of the human race, not already protected, could all be brought within the circle of the contagious emanation. It would, however, reverse all that is known as fundamental in contagion or fomites, to assume either that a cotton bale which had never imbibed the contagion or fomites of small-pox, could nevertheless originate or communicate that disease; or, that while the garments of a small-pox patient are dangerous, and should be detained, washed, fumigated, or burned at quarantine stations, the patient himself should be sent into the bosom of society without detention, as being incapable of fomites. The same reasoning applies to the assumed fomites of yellow fever, in order to give consistency to this conventional logic.

It is reasonable to assume that the fomites of yellow fever, when discovered, will not prove to be either ordinary filth or simply impure air, but some specific, peculiar local agent, which produces a specific or peculiar disease—not any disease indifferently, as cholera, intermittent, rheumatism, small-pox, typhus, etc. If the material cause or fomites of yellow fever (the auxiliary influences of locality being unknown) were appreciable and could be readily identified by the naked eye, by the microscope, by chemical or other criteria, as a concrete, gaseous or mixed substance or ens, whether vegetable, animal, mineral, or something else, it might happen that these fomites, thus occasionally or periodically developed in one locality, would not flourish, though transported to another, as is known of many plants and animals. A remarkable fact adverse to the doctrine of transmissible fomites, (of which cotton is alleged to be one of the most certain carriers,) is witnessed in every year, namely, the continued shipment of cotton from New Orleans to the great *emporia* of the world, where this cotton from this port is manipulated and worn by, perhaps, one-half of Christendom, without having as yet carried yellow fever in that direction. As the exportation of cotton increased yellow fever declined in peninsular Europe, where it formerly prevailed with unexampled violence. It is not known that cotton extinguished those great epidemics; but it is known that they have not increased at the ports where New Orleans cotton has been sent in a constantly increasing quantity, (as at Liverpool, Havre, etc.,) and that, too, during the period in which yellow fever has been most active and deadly in this city. Fomites thus harmless need no fumigation, not even resolutions nor provisos by which useless quarantines are maintained, for the sole benefit of their officers, dependents and appointees in convention assembled, or elsewhere. Long ago I alluded to another remarkable circumstance or coincidence which has a bearing on the fomites of yellow fever, namely, that during the most stringent enforcement of quarantine, as in the peninsula of Europe and in Louisiana, this disease prevailed most. This may have been wholly accidental; but it shows that quarantine, as it regards things as well as persons, is not known to be useful. This accidental parallelism between quarantine and yellow fever in New Orleans continues.

Hypothetical phrases, as fomites, constitution of the air, epidemic constitution, malaria, *ens epidemicum*, etc., are worse in a scientific point of view than the personification of yellow fever under the name, YELLOW JACK, as the former terms virtually assert that the cause is known substantively, having physical, chemical, or sensible properties, as if it were an animal, vegetable, mineral, gaseous or liquid substance. Such evidence would be rejected at once in a court of jurisprudence, and, *à fortiori*, in a court of science. Analogy, it is true, teaches that yellow fever, as well as small-pox, has a cause, and that this cause may possibly be discovered and prevented. Among the many causes to which this fever has been ascribed, some may be the *causa vera*, but until the latter shall be proven, nothing will be discovered, even though both houses of Congress and the Convention should unanimously pass the strongest resolution to the contrary. Physical causes must be established by physical evidence, and not by a majority of votes.

Of the great majority of diseases of a purely epidemic character which sweep over the earth rapidly, from the rising to the setting sun, even the antecedents or forerunners are wholly unknown, and, consequently, cannot be determined by pathogenics consisting of resolutions or words only. Many of the ancients, and moderns, too, ascribe epidemics to Divine wrath, to human passions, to astral conjunctions, to earthquakes, etc.; some to saline, sulphurous, alkaline, acidulous, and the like matters diffused in the air; to predispositions not known; while the best of modern meteorologists utterly fail, not only in determining the causes, but even the precursors of an epidemic. Hippocrates has not been surpassed. He assumed an epidemic constitution to account for epidemics—a proposition which it is not safe to deny, seeing it is generally conceded, that effects have causes, though they may not be discovered in all cases, not even by a unanimous vote. Spontaneous epidemics, spontaneous generation, and the like, find few advocates.

The rise, extension, and decline of these yellow fever fomites in things do not run parallel with, or conform to any other variety of fomites yet known, at least in New Orleans, where, for the most part, epidemics attack the unacclimated in all parts of the city simultaneously. It exceeds the bounds of probability that the things imported, which are supposed to be the exclusive carriers of fomites, could thus suddenly be diffused for seven miles in the city. Things other than mail-matter are usually stored in warehouses, and the quantities which arrive on the approach of the yellow fever season of the year are inconsiderable.

A truce to logomachy and verbal dialectics History, that true logician, indicates an era not long past, when New Orleans was exempt, and New York suffered from yellow fever. Passion and interest, all powerful in swaying the present, are often but too forgetful of the landmarks of the past. There is nothing known in the sanitary conditions of these two great *emporia* of this Republic, which can give any assurance that what has happened may not . happen again. One advantage New Orleans may claim. She has a large resident population not susceptible to yellow fever. Should the Northern cities be again visited with this disease, as were Norfolk and Lisbon lately, and the peninsula of Europe at the beginning of the present century, the mortality would probably be far greater than ever occurred in New Orleans. What is called acclimation does not appear to exist, so far as exemption from this fever is concerned, only within, or near the tropics.—*N. O. Med. and Surg. Journal.*

INTRODUCTORY LECTURE UPON MILITARY SURGERY.

By CHARLES S. TRIPLER, M.D., Surgeon U. S. Army, Newport, Ky.

Delivered at the Ohio Medical College, at its session of 1858-59.

GENTLEMEN—During the last session of this college, by the invitation of your Professor of Surgery, I had the honor of addressing the class some half a dozen times upon various subjects in military surgery. These discourses were necessarily very desultory and imperfect, as they were simple, unpremeditated efforts, without adequate preparation or elaboration. An invitation to repeat these lectures having been extended to me, I have consented to do so, and shall therefore address you from time to time, as my engagements and your leisure will permit; hoping to interest you in this department of our common profession, and to profit you as well as myself by the labor this duty will impose.

It is to be regretted that a chair of military surgery has never been instituted in any of the colleges of the United States. I suppose, if my occasional remarks of last winter can be called lectures, they were the first ever delivered upon this branch of surgery in this country. We are, however, not so far behind our relatives over the water in this respect as might be imagined; for, with the exception of the chair in Edinburgh and one in Dublin, I do not know of any that have been officially recognized. Still, the labors of Hunter and Guthrie and others have not left the field entirely uncultivated.

Recent events, however, have so aroused public attention to the necessity of a well-organized and thoroughly instructed sanitary corps in every army, that we have reason to believe, ere long, no reputable college will be without such a chair. I shall not pretend, gentlemen, to offer you anything like a complete course of lectures upon military surgery. Such a course would occupy much more time than I have to spare, and would require, to meet my views of what it would exact, a full year's undivided labor in its preparation. For obvious reasons, I cannot devote so much time to it. It would give me great pleasure to do so, were it compatible with my public duties; but it is not. I shall endeavor, however, to touch upon the most important points.

In the history of the world, the wars waged by the several nations upon each other are the salient points; they fix the dates to which chronologists refer all other events, and they are the landmarks of each advancing step in the world's progress. For a thousand years we hear of nothing but fighting men among the myriads composing the armies engaged in these wars. Of the present well-ordered staff departments for supplying the wants of the troops in the field, we find no trace in the armies of old. Every man was his own quartermaster and subsistence officer. But the military surgeon early finds a historian and a poet to record his worth; and just in proportion to the civilization and cultivation of the age has been the degree of honor and estimation in which he has been held.

I shall not occupy your time in tracing the history of military surgery; that has already been done by abler hands. But I cannot forbear, by way of justification of the remark I have just made, to recall to your memories the sensation produced in the Greek host before Troy, when it was known that Machaon was wounded, and of the care with which he was removed on shipboard from the field. This was in the heroic age of Greece, when Agamemnon, and Achilles, and Ajax were the leaders, and Nestor and Ulysses the counselors of her armies; and which could find in Homer alone a poet qualified to celebrate their achievements. Of the army surgeon Homer thus speaks:

" Ιητηρ γαρ ανηρ πολλων ανταξιος αλλων,"--

miserably and inadequately rendered by his translator:

"A wise physician, skilled, our wounds to heal,
Is more than armies to the public weal."

If we pass to the age of Henry V., and thence on, including the reign of Elizabeth—an age of midnight darkness—and at the latter period just emerging into dawn, we find the army surgeon a miserable leech, the peer of drummers and fifers, and, as a necessary consequence, the lives of the soldiers in the hands of a pack of vile cheats and quacks. "I remember," says Gale, "when I was at the wars at Muttrel, in the time of that most famous Prince, King Henry VIII., there was a great rabblement there that took upon them to be surgeons. Some were sow-gelders, and horse-gelders, with tinkers and cobblers. This noble sect did such great cures that they got themselves a perpetual name; for, like as Thessalus' sect were called Thessalians, so was this rabblement, for their notorious cures, called dog-leeches; for in two dressings they did commonly make their cures whole and sound forever, so that they neither felt heat nor cold, nor no manner of pain after." He goes on to tell us that the Duke of Norfolk caused him and some other surgeons to inquire how so many men perished of such small wounds, when the knavery of this rabblement was detected, and they were imprisoned and threatened to be hung for their misdeeds. If the Duke of Norfolk and his master had been hanged for *their* misdeeds, in committing the care of their wounded to such men, justice would have been more fully vindicated. For when such abuses exist, those in authority are, in my opinion, alone responsible. But the fact shows the degraded status of the military surgeon at that period; and this not of necessity, for Gale himself was a competent and an eminent man, and had many worthy compeers. And we must recollect that Henry V. could employ, with a suitable stipend and suite, a competent surgeon to see to his *own* person, while his subjects were left to the mercy of the sow-gelder. Indeed, for selfish purposes, the basest of tyrants have seldom failed to appreciate the military surgeon. Even Charles IX., of France, while indulging personally in the agreeable pastime of shooting Huguenots, at the massacre of St. Bartholomew could take efficient measures to preserve the life of Parè.

"It was not, however, until the wars in which France was engaged, between the years 1732 and 1743, that the subject of military surgery began to assume its present systematic form. Hitherto the States of Europe had been content to enjoy the benefits of the labors of military surgeons, without having taken any direct part in the honor or advancement of this art." (Ballingall.) From that time to this, keeping pace with the progress of science, literature, and civil liberty, the department of military surgery, as an essential element of the military body, has been increasing in interest and importance, the sphere of its duties and scope of its authority constantly extending, its resources and usefulness regularly developing themselves, as one disability after another has been removed, and although it has not as yet reached the position necessary to secure its highest degree of efficiency, still events are rapidly advancing towards that consummation. I verily believe the day is not far distant, when to this department will be conceded by universal assent a military position and importance, second to none among the staff departments. The experience of the nations of the world, within the last fifteen years, has demonstrated the necessity of its emancipation from its absurd and irrational dependence upon other co-ordinate branches of the service. The moral courage of Florence Nightingale has shown the practicability of this, and its entire congruity with necessary military discipline. Humanity, the age, public opinion, political necessity, and true military policy and economy, are all converging to the same point. But before that time shall have fully arrived, a deal of prejudice and ignorance, remnants of a barbaric age and system, traditions of military hierarchies, developed under political organizations, as antagonistical to our own as the poles to each other, will have to be overcome, by patient perseverance in well-doing, and by demonstrating, from the statistics of war and well-ascertained facts and observations, that by erecting the medical department into a corps charged exclusively with the sanitary condition of an army, and vested with the military power to execute its functions, not only hundreds of lives of the common soldiers must be saved, but hundreds of thousands of dollars besides.

These facts and figures are now accessible. It remains to be seen what nation will first avail itself of the lessons they impart, and profit by the example they teach. The necessity for a thorough reorganization of the medical department of the British army so forced itself upon the attention of the British Government, by the events in the Crimea, that a committee of inquiry into the matter was instituted by the Queen. I regret that I have not been able, as yet, to procure a copy of their report; but from various notices of its result and purport that I have seen in the Reviews, I am persuaded that its facts, rightly interpreted and justly weighed, will force, even from that conservative Government, the speedy emancipation of their sanitary officers from the subordinate position in relation to all other officers in which they have hitherto been kept, and which has so crippled their efficiency, at the cost of thousands of lives and millions of money. But however reluctant those who sit in high places may have been, to admit the military equality of the medical officers, the estimation in which they, as a corps and as individuals, have been, and are held by the rank and file—the men who do the fighting and bear the suffering, in all armies—can neither be ignored nor denied. To the confidence inspired in the men, by the certainty that if wounded they will be zealously and ably cared for by their surgeons, *how much* of the bravery they show in the fight may be attributed! Sir George Ballingall tells us that in such repute was Parè among the French soldiers, " that we find their princes and generals willingly took the field, when they could prevail upon Parè to go out with them; and at the time when all the noblesse of the kingdom were shut up in Mentz, which was besieged by Charles V. in person, at the head of 100,000 men, they sent an embassy to the king, their master, beseeching him to send Parè to them. An Italian captain, for a great reward, introduced him into the city. They instantly sent, at midnight, to awaken the prince who commanded the garrison, with the good news of his arrival. The governor begged of him that he would go out next day, and show himself on the beach. He was received by the soldiers with shouts of triumph. 'We shall not die, though wounded—Parè is among us.' Mentz was at this time the bulwark of France, and it has always been ascribed to the presence of this single man, that they kept the city, till the gallant army that lay around it perished beneath its walls."

In the British army in the Crimea, that the same feeling obtained, we have a witness in Mr. Rawlinson, a civil engineer, sent out by the British Government as a member of the sanitary commission. "Having been wounded, he had to be surgically treated in the front—an opportunity which a civilian rarely obtains, or is anxious to obtain—and he says, ' I can state, that in the division in which I lay, from the officers to the men, the medical officers, if I may use so strong a term, were almost worshiped and idolized.' And again he says, 'I cannot find language strong enough to express what I think of our surgeons. I thought they were laboring under some disadvantages, and I do not think they are in a right position in a regiment. I do not think their feelings for their men are consulted sufficiently.' " (Blackwood.)

If it were becoming, or necessary, I might corroborate all that Mr. Rawlinson has said, from my own observation. In our own service, the medical officer has no reason to complain of the estimation in which he is personally held, by either officers or men.

But, although we have taken one step in advance of any other nation, in the right and only direction to promote his military efficiency, this very step ran counter to so many time-honored but worm-eaten traditions and prejudices, and provoked so much opposition, that the very limbs that took that step were half palsied by the effort, and now shrink in hesitation and doubt from the one step still remaining to be taken to reach the goal—that of the greatest efficiency the state of medical science will admit.

The necessity for a systematically organized sanitary corps, as an integral element of an army, all nations admit; and, all have endeavored, in one way or another, to secure that element, and to make it as efficient as possible; and all, without exception, have failed in making these corps as efficient as the confessedly able personnel composing them is capable of being made. The reason of this failure, to my mind, is obvious. It is, that in these organizations, governments have attempted to combine incongruous ideas—like certain equations in mathematics, that give imaginary roots, thus showing that incompatible conditions have been introduced into the problem. They are expected to keep the troops in health, and are denied the necessary authority to enforce obedience to the measures indispensable to that end. The radical idea in their organization seems to have been, to provide a body of medical men to prescribe for the sick, and perform the necessary operations upon the wounded of an army; and for that purpose alone, *any* plan of organization is sufficient—in fact, none whatever is necessary. To employ any competent physician, as individuals do in civil life, would answer this requirement. This, however, is but part—and that the less important part—of the duty of the military surgeon; and if this only were attempted or accomplished, neither the public expectation nor the demands of the service would at this day be satisfied.

Within our own times, the improvements in the *matériel* of war have effected almost an entire revolution in the profession of arms. To the exercise of ingenuity and talent in the construction of fire-arms the warmest encouragement has been constantly extended by all governments in Christendom, and by none more liberally than our own. Our own countrymen have contributed their full quota to these improvements. The percussion lock for ordnance, the repeating pistol, and what is called the Paixhan gun, are our own inventions. Improvements in pontons, for crossing rivers, and increased facilities for transporting troops and supplies, have also sprung from the active and fertile minds of our military men. We may say, generally, that we are not a whit behind any nation in anything required for attack or defence; and (without boasting) we may add, our arms have been as successful as those of any other nation, whenever an occasion has called for their practical exercise.

But however perfect and efficient may be our military engines, and however complete our facilities for the speedy transportation of troops and supplies, unless the *men* who are to use and give effect to these engines are correspondingly effective, our workshops will only be employed to furnish our enemy with the means of annoying ourselves. And *here* is the great and important duty of the medical corps: to *keep* the personnel of the army in effective working order—to preserve the health of the troops—to guard *against* sickness, not simply to treat it when it has occurred. What would be thought of the engineer who should neglect the means of keeping his works in order, by the timely use of all the means that science, experience, and skill afford, and should consider his duty discharged, by patching up a crumbling wall, or repairing the effects of decay? The ordnance officer is expected to keep his arms in order, as well as to repair them when injured. The quartermaster must keep his means of transportation in order, as well as repair defects in them, the result of accident or service. But of what use are all these things, unless the men to use them are kept in condition to use them effectively?

Now I maintain that an efficient sanitary system can be instituted and conducted only by the corps of medical officers, and that for this purpose these officers must be provided with the military authority, and the means to execute the measures they know to be necessary to secure this grand object.

It is not necessary for me to go into an argument to prove to medical men that outside of the medical profession there is no class of men who make the laws of hygiene a study, or who are competent to adapt and apply the laws of health to the ever-varying circumstances and emergencies that beset an army in the field. It will not do to say that the medical officer can suggest to the officer in command his hygienic plan, and *he* will give the necessary orders to carry it into effect. The best and plainest sanitary system has still in it so much that is incomprehensible to any but the professional man, that it cannot be made plain to any other; and, however well disposed an officer may be to institute and carry out such a plan, he cannot do it intelligently. Moreover, a modification of the details of the system may become necessary at any moment, from unforeseen circumstances; some parts of it may prove to be impracticable, without grave inconvenience; and in this emergency the professional man only can judge whether it may not be neglected without injury to the general design, or, if it be absolutely impracticable, what substitute can be found to remedy or prevent the evil that will probably arise from its neglect. The details of the sanitary system must be superintended by the sanitary corps; and for this purpose its officers must be clothed with military rank of a grade sufficient to defend them from the interference of other officers of a lower grade.

There are some propositions that seem, when stated, to be so clear and indisputable, that by almost general consent they are set aside as demonstrated truths, and therefore not fit subjects for examination or discussion. Among these is the proposition that the commanding officer of a body of troops must command all persons serving with that body of troops. To this dogma we owe it that the medical department of the army has never yet been in a position to fulfill its natural mission. Tradition and established usage, among the nations of Europe, have given this dogma its currency; and without any investigation of its logical truth or its necessary results, so far as the medical department is concerned, it is now held and applied in direct violation of a law of Congress by our military men. The spirit of the age, however, is at last disturbing the ancient, solitary reign of these dust-covered antiquities, and the world is no longer disposed to put up with mischievous practical results for the triumph of ideas, however venerable they may claim to be. Statesmen disturb and brush them away without the slightest remorse, when they stand in the way of political progress. "Our veneration for what has been," exclaims an eloquent Senator, "is too frequently made the excuse for what is; we are too ready to suppose that what has *been* done, has been well done and ought to be done again." (General Cass.)

I am not one of those who are disposed to claim that all innovation is improvement; on the other hand, I would insist upon cautious deliberation and the most thorough investigation, before I would consent to an important change in the economy of any public institution. But when a change is proposed, claiming for itself that it *is* an improvement, I do not consider it is a sufficient reason to condemn it, to say "that they don't do so in Europe." The timid reluctance with which any innovation was ventured upon, in our service, that had not received the sanction of European precedent or example, is, I think, gradually wearing away; and whenever such example is now appealed to, it is usually to sustain some favorite project or design;

and to this end, that particular notion is selected whose practice chances to correspond with the views of the projector; for among the whole number of kingdoms and empires of the Old World, two can seldom be found whose systems coincide exactly as to any given point. The United States is now old enough and powerful enough to select and construct its own systems, whether civil or military; and while we would not refuse to avail ourselves of an improvement because it was European, we would not perpetuate an error for no better reason. While we would avail ourselves of their experience to increase the efficiency of our own institutions, we would also be warned, by the same experience, to avoid their mistakes.

A glance at the military position of the medical officer in the French and English armies, during the war in the East, and a comparison of the results of the two systems, will serve to illustrate our views.

In both armies the medical officers were without military rank; they had rank assimilated to other officers, which gave them certain privileges, as in the choice of quarters, for instance, but they were entirely subordinate to the officers in command, whatever might be their rank. The British medical officer, however, had command of the orderlies in his hospital, regulated its police, and had authority to carry out his own orders, as regarded the treatment and subsistence of the sick. The apothecaries were also under his control. In the French army, the medical officer simply prescribed for the sick, performed operations, etc.; but had no control whatever over the nurses, the cooks, or the apothecaries. He had no military authority over the men in his hospital; was not responsible for its good order or its dicipline, and could only indicate to another officer what he considered to be necessary in any of these respects. This officer is called the Military Intendant. He is generally an ineffective officer of the line, who is incapable, from age, wounds, or other disability, of doing duty with his corps. He, however, has military rank, and is hence qualified to perform duties about which he knows little and frequently cares less. It is by his orders and under his authority that the nurses are kept at their duties, the patients are kept quiet in the wards, the police of the buildings preserved, etc. The French system is very elaborate, and is regulated to the minutest detail. In theory, it seems to be almost perfect, and contrasted with the British, where little seems to have been prescribed except that the surgeon should not spend any money, should see to the sick and wounded, and be subordinate to the military hierarchy, it is well calculated to excite admiration and invite imitation. But when we look into the results of the two systems, as developed in the late war in the East, we shall probably hesitate before we accord the French system the one, or sanction it by the other. The English are a *practical* people, and will not long allow a bad system to prevail when their native good sense shows its defects; and with all their con-ervatism and veneration for established custom, they seldom hesitate long in tumbling any institution over, if it is found to stand in the way of a practical good. So in Scutari and the Crimea, the lumbering old machinery of their venerable supply system was not long suffered to obstruct the effective administration of their hospitals, when the emergency demanded that it should be disregarded. And when the effects of consecrated error were made palpable to the public sense, they lost no time in taking steps to remedy that error, and to devise means for avoiding it in future. The French, on the other hand, abided by their beautiful theory, and found themselves, in consequence, under the absolute necessity of making peace when they did, because their army was so crippled by disease that they could no longer keep the field. The results of their military medical system, so far as regards the effectiveness of their army, reminds us of the scientific tailors of Laputa, who cut all their coats by the use of the sextant and theodolite, but yet Captain Gulliver says he never saw such ill-fitting garments in his life. To the statistics of the armies I appeal for my facts; and I must here state that honest, truth-loving John Bull confesses the whole truth, while imaginative, theoretical France, under cover of terms perfectly unintelligible outside of France, endeavors to conceal the significant facts that explode her system. Enough, however, is exposed, to show the radical defects of that system, and at how great an expense of men and money the absurd notion that the fighting men must have complete control of all the varied employments that make up the military whole, have been maintained. By a lucky chance, with a thoroughly disintegrated army, they escaped from a most perilous position; and as regards the most important element of their embarrassment, so far as we know, they have learned nothing.

But to the facts; and I wish you, gentlemen, in listening to them, to fix your attention upon the figures, not only in reference to this matter, but also in relation to the frightful disproportion of the deaths from disease, and those from the effects of the shot of the enemy, in both armies; for nothing can illustrate, in more speaking language, the necessity of what I am contending for—the pressing necessity for an entire *remodeling* of the sanitary department of armies.

I quote now from Dr. Bryce, whose statistics were obtained from the director-general of the medical department of the British army:

Total number of men sent to the East................93,959
Deaths from wounds and injuries 1,761
Killed in action 2,685
Deaths from disease................................ 16,298
Number invalided 12,902

The losses, then, from the casualties of battle, were 4,446, or about 3½ per cent., while the losses from disease were 29,201, and of these 16,298 were deaths, or 19.22 per cent. Here is a ratio of deaths exceeding that in the Walcheren campaign, under Castlereagh's administration, and almost equal to the total number of sick at the close of Pringle's campaign, in the same country, which he tells us was "above 4,000, or somewhat more than one-fifth of our whole number." But in the Walcheren campaign the loss was due to endemic disease, the aggravated bilious fevers and dysenteries of low and marshy countries. While in Turkey and the Crimea, Tuffnel says, "England landed 93,901 men, of whom 30,000 were lost to the country or invalided within the short period of eighteen months; and of these only one of every thirteen admitted into hospital was placed there in consequence of wounds. Of those who died, comparatively few were carried off by epidemics; the rest perished by disease which was capable of mitigation, if not entirely of prevention." Of the 23,392 English in the Crimea, 12,025 were sick in January, 1855; exceeding by 658 the number fit for duty; and in February of that year there were 427 deaths in the hospitals at Kulalee and Scutari. But fearful as this decimation of the British force appears to be, we shall find it very materially exceeded by that of the French.

According to an official return published in the *Moniteur*, and by order of the Emperor,

There were taken to the East........ 309,268
Lost there 69,299
                                                    ———————
There should have been left 239,969
But there re-entered France and Algeria............227,135
                                                    ———————
Leaving... 12,834
who are not accounted for at all.   ·

In this return the number of the killed in action is not distinguished from the deaths by disease. In addition to the deaths, however, there were invalided 65,069 during the war.

Comparing as near as this imperfect statement will admit, we find the relative loss of the two armies to have been:

	ENGLISH.	FRENCH.
By death	22.07	22.99
By invaliding	17.34	21.04

The English had two-thirds, and a little more, of their total number in the East, at the close of the war, while the French had less than one-half.

(To be concluded in September No.)

The Black Doctor of the Artesian Well.

The Colored Philosopher on the Great Bore.—Our reporter has taken down *verbatim* " Doctor" Charles Saunders' lecture on the Artesian Well of Louisville, Ky. He gives an account of some remarkable cures, which we are assured were actually made. Our city readers all know Charley too well to require note or comment for his text, but non-residents may be happy to learn that, under the Dred Scott decision, he is nowhere in a social or civil point of view, but that he is one of those kind-hearted blacks beloved by everybody, while his profuse use of the biggest dictionary words renders him one of the standing objects of interest in our city.

With this preface we proceed to the lecture, word for word as he gave it.

Mr. Kellogg, being political thorough born, he dissolved to Mr. Dupont that he would excommunicate the bowels of the earth—feeling that he would have the smiles of Providence through his exploration.

He spontaneously and judiciously probed the bowels of the earth. He first excommunicated Congress water—the stream wasn't unanimous enough. He still progressed through, finding a domestical stream of Saratoga water. Her virtues wasn't substantial enough. He still continued to exonerate the earth. After succeeding two thousand and thirty-six foot, the stream was judiciously toploftical. The judicious powers threw up all the cuttings. The stream seemed to be very spontaneous in her invigorations, which become unanimously animated, seeing the brilliancy of these melodious white waters rolling up. We have a great many invalids. Viewing these flowing waters induced

them to drink of it. Many cases past cure by any physician, these
waters unanimously healed up. Cured so profectionately, caused the
notice of the community. Debilitated cases in families were said to
be the most effectual cures that ever could be legally interpreted.

We did believe that this was the healing spring of ever living
waters. Behold how marvelous the hands of Providence, through
the administration of his goodness, in sending this melodious water!
The profects of this water is of salt excommunicated with very little
lime—projected through the sulphate of iodine and alumina through
the profects of carbonic acid, which substantiates the body of this
water. This causes it to penetrate legally through the nervous system, excommunicating all the bile from the kidneys. We can, through
political respect, address our obedience to all settled ladies, calling
them to notice the brilliance of young ladies—seeing their appearance
dissembling the lily so melodiously unanimous by drinking small dona-
tions of this artesian water. Doctor Saunders' respects to the young
ladies for beneficial purposes. Take from a glass and a half before
breakfast to two glasses; you'll find yourselves politically irrelevated.
This water has raised all ladies above the skill of superstition.

Gentlemen, profected by debilitation, are here unanimously invited
to a special attention of the Artesian well, where you can have your
nervous affections substantiated. Come without superstition and I
will give you the details.

I have had some very spontaneous cases of scrofula, bathing their
faces well of a morning and taking two glasses of the water. In a
short time this disease was completely discomboberated. Evaporated
domestically from the well in the condition of good health.

Cases of dyspepsia, lasting from five to ten years, with inflammatory rheumatism, profected with dropsy, this water has discomboberated in a short time. This water acts very obstropolous on dumb
ague—or chills and fever, which we have many ladies here profected
with, or sick headache. I have asked them to bathe their faces for
about a half a minute. taking one glass of water, after which, domestically seeing the effect of the disease evaporate. See how brilliant
their complexion appears afterwards. Please examine the ladies'
teeth after washing them with the artesian water with their brushes!
See the dissemblement of their ivories from their occupation and examine their political appearance—you will either see the profects of
white lilies or the dissemblement of geraniums. I would almost be
tempted to say weeping willows; as it is not a fruit tree, I will leave

that out. It is judiciously inexpressible to prescribe this harmonious address to the young ladies of Louisville.

A blind lady from Pittsburg had been under four doctors eighteen months. She went to the well at White Sulphur and thence to Blue Lick; from there she absconded very personally to New Orleans. The disease was not affected. Her father taking her home from New Orleans, hearing of the Artesian well of Louisville, induced her to come here. She then came to the Artesian well, inquiring for Dr. Saunders, who sold water to a friend of hers in New York. I came forward and met her; she told me her wants. She wished to know if this was the Dr. Saunders. I told her that I was the circumstance named. Another lady asked me, did I think she could be cured at this well. After raising her veil and examining her face, I told her she was very thin-skinned, and this was the place she ought to have come to first. I very cordially invited her to take a, cheer before the spout, and handed her a towel to hold under the spout, and to take and bathe her eyes well. Then I asked her domestically not to wipe her face, but set by the stove and let it dry itself away. She done so. After which I imposed on her domestically four glasses of water. Filling of a bottle afterwards, asking her, communicatively, to excommunicate one glass just as she was going to bed at night. That water acted judiciously upon the kidneys. Four days after which she said that coming to the well she discovered something red before her. Finally, this water discomboberated all the bile and cold from her kidneys. One week and four days afterwards she stated she could see as far across the falls as any person who was in the yard. Which afterwards she wrote her name in our day book, requesting us to show it to the world, and she would answer for it. Another case of blindness, the wife of Dick Moore, of this city. This water has excommunicated the blindness from her eyes. She had been blind for about 4 years. She is now able to pick up her needle and thread it with Coates' fine cotton, and she can hemstitch as beautifully as any lady in the State of Kentucky. The brilliancy of the candle doesn't effect her within the least. Her sight is better and stronger than it ever was since she knew herself. And she is one of the most conscientiously happy ladies in the United States. All from the benefits of the Artesian water.

Mr. O'Hallan, who lives in this city, had been for more than ten years struck with blindness. I persuaded him unanimously to visit the well. He said he was afraid to drink the water. I told him he needn't fear it, he couldn't throw it up after drinking it. He asked me what would it do to him. I told him this water—he was badly diseased—would raise the envelopment of his abdomen and excommunicate all the bile from his kidneys. His blindness would evaporate spontaneously, and he would have the most harmonious eyesight he ever had. He very personally then went in to drinking of this water and bathing his face. He very shortly after imagined, on coming to the well, he saw something white before him. He said he raily believed he would get to see once more. The next morning when he came he said it was the size (the white spot) of a cream-colored house. Two days after that he came to the well. I asked him where his boy was. He said, "Thank God I have left my boy and stick at home; I can see well enough." And of all the happy men that ever was interpretated, I think he was one of the most conspicuous.

Charley advises the water drinkers not to infringe on their nervous systems by drinking too much at a time, but to take it piously till they get acquainted with the proceeds of it.

The colored philosopher closed his lecture with the following toast for the benefit of editors:

Hoping the predominating power of superstition may not predominate through the editors to the inculcation of Congress. Superstition may debate currency originally to the aid of the colony, and should flow beneficial through the legality of the human family. Currency should flow beneficial and become unanimously systematic. Hoping the projects of the neutralized spirits may never varigate, but may rise harmoniously through this molestation of all of our healths. Varigating of all cumbustions—and bringing out harmonious interviews.

AMERICAN MEDICAL ASSOCIATION.

We take pleasure in giving publicity to the following circular prepared by the committee appointed by the Convention of Medical Schools, held in Louisville on the second Monday in May last; and which explains the course of action which that committee have agreed to present for the adoption of the Convention at its meeting next year at New Haven:

"A committee was appointed at the meeting of the Convention of the Medical Schools of the United States, held in Louisville, Ky., on Monday, the second day of May, 1859, to consider the matters brought before the Convention, so as to propose a definite course of action at the adjourned meeting of the Convention to be held in New Haven, Ct., on Monday, the fourth day of June, Anno Domini 1860.

"At a meeting of this committee, held in Louisville, soon after their appointment, it was unanimously agreed upon to propose the adoption, by the Convention of Medical Schools, of a rule, requiring from every candidate for the degree of Doctor in Medicine, certificates of attendance on two full courses of lectures, at a regularly organized medical school, and of the study of medicine during a period of at least three full years, under the direction of a regular practitioner of medicine, who shall certify to the same under his own hand.

"It was proposed, also, that a resolution be passed, that any school which does not adopt and enforce this rule shall not be allowed to send delegates to the Convention of Medical Schools, nor to the American Medical Association, and that its graduates shall not be recognized as regular practitioners of medicine.

"It was thought advisable to recognize the deficiency in preparatory education on the part of many who offer themselves as students of medicine, and that all practitioners of medicine, as well as all professors, should be exhorted to do all in their power to impress upon those wishing to study medicine, the importance and great advantage of intellectual and moral discipline and culture, as well as of a good knowledge of their own mother tongue, and of some acquaintance with the Latin language, and with the elementary truths of mathematics and physics.

"The members of the committee have undertaken to put themselves in communication with all the regularly organized medical schools in the United States. The committee is charged with asking the attention of the faculty of which you are a member to the subject-matter of this communication, and with soliciting an expression of your opinions and views."—*Med. News.*

Homœopathy in Connecticut and Massachusetts—The Difference.

We have been furnished, from an entirely reliable source, with full accounts of the late proceedings in the case of Dr. J. S. Curtis, of Hartford, Conn., and which were instituted by the Hartford County Medical Society, and subsequently by the State Medical Society, for alleged infringement of their By-Laws.

Before commenting upon the matter, we wish to state that we notice it *by request,* both from medical gentlemen here and elsewhere;

and not because we delight in the topic, or have any personal p
whatever. The sentiments we may express, therefore, must
stood as being directed to *the subject*—not against individu
are constrained to add, that we think the subject is one whic
be considered in medical journals and by the profession
More especially should the medical press examine and spe
premises, because, as we are reliably informed, the newspape
of the procedure is a garbled one, furnished by an interest
It is time a full and definite understanding and verdict shoul
upon the points at issue. We have no need to declare our o
ions upon the general relations of Homœopathy to the profess
we have already freely and fully done so, on several occasio
Journal. Whatever we may now say, will at least prove
views are unaltered.

During the session of the " Connecticut Medical Societ;
Annual Meeting, holden in Middletown, May 15th, 1869, a
passed, expelling Dr. Curtis from the State Society for vie
the By-Law which forbids members of the Society to hold co
with irregular practitioners. This vote was a full endorsen
confirmation of the previous analogous action against D
taken in the County Society.

Now we are constrained, with our views of the matter, to
we think the County and State Society were abundantly ju
taking the course they did. It appears by the long and abl
a large number of the most respectable members of the Stat
to the statement of Dr. Curtis—and which were both publish
local newspapers—that Dr. Curtis had long been in the habit
what the Society construes as an infringement of one of its
viz.: that which forbids consultation with " irregular pract
Moreover, we are informed, in the same " Reply," that rep
monstrances were made to Dr. C. upon this ground—all of
systematically disregarded. The merits of the case, then, se
to lie in a very few propositions; thus—Dr. Curtis voluntaril
a member of the medical associations mentioned; he bound
therefore, by his own free act, to observe their By-Laws, h
right to interpret those jaws for himself—every member of
is, on the contrary, bound to take that signification of the la
is held by the Society at large—the universally admitted se
regulations, which, as a Society, it adopts. Dr. C. did not
the Societies mentioned being his judges—and bearing in

they alone had the right of interpretation and jurisdiction in these and similar premises—if not, of what use is a Society, and how does it protect its members? The By-Laws having been violated by Dr. Curtis, the Societies which framed them and are governed by them have the undoubted right to inflict the penalty deemed proper and just. In the case of one violation, or two, or three, even, it might be well to temper justice with mercy; but where a member shows himself determined to hold out against law and remonstrance both, there can be but one course. It will never do to have insubordination in the ranks of any army.

As for members of the community at large, or its entire body, being called to sit in judgment in cases of this nature—as some well-intentioned, but very shallow-brained, newspaper editors declare should be the course—it is not only a useless, but an absurd proposition; they are not competent to decide upon the questions at issue. The arbitration is properly vested in the associations where those questions arise.

The peculiar behavior or management which constitutes what the profession terms an "irregular" practitioner, the profession has a legitimate right to determine. If the medical body does not meddle with the rules, orders, and general management of other organizations, and if such meddling, did it take place, would be rebuked or laughed at—why should it, in its turn, be subjected to interference and outside, *ex cathedra* opinions and decisions upon matters properly under its control alone? The people. as a body, should be content to allow physicians to legislate for themselves, and to hold their own courts when necessary, unmolested, even by comments upon subjects about which the commentators are wholly ignorant.

At other times, we have expressed the opinion that no physician who practices his profession upon the broad ground of honesty and the legitimate and earnest seeking to benefit humanity, can, in justice to his fellows of the same stamp, rightly consult with a homœopathist. And we take this ground, in the conscientious belief that the latter, who bases his practice upon an exclusive dogma, cannot practice in an enlightened and efficient manner; that he is, consequently, obtaining money under false pretences—not being a physician in the true sense, but a dogmatist, the partisan of a specious, and, in the case of homœopathy, an absurd and unreliable, as well as, a partial and confined theory—for it does not merit the title of *doctrine.*

Now, as the Connecticut physicians very truly say, in their "Reply," the public have a right to employ whatever class of practitioners they choose, and also to change their physician when they like—the risk being wholly theirs, we would add: Conceding to them this right, however, how does it follow, as some would have us believe, that those physicians who repudiate humbug, should have no right to exclude those from their ranks who practice or who encourage incompetent pretension and one-sided dogmatism? The truth is, they *have that right*, and they ought always to exercise it. We honor the bold, honest, and straightforward interpretation of their By-Laws, and their enforcement of them—after due remonstrance with the violator— which has characterized the movements of the two Connecticut Societies above referred to; and we could wish that Massachusetts Medical Societies might be content—yes, might dare—to follow in the steps of those of their sister State. By such a course—and we here take occasion again to say, distinctly, that we are contending against *abuses*, not condemning *individuals*—that is not our province, but the other is; and we are not afraid to avow it and act accordingly—by such a course, we repeat, honest men would be protected in their rights, quackery of all sorts would be discountenanced, and Medical Societies would wield that just power which would render them worth belonging to. We should not be obliged to sit down, cheek by jowl, with those who are glad enough to avail themselves of all our legal rights, privileges, and pleasures, but who are ever ready to decry our motives, our tenets, and our practice, behind our backs. We cannot repress an expression of utter surprise at the course of any in our profession—entitled, either during a long, or for only a short period, to its honors and emoluments, and likewise, by their qualifications, to the esteem and confidence of the community—which leads them by word, look, or act to countenance those whom they know are acting in opposition to the salutary rules adopted by the profession; and who also will not scruple to ridicule them for fraternizing with them. The homœopathists have a Society of their own; why do they not retire within their own party lines? Why do they still continue to attach themselves to us—their antipodes in thought, feeling, and action? The reasons are sufficiently evident, to every one who is familiar with the relative positions of the parties. We need not specify them. *Self-interest* combines all the motives, in one expression.

One word, before we close, in reference to a point of which a great deal is said by those who make a practice of consulting with homœopathists and other quacks—we refer to the plea of " humanity"—and which has been advanced by Dr. Curtis. It is alleged to be a very inhuman and cruel act to refuse to administer to the urgent necessities of a patient for whom the homœopathist or other empiric avows himself unwilling to attempt to do anything more—or for whom he is not able, by reason of lack of skill or information, to undertake a surgical operation. The assertion is a *non sequitur*. If the empiric in attendance on so serious a case acknowledges his incapacity and solicits interference, *the friends of the patient have the responsibility thrown upon them*, as we, conceive, entirely. If the honest, regular practitioner, from a *bonâ fide* conscientiousness, does not feel that he can meet the former attendant in consultation, and the latter has admitted himself useless, the friends are to·decide whether they will have their suffering charge relieved or not. They can do it, by discharging the first practitioner, who cannot be benefited by a consultation with the desired new-comer, simply because the two cannot consult—they are wholly opposed in their remedial notions. So, then, it is, and ought to be, a sort of *experimentum crucis* with the friends of the invalid—will they have the patient relieved, or will they retain the person avowedly incompetent to relieve him, and so allow him to die? We imagine that these sort of instances, when brought to this test, will be easily provided for.

In conclusion, we quote the following resolution of the Connecticut State Society, and which, say the members who prepared the reply to Dr. Curtis, gives "a true statement of the opinion of the profession" there, and, we may hope, in many other places:

Resolved, That it is in violation of the letter and spirit of our By-Laws and Code of Ethics, both National and State, to hold any professional consultation, either surgical or medical, with any practitioner of any irregular sect in medicine.

This resolution, unanimously adopted, *was voted for by Dr. Curtis himself;* who, however, took upon himself to except from its provisions those homœopathists who had "received a degree from a medical college." "But what," add pertinently the writers of the Reply, "becomes of his [Dr. Curtis's] excessive humanity towards those of our citizens who, when sick, are under the care of the other various practitioners in this city? His 'humanity' fails to reach them, for here he stands upon the same platform with us." The same writers then go on to say that it is not one transgression of the sort specified, which would subject a member to expulsion; and they moreover aver that they never would "stand by and permit a patient to die," if their

efforts could save him. It is the "animus or spirit" which uniformly
and constantly governs any physician of their body, which they regard as so important, both to the integrity of the latter and to the
well-being of the community; and in this they are right, and our
sympathies are cordially with them. Would that as laudable a spirit
and as efficient an action ruled the councils of our own State Society,
when called upon to consider and adjudicate in similar cases.

IS SCARLATINA CONTAGIOUS?

Scarlatina has been quite prevalent during the last two or three
years in this locality (Queechy,.Vt.) It has made its invasions alike
in very elevated and low situations. The question of its contagiousness constantly arising, let me observe it as carefully as possible, with
a view of noting the evidences *pro* and *con;* and it has seemed to me
that the testimony decidedly preponderates in favor of its non-conta-
giousness.

This question is not only important in a scientific view, but the interests of humanity require its solution. I have repeatedly seen a
family almost entirely deserted by the neighbors, because they feared
the disease was *catching*, which is the popular belief.

In two of our standard works on Theory and Practice, by Dr.
Watson and Dr. Wood, we are told that scarlatina is contagious.
Having the highest respect for these two eminent men, and remembering a few words of that celebrated aphorism of our father Hippocrates, "*Experience is deceptive, and judgment difficult*," I feel like stating my own observations with great modesty.

In a family numbering ten, including servants, there have been
three or four cases of scarlatina, at different periods, with intervals of
several months or a year, and no other member of the family took
the disease, though all were exposed to it.

D. C. was attacked with the most severe form of scarlatina, and
died in five or six days. Several children in the family were often in
the room, and constantly exposed to whatever contagious influence
there might be, but not one of them had the disease; while two families,
one-fourth of a mile on each side, who carefully avoided going near
the residence of the patients, had several children attacked with it.
Numerous instances like the foregoing would seem to prove its non-
contagious character. What has been the observation of others?—
Boston Med. and Surg. Journal.

[From the New Orleans Medical and Surgical Journal.]

Wonderful Effects and New Application of the "Ready Method" of Marshall Hall.

By HUMPHREY PEAKE, M.D., Arkadelphia, Ark.

On Tuesday evening, August 23d, 1858, between eight and nine o'clock, I was called to see William A. Dickinson, of about the age of twenty-two years, a resident of this place. The messenger, a negress, came to me in great haste, saying that Billy was dead—that they had found him so in the garden. Suspecting that there might be some mistake, I ran, with all my might, to the house of his brother, a distance of three or four hundred yards, where the patient was. I was informed, as I entered the house, that he was not dead; and on going to the room in which he was, I found him tossing wildly about the bed, apparently in the very greatest agony, uttering cries and groans indicative of the most intense suffering. The report of his condition having spread rapidly, a number of persons had collected at the house. He seemed conscious, but returned no answers to my questions. His feet and hands were very cold, the coldness extending a considerable way up his arms and legs. The pulse was feeble, and beating about one hundred in a minute. I gave him half a drachm of McMunn's elixir of opium, with two drachms of aromatic spirit of ammonia in a draught of brandy, which he swallowed, it seemed, with some difficulty. I ordered his legs and arms to be rubbed with flannel cloths, wetted in brandy containing Cayenne pepper; sent immediately for mustard, and had a hot bath prepared. I noticed that he had cramps in the muscles of his feet and legs. I now got the following history of the case: He had been in the river, seining, during the whole of the afternoon, exposed to a very hot sun. The day was a very warm one. He came home in the evening after dark, and ate his supper alone, the balance of the family having already eaten. Nothing unusual was observed of him. Shortly after eight o'clock, on the family's retiring to bed, his absence was noticed. Nothing, however, was thought of this; it was merely supposed that he had gone down town, which was nothing unusual with him. Shortly after this, a negro woman happened to go in the garden, where she found him lying upon the ground—speechless, senseless, and she thought dead. This negress was dispatched for me, and a general alarm given.

I regarded the case as one of pernicious fever. The rubbings seemed to afford little relief; when, the bath being ready, he was put

... him as I prepared
... I went in the room
... before that his moaning
... some of whom were ap-
... enough to observe him, as they
... convenience in which they placed
... being towards the wall, against
... at him for some time—he seemed
... him breathe, but could not. All this
... at least, of more than a minute. I
... to get away, and I took hold of his
... had not yet been applied. The pulse was
... temporal artery, but could not feel it pulsate,
... the while. Then said I to those around, "He
... straightened him out in bed, placing him lengthwise
... lumber as a wet rag. I re-examined the pulse, but
... A thought of the "Ready Method" passed
... and at once, without any explanation, put it in exe-
... continued my efforts, as directed by Marshall Hall, for at
... two minutes—by-standers thought longer. Then, think-
... around would consider it foolishness to be thus handling
... I was about desisting, and said, "Poor fellow, he is dead;
... believe I can do anything for him," still, however, continuing
... turning, etc., when a man at my elbow, who seemed to understand
... better, said, "Doctor, keep on a while longer, don't quit." Some-
... encouraged, I still continued the turning. In something over a
... minute more, he made a feeble inspiration. while in the supine position.
I continued the turning, and in a few seconds this was succeeded by
another of considerable depth. They became more frequent as I continued the operation, and in the course of about ten minutes, the
breathing was fully re-established, and the senses had returned. He
spoke a few words, in answer to questions loudly propounded, and
moaned piteously. I got him to swallow some brandy. The pulse,
which was very feeble when I left off turning, became more full, and

gained strength. I now had the sinapisms applied to the forearms. All seemed to go on well for about half an hour, when the breathing became suddenly feeble and frequent, and in less than a minute ceased altogether. I did not take time to feel his pulse, but began immediately the posturing. At the least calculation, five minutes must have elapsed before my efforts were rewarded by his gasping feebly while supine. This was soon followed by others, and the breathing, the posturing being continued, was gradually re-established, with partial return of the senses, and evidently of great suffering.

To cut a long, and to me astonishing story, short, he *died*, and was brought to life *six times*. I say died, because I know no other word to express his condition. It sounds badly, I know, but I use it for want of a better word. If I had left him when I said he was dead first, no one would have doubted that he "died." I know that he would have been buried the next day. So say twenty witnesses who saw what took place.

But to return. Until he had "died" the fourth time, I had not the faintest hope of his ultimate recovery. It then occurred to me that if he could, by any means, be kept alive during the night, or until reaction should take place, that he might get well. I now determined to try electricity, with, I confess, no very clear idea of how it was going to effect any good; and, in the absence of anything better, I had procured, in a few minutes, a plate electrical machine. For this, and much kind assistance, I am indebted to Professor Samuel Stevenson, of the Young Ladies' Institute. A Leyden jar was charged, and the contents passed through myself and the patient. The charge was a moderate one, yet lightning could have had no more instantaneous effect—the breathing stopped at once. The machine was immediately put aside, and "Marshall Hall's Method" resumed. In about four minutes, it was supposed, an inspiration took place; this was followed by others, and the breathing was, for the fifth time, restored. Still regarding the case as one of pernicious fever, I had been thinking all the while about giving quinine, but had thus far foregone doing so. I determined now to do so at once, and accordingly fourteen grains of the disulphate were given at a dose. My father, who is a physician, and was distant one mile, was now sent for. Before he arrived the breathing again ceased—the sixth and last time. I did as I had done before, and persisting, even after we had all given up hope, was rewarded with like success. It most certainly was eight minutes from the time he ceased to breathe until he made the first effort at inspiration. It was a very feeble one, and it was a long time before the breathing was satisfactorily re-established. I was completely tired out.

My father now arrived, and I told him what had taken place and what I had done. On examining him now, we found the pupils somewhat contracted and insensible to light. The light of a candle, however, seemed to hurt his eyes, from which tears flowed freely, though the pupils did not obey the stimulus. My father regarded the case as one of the forms of *coup de soleil*, named by Dr. Bennet Dowler, of New Orleans, *solar exhaustion*. He proposed that he should take fifteen drops of tinc. opii., and have sinapisms on the back of the neck. Both were immediately complied with. I had sent and got my apparatus, intending to cup him, but had deferred doing so. It was now, however, thought proper, and, as preparatory, to shave the temples. He seemed to be getting better, and wanted to know what was going to be done. When told, and I ready to do so, he objected stoutly and jocosely. He did not like the looks of the scarificator; he had seen persons cut with them, and thought he could get along without it. Said he wanted to go to sleep. After much persuasion, he still objected; and, as he seemed so much better, it was concluded not to cup him.

He was soon in a sound sleep. This was about three o'clock, A. M. I remained with him until 5, when I left him, still asleep, and doing well.

At six o'clock, he began taking the disulphate of quinine, in four-grain doses, every hour. This he continued until 12 M.; after which time, he took two grains every hour until night. He also took, during the day, some fluid extract of senna, to move the bowels. He slept nearly all day, and generally had to be waked to take his medicine. At bedtime he took eight grains of blue pill, and six grains of quinine. He slept well during the night, and when he awoke, generally called for water. This he also did the previous day.

On Thursday, he took two grains of the disulphate of quinine every hour during the day, and until bedtime at night. On the Sunday following, I met him on the street, well. There was a complete blank in his memory from the time he ate his supper on Tuesday evening, until the following morning.

REMARKS.—Whether the foregoing case was one of poisoning from, as I regard it, or one of *solar exhaustion*, or whether it was either one, I leave to the readers of this paper to determine. It may not have been either one. Possibly, it was a complication of both. To describe the various forms in which this cousin-german of Proteus, pernicious fever, may appear, would transcend the contemplated limits of this article.

These remarks are appended mainly for the purpose of offering a suggestion in the treatment of *ictus solis, coup de soleil,* or sun-stroke. All standard works, so far as I know, are meagre as to information on this subject. The only paper on this malady of any value, in my estimation—and that is a really valuable one—is from the pen of Dr. Bennet Dowler, of New Orleans. This may be found in volume xii. of the *New Orleans Medical and Surgical Journal,* page 474, *et seq.,* to which I beg to refer the reader. Dr. Dowler, in his pathological investigations on this disease, has shown no lack of that indefatigable industry which characterizes all his labors. The result of his inquiries proves conclusively that the theory which regards *ictus solis* as a cerebral apoplexy, is an erroneous one, and that the organic lesions are found in the lungs.

In regard to the cause of death, Dr. Dowler says: " Be it what it may, the cause of death begins, continues, and ends in the breathing apparatus." But the most remarkable fact which his investigations have developed is the post-mortem circulation of the blood. He says: "After the death of the lungs, or the cessation of respiration, the heart and arteries will, in some instances, continue to act." Again he says: "Mr. C. died of solar asphyxia on the evening of the 24th of July, 1836. About an hour after he had been laid out, two messengers called upon me to visit the corpse, which was supposed to be alive. I found the body as warm as at death, though it had since been washed. I found a slight pulsation at the wrist and a feeble motion of the heart."

The suggestion which I set out to offer is, the application of the "ready method" of Marshall Hall to the treatment of *coup de soleil* in its worst form, *i. e.,* the *solar asphyxia* of Bennet Dowler. The remedy is so simple and easy of application, under all circumstances, that it seems unnecessary to urge its trial An argument in its favor, however, may be found in the fact that, so far, no other remedy has effected any good.

There is one important fact, I admit, as noticed by Dr. Dowler, that would rather lead to the conclusion that this means must fail. From his observations, it would seem that congestion or hæmorrhagic infiltration of the lungs, always present, precedes death. But from other important facts noticed by the observer, may it not be possible that in some cases, at least, this condition is the effect of the post-mortem circulation or exudation of the blood? Does it not seem probable that the "ready method" of Marshall Hall would have re-stored to life the man seen by Dr. D., in whom, an hour after death, there was " a slight pulsation at the wrist and a feeble motion of the heart?"

On the Artificial Production of Bone by Means of Displacement and Transplantation of the Periosteum.

By M. L. OLLIER.

The researches of Duhamel, and more recently those of Heine and M. Flourens, have demonstrated the importance of the periosteum for the reparation and reproduction of bone. Our own experience has led to similar results, and we have endeavored by experiment still fur-ther to demonstrate its truth.

We have dissected up portions of periosteum, and transplanted them in the midst of tissues normally foreign to ossification; and wherever we have engrafted them, new bone has been developed.

We have made three series of experiments. In the first series, we dissected long bands of periosteum from the tibia, (leaving one end adherent to the bone,) which were entwined in various ways around muscles of the leg. The result was the production of so many circu-lar, spiral, and figure of 8 formations of bone.

In a second series we excised the adherent end or pedicle of the band of periosteum three or four days after the operation, and in spite of this interruption to the primitive circulation of blood, the trans-planted periosteum continued to produce bone.

In a third series of experiments we completely detached the bands of periosteum from the bone at the time of the first operation, and immediately transplanted them in regions more or less removed—under the skin in the groin, on the back, &c., and even under such circum-stances ossific secretion was obtained, and true bony tissue was the result.

These experiments were made upon rabbits of different ages. Ad-vanced age diminishes, but does not destroy, this property of the peri-osteum. The osseous tissue thus obtained possesses the structure of true bone; the fundamental elements consist of bone corpuscles, in every way similar to normal bone. On the surface is a layer of compact substance studded over with Haversian canals. On the interior is found, at the end of a certain time, a medullary cavity, containing a reddish substance of similar anatomical characteristics, under the microscope, of normal marrow; and one or more foramina are seen to transmit blood-vessels.

This new bone is formed from the sub-periosteal blastema, which is in part carried away, attached to this membrane, when it is dissected from the bone.

Our experiments demonstrate that bone will be obtained wherever one succeeds in engrafting the periosteum; they prove that a membrane may preserve its essential properties in spite of its removal and transplantation in the midst of foreign tissues; and, as a practical consequence, it extends the field of anaplasty.—*Gaz. Medicale de Paris*, and *Nashville Med. Record.*

A Suggestion to Life Insurance Companies.

We have long been of the opinion that it is the duty of those having charge of the business of life insurance to inquire somewhat into the character and standing of the medical attendants of those applying for risk on their lives. It needs no argument to prove that the lives of those who place themselves under the care of well-educated and scientific physicians, are, humanly speaking, safer than those who employ ignorant empirics or unscrupulous mountebanks. This must necessarily be the case if medicine has conferred any benefit whatever on mankind, and there are few, we presume, stupid or prejudiced enough to deny but that it has.

Not only are these remarks true of the grosser forms of empiricism, but they apply equally to the more refined and popular systems of modern quackery; and it is to the latter that we more especially allude, as those who insure their lives are more apt to become the dupes of these than of the former.

Practitioners of Homœopathy are ordinarily ignorant of the very first principles of medical science, and their treatment generally inefficient—absolutely so, if they adhere to their system. So that a person in good health, who takes out a risk on his life, and subsequently becoming diseased, places himself under homœopathic treatment, necessarily cuts himself off from all the benefits to be derived from judicious medication, and in some instances may even suffer a loss of life for the want of timely and proper medical attendance.

We submit it, therefore, whether it would not be wise in life insurance companies to direct their inquiries into this matter, and require applicants to state whether they are in the habit of being attended by regular physicians, homœopaths, or other irregular practitioners; and if one of the latter, it seems to us that this fact should at least be taken into account in passing on the application. This would certainly be as pertinent and as pregnant an interrogatory as many that are insisted on, and would put the company in possession of a fact which they have a right to know.— *St. Louis Med. and Surg. Journal.*

COMMUNICATIONS.

The Connection of the Nervous Centres of Animal and Organic Life, with the Results of Vivisection.

By John O'Reilly, M.D., etc.

—" Scire tuum nihil est, nisi te scire hoc sciat alter—
At pulchrum est digito monstrari, et dicier, *Hic est!*"   Pzz.

Few articles of the present time have arrested the attention of the medical world so effectually as the one bearing the above caption.

Brief in its outline, clear and precise in its statement of the objects to be attained, adorned with a fervid and vigorous style, logical in its deductions, predicated upon premises that outwing objection, its conclusions are irresistible.

It reveals the mysteries of that system which, from time immemorial, has strung the energies of the most enlightened intellects to their utmost tension; and elucidates them in such a manner as to place them within the grasp of the most obtuse comprehension.

Truly, such an achievement is brilliant, in the widest sense of the term: whether we take into consideration the mystic influence the nervous system exercises over the functions of organic life, and its intimate connection with most of the pathological changes of the human frame, or the multiplicity of anomalous theories it has given rise to.

Such is, in "paucis verbis," a summary of the leading features of an article that bears the impress of a great mind—an article that bids fair to outlive the flimsy, verbose dissertations on "doctrines fashioned to the varying hour"—an article that shall embellish the brightest page in the historic annals of medicine.

No one of any pretensions to scientific acquirements, and who has been fortunate enough to peruse the article referred to, but must have been struck by the facility with which the most abstruse problems in physiology are solved. There is no metaphysical speculation, no windy satisfaction of the brain, no theoretical vagaries to be encountered in the article—it is void of such blemishes. It is based upon truth—and upon such truth as is the result of observation and experience—vivisection and logic. How, then, I am forced to interrogate, are we to estimate the advantages held out by so remarkable a production? By the immense facilities it affords the physiologist and pathologist in the exposition and amelioration of most of the " ills that flesh is heir to." Disorders, heretofore the "opprobria medicorum," are now susceptible of a satisfactory explanation, and the proper adaptation of remedies suggested.

The learned author has drawn aside the veil which for ages has concealed the sublime operations of the nervous system, that stage upon which all the phenomena of animal life are transacted, and illustrated its manifold beauties with a vigor and richness of thought, a rapidity and strength of language, which manifest the industry and perseverance of the man, and that scholarship and practical sense which embody his other numerous contributions to science.

It were useless to recapitulate the number of facts he has adduced in support of his doctrine. Sufficient be it for me to direct especial attention to that " small, pale, yellowish-red body," the utility of which is now clearly demonstrated, which for centuries has slumbered in undisturbed repose between the corpora quadrigemina, unmolested either by the physiologist or psychologist, silently acknowledging the empire of the will, and transmitting with electrical celerity its mandates throughout the indefinite ramifications of the human structure—the Pineal gland or central ganglion, the president of the ganglionic system. It is the focus from which radiate vitality and power—the concentration of existence and activity—it presides over the functions of organic life, and is the locket of the " vital spark of heavenly flame."

The variety and number of successful experiments performed by the author substantiate beyond a doubt the truth of his doctrine respecting the functions and importance of the central ganglion; but, independent of the experiments alluded to, the syllogisms contained in the latter portion of the author's first paper, on the connection of the centres of animal and organic life, are in themselves sufficient evidences of the paramount value of this seemingly insignificant gland—they are incontrovertible, and must be admitted.

Fortified, then, as they are, by a careful collection of facts, and a rigid induction of particulars, they are calculated to convince any one, not destitute of understanding, of the views entertained and promulgated by the illustrious author.

But as there are at all times individuals who close their ears to reason, and suffer prejudice and national antipathy to lord it over their minds, in the emphatic but indignant language of the great Sir Astley Cooper, "such persons, who object to a proposition merely because it is new, or who endeavor to detract from the merit of the man who first gives efficiency to a new idea by demonstrating its usefulness and applicability, are foolish, unmanly, envious, and illiberal objectors; they are unworthy of the designation either of professional men or gentlemen."

Among the many gems of that literary casket, we call particular notice to the *modus operandi* of belladonna, the janitor of the visual portals, the explanation of which, up to the publication of that pamphlet, remained a profound secret. It is applied to the eyelids; "it exercises a sedative action on the organic nerves in the skin, which inosculate with the nasal branch of the 5th pair, and is conveyed by the latter to the brain, central ganglion, and by reflex action from the ganglion to the brain, 5th nerve, ophthalmic division of the 5th, nasal branch of the latter, and lenticular ganglion by its communicating branch, and thence to the ciliary nerves that go to the iris." What an admirable exemplification of reflex action!

Time and space do not permit any further expatiation upon or citation of other equally beautiful illustrations of reflex action, according to the author's theory; but if the reader have any philosophical propensities, they may be gratified by a recurrence to the essay itself; for the comprehensive definition of vital action, the unique rendition of apnœa, and the interpretation of the virgin's crimsoned cheek when spoken to, or in presence of her "dimidium animæ," are truly deserving of attention for their great merit and originality, and will well repay a studious perusal.

But more than all, we admire the independence of the author, who divests himself of that servility which eminent minds are prone to pay to genius; and who, fearless of criticism, grapples with the arguments of a Bell and a Hall, saps to their very foundation the theories framed upon them, discloses their inconsistencies, explodes their doctrines, shatters to atoms the fabric raised by Brown-Séquard upon the titillation of a baboon, and upon their crumbled remains establishes his own by the force of facts and logic; which, beautiful in its conception and perfect in its execution, is destined to replace theories hitherto deemed forever fixed, but which ere long shall have "gone glimmering through the dreams of things that were." In nowise intimidated by the host of opinions that clash with his own, he heeds not, but argues into conviction; and, like the warrior resting on his battle-axe, he knows where his strength lies, and cares not to look beyond it.

Here, then, before concluding, it is befitting to pay the tribute due to this indefatigable laborer in the field of science, whose penetration enabled him to unravel the intricacies that have so long entangled the physiology of the nervous system, and which now is clearly illustrated in his elaborate and elegantly wrought essay, which shall long remain a master-piece of logical inferences, a lasting mausoleum of its author's erudition and industry, and the greatest scientific achievement of the age. AN INDEPENDENT AMERICAN.

BOOK NOTICES.

ANATOMY, DESCRIPTIVE AND SURGICAL. By Henry Gray, F.R.S.. Lecturer on Anatomy at St. George's Hospital. The drawings by H. V. Carter, M.D., late Demonstrator of Anatomy at St. George's Hospital. The dissections jointly by the author and Dr. Carter. With 363 engravings on wood. Philadelphia: Blanchard & Lea. 1859.

In no department of our science, so much as in anatomy, has there been so urgent need of a new book; nor, until the appearance of this work of Dr. Gray, has there been any British or American publication at all adequate to meet the wants of students in this important science. The plan adopted by Dr. Gray strikes us as possessing great merit and no little novelty.

The descriptive portion of the work is plain, simple, minute and accurate in a high degree, and seems to include all the details of human anatomy in all their varieties and intricacies. The classification of topics is admirable, and the surgical anatomy of each division of the body is separately given; and a separate chapter in this department is devoted to the special subjects of inguinal and femoral hernia, the perineum and ischio-rectal region and other complicated regions of the body, the surgical anatomy of which presents intrinsic difficulties to the student. Practical men in operative surgery will know how to appreciate the value of such a work, for study and reference.

The drawings are, for the most part, original, and superior to those found in any of our other anatomical works; for the names and references, instead of being in figures, are plainly written on the face of the wood-cuts, the advantages of which must be obvious. Moreover, they are artistically executed, and surpassingly beautiful and graphic.

It is due to the worthy American publishers to add, that they appear to have appreciated the great value of this elaborate work of Dr. Gray, for they have excelled themselves in bringing it before the profession. The style and finish of this huge volume of 750 royal octavo pages, the paper, typography, binding and engravings, are all super-excellent; and its intrinsic merits will render it the text-book of anatomy in all the colleges of the land.

CONTRIBUTIONS TO MIDWIFERY AND DISEASES OF WOMEN AND CHILDREN; with a Report on the Progress of Obstetrics and Uterine and Infantile Pathology in 1858. By A. Noeggerath, M.D., and A. Jacobi, M.D. New York: Baillière Brothers. 1859.

These two authors have here combined their efforts in the kindred field of research, to which they are devoting themselves with laudable ardor and industry; and the result is a volume of very great interest and utility. alike scholastic and practical, highly creditable to them both. We predict for them a career of honorable usefulness in the country of their adoption, and the profession will be under strong obligations to them for their *résumé* of German medical literature, which is a *tabula rasa* to too many of us. The publishers have issued it in very handsome style.

A HISTORY OF THE DISCOVERY OF THE CIRCULATION OF THE BLOOD. By P. Flourens, Professor at the Museum of Natural History of Paris. Translated from the French by J. C. Reeve, M.D. Cincinnati: Rickey, Mallory & Co.

This little book comprises a vast amount of historical information, on a subject too little understood, and very inadequately treated in any of the so-called histories of medicine. It illustrates one of the most important events in medical science; an epoch, indeed, upon which turns the success of most of the modern discoveries and improvements, which, but for Harvey and his co-laborers, had never been made, unless some other genius had thrown this luminous discovery upon physiology, which else had never become a science. The translator and publishers merit the thanks of the profession.

URINARY DEPOSITS; their Diagnosis, Pathology, and Therapeutical Indications. By Golding Bird, M.D., F.R.S. Edited by Edmund Lloyd Burkett, M.D., &c. A new American from the 5th London edition, with eighty illustrations on wood. Philadelphia: Blanchard & Lea. 1859.

The late Dr. Golding Bird, by his extensive knowledge and toilsome researches into urinary maladies, has earned a name which can never die. His friend, Dr. Burkett, has prepared this new edition of Dr. Bird's work since his decease, and has greatly improved it. Every physician and student will find the study of this book indispensable, if he would meet his responsibilities in practice. The publishers have done good service in bringing it out so promptly.

MANUAL OF ELEMENTARY CHEMISTRY, Theoretical and Practical. By George Fownes, F.R.S., &c. Edited by Robert Bridges, M.D., &c. Philadelphia: Blanchard & Lea. 1859.

This work is so well known and highly esteemed, that it is only necessary to say that a seventh and revised edition having appeared in London, the American publishers have promptly reproduced it here in superior style. Dr. Bridges has availed himself of the opportunity to add to its merits. We commend it as the best book for students.

EDITOR'S TABLE.

THE LONG AGONY IS OVER.

The office of City Inspector is at length filled by the appointment of Daniel E. Delavan, Esq., a gentleman every way better qualified for its multifarious duties than either of the batch of nominations which the Mayor had successively made. We have little doubt that he will prove to be a good officer.

But Mr. D., though a good *Democrat*, is not a *physician*, and a numerous meeting of the profession last fall affirmed that none but a thoroughly educated medical man was competent in this department. In deference to this judgment, our worthy Mayor gave his first nomination to a physician, but his experience with the medical men who obtruded themselves into his counsels, and betrayed him into a blunder, deterred His Honor from any other *medical* nomination, and hence our Health Department is still in the hands of politicians, who are in blissful ignorance of sanitary science. The would-be "heads of our profession," in New York, have here a lesson which should take the gas out of their self-inflated brains, for they can neither get office for themselves or others. They have defeated the work of reform, and put back the hopes of the profession for sanitary improvement for years, by their officious and arrogant selfishness.

Neither the City Inspector, Health Wardens, nor indeed any other of the multitudinous corps of officials to whom the *Health* department of this great city is committed, has been taken from the ranks of the medical profession. Even the Board of Health, which certain medical dignitaries undertook to revolutionize, by lobbying through the Legislature, at Albany, a Sanitary Bill, from among the batch of bills got up for the purpose, has been left, as aforetime, with the chosen three of political doctors, viz.: Dr. Jedediah Miller, Dr. William Rockwell, and Dr. Alexander Gunn, the only change being the substitution of the last named for Dr. Thompson, which is an even swop.

And yet, there is reason to fear that even after such an experience of the utter impotence of medical men in the race of politics, the lesson will be lost. Certain incorrigible office-seekers will next year again call upon the Academy and the profession to agitate anew in their behalf, under the banner of Reform. But the selfishness of the parties will again be betrayed to the constituted authorities, and politics will perpetuate the spoils of office in the hands of the dominant party. When will our profession learn to maintain its dignity and preserve its self-respect ?

---•◦•---

Notes on the late Quarantine and Sanitary Convention at New York.

Convention of 1857, in Philadelphia.

Yellow fever can be introduced (imported) by *persons* and *things* (fomites!)—that its action upon individuals is limited, and *cannot produce* an epidemic in the community, unless there exist in the latter circumstances which are calculated to produce such disease *independent of importation.*

Convention of 1859, in New York.

Resolved, That in the absence of any evidence establishing the conclusion that yellow fever has ever been conveyed by one person to another, it is the opinion of this Convention that the personal quarantine of cases of yellow fever may be safely abolished, provided that *fomites* of every kind be rigidly restricted!

The creed of the *Philadelphia* Convention may be thus translated, viz.:

" Yellow fever is communicable [contagious] by persons and things, but cannot become epidemic anywhere, unless local causes exist capable of generating yellow fever, *independent of importation or contagion!*"

This last was condemned as vague, indefinite, and contradictory, if at all comprehensible, and this by the Charleston Common Council—to say nothing of its logical fallacy in ascribing more causes for an effect than are necessary to produce it. The physicians of Charleston, of over 25 years' experience, appealed to by the Board of Health in 1858, declare adverse opinions to the contagiousness of yellow fever, as do also, with wonderful unanimity, the medical authorities of New Orleans.

But now turn to the creed of the *New York* Convention of 1859, which may be condensed thus:

" Yellow fever is not communicable (contagious) by *persons*, and hence the sick need not be detained at Quarantine—provided *things* are rigidly restricted—or in their precise language, *things*, not persons, being the cause of the *communicability* of yellow fever."

What a marvelous change within two years, and in the same men! Or is it the *latitude* of Philadelphia and New York that explains how *persons* can give yellow fever to *things*, and cannot infect *persons?* Do they mean that the persons sick with yellow fever cannot spread yellow fever if in a state of *nudity;* but that a *jacket* or *shirt* from such patients is a source of danger? Pray how do the clothes become infected, unless from the *persons* wearing them? And if the *persons* infect the *things,* and these *things* can infect *persons,* and vice versa indefinitely, on what grounds can they affirm that the Quarantine against *persons* may be safely abolished, provided *fomites!* things, are rigidly excluded? This reasoning in a circle is the very sublimation of folly. The contagionists of the last century were consistent, and so are their successors and Dr. Francis, who denounce the late assemblage of medical savans at New York, an "IN-sanitary convention." Dr. Hosack was a consistent contagonist, and maintained that a peddler's pack filled with earth taken from the seat of an epidemic yellow fever, and carried upon his shoulder from one city to another, would engender the pestilence. And the venerable mover of this insane resolution but a few years since publicly declared his belief that the contagion adhered to the *walls and furniture* of the houses in which the sick and dead had been found, not merely for months, but for *years afterwards!* despite of all purification. He has now been driven to give up personal contagion, but takes refuge in *fomites!* with his old heresy.

Well may Dr. Dowler exclaim:

"Among the 91 votes cast on this memorable occasion, it is highly probable that not 10 of the voters ever witnessed an epidemic of yellow fever, although some of them professed to have read as high as 300 volumes on this disease. *The proviso stultifies, and even flatly contradicts the resolution!*"

What are *fomites?*—literally, "anything that kindles or keeps the fire in." Lexicographically—"a term applied to substances which are *supposed* to contain contagious effluvia, as woolen goods, feathers, cotton, &c."

But the New York dogma and that of Philadelphia are both alike in this: both were adopted by theoretical *contagionists,* and the old leaven ferments, notwithstanding their spasmodic efforts to purge it off, or at least to conceal it; verifying the old adage, that "it is hard to teach old dogs new tricks."

Yellow fever is *catching* from *persons or things!* and both must be excluded, says Philadelphia!

Not so, says New York; yellow fever is not *catching* from *persons,* but only from *things,* and these last only need be excluded.

But Philadelphia replies, yellow fever will not spread anywhere, unless there are local causes adequate to produce it, independent of importation of either persons or things!

Nay, says New York, FOMITES! there lies the danger; *things*, not *persons*, will breed the pestilence.

But all agree that yellow fever is catching some how or other, and the ultimatum of both alike is—Quarantine against yellow fever!

But alas for the benighted people of New Orleans! "They have not discovered *fomites* in things, and hence, when they run away from Yellow Jack, they carry their *things*, clothing, boxes, and baggage, all *fomites* with them, and nobody catches it. And when the epidemic declines, they return by thousands to houses depopulated by death, houses shut up for weeks, after all their tenants have been carried to the grave, and from which no one has attempted to remove the dreaded *fomites!*—50,000 living experiments against contagion!—50,000 exposures to fomites! and nobody catches it! What means the immense shipment of cotton (fomites) all over the world from the midst of yellow fever epidemics? as to Havre, Liverpool, &c. Has yellow fever ever been suspected in that direction? And yet *cotton* is one of the worst of *fomites*, the most susceptible of the suspected articles!" See Dr. Dowler's withering review of the late New York Quarantine and Sanitary Convention, in this number of the GAZETTE. It will repay perusal. We commend it to Dr. Alfred C. Post and Dr. Jedediah Miller, and the other enlightened and experienced counselors chosen by the N. Y. Chamber of Commerce. *Vive la bagatelle!*

DR. J. S. CURTIS,

Of Hartford, Ct., has been expelled from the profession, by the County and State Society, on the charge of habitually consulting with Homœopaths, and persisting in such irregularity after due remonstrance. He appeals, as do all the quacks, to the newspapers, under the caption of "Bigotry of the Medical Profession," and publishes what would have been his defence, had he made any, an unspoken speech, but, like all bunkum oratory, coming to a "lame and impotent conclusion." We wonder whether he will carry up his case to the American Medical Association, which happens to meet in Connecticut next June? If so, may we be there to see.

We have long since expressed our opinion, that every physician who degrades the craft by meeting any Homœopath in consultation should be forthwith indicted under the statute of frauds, for obtaining money under false pretences, as he unquestionably does if he receives a fee for such consultation. Our rule has been invariably, to refuse to see a patient who has been treated by a Globulist, until he was discharged and paid. A consultation by a regular physician with a Homœopath is a farce not merely, but a fraud. Hence Dr. Curtis's "offence is rank, and smells to heaven." No plea of "humanity," such as Dr. Curtis hypocritically urges, can avail. It is the *fee*, and this only, not humanity, which is the tempter. Everybody has the right to choose a Homœopath, instead of a physician, when he is sick, but he does this under no less a penalty than to exclude himself from all benefits which the counsel of a physician can afford him, in any exigency; and the sooner this is understood, the better for all parties.

We know nothing of the Homœopaths of Connecticut, but presume they are all alike. Here the very chiefest among them has a "weak sister" or "female brother," on whose mesmeric or clairvoyant skill he relies for diagnosis and treatment; and in urgent cases he holds a "spirit circle" for rapping out the disease and remedies, for either of which humbuggery he receives an exorbitant fee. Shall a physician consult with or recognize such a mountebank? However many reasons he may assign for such offence against the Code of Ethics, the only true reason is the money he makes by it, for "by this craft we have our gains," and the "wages of unrighteousness" are his reward. This is a free country, and every man has the right to do as he pleases; but we must have the right in our profession to choose our own company, and to refuse recognition of any Homœopath, or those who consort with them.

The physicians of Hartford have published a reply to Dr. Curtis's defence, which places them *rectus in curia*, by defining their position. Let them still stand to their principles, and repudiate treason to the profession, by ostracizing the traitors, and refusing to work in partnership with the devil.

DR. FRANCIS'S ORATION,

Before the Historical Society, itself a volume of research into modern antiquarianism, seems destined by its popularity to furnish materials for an indefinite number of volumes, and to be everywhere read; portions of it having appeared in many of the journals and magazines, at home and abroad. We have already referred to one of these volumes, viz.: "Old New York, or Reminiscences of the past

Sixty Years;" and now we chronicle another publication based on the former, viz.: "Reminiscences of Samuel Latham Mitchell, M.D., LL.D., &c.," which the author has found time to rewrite and enlarge, from the article in the "Manual of the Corporation of the City of New York, by David T. Valentine, Esq., for 1859." Having enjoyed the personal acquaintance and friendship of the illustrious Dr. Mitchell, we can testify to the fidelity of this memoir by Dr. Francis.

THE MEDICAL AND SURGICAL REPORTER

Has needlessly volunteered both sympathy and counsels to our brethren at New Haven, in anticipation that the meeting of the American Medical Association, in that city, in June, 1860, will prove an inconvenient infliction. The editors may spare themselves and their readers the apprehensions their article on this subject is calculated to awaken, for our Connecticut brethren understand their own business, and will be prepared to extend the delegates, and the ladies who may accompany them, a genial and hearty welcome. The City of Elms, and its vicinity, will not be so thronged at the time from any cause, as to be incommoded by the gathering of our Medical Congress, and their guests will not fail to be met by a generous reception and cordial hospitality, in which the Committee of Arrangement will have the active participation of the State Medical Society, including representatives of every county in the State.

FEMININE DOCTORS.

The Pennsylvania State Medical Society has condescended to take formal notice, by a denunciatory resolution, of the Female Medical College of Philadelphia, and the "woman-doctors," which the male and female professors of that school are annually manufacturing. This appears to us rather small business for a State Society, and this folly has brought upon the parties concerned the censures of the daily press, which, of course, defends the feminine doctors and their masculine teachers. The women "pitch in" to the "Jewell" of the Philadelphia doctors, who is the supposed father of all this mischief, and handle him without gloves. He had better take the advice of Samuel Weller hereafter, and "beware of widders," and learn the lesson, "Barney! let the girls alone." The Reporter "advises the men-doctors of Philadelphia to let the women-doctors alone severely!" What

do our ungallant neighbors mean by *severely*? Do they mean to in-
timidate the dear creatures? We hope Dr. Edwin Fussell, the
worthy Dean of the College, and who teaches the feminine pupils the
art and mystery of " midwifery and the diseases of women," will keep
an eye on our brother editors who utter this menace. He and his
brother professors in this Female College, if all four are of the masculine gender, are bound, by all the laws of chivalry, to protect the
only two weak sisters in the Faculty, viz.: Miss Ann Preston and
Mrs. Emeline H. Cleaveland, from the " severity" of Drs. Butler and
Levis, who dare to threaten them.

The former of these ladies is a tender plant, and could not bear
" severity," for lack of physical strength: as we infer, from having
heard her lecture in this city before a promiscuous audience, on physiology and hygiene, and were grieved to witness in her person a sad
and sorry compound of morbid anatomy, pathology, and the very antipodes of hygiene or physiology either. We longed to prescribe for
her *beef-steaks, porter, and chalybeates*, which her physical condition
demanded. Her mental status could not be judged from the string
of commonplace axioms she uttered about the laws of health and
life, all of which she must have practically ignored during her long
life, else she had proved them to be of none effect, as may be inferred
from her corporeal imbecility. Possibly she doomed herself to celi-
bacy, for the purpose of becoming a doctor; but if so, we fear she
will be a martyr to her professional ambition. Let her "throw physic
to the dogs," and choose a husband—better late than never.

On the general question of feminine doctors, we have an opinion
that is an opinion, but we forbear to express it; warned by the fate
of our pseudo-friend, Dr. Jewell. As, however, we perceive there is
a vacancy in the chair of surgery in the Female College of Philadelphia, we have a candidate, in a certain female surgeon and obstetrician, of Brooklyn, who has proved her surgical skill, by destroying a
mother and her unborn twins, by female doctoring, a few days since.
Her name is Mrs. Lodge, M.D., and she may be found in jail for this
triple murder, on the commitment of the Coroner.

We have female M. D's in New York, who have been regularly
graduated, and they too have a college, and a hospital, and a dispensary, and a lying-in infirmary, and a school for *nurses*, which latter is
the true mission of the sex. But our State Medical Society has not
declared war upon the windmill, nor shall we. If we were sick, and
could be treated *secundum artem* by a female doctor, we should say,

"Avaunt, you horrid men!" We cannot, therefore, find fault with others for doing as we would do ourselves, by giving preference to the tender sex in any capacity. This would conform to Dr. Bigelow's doctrine, viz.: " *Nature and art* in the cure of disease," for one touch of nature makes the world akin.

We remember an anecdote which we heard of an old friend who expressed his opinion that to see a dog walking on his hind legs, was *wonderful*. "The *wonder* is, not that he does the trick so *well*, but that he can do it at all!" So when we see or hear a *woman* lecturing on the rostrum on any subject, we do not expect her to do it *well*, but our marvel is that she can unsex herself by doing it at all, in a promiscuous audience. How any *man* that has bones in him can degrade himself by obtruding into a female college to teach midwifery to women and girls, passes our comprehension. Granted that there is no one of the opposite sex to be found in the country, who is capable. Then let the women import Madame Boivin or Lachapelle, from Paris, if they must have a school for old or young " women-doctors," for these feminines have unsexed themselves, for the purpose of acquiring the knowledge in the Parisian hospitals to teach and practice midwifery. But none claiming to be of the opposite sex, unless he can prove himself to be a *neuter*, should be thus employed in a female college, as a matter of *taste*, to say nothing of morality, which may be excluded from a question of comeliness and propriety.

Our neighbors of the *Reporter*, at Philadelphia, it seems, have " shown the white feather," in the war they have provoked on this subject, for by their pacific proposition to ignore the existence of women-doctors, they find themselves between two fires. In front, they are met by a phalanx of the Amazons, who refuse to " let *them* alone," and are backed by an army of defenders and the public press. While a " fire in the rear " has been commenced in behalf of the belligerent and venerable Jewell of a doctor, who attacks them in their own columns. We regret to see these symptoms of " backing down " on a question upon which they are clearly right. As hostilities are but just begun, however, discretion is perhaps the better part of valor.

> For he who fights with *women*, and runs away,
> May live to fight the *men* another day.—Penn.

------•◦•------

Dr. Sanger has published an elaborate Report of the several hospitals in his charge on Blackwell's Island, New York.

A CASE OF TWINS, IN WHICH ONE WAS BORN JUST TWENTY YEARS AFTER THE OTHER! ♦

Prof. J. B. Flint, of the University of Louisville, in a very able address, as President of the Medical Society of the State of Kentucky, deprecates in very strong terms what he calls "star lecturers," who go from place to place, like star actors, their employers expecting to be reimbursed by *full houses*. He dislikes the modern attempt to engraft this invention of stage managers upon medical colleges. If we must have "stars," however, we think the idea a good one to imitate nature, and have them of two classes, the "fixed" and the progressive. We think some of our friends out West prefer the "fixed."

Dr. John Frederick May certainly has indisputable claims to the latter class. In 1839 he delivered an introductory before the class in the Columbia College. This he gives no particular name. He is called on in due form by his admiring pupils for a copy for publication, and it is accordingly published. In 1859, *just twenty years after*, he delivers an introductory lecture before the class of Shelby Medical College, at Nashville, which he dubs "INDIVIDUAL EFFORT." How much *individual effort* it required to produce this essay we propose to indicate, as this also was called for by admiring pupils for *publication!* and gracefully handed over by the Professor for that purpose.

THE TWINS!

FIRST BORN.—**1839.**   LAST BORN.—**1859.**

Page 5.

We are about entering its various departments, in each to separate the glowing truths of scientific research from the erring theories and false hypotheses which have mingled with them; to unfold to your admiring gaze the beauties and the wonders of the human organization; to explain to you the aggregate of those phenomena which constitute life, and the admirable perfection and harmony of the laws which preside over and govern them; to make you acquainted with the perversion of these laws, and the various diseases which are consequent upon their derangement; to bring before you the numerous remedial agents by whose means these same laws may be readjusted, and the integrity of the organization be restored; to expound to you those conservatory principles by a knowledge of which the hand may be safely carried through parts where le-

Page 3.

We invite you to enter with us into its various departments, in each to separate the glowing truths of scientific research from the erring theories and false hypotheses that have been mingled with them; to unfold to your admiring gaze the beauties and the wonders of the human organization; to explain to you the aggregate of those phenomena which constitute life, and the admirable perfection of the laws that preside over and govern them; to make you acquainted with the perversion of these laws, and the various diseases which are consequent upon their derangement; to bring before you the numerous remedial agents by whose means these same laws may be readjusted, and the integrity of the organization be restored; to demonstrate to you the beautiful truths of that science whose laboratory, though the universe itself, yet draws renovat-

40

sion would be fatal, to stay the aneurismal flood, or extirpate the forming seeds of death; and to demonstrate to you the beautiful truths of that science whose laboratory, though the universe itself, yet draws renovating principles from even the sponge of ocean's depths, or the fragile weed which is borne upon its billows' foam!

ing principles from even the sponge of ocean's depths, or the fragile weed which is borne upon its billows' foam; and to expound to you those conservatory principles by a knowledge of which the hand may be carried safely through parts where lesion would be fatal, to stay the aneurismal flood, or to extirpate the forming seeds of death.

Page 6.

It requires no deep research, no philosophical analysis, in order to be convinced that the spirit of improvement is abroad, and is steadily working great and salutary changes in the general face of affairs; and it would indeed be evincing great ignorance of the present state of medical science not to perceive that it has most deeply felt the influence of this spirit, and most extensively participated in these changes. Within less than half a century, its whole aspect has been revolutionized. Branches which formerly were unknown, have been in this short period created; and others which, although in existence, exercised but little influence over the progress of medicine, have assumed the highest importance, and become the very basis of its advancement. The practice of medicine at the present day is something more than a simple routine of measures subject to the visionary and ever-fluctuating theories of the imagination. It has assumed in "the circle of the sciences" a high and independent station. It has become a profound philosophy, whose principles can be determined and understood only by rigid induction and untiring investigation, and which can be put into successful practice only by means of close observation. extensive information, and a well-disciplined and discriminating judgment.

Page 5.

It requires, then, no deep research to be satisfied that this spirit of improvement is abroad, and is constantly and steadily working great and salutary changes in the general face of affairs; and it would indeed be evincing great ignorance of the present state of medical science, not to perceive that it has most deeply felt the influence of this spirit, and most extensively participated in these changes. Within little more than half a century its entire aspect has been changed. Branches in this time have arisen to importance which before were not understood; and others, which exercised but little influence over the progress of medicine, have become of the highest importance, the very basis of its advancement. Medicine has, in fact, assumed in the circle of the sciences a high and independent station. It is no longer a simple routine of measures, subject to visionary and ever-fluctuating theories of the imagination; it is a profound philosophy, whose principles can be determined and understood only by rigid induction and untiring investigation, and which can be put into successful practice only by means of close observation, extensive information, and a well-disciplined and discriminating judgment.

Page 8.

Forty years have not yet rolled by since the immortal Bichat published his treatise on the membranes and delivered his lectures on pathological anatomy. Prior to him, its study had only been prosecuted at intervals, and in the most vague and irregular manner. Bonetus, it is true, at the close of the seventeenth century, endeavored to collect in a systematic manner the imperfect anatomical observations which had been made up to his time,

Page 7.

But little more than half a century has rolled by since Bichat published his immortal Treatise on the Membranes, and his Memoir upon Life and Death. Before his time the study of morbid anatomy had only been prosecuted at intervals, and in the most vague and unsatisfactory manner. Bonetus, it is true, at the close of the seventeenth century, endeavored to collect in a systematic manner the imperfect anatomical observations that

in regard to the causes and seat of diseases. But his work was filled with erroneous theories; for all that existed of pathological anatomy in his time, were a few isolated facts, almost lost in the voluminous works of theory and error, to which they had been occasionally consigned. His labors, however, formed a point of departure for Morgagni, who, entering more profoundly into the views contained in them, and multiplying autopsic examinations, has transmitted to us a work replete with sound pathological remarks, drawn from the most exact observations of nature. After Morgagni, we find Walter, Sandifort, Lieutaud, Portal. Vicq D'Azyr, Baillie, and a few others, contributing, by some useful discoveries, to augment the knowledge relative to pathology. But their works, as well as those of Morgagni, can scarcely be considered more than memoirs—the disjointed fragments of the foundation scattered about promiscuously, which it required the hand of a master to collect and cement before the grand and systematic structure could be raised. Bichat saw this deficiency, and his vast mind, guided by the torch of physiology and inductive philosophy, classified the tissues according to their analogies, and having thus created *general* anatomy, he sought, by continued examinations, to elucidate their pathological states. Thus, he may, in truth, be said to be the founder of the system with whose importance I wish to impress you. What had been done before him was disjointed, uncombined, and vague. His genius breathed upon the commingled elements, and system and order were produced. Like the solar lens, it drew together the few and scattered rays that were visible in the horizon, and adding to them the coruscations of his own mighty intellect, it conveyed the whole. until, from the intensity, light, and truth, and form, and harmony burst upon the profound obscurity.

had been made up to his time in regard to the causes and seat of disease; but his work was filled with erroneous theories; for all that existed of morbid anatomy in his day were a few isolated facts, almost lost in the voluminous works of theory and error to which they had been occasionally consigned. His labors, however, formed a point of departure for Morgagni, who, entering more profoundly into the views contained in them, and multiplying autopsic examinations, has transmitted to us a work replete with sound pathological views, drawn from the exact observations of nature. After Morgagni, we find Walter, Sandifort, Lieutaud, Portal, Vicq D'Azyr, Baillie, and a few others, contributing by some useful discovery to augment the knowledge relative to pathology. But their works, as well as those of Morgagni, can scarcely be considered more than memoirs—the disjointed fragments of the foundation scattered about promiscuously, which it required the hand of a master to collect and cement before the grand and systematic structure could be raised. Bichat saw this deficiency, and his vast mind, guided by the torch of physiology and inductive philosophy, classified the tissues of the human organization according to their analogies, and, having thus created *general anatomy*, he sought by every opportunity to elucidate their pathological states. Thus he may in truth be said to be the founder of the system which has since exercised so much influence upon the progress of medical science. What had been done before his time was disjointed, uncombined, and vague. His genius breathed upon the commingled elements, and system and order were produced. It drew together the few and feeble rays that were visible in the horizon, and throwing upon them light from his own mighty intellect, he deduced fact after fact, and principle upon principle, until truth, and form, and harmony burst forth upon the profound obscurity.

Page 13.

The practice of medicine, and every rational theory in regard to disease, must be derived from the cultivation of Pathological Anatomy, aided by clinical observation. Select any dis-

Page 9.

The practice of medicine, in fact, and every rational theory of disease, can only be derived from a thorough knowledge of the general anatomy of the tissues, and the deductions which

ease that you please, and what does it present to you? A problem, placed before you, which you are called upon to solve; and as data to enable you to do this. you have symptoms, some of which are perceptible to yourself, and others to the patient only. These symptoms are nothing more than "an expression of suffering on the part of the organ which is diseased." But in the animal economy one diseased part will frequently, by *means of sympathy*, produce a train of symptoms, in various and more important parts; sympathetic symptoms, which I have already told you, are often so prominent as to obscure those which emanate from the true seat of the disease, and thus completely blind you as to the nature of the affection you are called upon to relieve. What will guide you in the chaos of symptoms, if I may so express myself, which are so confusedly blended, and which. nevertheless, it is so necessary you should understand? Will you rely upon your anatomical information for obtaining this knowledge? However precise and perfect this may be, and however important, as I have already declared, it is but a history of the relations of parts as they exist in the inanimate frame after the vital spark has fled the tenement; it is the science of the dead, inanimate machine merely. It does not explain to you one single phenomenon of life. It tells you of the position, the size. and the texture of the various component parts of the human body, but it does not present to you these parts acting. It does not show them to you animated, and fulfilling the various functions whose aggregate constitutes life, &c.

are drawn from this knowledge by morbid anatomy. Select a disease, any disease that you please. and what is it? A problem, which you are called upon to solve; and the data that are before you to enable you to do this are the symptoms which it presents, some of which are evident to yourself, and others to the patient only; symptoms which, as has been truly observed, are the "expression of suffering" on the part of the organ which is affected. But how often do symptoms alone deceive us in regard to the solution of disease! How often do they mask and conceal from us by means of sympathy, as I have already said, or of similarity of function. the part or organ that is really in a morbid condition! How often do we see, by merely sympathetic influence, a morbid condition of the liver manifest itself by sympathetic symptoms at the shoulder. or an affection of the hip-joint express itself by suffering at the knee! Nothing, in fact, is more common in the animal economy than for an organ, when afflicted, to show it by symptoms in distant and sometimes more important parts of the system. What is to guide you. amid this chaos of confusedly blended symptoms, in regard to the diagnosis you may wish to form? Can you rely upon descriptive anatomy to enable you to arrive at a correct result? However perfect your information may be here, however precise your knowledge of the human form, it is but a history of the relation of parts as they exist in the inanimate frame, after the vital spark has left the tenement; it is merely the science of the dead, inanimate machine. It does not explain to you one single principle of life ; it tells you of the position, the size, and the relations of the various component parts of the human organization, but it does not present to you these parts animated and active; it does not show them to you fulfilling the different functions whose aggregate constitutes life, &c.

Page 15.

Etiology, or the history of causes, may often provide for you "prophylactic indications," but it will as often mislead you. if it is your only method of ascertaining the nature of disease. And if you rely upon the other means

Page 10.

From etiology, or a knowledge of the causes of disease. you may often draw prophylactic indications, but you may rest assured that it will frequently mislead you if you rely upon it to ascertain the nature of disease.

that I have mentioned, I have only to say that you descend at once to the level of the miserable empiric, who at hazard administers his nostrums, and blindly relies upon chance.

And if you trust alone to the therapeutic action of your remedies, you trust, in other words, to chance, and you descend at once to the level of the miserable empiric, who at hazard administers his nostrums, and blindly hopes for success.

Page 19.

Our profession has felt too long and too deeply the retarding influence of "false facts," based upon theoretical delusion; and even at the present day it numbers many minds who are never at ease unless they are in the world of abstractions; who are inspired with the pen, but lost when in the presence of disease; generalizers, who are unable or unwilling to endure the slow and patient march of observation, finding it easier to *invent* for Nature, rather than to *learn* from her teachings. For them, an idea *à priori*, is a point of departure, "and one induction, a principle demonstrated." They are, in truth, the *poets* of our science; and though their theories may dazzle by their brilliancy or excite the admiration from their ingenuity, their *practical* influence in our profession is as evanescent as it is visionary. Like the phosphorescent spangles that are turned up by ocean's wave, they glitter in the track of the noble bark as it courses on, but emit no ray to warn her of the sunken rock—no light to guide her onward to the destined haven of her voyage!

Page 14.

Medicine, in fact, though eminently practical in all its aims, has felt too long and too deeply the influence of *false facts*, based upon mere theoretical opinions, and even at the present day it numbers many minds that are never at ease unless they are in the world of abstractions; who are inspired with the pen, but who are lost when in the presence of disease; generalizers, who are unable or unwilling to endure the slow and patient march by which truth is found; finding it easier to *invent* for Nature, rather than to learn from her teachings; for whom "an idea *à priori* is a point of departure, and one induction a principle demonstrated." Such may, in truth, be called the *poets* of our science, whose views, although they may dazzle by their brilliancy or produce a sensation by their ingenuity, are in our profession, indeed, in every practical profession, as evanescent as they are visionary. Like the phosphorescence that is turned up by the ocean's wave, they glitter in the track of the noble bark as she courses on, but they emit no ray to warn her of the sunken rock, no light to guide her *onward* to the destined haven of her voyage.

Page 23.

Enter then not lightly, I entreat you, upon the preparatory labors of this school, which are to qualify you for the faithful and honorable discharge of this high trust; but come fully impressed with the magnitude of the contract which will be created by it between yourselves and society, and with the determination to lay *now*, well and deeply, the basis of those studies which may enable you to meet these responsibilities calmly and conscientiously. Come with a deep sense of the high and noble nature of the profession you have chosen, and with an ardent thirst for its truths, and by patient investigation and zealous research, you will obtain them, &c., &c.

Page 16.

Come, then, to the studies which are before you with a deep sense of the magnitude of the contract which will be formed between yourselves and your fellow-men, and with the determination to lay now well and thoroughly here in this school, that foundation upon which you may base the power and knowledge to meet these responsibilities calmly and conscientiously hereafter. Approach them not as belonging to a speculative, but to an eminently practical science; not as studies from which may be acquired a routine of superficial knowledge that may enable you to make *merchandise* of the sufferings of your fellow-men, but as belonging to an elevated and inductive

Guided by such principles, you will uphold the honor of your profession, and be rendered worthy of entering its temple; principles which glowed in the mind of the eloquent Roman when he uttered that beautiful, yet just sentence. "*Homines ad Deos nulla re proprius accedunt, quam salutem hominibus dando.*" Let *your* aspirations be elevated like the sentiment contained in it. and your reward will be commensurate.

science; a profound philosophy, whose principles can only be acquired by the most persevering industry, and can only be truly practiced in a spirit of enlightened philanthropy.

Animated by such views, and sustained by such principles, you will become worthy to bear the honored title of physician; worthy of that eloquent tribute which the greatest of Roman orators has paid to the *true* physician: " Homines ad Deos nulla re proprius accedunt quam salutem hominibus dando." Worthy, &c., &c.

In truth, we are right sorry to see this. Our friends out West are not so sharp as they claim credit for. What has become of the "Bound Book" of our friend of the *Nashville Journal,* in which he keeps so many old documents stored away, as rods in pickle, to draw on as occasion offers? He praises Dr. May's lecture, and, it would seem, believed, with the "boys," that it was very new and very nice! Dr. May is a fixed "star," and Dr. Bowling one of his wrapt admirers.

MEDICAL JOURNALS.

Several of our exchanges have been discontinued lately because of *non-paying* subscribers, who have thus deprived all who *did pay* of the luxury and profit of reading good journals, which they would be glad to continue to pay for, if the publishers had not been driven from the field, by having so many delinquents on the *black list.* The *Montreal Chronicle* and *Maine Medical Journal,* both ably edited by laborious and gifted men, have been thus sacrificed, to the regret of many, and to the loss of us all; and these are not alone.

Still, however, we have to announce that our old friend, Professor Weber, of Cleveland, Ohio, has ventured on the experiment of a new monthly, at *one* dollar per annum, and, as we know him to be a capable editor, we wish him better success than his neighbors, notwithstanding he has trespassed upon our patronymic name, to which for eleven years we have claimed the exclusive right. We marvel that he was not deterred from this plagiaristic enormity by the fate of the *Louisville Medical Gazette,* which is already defunct, a melancholy example of *infant* mortality, a just retribution upon its parent for pirating our *good name.* But "*de mortuos,*" &c. Better luck for our new neighbor in Cleveland, who excels us all in cheapness.

To all our non-paying subscribers, and their name is Legion, we would say, send Dr. Weber a dollar in advance for his journal, and on notice that you have done so, we will discontinue ours, and forgive our debtors, hoping to be forgiven for having trusted them so long. We have been urged to publish our black list, but it is so long that it would fill this number, to the exclusion of everything else; and we have decided that if we hereafter send our GAZETTE without *payment in advance*, we deserve our fate. Let our confrères all say Amen.

DR. EDWARD JENNER COXE,

Of New Orleans, has just published "Practical Remarks on Yellow Fever, having special reference to its treatment." His knowledge and experience qualify him to write on this important subject, and his essay is eminently sound and practical. We observe that contagion has no countenance from the author, who knows the local origin of yellow fever by mathematical demonstration on the spot.

THE SEMI-MONTHLY MEDICAL NEWS,

Of Louisville, Ky., is out with a spirited article denunciatory of the Kappa Lambdas, for whom, it seems, nobody has a word, as they are confessedly indefensible, and hence their ominous silence. But we are tempted to remind the Dr. *B's*, our confrères, that the newspaper puffs of a certain Louisville professor, who shall be nameless, for the radical operation in hernia, and claiming for him, so flippantly, merit, and even novelty, apart from being ludicrous, are quite as unprofessional as K. L.-ism, or any other of our New York delinquencies. We pause for a reply.

PRIZES.

The Editors of the *Medical and Literary Weekly* will award, through a committee appointed for that purpose, on the first of October next, to successful competitors, the following prizes:

For the best original Romance.......................$200.
For the best Poem...........................Silver Cup.
For the best Article on Quackery................ "   "
For the best Hygienic Article................... "   "
For the largest List of Subscribers........Not less than $100.
For the next largest List........................... 50.
For the next largest List................. .... 25.

Competitors for the Literary and Hygienic prizes will send in their articles by the first of September next—the paper to be enveloped by itself, with a motto on the envelope; the name of the author in another envelope, bearing the same motto on its outside. The envelopes containing the names will not be opened until the awards have been decided upon.

Competitors for the prizes for the largest lists of subscribers can send in their lists by the first of October, or in installments from this date till that time, with their own names appended. The money must accompany the lists in all cases.

Price of the Medical and Literary Weekly, $2 per annum.

Address Taliaferro & Thomas, Atlanta, Georgia.

MEDICAL VOYAGERS TO EUROPE.

Professor Paul F. Eve, of Nashville, Tenn., and family, are off in the Persia, from New York, on the 6th of July; and they were followed by Professor J. B. Lindsley, also of Nashville, with his family, on the 13th, in the Arabia, from Boston. We should not be surprised if the former gentleman should commission the latter to take charge of the ladies of his party, while he, true to his instincts, makes a flying visit to the "seat of war," to look after military surgery, of which Baron Larrey, the 2d, seems likely to have enough and to spare. Having served under the father, Baron Larrey the 1st, in a former war, Dr. Eve has not lost his penchant for the camp and tented field, and might be tempted to renew his commission after "seeing blood in Italy," if he were not under bonds to return to Nashville in October, for his duties in the University, and which his traveling companion, "the Chancellor," will see that he does not escape. Dr. Coleman, of Augusta, Ga., who is of the party, will probably enlist during the war, under the impulse of patriotic and professional motives. We wish all a prosperous trip, and a safe return.

MISCELLANEOUS ITEMS.

Episcopal Hospital of Philadelphia.—Dr. Henry Hartshorn has been appointed Attending Physician, in place of Dr. J. B. Biddle, resigned. It is to this institution that the surgical instruments of the late Professor T. D. Mutter have been presented, by his widow.

Dr. D. Francis Condie has been elected to the Presidency of the State Medical Society of Pennsylvania. The Society honors itself in thus conferring its highest dignity on one who is worthy of the loftiest position which our profession can bestow, for the fidelity, industry, and ardor with which he has served his generation, by his contributions to the medical literature of our science and art. There are few men more widely known, or so universally esteemed by the profession of the whole country, as the very "soul of honor." We congratulate him on this new token of appreciation by those who know him best.

Savannah Medical College.—Dr. W. R. Waring succeeds Dr. Howard in the chair of Anatomy, the latter.having resigned.

The New York Medical College is making progress in the right direction, by reorganizing and strengthening its faculty. In addition to the transfer of Prof. Peaslee to the Obstetrical chair, they have made the following new appointments, viz.: Dr. Austin Flint, Jr., to the chair of Physiology. &c.; Dr. James Bryan, Professor of Anatomy, and Dr. Meier, Associate Professor of Anatomy. Other changes and new appointments are rumored, but those mentioned are consummated, and they are all able men and fitly chosen.

College of Physicians and Surgeons.—We were in error in announcing the new appointments in this school as Adjunct Professors, their designation being "*Lecturers* adjunct to the Professors of Surgery and Midwifery" respectively. They are not yet professors, but must tarry a while as Lieutenants before they can be made Captains.

Dr. Edward Hartshorne has been appointed to the Surgical staff of the Pennsylvania Hospital, in place of Dr. Neill, who has resigned.

Dr. Joshua B. Flint has published his address before the Kentucky State Medical Society, as its President, in which he fully endorses the heresies of Drs. Forbes and Bigelow, upon which we have recently had occasion to comment. His plea for conservatism in surgery, some years since, seems to have led him into ultra-conservatism in medicine, and we only regret that so much ability as he undeniably possesses should be employed in propagating error and multiplying skepticism. More anon.

Pharmacopœia Convention.—The notice of the meeting of this important body, in May next, should not be overlooked by the authorities entitled to representation. There is an absolute need of radical improvement in the U. S. P. published by this Convention ten years ago. *Verbum sat.*

Mortality.—Among the recent deaths in our ranks, we find the names of Dr. Ackley, of Cleveland, and Dr. Bond, of Philadelphia, th able men.

Honorary Degree.—The Castleton Medical College of Vermont has conferred the degree of M.D. on Dr. S. N. Marsh, of this city, the well-known inventor of the Radical Cure Truss, and other improvements in Mechanical Surgery.

CONTENTS.

UNIVERSITY OF NEW YORK.
MEDICAL DEPARTMENT.
SESSION, 1859-60.

The Session for 1859–60 will begin on Monday, October 17, and will be continued until the 1st of March.

Faculty of Medicine.

REV. ISAAC FERRIS, D.D., LL.D., Chancellor of the University.

VALENTINE MOTT, M.D., LL.D., Emeritus Professor of Surgery and Surgical Anatomy, and ex-President of the Faculty.

MARTYN PAINE, M.D., LL.D., Professor of Materia Medica and Therapeutics.

GUNNING S. BEDFORD, M.D., Professor of Obstetrics, the Diseases of Women and Children, and Clinical Midwifery.

JOHN W. DRAPER, M.D., LL.D., Professor of Chemistry and Physiology, President of the Faculty.

ALFRED C. POST, M.D., Professor of the Principles and Operations of Surgery, with Surgical and Pathological Anatomy.

WILLIAM H. VAN BUREN, M.D., Professor of General and Descriptive Anatomy.

JOHN T. METCALFE, M.D., Professor of the Institutes and Practice of Medicine.

J. W. S. GOULEY, M.D., Demonstrator of Anatomy.

J. H. HINTON, M.D., Prosector to the Professor of Surgery.

ALEXANDER B. MOTT, M.D., Prosector to the Emeritus Professor of Surgery.

Besides Daily Lectures on the foregoing subjects, there will be five Cliniques weekly, on *Medicine, Surgery, and Obstetrics.*

The Dissecting-room, which is refitted and abundantly lighted with gas, is open from 8 o'clock, A. M., till 10 o'clock, P. M.

Fees for a full course of Lectures, $105. Matriculation fee, $5. Graduation fee, $30. Demonstrator's fee, $5.

UNIVERSITY OF BUFFALO.

Medical Department.—The Annual Course of Lectures in this Institution commences on the FIRST WEDNESDAY IN NOVEMBER, and continues sixteen weeks. The Dissecting-rooms will be opened on the first Wednesday in October.

Clinical Lectures at the Buffalo Hospital throughout the entire term, by Professors HAMILTON and ROCHESTER.

FACULTY.

JAMES P WHITE, M.D., Professor of Obstetrics and Diseases of Women and Children.

FRANK H. HAMILTON, M.D., Professor of the Principles and Practice of Surgery and Clinical Surgery.

GEORGE HADLEY, M.D., Professor of Chemistry and Pharmacy.

THOMAS F. ROCHESTER, M.D., Professor of Principles and Practice of Medicine.

EDWARD M. MOORE, M.D., Professor of Surgical Anatomy and Surgical Pathology.

THEOPHILUS MACK, M.D., Lecturer on Materia Medica.

SANDFORD EASTMAN, M.D., Professor of Anatomy.

AUSTIN FLINT, JR., M.D., Professor of Physiology and Microscopy.

BENJ. H. LEMON, M.D., Demonstrator of Anatomy.

Fees—including Matriculation and Hospital Tickets, $75. Demonstrator's Ticket, $5. Graduation Fee, $20

The Dean is authorized to issue a perpetual ticket, on payment of one hundred dollars.

Students who have attended a full course of Lectures in this or any other institution, will be received on payment of $50. The fee from those who have attended two courses elsewhere is $25

For further information or circulars, address,

THOMAS F. ROCHESTER,

BUFFALO, 1859.   Dean of the Faculty.

ATLANTA MEDICAL COLLEGE.

UNIVERSITY OF VERMONT.

THE DRUG STORES,
510 Grand Street and 32 Catharine Street.
EDWARD C. PASSMORE

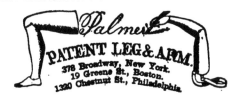

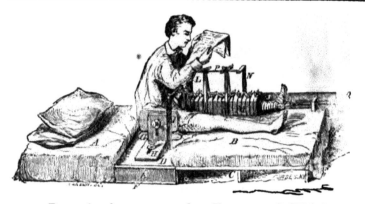

Burge's Apparatus for Fractured Thigh,

INVENTED BY

J. H. HOBART BURGE, M.D., of Brooklyn, N.Y.,

AND

WM. J. BURGE, M.D., of Taunton, Mass.,

has been thoroughly tested in actual practice, and has produced the most gratifying results. It is remarkably simple in its construction, easily applied, comfortable to the patient, adapted to fracture of either limb and to patients of any size. It is free from all the objections to which the ordinary straight splint is liable, and possesses other new features of great practical utility. By it the counter-extending pressure is confined to the nates and tuberosities of the ischia, and does not at all impinge upon the front of the groin, by which means one of the most frequent sources of annoyance and danger is obviated. No part of the body is confined except the injured limb and that to which it is immediately articulated, viz., the pelvis; thus the chest is left entirely unrestrained, and entire freedom of motion granted to the whole upper part of the body, which tends greatly to the comfort and health of the patient.

The pelvis is so secured as not to be liable to lateral motion or to sink in the bed.

Provision is also made for facility of defecation, thus insuring the greatest possible cleanliness, and preventing the necessity of disturbing the patient when his bowels are moved.

☞ Members of the profession may obtain this apparatus, complete in all its parts and nicely packed, by sending FORTY DOLLARS by mail or express to the address of

GEO. TIEMANN & CO.,

63 Chatham St., New York,

C. E. BORDEN,

Taunton, Mass., or

HIGBY & STEARNS,

162 Jefferson St., Detroit, Mich.

For further particulars see Transactions American Medical Association, Vol. X., and New York Journal of Medicine, May, 1857, and September, 1858.

AMERICAN
MEDICAL GAZETTE.

Vol. X.   SEPTEMBER, 1859.   No. 9.

ORIGINAL DEPARTMENT.

On Recto-Vesical Lithotomy, with the Report of a Case in which this Method was successfully employed.

By Prof. Louis BAUER, M.D., M.R.C.S., England, &c.

A close investigation of the various structures annexed to the urinary bladder, and the different practicable channels by which the latter may be entered for the purpose of removing urinary calculi or foreign bodies in general, cannot fail to impress us with the advantages of recto-vesical section. Aside from the facility with which the bladder can be reached through the rectum, and the simplicity of the operation itself, we almost entirely avoid any important structure appertaining to the discharge or retention of urine, the ejaculation of semen, and other subordinate organs belonging to any of these functions. We encounter, moreover, no blood-vessels of any account, and have, therefore, no apprehension of hæmorrhage.

These considerations suggest at once both the feasibility and superiority of this recto-vesical lithotomy, and it is surprising that this operation has not been resorted to and preferred to other methods now in vogue, though evidently of less operative value.

Although tradition has handed down the intelligence that the ancient Egyptians had already performed lithotomy per rectum, we are yet without accounts as to the manner of its execution or the results attained.

Certain it is, that if the operation was ever known or practiced by the ancients, it had become entirely obsolete and been forgotten when C. L. Hoffmann, in the year 1779, again suggested it. But, in the

41

enthusiasm arising from the comparatively good results attained by lateral section, his proposition was utterly disregarded.

Sançon, led by similar reflection, caught the idea likewise, and had the boldness not only to suggest, but also to execute, lithotomy per rectum; his thesis on this subject was published at Paris in the year 1815.

Sançon's operation, although a decided step in the right direction, is, strictly speaking, not recto-vesical section itself, for he appropriates *only* the external sphincter muscle, exposing thereby the prostate gland, and, working his way between the latter and the anterior wall of the rectum towards the basis prostatæ, he incises the corpus trigonum.

The only surgeon who ever conceived a correct idea of recto-vesical lithotomy was Sleigh. He suggested the dilatation of the external sphincter by Weiss's three-bladed speculum, and the incision of the bladder through the rectum immediately behind the prostate gland; and this process it is which we must consider as genuine recto-vesical section.

Both operations, however, have made but little headway in professional favor; and the few surgeons that adopted Sançon's method were the more justified to lay it aside, since the author himself relinquished it in favor of Vacca Berlinghieri's modification. With reference to Sleigh's operation, we are unable to say how often and with what success, or indeed whether it was performed at all. Thus, we may fairly assume that recto-vesical section, as a legitimate and generally recognized method, had no practical existence; for all our careful research has not revealed a single instance in which Sleigh's operation had been executed, and at any rate, not within the last thirty years. So much so had his process been disregarded or undervalued, that most authors and the most complete works on surgery do not even mention his name in connection with lithotomy.

All that has been said in favor of or against recto-vesical section exclusively refers, therefore, to the method of Sançon; but it is evident that the *pro* and *con* appertain in a still higher degree to Sleigh's process.

Most surgical authors ascribe to lithotomy per rectum the decided advantage of easy execution, directness of application, the smallest practicable wound, and the least possible hæmorrhage; the correctness of which advantages may be readily proven by experimentative operation on subjects. Many difficulties in connection with the operation are, however, alleged, tending to annihilate so completely all the advantages enumerated, as to exclude the inducement of ever again resorting to the operation.

The truth, however, is, that all sorts of difficulties, how insurmountable they may have appeared or actually been in a former epoch of surgery, have, for our time, lost all practical significance, as we presently shall proceed to show.

First of all, it was said, that the space between the basis of the prostate gland and the *cul de sac* of the peritoneum be too small, and that its injury was inevitable on making a sufficiently large incision into the corpus trigonum of the bladder. This objection cannot be maintained, having found this space of the length of $1\frac{3}{8}$ inch—consequently larger than what under ordinary circumstances is required. For the extraction of a stone of medium size, a wound of three-fourths of an inch suffices; and if a larger aperture should be desirable, its extension into the prostate gland is practicable. The superior angle of the wound is thus more than half an inch remote from the peritoneal duplicature. But even under the worst supposition, that the peritoneum should be injured, it follows not, that any particular danger would thereby prejudice the ultimate result of the operation, since we have become acquainted with the means by which simple peritoneal wounds may be rendered almost harmless. We may but put the reader in mind of the many successful operations of ovariotomy, and especially of a case operated on by our distinguished friend, Isaac Baker Brown, Esq., at St. Mary's Hospital, of London, some years ago, in which the abdominal cavity had been exposed to the atmosphere for fully 45 minutes without producing inflammation of the peritoneum.

It has been furthermore insisted on, that injuries to the vasa deferentia, the seminal vesicles, and the ureters could scarcely be avoided. This objection, also, does not hold. We have made this operation on subjects, and, without exercising any particular care, did not touch either the peritoneum or any of the other parts named. The ureters can hardly be taken into account, as they are farthest removed from the line of incision. And the vasa deferentia, being of more immediate importance, leave, in the empty state of the bladder, an intervening space of half an inch at the closest approximation. But if the bladder is properly distended with water, that space is considerably enlarged thereby, and an incidental injury to either vas deferens totally out of question. The staff should, however, be dispensed with, not only as unnecessary, but likely to be mischievous in misdirecting the line of incision; for the operator has ample space and access to choose the point of puncture, and to give the knife the intended direction without the aid or incumbrance of the staff.

Another objection raised, is the entering of fæces into the bladder, and the continual irritation of the wound by their passage. This difficulty is, to modern surgery, of no particular consequence, as it is in the power of the surgeon to protect both bladder and wound from contact with the excrements.

It is, of course, necessary that the intestinal canal be evacuated prior to the operation, by both cathartic and injection, and then so completely to constipate it by large doses of opium, and eventually by acetate of lead, that no fæces can descend deep enough to come in contact with the wound.

Infiltration of urine into the cellular tissue of the pelvis, and its subsequent inflammation, or the formation of pus or gangrene in the organs of the pelvis, also incurable recto-vesical fistulæ, are additionally enumerated as the most frequent attendants of this mode of operation. But since Dr. J. Marion Sims has introduced his incomparable suture into surgery, with which he daily attains the happiest results in vesico-vaginal fistula, the last-named objection has lost all its force. No one can, indeed, doubt the successful union of a recent wound in comparatively healthy structure, when finding that the silver suture closely unites the irritated and callous edges of old vesico-vaginal fistulæ.

The unceasing labors of this highly meritorious surgeon have indeed initiated a new era in surgery, and his improvements are doubtless calculated to impart a new and lasting impulse to lithotomy.

We have thus argumentatively disposed of the principal difficulties as regards recto-vesical section, and have thereby paved the way for its practical introduction.

The opportunity to see our favorable opinion of the therapeutic value of this operation fully realized by practical results, has been meanwhile afforded us.

Mr. James Titus, a merchant, twenty-six years of age, of good and robust constitution, and enjoying at the time general good health, consulted us in reference to some trouble about the urinary bladder. The examination revealed a moderately large and hard stone. We proposed an operation, and the patient acceded.

Though having almost certainly resolved on the recto-vesical section, we did not fail to avail ourselves of the counsels of some of our professional friends. They all agreed with us, that the operation would in every respect be fully justified and practicable, and they shared our expectations of a complete and speedy result.

Dr. J. Marion Sims, to whose high-minded and benevolent conduct towards us on many former occasions we felt already deeply indebted, immediately proffered us the assistance of his valuable experience; and Drs. Louis Sayre, Palmedo, Whaley, Emmet, and others, kindly tendered their aid.

To guard against any unforeseen contingencies, the patient was first carefully examined by Drs. Sims, Emmet, Whaley, and ourself; and it was thereby established that, by means of Sims' speculum, sufficient room could be secured for operative proceedings. The inferior hæmorrhoid artery was found to lie in a deeply descending position, approaching almost the median line and the basis of the prostate gland, where its pulsation could be distinctly felt.

The parts surrounding the external sphincter appeared healthy, whereas its mucous membrane was coarsely wrinkled, and studded with varicose knots. The water injected into the bladder, as well as Sims' speculum, caused such irritation, that the patient protruded the base of the bladder with the anterior wall of the rectum—a circumstance which had frequently attended his alvine evacuations. The prostate gland appeared of normal size, and was from all sides accessible to the touch. There was, therefore, nothing of an untoward nature about the local condition of the case.

The 18th of July, of the present year, was fixed upon for the operation. About twenty members of the profession, who had manifested a lively interest in the undertaking, were assembled, and by their presence bore witness to the importance they attached to the operation. Besides the gentlemen already named, there were present Drs. Carl Th. Meier, Green, Krakowitzer, Ostrander, Voss, Maebert, Valentini, Lee Jones, and others. The patient, prepared by cathartics and enema, was laid upon his left side, with his legs crossed and drawn up, but not fastened. By means of an elastic catheter the bladder was injected with water, and the former left in position Chloroform was not administered, partly because the operation was not a very painful one, as well as for the purpose of securing a perfectly quiet and unaltered position. Thereupon we introduced Sims' speculum, firmly drawing the sphincter backward and upward, by which means the operative field, with all its contours, was freely exposed. We next fixed the left

forefinger into the middle of the posterior margin of the prostate
gland, and inserted the point of a small two-edged scalpel of Luer on
its median line, through the rectum into the bladder, slightly directing
the knife anteriorly and superiorly to a supposed point, about one and
a half inch above the symphysis, in the linea alba. The wound was just
large enough to admit the left forefinger; the hæmorrhage consequent
on the incision was very slight, and scarcely exceeded half an ounce.
We had presumed that the pressure of the water in the bladder would
have been of sufficient force to press the stone towards the wound, if
not to eject it.   But this was not the case, principally owing to the
fact that the patient was not able to bear a more copious injection.
The wound being too small to extract the stone with the finger,
we introduced a straight stone forceps, in doing which we unfortunately got hold of the catheter as well, (which, as already stated, we had
by way of precaution retained there, so as not to injure the sutures upon
its reintroduction;) and the assistant's attention being absorbed in the
operation, failed to notice that the catheter had moved.   Having
thus vainly tried for several seconds to extract the stone, we conjectured that the difficulty rested upon the relative disproportion of its
size and that of the wound, and hence we increased the length of the
latter by about two lines, in the direction of the prostate gland, without, however, relinquishing our hold on the stone.   On renewing the
tractions we succeeded in bringing the stone into the wound, and discovered that the catheter likewise had lodged there.   This difficulty
being removed, the stone was withdrawn with great ease, and the
act was thus consummated within the space of fifteen seconds.

It may be readily comprehended that the difficulty arising from the
retention of the catheter could have been averted, as the subsequent
introduction of another catheter met with no obstacle.   We are equally
convinced that the wound would have sufficed, without lengthening it,
to allow the withdrawal of the stone, the length of the latter being
$2\frac{1}{4}$ inches by $1\frac{1}{2}$ wide, and 1 inch thick, and weighed $1\frac{1}{2}$ ounce.

Beyond the delay of several seconds in the performance of the
operation, no other disadvantage was thereby occasioned. .

That the hæmorrhage was slight, is satisfactory evidence that we
were fortunate enough to avoid injuring the hæmorrhoid artery.

The second act of the proceedings consisted in uniting the recto-vesical wound, an operation which we could not have intrusted to more
skillful hands than those of our excellent friend, Dr. J. Marion Sims.
The doctor inserted, with great elegance, five silver sutures, and

his complete success may be judged by the fact that on injecting the bladder not a drop of fluid escaped into the rectum. This completed the operation. Two grains of opium were at once given to the patient, who was thereupon put to bed. An elastic catheter was then introduced, and secured. The patient assured us of his entire comfort; that he had experienced almost no pain from the operation, and that the only inconvenience he suffered had arisen from the peculiar position in which he had been placed. Ice-water and iced milk were ordered for his diet.

July 18th, 6 P. M.—Patient is comfortable, free from pain; his urine, which passes freely from the bladder through the catheter, is dark red, as if containing blood, and of sour reaction. The effects of the opium are very moderate. Prescribed another dose of opium and oil emulsion, with liq. potass. carbonatis.

July 19th, 2 A. M.—We were called to the patient. The urine had ceased to pass, and severe pains in the bladder had set in, while he also complained of headache. The catheter, which was found to be choked, was removed, and another introduced, when the urine streamed out with great force. No urine in the rectum. Patient greatly relieved; atmospheric temperature about 82 degrees Fahrenheit; the patient was in a feverish condition, and cold applications were thereupon made to the head and hands.

Having introduced a tube into the rectum, to allow the escape of flatulent gases, we left him at 4 A. M. in a comparatively comfortable condition.

10 A. M.—Patient had slept several hours. Pulse, temperature, and thirst moderate. The urine being of a brown-red color, and seemingly containing much blood, passes freely through the catheter; abdomen distended by gases, but not tender; bladder and rectum free from pain; slight discharge of bloody mucus from the rectum.

The urine, microscopically examined, shows neither blood nor pus, but an abundance of uric acid, some urate of soda, traces of phosphates, mucin, mucous corpuscles, epithelium, and vibriones.

6 P. M.—Pulse good; patient has slept twice, about three hours each time; has discharged 1½ pint of urine, which reacts but little acid; suffers no particular inconvenience from the catheter; no pain in bladder or rectum, nor even the slightest irritation; moderate disposition to evacuate bowels. Prescribed two grains of opium.

10 P. M.—Patient sent for me in haste; he felt uncomfortable in consequence of the retention of urine, caused by the obstruction of the

The patient experienced no inconvenience whatever, and he enjoyed the exercise, without feeling any inclination to urinate.

Thus, on the eighth day after the operation, the patient had completely recovered, and was dismissed from our treatment.

It is scarcely necessary to add any closing remarks to this communication, inasmuch as we have in the introduction sufficiently indicated our views in regard to this method of operation. The result obtained requires no further comment. Nevertheless, it appears desirable to refer to some points which presented themselves, both during the operation and in course of the after-treatment.

1. The operation, as we have elsewhere stated, was, for sufficient reasons, performed without administering chloroform, and we have the less cause to regret this, as it was painless throughout—a circumstance the more surprising from the fact that the patient is naturally of an easily excited, nervous temperament, his pulse at the time of the operation being 150; and that, on the other hand, the lower portion of the rectum is on the slightest irritation exceedingly painful and troublesome. The simple wound seems to be exempt, however, from pain, as the concrete case demonstrates.

2. The retention of the catheter during the operation is entirely unnecessary, and in this instance proved itself an obstacle to the speedy execution of the operation. If it be apprehended that the patient could not retain the injected water, we should prevent its discharge by the application of an india-rubber ring to the penis, in preference to the catheter.

3. The infusion of air as well as water into the bladder during the after-treatment we do not commend, because of the proneness to alkaline fermentation of the organic components of the urine, (mucin, mucous corpuscles, and epithelial cells,) which would be additionally stimulated by the entrance of atmospheric air. In our case, putrid gases were thus generated in the bladder, which, on escaping through the urethra, caused a burning sensation. The chemical action of the gases on the wound was also to be apprehended; and although this was not evidenced in this instance, caution demands that, in future cases, surgeons should seek to prevent the accumulation of putrid gases, as much as may be in their power. It should be understood, however, that in clearing the catheter we infused but little air, so as not to expose the patient to the danger of bursting the wound by its pressure.

4. Liquor kali carbonici proved not only to be of excellent effect in

neutralizing the uric acid of the urine, but also in checking the foul fermentation of the fæces.

5. For the purpose of constantly keeping the wound free from contact with the urine, we allowed the catheter to remain, no doubt, longer than necessary, which caused a traumatic gonorrhœa. We are of opinion that our caution carried us too far, and that two days would have sufficed to fully close the wound; while, on the other hand, there was danger that the gonorrhœa might have communicated serious inflammation to the bladder.

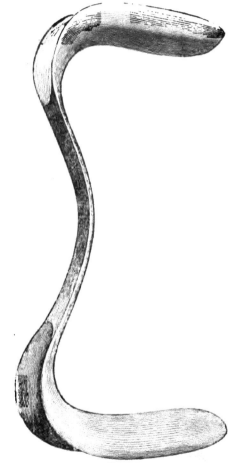

Fig. 1.

In our procedure during the operation, as well as in the after-treatment, there is nothing that is new or unknown, and it is scarcely necessary that we should further enlarge on it. For the better understanding of those, however, who are unacquainted with Sims' suture and the instruments used by that gentleman, we add several engravings.

Fig. 1 represents the speculum, originally intended for the vagina, but equally suited for recto-vesical section.

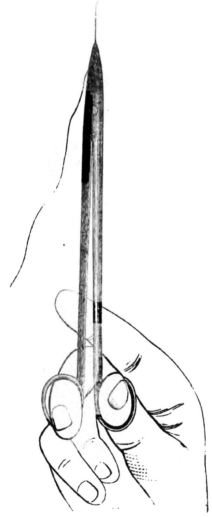

Fig. 2.

Fig. 2, Sims' needle-holder, with a needle one inch in length, attached to which is a loop of silk thread. The margin of the wound is held by a sharp hook, and drawn up when the needle is passed through it. The same process is followed with the opposite margin. The needle should be held in a right angle with the forceps, and then the silver wire, hooked in the silk loop, is drawn through.

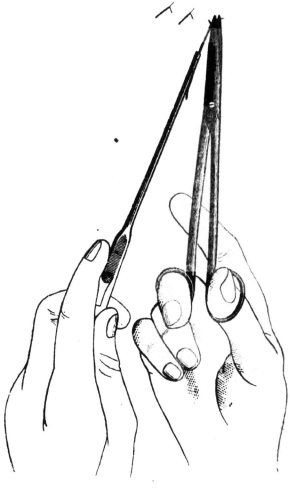

Fig. 3.

Fig. 3, the process in which the wire, held by a long pair of forceps, is, by means of a small director, bent over the wound; and next, the closure of the latter by torsion with the forceps.

Fig. 4, silver suture after removal.

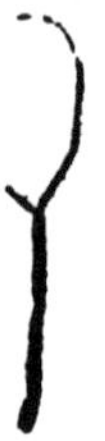

Fig. 4.

The author is well aware that vesical suture has been repeatedly employed, but only in high lithotomy; and even recently, Dr. Lotzbeck, of Tübingen, communicated a case from the clinic of Professor Von Bruns, in which it was applied with good effect; but, to our knowledge, it has never been resorted to in low section, and Sims' suture is by far better qualified than all others.

In conclusion, it may be remarked, that we should not commend recto-vesical section in young patients, on account of the peritoneum descending deeply into the small pelvis, and sometimes as low as to reach and cover the prostate gland.

Cor. Warren and Clinton Sts , Brooklyn.

THE UTERINE SOUND.

By ADRIAN T. WOODWARD, M.D.,

Professor of Obstetrics and Diseases of Females, in Castleton Medical College, Vermont.

This is an instrument of very great value, and is indispensably necessary to the formation of a correct diagnosis in many cases. It has been highly extolled by Professor Simpson, as the only medium by which a reliable knowledge of the situation, character, circumstances, and even the existence of tumors of the uterus, can be attained, when they are of small size; and likewise as the only means of determining the exact situation and relation of the pelvic viscera, the length of the womb entire, and the relative measurement of cervix, body, and fundus; all of which we fully endorse, having had many opportunities to verify the testimony afforded by the instrument upon the above-mentioned points. It is, however, to present to the profession another important use to which the uterine sound may be applied that I lay this article before your readers. I shall not attempt further preface, as the uses of the instrument under consideration have been ably discussed in text-books and journals. In *all* cases of uterine affection, the condition of the organ as relates to size, color, and consistence, is as important as its position; and, in the vast majority of those presented to the physician, it is of greater consequence that these be understood.

No one familiar with the use of the speculum will need to be assured that the *taxis* is not a certain guide to the knowledge of the existence or non-existence of *ulceration*. Any physician can verify this by an instrumental examination of the womb he has just *touched*. So, too, will he find that he has been misled in regard to the presence or absence of *induration* of the cervix, if he will introduce a bi-valve speculum, and pass the uterine sound through it up to the neck of the womb; by pressing it upon the lips at various points, he will be at once accurately informed of its consistence, by the degree of resistance offered to the instrument. If the organ is not indurated, it will be indented by the sound, which will be received into a cup-like depression, very distinct to the eye of the operator, from which it will not slip, even when considerable pressure is applied at a right angle to the plane upon which it strikes against the organ. On the other hand, if the cervix be indurated, the cup-like depression will not be produced, and the instrument will glide off into the angle formed by the contact of cervix and the speculum, or cervix and vagina; it being impossible to imbed the instrument in the resisting lips sufficient to prevent its slipping off at the slightest pressure applied, as in the former instance.

To determine the existence of induration in a case of inflammation of the uterus requiring local applications, is of the highest importance to the practitioner, as a safe and sure guide to the proper use of the various antiphlogistic agents now in vogue.

If, in local inflammation of the uterus, we find the cervix indurated and enlarged, we understand that exudation has exceeded assimilation and absorption; for it must strike the mind of every one that exudation into the substance of an organ cannot long exist unassimilated without the plasma taking either a higher or lower grade of organization: if the lower, suppuration will ensue—a condition rarely met with in this region; if it assumes the higher grade, then the part becomes indurated. If we find the cervix inflamed, increased in size, and soft, (*not indurated*,) we suppose that assimilation keeps pace with exudation, and that the nutrition of the organ is augmented; and, under the influence of such a change in the nutrition of a part, we should look very properly for enlargement, and, indeed, shall seldom fail to find it.

But can every one—nay, can *any one*, in all the cases presented to him, invariably determine the extent of induration by *taxis*? I say he cannot. I am aware that I am making a bold assertion, yet I venture it, and ask of any one who questions it to use the uterine sound, as I have directed, in the next six cases which come under his observation, and learn thereby how he may have deceived himself in the cases heretofore examined.

There are two kinds of enlargement of the cervix uteri to be recognized as dependent upon existing inflammation in the part.

1st.'Hypertrophy, which I recognize as a growth of the normal structure, and met with in those cases in which exudation is in excess over the healthy standard, assimilation keeping pace with it, (i. e., excessive nutrition.) In this, we find enlargement without induration, attended by the usual general symptoms of inflammation of the cervix.

2d. When enlargement exists, attended with induration, it is dependent upon the organization of exuded plasma, which of course is not connected, as far as we can judge, with growth of the normal structure, which alone constitutes hypertrophy. Without insisting upon the choice of terms to be applied to these changes, we will pass to a consideration of the importance of distinguishing in practice the difference between the two varieties of enlargement. The cautious practitioner will feel his way with the milder, before resorting to the more potent cauteries, and it may at first sight seem useless to advise in the matter; but when we consider that valuable time is often wasted in waiting for the milder caustics to do the work which can only be accomplished by the more potent—or that, after waiting what may seem to be a reasonable time for them to work a cure, we may recklessly doom the patient to protracted misery by too readily resorting to powerful escharotics—it may not appear altogether unimportant to record the experience of even an humble observer.

After an experience of several years in the treatment of these affections, which has not been limited to a few cases, I am convinced that *true hypertrophy*, with the attendant inflammation of the cervix uteri, can in the great majority of cases be subdued by the arg. nit., without the aid of potass. fusa or the *actual cautery;* and that, when these are resorted to in this variety of enlargement, a rapid wasting of the vaginal cervix ensues, attended by hardening, similar to the induration of a cicatrix, smooth, shining, and often fissured occasionally, radiating from the os in more than one direction, and giving to the cervix somewhat the appearance of incipient carcenoma. This condition, when once developed, will defy all attempts to eradicate or modify it, time alone being equal to any amelioration of the condition of the party. Every one will see how this hardening will affect dilatation of the os in parturition. I have yet to learn that it favors the development of cancer, if, indeed, there can be any possibility of its doing so; still, for many other important reasons, which will at once present themselves to the practitioner, this condition ought by all means to be avoided. A single application of potass. fusa will occasionally, though rarely, effect this change; the second quite frequently; and the third almost invariably results thus. Enlargement, attended with induration, will, however, frequently demand for its reduction the use of potash, and in this condition the cervix tolerates the remedy, losing with every application more or less of its hardness.

I have not intended to give a dissertation upon the treatment of uterine inflammation, for the limits of such an article will not permit it; I have alluded to it simply to demonstrate the importance of an examination of the case by the uterine sound.

CASTLETON, VT., *July 25th*, 1859.

A Case of Successful Delivery, by a Transverse Section of the Fœtus, wholly within the Uterus.

By T. RAYMOND. M.D., of St. Catharine's, Canada West.

On the 9th of March, 1843, an Irish woman, Mrs. Shay, had been in labor about four hours before I saw her. Said she had had three children without suffering extraordinary pain. Upon examination, I found that the fœtus was lying across the pelvis, its head right side, and the nates on the left pelvic rim, presenting the back a little inclined to its right side, so that the lowest dorsal vertebra was nearly above the axis of the pelvis, which I could by manipulation clearly ascertain; long and repeated attempts to alter this position were fruitless. After administering 35 drops of laudanum, combined with 15 drops of spts. camphor, there was no cessation to her pains, nor muscular relaxation. The fœtus could not be moved. The opium, camphor, and swt. spts. nitre that she took only aggravated the case, and made the safe delivery more and more hopeless, although the uterus all this time was sufficiently dilated to admit easy parturition.

In this situation she continued about four hours, and my best exertions were used to move the fœtus. In the mean time, I discovered that the funis lay across the child, beneath its right arm, and the circulation had ceased; the fœtus was dead, and I abandoned the idea of attempting to deliver her by any prescribed means. I wound a piece of broad tape around the handle and blade of a scalpel to within one-

42

fourth of an iuch of the point, and commenced dividing the lowest dorsal vertebra from the upper lumbar, with the design to follow the rib to the sternum, which I performed, finding, as I proceeded, the dissected extremities protruded, which I found assisted me in the operation. When my scalpel was of no more use, on account of its straight form, I took a knife, exactly the shape of a gum-knife, and wound it in the same manner that I did the scalpel, and, with great caution, proceeded to divide the fœtus through its whole extent, till the division was complete; I then took, without much difficulty, the separated parts, first the inferior. I was about six hours in performing this operation, and am of the opinion it is quite practicable when the presentation is favorable to the operation.

CASE OF STRANGULATED HERNIA.

The following case of strangulated hernia conveys a practical lesson, which may be of service to the junior members of our profession, and for that reason I report it:

A few mornings since, Dr. Nelson, my partner in business, and myself, received a message from Dr. R. Esselstyne, of the adjoining town of Red Hook, to meet him at 10 o'clock, A. M., at the house of Mr. A., a respectable and wealthy farmer, whose wife, he stated, had a strangulated hernia, which, with all his efforts, he had been unable to reduce, and which most probably could not be reduced, except by an operation. We accordingly met him at the appointed hour, and learned that the rupture of Mrs. A. had been produced by a fall some ten or twelve days previous, and had been strangulated a few hours. There was a tumor in the groin, just without the external ring, about the size of a large hen's egg, not very painful, but as hard as a brick. There was of course obstinate constipation and vomiting, but, as the symptoms did not seem to be so dangerously urgent as to require an immediate operation, we decided to make one effort more at the taxis before commencing it.

As she was not then under the influence of opium, we gave her at once five grains, and applied a bag of pounded ice to the tumor, and, after waiting an hour or two for these to produce their full effect, we placed her in the proper position, with her hips elevated to an angle of about 45 degrees, and her thighs drawn upward and inward, and commenced our efforts at reduction, and, by gentle but persevering efforts, we gradually pressed out from the tumor the impacted fæcal matter, sufficiently to enable us to slip back the intestine into the abdominal cavity. This success gave us very great satisfaction; and, as we had carefully abstained from all violent efforts, and there was no evidence of a high degree of inflammation in the returned bowel, and none of gangrene, we supposed that we had saved the life of the patient, and with great confidence told her that she was safe. We then had her removed from the low bed, on which she had been placed for our convenience, to another, and in an hour or two we left her in a very comfortable state. The opium had not narcotized her excessively, and there was not one alarming symptom.

Under these circumstances, what was our surprise to learn the next forenoon that the patient was dead! We could hardly credit the fact, but it proved too true. We were informed afterwards from Dr. E. that when he left, which was at about two o'clock, P. M., the patient was comfortable, and apparently doing well. Early in the evening he was sent for in great haste, with the message that her friends feared she was dying. He went immediately, and found that she had continued to do well until evening, at the time when the family took their tea. As she had eaten nothing for a day or two of any consequence, and as she seemed to be able to get up, they encouraged her to do so, which she did, and whilst sitting at the table she became faint, had a chill, her face and extremities became very cold, with great weakness. She was immediately put to bed, and soon after, when Dr. E. arrived, he found her in this state, and also insensible.

By warmth, frictions, &c., he succeeded in partially producing reaction, and she was so far restored to consciousness as to be able to speak and reply to questions. Being compelled to leave, he left directions to have the frictions, warmth, &c., continued. Soon after he left, however, she relapsed into her former state, and in an hour or two thereafter died. Like ourselves, Dr. E. had been entirely confounded by the result, and wished to make a post-mortem to ascertain the cause. When he called, however, next morning, the body was in the hands of the undertaker, and he was permitted to examine the state of the intestine and abdomen only, which he did, but could not examine the brain. He found nothing in the state of the returned intestine or the peritoneum to account for the death of the patient. There were no signs of gangrene, not even a bad smell on opening the abdomen, and the intestine had not been very much inflamed.

Now, the interesting question in this case is, What was the cause of death? The above examination shows most conclusively that it was not in the abdomen.

One dose only of opium, five grains, had been given on the day of her death. She was not much narcotized, and there was no evidence of congestion of the brain until after the faintness on getting up and sitting at the table, and, in our opinion, it was this ill-advised act that was the cause of death. Had she continued quietly in bed until she had taken food and her strength somewhat restored, she would in all probability have soon recovered. She was old—over seventy—feeble, and much exhausted from the effects of her fall, as well as the hernia; and it is a well-known fact that persons in a state of great exhaustion, on being placed in the erect position, sometimes die suddenly. This was the great and fatal mistake committed in this case.

On the pathological condition of the brain and heart in these cases I have no time to speculate.. E. PLATT.

RHINEBECK, 18*th June*, 1859.

— — —•••— — · —

On the Causes of the Excessive Mortality attending Amputations.

By Prof. A. BUROW, M.D.

[Translated for the AMERICAN MEDICAL GAZETTE, by Prof. BAUER, M.D.]

The number of amputations which occur in a surgeon's practice, be it ever so extensive, must necessarily be limited; so much so, that the comparatively small number of cases which are thus brought to his notice cannot properly be taken as a reliable basis for a general statistical average. External circumstances beyond his control may favor or prejudice a small number of cases, and thus lead to extraordinary results. The axiom in statistics, that from large quantities only reliable conclusions may be drawn, is obviously correct.

Pauli has collected 7,678 cases of amputation of the extremities, which show an average ratio of mortality of $33\frac{1,618}{7,678}$ per cent. In our surgical practice, which extends over the space of twenty-five years, we have performed but sixty-two cases, only three of which resulted in death—equal to $4\frac{8}{6}$ per cent. The comparison of this mortality with that ascertained by Pauli shows such an extraordinary difference, as to justify our examining the causes of the mortality.

With reference to the locality of our amputations, they were performed:

On the lower third of the forearm ....12 times.
" 	middle and upper third...................... 3 "
" 	humerus:
" 	 " 	 . lower third......................... 7 '
" 	 " 	 middle .... 5 '
.. 	 " 	 upper third.... .... 4 · '
" 	 " 	 near the shoulder-joint................. 4 '
" 	 " 	 on the metatarsals................... 1 '
 	leg ....11 '
 	thigh:
" 	 " 	 lower third (with two deaths)............ 8 '
" 	 " 	 upper third (with one death)............. 7 '

 	 	 	 	——
 	 	 	 	62 cases.

Causes for which amputation was performed:
 	Crushing of the hand by blasting and gun-shots........ 9
 	Other lacerations and injuries...................... 2
 	Extensive caries of the hand....................... 1
 	Neglected onychia............................. 1
 	Carcinoma of the hand, (the disease relapsed after com-
 	 	plete closure of the wound, and caused the death of the
 	 	patient fourteen months after amputation,).......... 1
 	Mortification of the forearm in consequence of onychia.. 1 "
 	Crushing of hand on the lower third................. 1
On the Humerus:
 	Caries and necrosis... 3
 	Gun-shot wounds................................. 5
 	Lacerations and injuries by machinery................ 5
 	Pseudarthrosis................................. 2
 	Comminuted fracture near the shoulder-joint, (late ampu-
 	 	tations,).... 2
 	Hæmorrhage and incipient mortification, consequent on
 	 	aneurism................................... 1
 	Humerus torn off............................... 1
 	Progressed gangrene after gun-shot wound, (six days after
 	 	injury,)..................................... 1
On the Metatars:
 	Gangrene, (frostbitten,)........................... ɪ
On the Leg:
 	Gangrene, frostbitten, (late operation,).............. 3

Comminuted fracture........................... 2 cases.
Caries.. 2 "
Traumatic injuries, (primary amputations,)............ 4 "
Thigh:
Comminuted.................................... 2
Extensive ulceration and caries, (with three deaths,)...11 "
Pseudarthrosis................................. 1
Pseudophasms.................................. 1
                                              ——
                                              62 "

The majority of these patients belonged to the lower classes of society, and their constitutions were more or less impoverished and vitiated. With few exceptions, the amputations were undertaken in our private hospital, sustained only by our slender means. The diet allowed was reduced to the most necessary articles of food, without extras; and even the room allotted to each patient was extremely limited. Sometimes five individuals, who had undergone various operations, were placed within the small space of 1,500 cubic feet.

Nor can we claim particular skill as the cause of our success, a great number of the amputations having been executed by our clinical students. In fine, the causes which demanded amputation were indeed such as not to favor a promising prognosis. We may be permitted to relate three instances in illustration.

A servant-girl had been caught by the cog-wheel of a threshing machine, and twice drawn under the cylinder, whereby the right arm was torn off, leaving a crushed stump, scarcely two and a half inches in length. Fragments of the nervous plexus and the pulsating brachial artery hung from the wound. The right thigh presented a double fracture, and the copious bloody expectoration indicated serious injuries of the thoracic organs. In this condition the patient had been transported ten miles over a rough road.

The laceration of the soft parts did not admit of equally and sufficiently large flaps, while the humerus had to be removed immediately below the tubercula. This patient recovered without either excessive reaction or remedies.

Michel, a Jewish peddler, eighty-two years old, suffered from cubital aneurism, caused by venesection. In order to relieve the aneurism, we resorted to moderate compression, ligatures being impracticable, on account of supposed atheromatous degeneration of the arterial coats. Sloughing of the aneurismatic sac and hæmorrhage ensued, demanding immediate amputation. The age of the patient, and the serious loss of blood, rendered the prognosis more than doubtful; but the general infiltration of the arm, and the signs of mortification, were sufficient to qualify the case as utterly hopeless. Amputation was, however, insisted on by the friends of the patient; and being, indeed, the only means of saving life, it was resorted to. The wound presented a bluish discoloration, and the veins were filled with thrombus. The patient nevertheless recovered, and left his bed on the fifth day; the reaction being slight only.

Quedwan, a farmer, while hunting, had shot himself in the wrist, in such a manner that the charge penetrated the arm to the elbow-joint. The attending physician had been unwilling to make an immediate amputation. On the sixth day after the accident, we saw the patient. Mortification had set in, extending upward to the shoulder-blade, without an attempt at demarcation. The inflamed veins extended towards the thorax, and the patient found himself, moreover, in a typhoid condition, with cool extremities, thready and frequent pulse, and delirium. The amputation was resorted to only at the urgent request of his relatives. Although we approached as near as practicable to the shoulder-joint, sufficient healthy structure could not be found to cover the bone. The flaps looked discolored, and the veins were obliterated by closely adhering thrombi. But notwithstanding these complications, and although sloughing of the flaps supervened, the patient recovered.

It is evident, therefore, that we had to contend with more than ordinarily difficult and highly aggravated cases in our operations. Under these circumstances, the limited mortality attending our amputations must justly surprise the professional reader, and the question is therefore quite natural: To *what* have we to ascribe the uncommonly favorable results of our amputations? And again, What are the causes that hitherto have led to the immense mortality of 33 per cent., as Pauli has elicited?

We are fully prepared to give a positive answer to both questions, and do not hesitate in maintaining, however bold and presumptuous it may seem to the unreflecting mind, that favorable or unfavorable results solely depend on the after-treatment of the stump.

In all cases, when circumstances permit it, the flap operation, and, excepting in case of the leg, the double flap operation, is preferable. All the indications (with the exception of one only) hitherto held as in favor of the circular operation are fallacious, and the exception is the want of substance for the formation of flaps.

According to the opinions of numerous surgical authorities, the wound of the circular cut is of smaller dimensions than that caused by the flap operation. But in either operation it should be sufficiently large to cover the bone. The surface of the wound is too small if it does not suffice to furnish a good bed for the bone, and the flaps are too large if projecting beyond the bone. It is clearly susceptible of mathematical demonstration that in the circular operation the wound is actually larger towards its angles than necessary for the purpose— an objection which does not apply to the flap operation; and the wound in the latter case is cleaner, owing to the drawing rather than the pressing of the knife.

Another indication in favor of the circular operation has been found in the locality, such as the lower third of the forearm and leg. We cannot comprehend, however, why these parts should not be equally suited to flap operations; all the objections that can be brought against the one hold good of the other. This, at least, has been our experience.

Numerous books on surgery teach that where suppuration is intended, the circular cut should be preferred. This indication is, to say the least, an absurdity, which unfortunately has been so thoughtlessly carried from time to time as to be discreditable to their authors. Every surgeon of any experience is fully aware that in flap operations the first intention is by no means a reliable mode of union, and that suppuration generally ensues; the latter can at all events easily be induced, and is therefore not to be looked upon as exclusively belonging to the circular operation. As an offset of such untenable indications, many advantages may be enumerated which prove the superiority of the flap operation.

With flaps only can we fully, and without inconvenience to the patient, close an amputated wound. Were we to suppose a case in which the soft parts equally surround the bone, they would form, when well united, the segment of a sphere. In double flap operation we accomplish the same object with half the material; and the same may be said of a single flap, which, of course, would have to be of double the size.

Another postulate for a good stump is a coniform wound, scarcely to be accomplished by circular operation, unless Von Graefe's fantastical operation (pyramidal cut) be adopted, and in that case the wound would be twice as large.

In a well-developed arm the length of the flaps required should be from $2\frac{1}{2}$ to $2\frac{3}{4}$ inches, to cover the bone without constraint; and in the thigh from $4\frac{1}{2}$ to 5 inches.

The result of an amputation, independent of the formation of the stump, depends, in our opinion, on the comfortable closure of the wound, and we have therefore given this point particular attention. In this respect we learn by observation that the bones in flap amputations invariably unite with the nearest portion of the skin, and the remaining soft parts form the cushion around the bone. The bone has moreover an almost centric position in the stump, being covered with a firmly adhering cicatrix from three to four lines in thickness. The same cicatrization takes place if the flaps have been cut too long; with this difference, however, that the cicatrix is drawn inward, and towards the bone, while the flaps bulge out. This formation of the stump is in no way prejudicial to its usefulness. But if the flaps be made too short the stump will be pointed, the cicatrix tense, and more or less wide. This condition of the stump is exceedingly inconvenient for the application of artificial means, the cicatrix being highly sensitive to atmospheric changes, and excoriating on the slightest provocation.

It does not appear necessary that the periosteum should be scraped from the bone at the point where the saw is to be applied; on the contrary, we have frequently seen it attended with necrosis of an annular piece of bone, which, of course, protracts the cicatrization. We have for these reasons always omitted it, and not met with necrosis in a single instance.

Having secured all the vessels, we expose the wound to the atmospheric air for the space of twenty to thirty minutes, to allow the copious discharge of plastic material, mixed with blood. This mode of treatment is the more necessary if the soft parts have been previously engorged, and infiltrated by an inflammatory process. The wound is then the more closely and accurately united, if *prima unio* is desired. Three straps suffice on the forearm and for the arm generally; the flaps of the leg, the thigh, and of a well-developed and muscular arm require from two to three sutures, with three to four additional straps. We prefer the ordinary suture, with a loop, for the convenience it offers of slacking or tightening it.

Compresses, rollers, or other articles of dressing we never apply, but reject them as inconvenient, because of the pressure or irritation they may cause. When the application of ice-bags is deemed useful, we protect the wound against immediate contact with them by first covering it with a linen rag. To attain the first intention without the slightest suppuration, the wound should be hermetically closed with collodium.

The dressing of amputation wounds with plasters, ointments, compresses, etc., with a view of excluding the atmospheric air, is a fallacy, and should be strongly reprehended. The purpose is not realized by these means; they admit the air, and subsequently impede the free discharge of liquid and gaseous secretions, and are, therefore, highly objectionable.

The application of ice to stumps, so generally adopted by surgeons, we consider of but limited utility, and should be confined to cases in which it gives actual relief to the patient. Only when the stump is much swollen and hot, and the patient rendered more comfortable thereby, the application may be judiciously resorted to. That ice-bags reduce the temperature of the skin only, and not the parts generally, is shown by the introduction of the thermometer into the wound; but they may seriously interfere with the capillary circulation, of the skin at least, and thus impede the healing process.

For these reasons, we do not indiscriminately apply cold fomentations, and certainly not immediately after amputation. If the stump becomes hot and painful, we use them only as long as this condition prevails.

A few hours after amputation, considerable changes take place in the appearance of the stump, indicating the active operations of restoring nature. The entire stump swells considerably, and not rarely attains the double size of the corresponding member. The swelling is occasionally so great as to render it necessary to loosen the straps and sutures. A good swelling is usually the precursor of a favorable suppuration, while we look upon its absence as an unfavorable symptom in the prognosis.

If the healing of the stump proceeds satisfactorily, there is little or no occasion for medications. The inflammatory process is but rarely so excessive that it cannot be restrained by judicious local treatment. The straps we renew as often as cleanliness requires it, and over the wound we spread loose lint to absorb the matter.

How moderate the local reaction occasionally may be, if the case has proper treatment, may be seen from the following:

A young man, whose forearm we amputated in a village three miles distant from our residence, paid us a visit on the following day. And a woman, whose forearm had been removed in the upper third, we, on the following day, found engaged in making up her bed, at which she had to use the stump to a certain extent.

Such has been our management of stumps; and having already

stated that all other external circumstances of the patients were against the favorable termination of the amputations, we may justly infer that the local treatment of the stump which was adopted had the most material influence upon the satisfactory results.

When asking for the causes of death after amputation, we are answered with the high-flown name, "Pyæmia." And what is understood by this term? *Purulent absorption*, or *poisoning*. The presence of pus in the blood has been rendered more plausible since the discovery of white blood-corpuscles. But nobody could, nor can, understand or clearly demonstrate the mechanism of its absorption. And since the most reliable microscopists have frankly admitted the utter impossibility of microscopical discrimination between pus and white blood-corpuscles, the whole doctrine of pyæmia has been sadly shaken.

Numerous experiments of a very conclusive character have tended rather to increase the mystery of this doctrine; for artificial injections of laudable pus into the veins of animals have, in many instances, failed to produce pyæmic symptoms. Nor could the pus-corpuscles be recognized in the blood a few hours after injection. The latter observations and experiments of Rud. Virchow, with reference to thrombosis and emboli, have established that the theory is totally untenable.

Nobody disputes the absorption of pus; for daily experience demonstrate the disappearance of large quantities from abscesses and serous cavities. At the same time, however, it has been ascertained that pus-corpuscles to be absorbed have to undergo fatty degeneration, and a process of emulsion, like that of fatty matter in digestion, in order to re-enter into circulation. In the absence of a fat metamorphosis the serum of the pus is absorbed, while the solids of pus undergo certain chemical changes to render them harmless.

Pus-corpuscles could enter the circulation in two ways: by the lymphatics or the veins. In respect to the former, Virchow's experiments have proved the fact that simple coloring matter injected into the lymphatics does not, and cannot, pass the adjacent lymphatic glands, and is retained in the injected vessel.

It cannot, therefore, be presumed that pus-corpuscles should pass the glands, as they are of larger size than pigment granules. The absorption of pus by veins could only be supposed to take place in two ways: either by perforation of the venous coats, superinduced by a neighboring abscess, or by purulent phlebitis.

The former mode of absorption may be thought possible, although it cannot be demonstrated. At all events, this process cannot take place as often as pyæmia is supposed to occur; while purulent phlebitis, irrespective of its rare occurrence, leads to the immediate formation of thrombus, closing the lumen of the vein, and self-evidently preventing absorption.   The thrombi formed under these circumstances have been carefully examined by Virchow, who found no pus in them; the soft material resembling, and therefore mistaken for pus, was nothing but decayed fibrin.

Thus every pretence of pyæmic absorption has been overruled as incompetent.

It is not within the scope of our purpose to enter upon the examination of the nature and morbid consequences of the so-called emboli, but it is nevertheless of great importance to show their connection with the mortality of amputations.

We should bear in mind that thrombus forms within the veins when they are in a state of inflammation, and that consequently the same agency is at work in those of an inflamed stump.   In all thrombi there is a possibility of their decay, and of their re-entering, in the form of particles, the circulation of the veins.   These particles may thus be removed to remote places, constantly growing by juxtaposition, finally obstruct other veins, and in that way cause, as Virchow and other reliable observers have clearly demonstrated, the so-called lobular or metastatic abscess—the most characteristic symptom of pyæmia.

We have already adverted to the fact that the stump, a few hours after amputation, materially increases in size, unless restrained by pressive bandages or dressings.   All the parts of the stump participate in the dilation; the lumen of the respective veins, and their thrombi in like proportion, are consequently more expanded, and the latter, therefore, less apt to leave their respective places of formation. If, on the contrary, the stump is constrained from expanding, the thrombi are comparatively smaller, and as they become detached after the principal inflammation has subsided and the veins are again permitted to expand, it is by sheer accident if the thrombi do not enter the circulation, and thus cause great mischief and death.

The treatment observed in our amputations has, in this respect, obviated one of the leading and most frequent causes of death in all capital operations, and it has now received its scientific commentary by the observations of Virchow.

In conclusion, we should state, that infection of the wound may result in a fatal termination; and this interpretation has been substituted for purulent absorption.   The possibility of contagious absorption is the less deniable, as the *contagion* is not only palpable, but gaseous even; hence the exposure of the wound should be carefully protected from contact with unclean material of any kind, the sponge used at post-mortem examination, and even the touch of the unwashed hand which has been employed on such material. Contagion by such means, however carried into the system of the patient, is yet of too rare occurrence that it should exercise any material influence upon the event of mortality; and even in this, embolus retains its pathological importance.

The extent to which we may by this examination of the causes of mortality after amputation have convinced our professional colleagues of the superiority of our local treatment of the stump, we leave to their impartial reflection, deeming the arguments adduced in favor of our treatment sufficiently strong to invite their adoption of a like proceeding.

COMMUNICATIONS.

OUR PHILADELPHIA CORRESPONDENT.

No. 14.

" Not for themselves did human kind
Contrive the parts by Heav'n assign'd
   On life's wide scene to play;
Not Scipio's force, nor Cæsar's skill,
Can conquer Glory's arduous hill,
   If Fortune close the way."   AKENSIDE.

" Oh! as the bee upon the flower, I hang
Upon the honey of thy eloquent tongue."   BULWER.

DEAR GAZETTE—A talented and educated pauper is a dangerous individual in the community; and such an individual in our profession is no exception to the rule. Every rich ass who wants to bray without being seen, has the aforesaid pauper at his command; and sometimes without asking him, the service being rendered *in hopes of reward*. Do you have many such in Gotham?

By-the-by, your exposition of the Kappa Lambdas of your city reminds me that there were, and doubtless are, still such animals in our own. I know some names, busy lately in transactions congenial to such an association, which were formerly the names of recognized members of such a society in our city. What would some learned authors of this ilk think if we were to mention their names in this connection, as we very easily could ? Does not the existence of this Association point to certain persecuting transactions in our city during the last *several* years? We are inclined to think so I I Shakspeare, I think, says something about a whip, to scourge such rascals through the world.

We have been a little amused at the quiet, not to say secret, manner in which a resignation and an appointment in the Pennsylvania Hospital have taken place lately. No Kappa Lambda business, of course.

Since writing the above, we have learned that the resignation was by invitation of the Board of Managers: and the appointment was unheralded, to prevent certain outsiders, who were supposed to have influence in the Board, from being acquainted with the vacancy.

Our Blockley Hospital (fruitful source of gas and gossip) is now in a state of tribulation; a number of the present Board desiring to abolish that large bone of contention, the chieftainship, and thus save themselves from trouble among the doctors, and the institution the expense of his salary. We think the movement impolitic, if not impracticable, and would recommend the Board to retain the office, and place in it a man who is qualified to fill it.

Our third College, with its new organization, has issued its announcement, and placed itself in position to benefit by all the patronage it can get. We predict for it an existence similar to that of the latter days of the Philadelphia College—viz., picking of the bones, and the gathering of the crumbs, from a table which, no longer having a good purveyor, gradually becomes bare of provender. 'Tis true that, in the affairs of colleges, as well as in those of men, there is a tide; 'tis also true, that Fortune, "blind goddess" as she is, generally refuses to bestow her favors on any but the brave and the worthy. In accordance with a remark of Cæsar, "*Viam aut veniam, aut faciam.*" This motto, I fear, is not the motto of the Faculty of the above-named school. The truth is, there is as much obsequious deference, not to say unmanly mental and moral prostration, to the powers that be, in our profession, as in any other. This feeling emasculates men of talent, and often sacrifices real ability, at the shrines of worldly interests and sordid fear. We once heard a lecture by the celebrated Graham, of "Graham bread" notoriety, in which he depicted popular sentiment as an army, drilled up to a certain line, (the line of expediency and popular propriety,) beyond which, if any, more daring than their friends or neighbors, presumed to pass, they were followed at once by a terrible outcry from the whole rank and file, and sometimes even shot down, by those who kept within the limits of the above-named line.

YARBS.—There is in our city, and doubtless elsewhere, a very considerable trade, traffic, and professional business done by a certain class, in the collection, preparation, and dispensing of vegetable medi. . cines, or, as some of the old-lady dispensers call them, " yarbs."

The business, as far as we can learn, may be divided into three departments: 1st. The collection of the plants, which is done by professed collectors, men, women, and children, white and black, some of them practicing, at the same time, extensively among the rural populations. This, we doubt not, was the beginning of Thomsonianism; a vigorous but uneducated mind taking hold of a few simple facts and extending them to the establishment of a system, which has, to counterbalance the many evils which have resulted from it, afforded the profession and the public much important and valuable knowledge on the toxicological and medical properties of the American Medical Botany. 2d. The drying and preparing of these simples are carried on extensively not only in our large cities, but all over the country, by persons who vend them to the people, to the druggists, and to the country practitioners. 3d. We have quite a large number of practitioners in the form of men, old women, negroes, and Indians, who rival our best physicians in Philadelphia and elsewhere, in some cases quite successfully, in the application of their simples, preparations, and nostrums, to the cure of numerous, particularly *incurable*, diseases. We know of an "Indian Doctor" and his wife who practice quite extensively in our city, and, from what we have seen of their cases, with considerable judgment, though evidently with a plentiful lack of knowledge in the science of anatomy, physiology, and pathology.

Some black practitioners among us, who generally combine the two offices of preacher and doctor, make considerable pretensions to medical and surgical knowledge, though the attempt made in Brunswick and elsewhere to endue the African with a sound medical education has as yet, we believe, been a failure. The negroes among their own population retain a vast amount of superstition, in the form of second-sight, witchcraft, etc., etc. They flourish among us chiefly among the simples and in obstetrics, and seldom aspire to important surgical cases. The white practitioners among the simples are either old women or old men—commonly the former. We have

visited lately several of their depots, and been surprised at the
amount of their practice and the extent of their trade. Mrs. Ryan,
in Locust, above Tenth Street, has a large store filled with plants,
hanging on clothes-lines across the room, tied up in bundles on shelves,
packed up in bags under the tables, and spread out in the window to
dry. She has her bottles of tinctures, her jars of salves, the most
sovereign of which, I believe, is the "Green Salve," together with
plasters, and other vegetable preparations. Her patients, who have
often spent all their money with, and been given up by, the regular
doctors, attend her daily clinic; and while undergoing her simple and
cheap course of treatment, loudly laud the efficiency of her skill and
the power of her *yarbs.*

Mrs. O'Rourke has a similar establishment in Eighteenth Street,
above Vine, with whom we held, not long since, a very edifying con-
fabulation. As usual with our profession, she complained of the in-
gratitude of her patients; said they would come to her shop, (which
was by no means filled with a beggarly account of empty boxes,) ask
for a box of her salve or a bottle of her tinctures, and when in possession of the medicine and asked for the money, would say that they
had left home without it; did not think of it; would call again to-
morrow; or make some other frivolous excuse to cheat the poor woman
of her advice and medicines. After reciting several similar cases, she
broke out in an indignant style—exclaiming that she would go any
lengths to assist a poor and worthy person, whose gratitude would be
an abundant compensation; but that the deceitful and worthless were
to her a pest and an abomination, robbing her both of property and
reputation. She had but few complaints against her fellow-practi-
tioners. (Very different from some of us, friend GAZETTE.) In order
to console her in her troubles, we recited to her briefly a case which
had occurred in our own practice, wherein a man (who owned the
house he lived in) was dropsical from head to foot; had been attended
by several skillful physicians; was considered, and thought himself,
incurable; made his will, which we signed as a witness; and placed
himself under our treatment. This man, instead of dying, gradually
improved, and gradually got well, and when we sent our bill in, indignantly denied the claim; said that we had done him no good, and
refused to pay us; and, indeed, took a few turns in a *water-cure* establishment, invited the water-cure man to his house, and made himself
busy all over town in slandering all the regular doctors who had attended him. This so amused our venerable female friend, that she

broke out in an ungovernable and hearty laugh, during which we left her.

Mrs. Lye has quite an extensive store, with all the dignity of printed labels, showy hand-bills, jars, bottles, painted shelves, with numerous preparations, all of a vegetable character, in Tenth, below Market Street. We believe she keeps all the Thomsonian preparations, and practices extensively, and sells large quantities of medicine.

In Market Street, below Tenth, is a large store—been there for many years. They sell nothing else but vegetable and Thomsonian medicines.

Another store seems to have a plethora of roots and yarbs, in Dock Street, above Second; it breaks out on the pavement in bundles and boxes in the form of dry plants, roots, barks, &c., &c. The presiding spirit here is a tall, thin, oracular gentleman, with an old pair of round glass, iron spectacles, long bony fingers, uncropped nails, dilapidated habiliments, and the general appearance of a pretty well-dried specimen of the class of Saurians, who dilates on the virtues of the yarbs, to his customers and the passers-by, in a tone which reminds one of Sir Walter Scott's " Old Domine," whose constant ejaculatory expression was *pro-digious!*

The last character which we shall introduce under this caption is one met with very recently; he was a man of about fifty-five years of age, well-built, fair-complexioned, laden with a large bag or wallet, containing roots, herbs, and " traps." The chief implement among the latter was an iron sauce-pan, with which the worthy man, in his peregrinations over mountain and valley—for he had carried his pack all the way from the Alleghany Mountains—cooked such scanty food as came in his way. He said the business was not very profitable, but necessity forced him to follow it. (Alas! how many of us who claim to belong to the higher order of the Sons of Esculapius have to acknowledge the same thing!) His worn-out and slipshod shoes, his scanty unmentionables, his soiled and dilapidated linen, and coatless arms, with unshorn face, " whose well-proportioned beard like to the tempest tossed," his matted hair, an old white hat, all—all bore testimony to the truth of his remark; yet, with all this, there was a certain dignity in his tone and manner, even while bending under his load of catnip, celendine, mint, pennyroyal, hoarhound, &c., &c., which gave positive evidence of the elevating influence of science on the very humblest of her votaries.

The mercury in this latitude has to-day been above 90 degrees;

43

the same thing has occurred several times during the last two weeks. The heat has been intense, the sudden intermission of temperature inducing a fall of the mercury to the extent of 30 degrees. These rapid changes from heat to cold, and the reverse, have produced their usual effects in the form of diarrhœas, dysenteries, cholera infantum, sunstroke, &c. These are the chief diseases of the season.

A large proportion of our citizens being out of town, our doctors are not very busy, and some of them will soon follow their patients. But it is becoming late and I am very sleepy, so good-night, and *au revoir*.   Yours,   SENECA.

[For the American Medical Gazette.]

AUDI ALTERAM PARTEM.

So numerous have been the discoveries within the last few years, in all the sciences, physical, medical, and especially physiological, that we are almost disposed to conclude that Nature, skillfully interrogated, or put to the question, may be made to disclose most, if not all, her secrets. Two or three years since, Dr. Blatchford reported a discovery, (see Transactions State Medical Society for 1856 or '7,) by means of adroitly getting admission into her "*arcanum*," or private workshop, getting a peep behind the curtain, and thus find out the method by which she manufactures the "*primum mobile*" of human beings; and very possibly, long ere this, in order to show that the discovery is no hoax, and to gratify the curious, he "has made a little *homo* all alive," and thus dispelled all darkness on this subject.

A learned Frenchman, too, M. Bouison, as the result of a long series of embryogenic experiments, has made another very interesting and very useful discovery, on a subject that previously was altogether in the dark—the cause of hare-lip. Here it is, for the benefit of your readers who may not have had the good luck to have seen it: " The same organic action that presides over the buccal aperture presides also over the formation of labial fissures;" * * * * " and as to the latter, it has variable limits, sometimes acting to a small extent, producing simple hare-lip; sometimes so extensive as to produce either partial or entire destruction of the superior lip." The reason why the upper lip is more frequently affected than the lower is, that " it is situated between the mouth and the nostrils, which are both the seats of an absorbent power." This is satisfactory; but it took years to find it out. How simple the most difficult problem, when once solved!

In the last GAZETTE, Dr. O'Reilly, in his article on the Nervous Centres and Vivisection, has shed much light on some subjects not before understood; and among others, the *modus operandi* of belladonna in producing dilatation of the pupil. "It exercises a sedative action on the organic nerves in the skin, which inosculate in the nasal branch of the 5th pair, and is conveyed by the latter to the brain, fifth nerve, ophthalmic division of the fifth nasal branch of the latter, and lenticular ganglion, by its communicating branches, and thence to the ciliary nerves that go to the iris." This, the author says, is a beautiful illustration of reflex action, according to his theory, and solves a difficulty that was never solved before   This we shall not take upon us to deny, but would like to know why hyoscyamus, aconite, veratrum, digitalis, conium, prussic acid, and other sedatives, do not produce a like effect.

That curious, and very interesting phenomenon, "blushing," the author thus explains. He says: "When a young lady is spoken to about her lover, she instantly blushes." "How is this accounted for? The mind communicates with the central ganglion; the latter by reflex action through the brain and facial nerve, to the organic nerves in the face, with which its branches inosculate." Very ingenious this; but let us look into it a little further, and perhaps we shall find that there is a good deal yet about it of which we know nothing. It is assumed, in the above explanation, that the mind, or soul, which is the same thing, is an entity, and has a "local habitation;" it *communicates* with the central ganglion; it does not, therefore, occupy the same part of the body, and is connected with it only mediately. *Where*, then, is its seat? and *how* does it communicate with the ganglion? Is it enthroned in or upon the "sella turcica," and does it from thence send its messengers to distant parts of the body, with its mandates, as was once supposed? What kind of messengers does it employ? A thought spontaneously arising in the mind may, and frequently does, produce blushing. This is a well-known fact. A *thought* has no substance, no parts, no extension, and is therefore immaterial; yet this thought either mediately or directly, no matter which, so acts upon the organic nerves of the face, which of course are material, as to excite "blushing." Indeed, in all cases, it is "thought" only that excites it. *How, in what manner*, does that which is immaterial act on that which is material? These questions are involved in the above explanation, and when solved, will make it complete. In the act of blushing there are a series of phenomena, each one of which must be explained, or the solution fails.

The inquisitive student of nature cannot fail to be interested also in the author's explanations of "*vital action.*"

"When a child is born it seizes the nipple of its mother in its mouth. How can this be explained? Answer: By vital action. What is vital action?

1st. "It is an *intelligent power* inherent in, and emanating from, the organic nervous system.

2d. "It is the breath of life, which, when blown out, leaves man an inanimate mass, such as he was when God made him out of the slime of the earth.

3d. "It is what is generally known as instinct.

"How can this be proved? By recollecting the part the lenticular ganglion plays in the regulation of the movements of the iris, and the otic, in the tensor tympani muscle."

This makes the matter plain. No one, or no student of physiology and nature who is so fortunate as to see these explanations and this last proof, can fail to understand what vital action is, heretofore one of the mysteries of nature; but, as I said at the beginning of this article, these are rapidly disappearing, and the present generation may expect, from the progress we are making, to see the last of Nature's "*Arcana.*" E. PLATT.

RHINEBECK, *July 15th*, 1859.

DEAR DOCTOR—Be so good as to announce that the first three volumes of the New Sydenham Society's Publications will be ready for delivery August 15th, and may be had by application to the undersigned. Subscriptions now due.

Respectfully,

C. K. HEYWOOD, 66 West 20th Street.

DR. D. M. REESE.

Dr. J. M. Carnochan has lately tied the common carotid on the opposite side, in the case of elephantiasis of the face, heretofore reported, and thus far with marked benefit.

He has since tied the external carotid, the facial and lingual arteries, for an aneurism by anastomoses in the roof of the mouth, which was congenital. We have heard of several other operations by the same gentleman lately, who promises to rival Dr. Mott in the number and extent of his ligations of arteries.

SELECTIONS.

INTRODUCTORY LECTURE UPON MILITARY SURGERY.

By CHARLES S. TRIPLER, M.D., Surgeon U. S. Army, Newport, Ky.

Delivered at the Ohio Medical College, at its session of 1858-59.

(CONCLUDED FROM THE AUGUST No.)

Dr. Bryce has severely criticised and successfully impeached the accuracy of the French return. He has shown that, in the month of March, there were more than thirty thousand men in the ambulances in the Crimea, and in the hospitals on the Bosphorus, who were rated as effectives by the French minister. But we have still the significant fact that but one-half the French army was left in the East at the close of the war, while the English were able to muster more than two-thirds of theirs.

But we find this further important fact: the British losses attained their maximum in the *first half* of the campaign, and then rapidly diminished till the close of the war, leaving *that* army in a better fighting condition at the *end*, than in the *beginning* of active hostilities; while with the French the very reverse is the fact; so that it has afforded Dr. Bryce the means of demonstrating that the peace of April, 1856, was a political necessity for France. Her army was rapidly becoming one vast hospital. That this deplorable result was but the natural consequence of the military Intendancy system of France, or, in other words, of the usurpation of medical functions by officers totally ignorant of hygiene, and who, by virture of the military authority they possessed, disregarded the suggestions and even entreaties of scientific men, I shall attempt to show by their *own* writers. I quote M. Baudens:

"It is undeniably a pernicious practice to crowd sick tents and huts into a confined area. Granted that the exigencies of the service necessitate such a proceeding in the Crimea, but the same overcrowding took place at Constantinople, where ample space was available; and it is to this condition of the hospitals that I ascribe the persistence of cholera, and the prevalence and ravages of typhus and hospital gangrene within them. When the surgeon asked for more room, it was answered that facilities for carrying on the ordinary work of the place deserved the first consideration; and hence, in order to economize a few paces, in passing from one hut to another, the most

simple and self-evident laws of preventing diseases were violated. Besides, the surgeon was not even *consulted* respecting the situation for
a hospital; and it happened that, at Constantinople, one was placed
in the immediate vicinity of a marsh, and had to be abandoned because of its febrific emanations." "But the army medical staff and
the Intendance functionaries rarely interpreted the phrase '*overcrowding*' in the same sense. The latter stuck to the strict letter of the
military rule: so long as a patient had the regulation allowance of
cubic feet, overcrowding was an *impossibility;* while the physician
saw it to exist from the moment when disease is aggravated, and its
fatality augmented by reason of too many sick being congregated
within a given space. It was under these circumstances that our
English ally offered to us the aid of their personal and material resources. General Storks proposed to build and completely furnish for
us hospital accommodation for a thousand patients, for whom he would
also undertake to supply food and medical attendance."

Gentlemen, can any Frenchman read the last paragraph without a
blush? Would the people of the United States tolerate, for a moment, such a military sanitary system in their own army, fraught with
such certain disaster, suffering, and death to their own volunteers and
soldiers, if they knew of its existence? and that, in order that the
venerable old idea of the unrestricted subordination of the medical to
all other officers should be perpetuated, even among us, who have no
princes of the blood, no dukes nor lords in our military hierarchy, and
in spite of common humanity and common sense?

Look, again, at the candid confession of Baudens as to the police,
etc., of the French hospitals—matters that the Intendants *were* capable of attending to, and which they would have been *compelled* to attend to, had they been, as they should have been, under the military
authority of the medical officer:

"The English hospitals were remarkable for cleanliness. We have
seen that this quality did *not* exist in ours. The difference is partly
due to the higher and more independent military position which the
English surgeon holds, and which entitles and enables him to exercise
greater authority in hygienic measures. His ordinary sick-diet table
is more ample and varied than the French, and the surgeon can order
what extras he thinks proper for the sick. Indeed, the English camp
was abundantly provided with stores and comforts of all kinds; to
which circumstance is to be ascribed its preservation from scurvy and
typhus in 1856. When we compare the conditions in which the

English soldiers were placed at the commencement of the war, which took them unawares, with those in which they were in 1856, we are forced to acknowledge the greatness of the British nation."

And with regard to the condition of the French army at this time, Baudens again exclaims: "We were threatened with a certain and frightful disaster. It was necessary to devise measures and to act promptly, under penalty of being reduced to impotence—the safety of the army was at stake." Baudens had recourse, in this emergency, to direct and fearless representations to the Emperor himself, who had the good sense to give him ample, but an exceptional, authority; and thus he was enabled to arrest the evil and save thousands of his fellow-soldiers. Had the medical corps been endowed with a suitable military rank, these disasters never could have occurred. Hecatombs of French soldiers were ruthlessly sacrificed, the success of a campaign hazarded, and the honor of France compromised, in order that a sous-lieutenant of the line might be the military superior of M. Baudens, the physician-general of the army.

The contrast here is too marked to be mistaken. We have a French army taking the field, thoroughly appointed and prepared—its sanitary corps perfect in its organization, so far as theory could perfect it—its functions well defined, and, in order that its attention might not be diverted from what was supposed to be its true mission, no other duty was imposed upon them than that of prescribing for the sick; all military authority was denied it; and because military command was as necessary to the discipline of a hospital as to that of a regiment, a *line* officer, called the Military Intendant, was assigned to this command, with the *personnel* of the whole sanitary machinery under his control. Nothing, apparently, could be more simple and effective; and there are not wanting intelligent officers in our own service, who see in it so much to admire, that, if it were possible, they would introduce the same system into our own hospital establishment. Well, it had a fair field in the East, and for a while all went well. The British troops for the first few months were fearfully afflicted by disease, while the French were singularly exempt; and the English press, and the English people, could scarcely find language strong enough to denounce the inefficiency of their own medical staff, and to contrast it most unfavorably with the French. But, gentlemen, at that time the British medical officer had scarcely any more authority than the French. His supplies were in the possession of the Commissariat, and to reach them a long routine of red tape ceremonial had to be gone through with, at the expense of time, opportunity, and patience, in their effect paralyzing the best efforts of the medical officers. The evil became at last too aggravated to be borne; routine, precedent, and the military dogma were cast aside; supplies were seized upon, from the necessity of the case. The medical officers *assumed* the necessary military authority to save their men, and we find the British army coming out of the contest stronger in men, and in infinitely better sanitary condition, than it was three months after it had landed.

And now what was the condition of the French ? An eye-witness sums it up in a few telling paragraphs, thus:

" 1. Two formidable epidemics—scurvy and fever—marked the beginning of the winter of 1855–56, both utterly ruinous to an army in the field, and *one* self-propagating to an illimitable extent, whilst the circumstances in which it acquired its first intensity continued to exist.

" 2. That the invasion of such an amount of disease at the above period was *unexpected*, and during several months continued *unprovided for*, as regards surgeons, hospital accommodation, and furnishings, clothes, and other necessaries for the sick.

" 3. That in these extraordinary circumstances, the form and functions of the medical staff were as closely restricted as *à l'art de guérir*, and on questions affecting the hygiene of the troops, and management of hospitals, as strictly subordinated to the *intendance militaire* as they are at the Val de Grace; by which means *the destruction of the army was still further insured.*"

I think enough has now been adduced to show the pernicious results of the French system, and I cannot perceive how it is possible that a nation, not stricken with judicial blindness, can permit it to remain an hour. Whether the French have profited by their disastrous experience or not, I do not know; that the British have done so, and essentially modified their system, I do know. The Queen has settled this matter by a recent warrant, in a manner which seems to have given satisfaction to the medical staff. As I understand it, it has given to the medical officer the same sort of rank that is accorded to other staff officers, and the same independent control of his special department. If it has not, it will fail of its full effect; for, as regards the officer himself, there will remain an invidious distinction between him and his brother officers, and hence dissatisfaction, discontent, and a sense of personal degradation will exist, thereby impairing his usefulness; and, as regards the service, any control *whatever* over the sanitary details of an army conferred upon an officer of any other corps, may at any time, through caprice, lack of judgment, or obstinacy, seriously impede the prompt and effective administration of the same, at the imminent risk of irreparable disaster.

Still, it must have required a strong and determined effort to break through, in such an army as the British, the authority of the old dogma, that an " officer must command or be commanded." A writer in *Blackwood's Magazine* has well remarked, " There is no doubt that it is extremely difficult, and in fact this difficulty is at the root of the whole of the difficulties of our army service, to get persons whose pursuits are not combative, to co-operate in military operations. The command and obedience to which our citizens are so little accustomed, are the vital spirit of an army. It is *sometimes* necessary, and oftener *natural*, that it should extend beyond the pure military body to whatever other class comes in collateral connection with it." And again, " The position and functions of the medical staff form the most important of all the matters to be adjusted between the combative and non-combative portion of our armaments."

We may remark parenthetically only, that the old distinction between *combatants* and *non-combatants*, as applied to the medical officer, has been roughly handled, and in not a few instances scouted as absurd, by officers of the highest rank in the British army. In our own army *they* are the *only* officers of the administrative branches of the general staff whose duties require them to be present on the field of battle. In the brilliant campaign of General Scott in Mexico, the medical staff was the only one that had an officer killed or wounded. No officer of the quartermaster or subsistence department was either killed or wounded. To any one who understands the meaning of terms, and the duties of these departments, to call one of them combatant in contradistinction to another, as a pretext for conferring military rank upon that one, and denying it to the other, the idea is simply absurd. We may say, as Cicero did of the Roman Augurs, "We cannot see how two men, maintaining that opinion, can look each other in the face without laughing."

Lord Dalhousie, in a memoir upon the medical service appended to the report of the Parliamentary committee, remarks:

" There are several particulars in which the medical service as a body lies under great disadvantages, and which they regard, justly in my opinion, as grievances that ought to be removed. I refer to the inequality which now prevails between the position of a medical officer, and that of his brother officers, in respect of pension, honors, and rank. I respectfully submit that such inequalities are founded on *no sound grounds of justice*, expediency, or policy; no *valid* reason ever has been, or can be, alleged for maintaining them. Their effect is to depress the spirit of the medical officers, to depreciate a profession and class of service which ought to be held in the utmost respect, and supported equally from motives of prudence and gratitude.

" But the most galling, the most unmeaning and purposeless regulations by which a sense of inferiority is imposed upon medical officers, is by the refusal to them of *substantive rank*. The surgeon and assistant surgeon rank invariably with captain and lieutenant, but the rank is only *nominal;* whenever medical officers and others are brought together on public duty, the former has no rank at all, and the oldest surgeon on the list must in such case range himself below the youngest ensign last posted to a corps.

" It is impossible to conceive how such a system as this can have been maintained so long on the strength of no better argument than that ' it has been, therefore it ought to be.' It is impossible to imagine what *serious* justification can be offered for a system which, in respect to external position, postpones service to inexperience, cunning to ignorance, age to youth; a system which gives a subaltern, who is hardly free from his drill, precedence over his elder, who, perhaps, has served through every campaign for thirty years; a system which treats a member of a learned profession, a man of ability, skill, and experience, as inferior in position to a cornet of cavalry, just entering on his study of the pay and audit regulations; a system, in fine, which thrusts down gray-headed veterans below beardless boys."

It was the combined consideration of such facts as these, brought out and verified by the labors of the Parliamentary commission, both as regarded the intolerable injustice of denying to the medical officers a suitable but *positive* military rank, and as regarded the money and life loss, demonstrated to be the natural consequences of so injudicious a system, that has resulted in the royal warrant of October 1, 1858. In speaking of this warrant, Mr. Tuffnel remarked, in a recent lecture in Dublin, that it was the intention of Lord Panmure's government to make the medical service of the army as perfect as means could make it, so that it should be a credit to the country, and an object of desire to the whole medical profession. Mr. Tuffnel also showed that, " instructed by the events of the past few years, England has now taken steps for the husbanding of her physical power; that she has been made aware that, even regarded merely in a pecuniary point of view, the most wasteful of all expenditure is the expenditure of men; and that she now knows that there is scarcely any conceivable amount that it may be necessary to pay for what is required to preserve the health and efficiency of the soldier, that is not advantageously laid out."

I do not doubt that a sincere and honest effort has been made in the recent action of the British Government to remedy the evils that have been so forcibly shown to exist in the sanitary department of their army. The extent to which they have advanced in achieving this object, I hope will prove adequate to the end in view. The exigency that demanded action was unmistakable, and will not be satisfied with any temporizing expedients.

But whatever they may have done in their own emergency, their facts are ours as well as theirs. Let us profit by their example, without being slavishly fettered by their precedent. Inveterate habit in the abuse of terms has drifted us, thus far unresistingly, with the notion that the commissary of subsistence who purchases provisions in Cincinnati for the subsistence of the soldiers, is a *combatant*, while a medical officer—(I use the language of a major-general of the army, in speaking of a medical officer at Molino del Rey: " The last mentioned, when the men of his regiment were almost deprived of commanding officers, assumed the duties of his fallen comrades, and was desperately, probably mortally wounded")—is *officially* a *non-combatant!*

The dogma of the necessary alternate of commanding or being commanded, that has been the fruitful source of so many mischiefs, and is at the root of the difficulty of securing the efficient co-operation of the different professions that are now combined in the organization of an army, has had its practical refutation demonstrated in our service by the experience of almost half a century. The law forbids the exercise of command, out of their own corps, to the officers of the engineers. Still, they are *not* subject to the orders of their juniors in the line. They cannot command, nor are they commanded except by a superior; and what has been the result of this *assumed* military heresy? Let the world produce their superiors as an efficient and scientific corps! Their independence of all outside interference, and their being exclusively intrusted with the means of performing their own duties, have made them what they are, and the country has reaped the advantage of its wise legislation in regard to them. This is the only corps in the army that has any analogy with the medical, as regards scientific acquirements, specialty of function, peculiarity of administration, and claims to independence of action, because it is not at all understood or comprehended by any other department. And I here assert, without fear of successful refutation, that the only possible means of reaching the maximum efficiency of the medical corps is by assimilating it by law in its military position to the corps of engineers. So long as we trifle, and temporize, and look to Europe for authority before we venture upon this self-evident, common-sense, practical plan, so long must the people of the United States agree to pay the cost in thousands of men and millions of money.

And now, gentlemen, in view of the important duties of the medical officer demanded by modern progress, it is plain that a corresponding degree and range of acquirement is necessary upon his part before he can presume to undertake them. He has duties to fulfill in relation to the mass, and in relation to the individual soldier. For the first, a competent knowledge of the laws of hygiene is indispensable; among its dependencies, this science enumerates geology, meteorology, and chemistry. Without a competent acquaintance with these difficult branches of science, the medical officer is neither fitted to investigate the cause of diseases, nor to devise means to obviate or to remedy their effects. For the second, he must be both surgeon and physician. He can select and cultivate no specialty; but in every department he must be ready to apply the resources of his profession whenever an emergency demands them. A superficial knowledge *may* pass a candidate through a scholastic examination, but it will avail him little before an army medical board, or the still more painful ordeal of the battle-field. By his conduct here, he is to stand or fall, if he select the military branch of his profession. And, my young friends, if any of you shall hereafter receive a commission in the army of the United States, you will then be an officer, and you will be expected to be a gentleman. The integrity and honor of the officer of the army *is* and *must* be above suspicion. A lapse in either expels the offender from that small but pure community; and you will there find yourself the associate of a highly-educated, cultivated, and refined body of young men of your own age, the graduates of the military academy at West Point; and among your seniors you will be brought into intimate association with men whose names and deeds adorn the history of our country. To live in such a community, a young man must be fitted by education and acquirement to sustain himself in it. From no class of officers is more expected, as well in special as in general information, than from the medical officers. I would advise you, then, if you think of embracing this profession, not to do so until you have a competent knowledge of classical and general literature, and particularly of mathematical and mechanical science. You will certainly find use for them at every step in your military career. If you have neglected these branches of learning thus far, do not permit your professional pursuits to be interrupted by an attempt to acquire them *now;* but devote a year or two to them assiduously after you shall have left these halls. You will never regret employing the leisure that all young medical men have on their hands at the commencement of their career in this way.

I am admonished, however, that upon this occasion I have said enough. At a future opportunity I shall direct your attention to the special professional attainment necessary for the military surgeon.

REINTERMENT OF THE REMAINS OF JOHN HUNTER.

Mr. Buckland, a son of the late respected Dean of Westminster, has lately been employed examining the vaults of St. Martin's Church, London, in search of the remains of Mr. John Hunter. After some search he found the coffin. It was in an excellent state of preservation, covered with fine black cloth, and studded with gilt nails and ornaments. Upon it was a brass plate with the family arms, and the inscription, "John Hunter, Esq., died 16th October, 1793, aged 64 years." The Royal College of Surgeons having obtained the sanction of the Dean and Chapter of Westminster Abbey, last March removed the coffin from St. Martin's Church and reinterred it among the illustrious dead of England. The following inscription was also placed on the lid: "These remains were removed from the Church of St. Martin-in-the-Fields by the Royal College of Surgeons of England, March 28, 1859." The funeral was attended by the Colleges of Physicians and Surgeons, the Apothecaries' Company, and others among them Dr. Baillie, a grandson of John Hunter. A movement is on foot to erect a monument in Westminster to the memory of the great surgeon, and the subscription list is being well filled up in England. Nor is America behindhand in paying her tribute to his memory, as the proceedings of the American Medical Association show.—*Nashville Journ. M. and S.*

OBLIGATION.

" Prof. Agassiz, in his eulogy on Humboldt, stated that the great savan had loaned him fifty pounds to pay his expenses as a student, and that the Professor in after-life, when he could have repaid the debt, wrote to Humboldt asking ' *the privilege of remaining forever in his debt*, knowing that the request would be more consonant to his feelings than the recovery of the money;' and he adds, ' I am now in his debt.' This anecdote has given rise to several disquisitions on nice points of honor, and however much of the heart's poetry there was in the request of Agassiz, we have heard a story which will bear narration as a companion, or a contrast picture. Years ago, when ' Old Drake' was the dramatic Napoleon of the West, and had his headquarters in Cincinnati, an actor by the name of Meer was attached to his company. Meer having been transfixed by Cupid's dart, shot from a pair of fine eyes, wanted to go to Philadelphia to get married. His funds being low, he applied to young Sam. Drake for a loan, which was cheerfully granted. Reuben—for Meer rejoiced in the name of Jacob's first-born—went East, and the next season brought back his blooming bride. He was so engrossed with his new domestic relations that he forgot to make restitution of the loan, until, at the end of the dramatic campaign, Drake reminded him of the existence of a little document in the shape of an I O U. Reuben looked surprised, incredulous, horrified ! For a moment he was speechless, but at last the pent-up volcano burst forth in these lava words: ' Sam. Drake, I thought you was my friend; I have loved you as a brother. But all's over between us, *for the man who reminds me of an obligation cancels the favor !* Which of the twain exhibited the most philosophy, Agassiz or Meer, is a question for casuists to settle."

The above was not written by us, but the writer leaves our sentiments to be inferred. No matter who wrote it, the heart of the man of honor brightens it with its genial sunshine. We will not treat the subject so gingerly. We sometimes like to be what magnificent and highly elaborated rascals call rude, when we know that we are right. Prof. Agassiz has published to the world a stain upon his moral character, that we would not leave as a legacy to our heirs for all the fame of Humboldt. The descendants of Agassiz will remain under pecuniary obligation to the descendants of Humboldt through all coming time.

Meer's moral obliquity was not more hideous than that of Agassiz.

Meer and Agassiz are types of a large class, and our deliberate judgment is, that in respect of this feature of borrowing money with an intention to keep it, a more rascally class does not exist upon the face of the earth. The man of honest impulses loathes and scorns every approach to dishonor. It is to him a fountain shut up and a book sealed. The lowest and vilest of these approaches is that of borrowing money, and failing under any pretence whatever to pay it. Poor Humboldt, we suppose, granted Agassiz the "privilege of remaining forever in his debt," because he could not help himself. Being himself a man of a high sense of honor, we may imagine his feelings upon the reception of the letter of Agassiz.

Agassiz is considered in the front rank of our great men. What an example he offers to the youth of our country, struggling for honorable position ! He will find that American soil is not yet prepared for such exotic plants. Agassiz, we suppose, would contend that he desired to continue under obligation to his illustrious patron. Would not the obligation of gratitude have continued when the pecuniary obligation ceased? Had he paid Humboldt honorably, still would not there have been left a vast margin for gratitude for help when he needed help ? Did he suppose that a few paltry dollars could cancel that obligation when he begged permission to keep them in his own pocket ? Bah !

[We honor the moral courage of the *Nashville Medical and Surgical Journal* for uttering the truth, which many felt, but dare not speak.]

CASTRATION IN EPILEPSY.

A paper was read by C. Holthouse, Esq., on this subject, before the Royal Medical and Chirurgical Society, founded upon the operations of Drs. McKinley and White, of Tennessee; Dr. Talbot, of Missouri; Dr. Hacker, of Louisiana; and Dr. Holly, of Germany—whereupon much discussion was elicited, evidently, and we think justly, opposed to the operation.

In the course of this discussion, Mr. Hale Thompson remarked that "he had heard more false logic in the paper than he had ever heard in the Society before; and he suggested whether it would not be better to follow the rules of practice laid down by eminent surgeons in this country, rather than adopt ill-understood American eccentricities."

We think it would decidedly, but still respectfully submit that Mr.

Thompson displayed bad judgment, and worse taste, in thus alluding to the opinions of a few individuals.

Mr. Holthouse thus concluded his reply: " It was said that the removal of a healthy organ was not justifiable. Nor would he justify it in a healthy individual; but in case of disease it was sometimes necessary, as in amaurosis, which had been cured by the removal of healthy teeth. If the teeth might be removed to save the eye, he did not see why the testes might not be removed to save the brain."

We see great objections to the argument of Mr. Holthouse, and cannot concur in his opinion, but we do not hence pronounce that opinion a British eccentricity, nor do we consider the conglomerated treatment of the case of traumatic tetanus at St. Thomas' Hospital a British eccentricity.—*Louisville Med. News.*

TRAUMATIC TETANUS.

A case of recovery from this disease is reported to have occurred in St. Thomas' Hospital. A girl aged eight years, received, in falling, a slight abrasion on her knee, two weeks before admission to the hospital. The symptoms seem to have been well marked and attended with emprosthotonos. The treatment consisted in colchicum, hyoscyamus, iodide of potassium, infusion of gentian, jalap, mercury, leeches to the spine, mercury with chalk, Dover's powder, wine, syrup of iodide of iron—all within a period of thirteen days, and yet she recovered. Verily, " there is a Providence that shapes our ends," etc.—*Louisville Med. News.*

Commencement of the Medical Department of the University of Louisiana.

The Annual Commencement of this institution took place at Lyceum Hall, on Saturday, March 19th, 1859. The degree of Doctor of Medicine was conferred on ninety-seven of the candidates for professional honors. There was also one graduate in the department of Pharmacy. Dr. Hunt, Dean of the Faculty, delivered to the class an address. Dr. J. W. Saunders next followed in a valedictory address.

It will no doubt be gratifying to the friends of the University to hear of its continued prosperity. The number of matriculates for the session of 1858 and 1859 was three hundred and thirty-three, being an increase of fifty-seven above that of the previous session.—*New Orleans Med. and Surg. Journal.*

EXCISED KNEES.

A most curious and novel sight occurred the other night, at the London Medical Society, which took my fancy very much. Mr. P. C. Price, a young surgeon of great promise, a protégé of my friend Mr. Fergnson, and who has at the same time performed most of the capital operations, read a paper on some of the causes of failure following the operation of excision of the knee-joint, in which he most ably considered the subject, and very satisfactorily showed that the want of a successful issue depended upon circumstances which might have occurred had amputation been performed. At the conclusion of his paper, some ten or more male and female persons walked into the room, each of whom had undergone resection of one of their knees, and who were living proofs of the value of a limb without a joint. One lad could walk his 14 miles a day, without inconvenience or fatigue—all were in excellent health. The sight was rather amusing, too, for both males and females had their knees exposed whilst walking up and down to show their anarthrodial agility. Mr. Price is engaged in the preparation of a treatise on excision of the knee, which will be copiously illustrated, and at the same time will contain an account of every operation that has been done, up to the year 1858.—*Montreal Chronicle*.

DISEASES OF THE AIR-PASSAGES.

The *N. A. Medico-Chirurgical Review*, in concluding an able review of Dr. Horace Green's late work on Diseases of the Air-passages, expresses the following just and liberal sentiments, viz.:

" From this brief survey of the history and literature of this interesting subject, it will be seen that the practicability and utility of Dr. Green's method have, at length, after the lapse of nearly a quarter of a century, been sustained and verified by unquestionable medical authorities in Great Britain, France, and Germany. In our own country, on the contrary, the views of Dr. Green have gained but few adherents. In the city of his residence these views are even violently opposed by some of the oldest and most influential physicians, as the recent proceedings of the New York Academy of Medicine, relative to the death of Mr. Whitney, amply testify. We are neither acquainted with, nor have we ever seen any of the parties concerned in the disgraceful transaction to which we allude; we therefore speak disinterestedly when we say that, having read attentively the reports

44

of these proceedings, as published in the *American Medical Monthly* for February, 1859, and in other journals, we are constrained, from the evidence therein set forth, to regard the arraignment of Dr. Green before the Academy as an undignified, impolitic, and badly-managed attempt to cast obloquy upon him, and to bring into disrepute his views concerning certain respiratory diseases, and the plan of treatment based upon these views."

THE PARISIAN CONFRERE AS DEPUTY-PHYSICIAN.

"To go away and trust your patients to a *confrère*, is to furnish a dangerous opportunity to one of the crying appetites of the day. I rather would shut my door, and tell the porter to say I was absent, than recommend my patients to a confrère. If the case is not urgent, they will wait till I return; if they will not wait, hazard perhaps will serve them worse than I should by handing them over to a *confrère*, whom they will appreciate less than they do me. The chosen *confrère* who supplies my place is sure to make himself very amiable, very attentive, *empressé* and *prévenant*, out of esteem and affection for me. He will discover that he has a conquest to make, and he will use his best means to gain it. An illustrious doctor, who lived at the beginning of this century, was wiser. He lived in grand style, and every year took two good months' vacation. And what sort of a man did he leave as his substitute? He himself was an 'elegant' man of the world, spiritual, lettered, catholic, or pretending to be so; all his clients were people of the court, noble dames, and bishops; and he chose for his substitute a very worthy *confrère*, to whom all the world did justice, but one who was timid, reserved, careless of dress, abrupt in his address, and but little of a Voltairien. The contrast was striking, and we may guess to his profit."—*L'Union Médicale*.

COPLAND'S DICTIONARY.

[From the report of Dr. Coale, Librarian to the Massachusetts Medical Society, we clip the following *jeu d'esprit:*]

"The remarkable, not to say startling event of the year—one which he trusts will cause his term of Librarianship to be *cum creta notata*—one that will make this an *annus mirabilis* in the history of the Massachusetts Medical Society—is the completion of Copland's Dictionary. Through twenty-five years, 'in linked sweetness long drawn out,' the publication of this work has been protracted. Empires have fallen, others have risen on their ruins, and these in turn given way to others—the political and scientific aspect of the face of the globe has been changed many times and oft—but Dr. Copland, with continuous and unflagging pertinacity, has progressed steadily through the alphabet. All things sublunary, or to put it more strongly, all things finite, have a termination; and to-morrow men who, in the prime of life and in the full flush of youthful hope, consulted the let⁺ A, may, in gray hairs and spectacles, improve their knowledg⸱ medical subjects commencing with U, V, W, X, Y & Z."

YELLOW FEVER USEFUᵀ

The old adage is, that all things are maᵈ
Until lately we have been at a loss to diᵣ
But we have found it out. He coᵣ
quacks, in the shape of Hoᵣ
Pile Doctors, *et id omne ᵖᵣ*
gins to shine betweeᵣ
calls northward.
yellow-fever
months ᵢ

⸱es ᵖ
⸱œopat
Aₛ
⸱nus. the shoulde
Their lives aₑ
At any ᵣ
grave. —N. O.
⸱n the year.
[Dr. Brickell, the edito⸱
too is off for more northe
censure the quacks?
Yellow Jack ⸱⸱

Case of Pseudarthrosis of the Upper Third of the Thigh, successfully treated by the Use of Silver Wire.

By E. S. COOPER, M.D.,

Professor of Anatomy and Surgery in the Medical Department of the University of the Pacific, San Francisco, California.

Wm. Mc——, æt. 50, applied for admission into the Pacific Clinical Infirmary, August, 1857, in consequence of an ununited fracture of the femur, just above the trochanter major, of two years' standing. His general health being feeble, he was sent away without an operation. Six months after, his general health becoming good, he returned, and I performed the following operation:

An incision eight inches long was made in a longitudinal direction, with the thigh commencing at a point corresponding to the upper part of the trochanter major. Incisions were then carried to the bone, and the fragments exposed, when the intervening substance was cut away, leaving two long surfaces looking towards each other.

A drill about one line and a half in diameter was then applied, and holes made through the fragments, when a silver wire one line in thickness was introduced, and the bony surfaces drawn together. A pledget of lint was then laid in the wound, so that no portion of the soft parts could heal by first intention.

A roller was applied to the limb, after which splints were put on, and the dressing completed.

The lint was removed in seven days, suppuration being fully established, and, as there was no great amount of tenderness, I began to move the wire, for the purpose of making the ultimate removal easy. At the end of two and a half months the wire was removed, when the bony union was perfect.

Notwithstanding this individual has been the subject of rheumatism, and suffers from it still in the knee and ankle of the same limb, he has no pain nor trouble of any kind in the region of the operation. The fragments are perfectly consolidated.

Remarks.—The successful operations for pseudarthrosis have of late become so common that their reports in medical journals may justly be regarded stale publications.

But, while very great improvements have of late been made in the treatment of these cases, still these improvements have not led to an exhaustion of the subject; and as the method above detailed differs somewhat from that ordinarily pursued, I think the case will not be altogether uninteresting, particularly as the treatment was in one respect carried out in opposition to the advice of most, or all, surgical writers, viz., keeping the wound entirely open, so that the divided soft parts could not heal by first intentions.

I am convinced by my own experience, and by observation in the hospitals of Europe, that the source of the greatest trouble and danger in these cases is due to the burrowing of purulent matter, and that it can nearly always be prevented by the above plan.

I am fully convinced also, from experience, that the admission of atmosphere to bones which have been fractured, or otherwise injured, is not a source of irritation, as is now universally acknowledged by surgical writers. The mistake, in my humble opinion, that has been made is this: viz., that in all cases of injuries of bone, when air is admitted to it, (take as an example a compound fracture,) there is more or less destruction of continuity of soft parts, and there is not generally a free opening constantly kept for the discharge of purulent matter; and this burrowing, producing inflammation, is often the cause of such dangers, and often fatal results, as so frequently occurs in this class of injuries. But for engrossing space, I would discuss this subject much further. I will, however, present it to the notice of the profession in the report of other cases directly bearing upon this point at an early period, giving statistics of results of operations, including those in which the larger joints, such as the knee, were opened freely without any untoward symptoms occurring.

By the application of lint to the entire surface of the wound, and a roller to the limb, as tightly as can conveniently be borne, for six or eight days, until the whole has become a granulating mass covering the surface, nearly all communication between the wound and the neighboring muscles is cut off, so that it is easy to perceive that burrowing of matter would not be very likely to take place between the neighboring muscles.

Further Remarks upon the Connection of the Nervous Centres of Animal and Organic Life.

By JOHN O'REILLY, M.D., etc.

"Quidquid præcipies, esto brevis, ut cito dicta
Percipiant animi dociles, teneantque fidelis."   HOR.

Every operating surgeon knows, to perform an operation on the dead subject, is quite a different thing to doing it on the living body.

The same remark is equally true with respect to exposing the Pineal gland in the living or dead animal. In the former there is great trouble; in the latter there is no difficulty.

By a simple experiment, any person can satisfy himself that the Pineal gland is a ganglion of the organic nervous system, as piercing the gland with a fine needle will produce the following phenomena:

Oscillation of the iris, contraction of the iris, rolling and fixing of the eyeballs, and tetanic spasm of the muscles of the body.

It should be observed, unless the gland is touched, no such effects are produced by puncturing any other part; which fact affords in itself, in the strongest manner, negative proof of the importance of the ganglion.

A glance at the annexed plates, drawn by my friend, Mr. William Henessy, from dissections made by myself, will show the mode of carrying out the vivisection, and demonstrate the relative anatomy of the ganglion.

A perusal of the first and latter part of my paper, to which I most earnestly and respectfully beg to refer, will convince any person of the truth of the deductions to be arrived at from what takes place when the ganglion is irritated.

If one line be drawn transversely, so as to allow the posterior lobes of the cerebrum to touch it, and another in the direction of the longitudinal fissure, the ganglion will be found in the median line, at a distance of three-quarters of an inch from the transverse, and at a depth of one inch and an eighth from the peripheral surface of the cerebrum.

In case an attempt is made to puncture the ganglion, and that it escape being wounded, the sheep will fall into a state of coma, and commence snoring.

If the gland is now cut down on, it will be found surrounded by a clot of blood.

It is a remarkable fact, that life should exist not only in the body of the sheep after decapitation at the articulation between the atlas and occipital bone, but likewise in the head, notwithstanding the mutilation of the brain, and the destruction of the Pineal gland or ganglion. Yet such is the case; and the mouth will shut and open once or twice. Here it will be recollected that the vital agent is in the spheno-palatine ganglion.

It will be recollected I maintained, throughout my observations, that each organic ganglion was the seat of vitality. If an eel be cut in half a dozen pieces, each part will be alive, because each part contains one or more organic ganglia.

Nutrition, assimilation, secretion, and absorption are the result of organic nervous influence. How are these important matters provided for in the encephalon? Where is the organic ganglion to be found destined to preside over these functions in the brain? I will answer, In the *sella turcica*, and is that body called the pituitary gland, which is composed of gray and white matter, incased in the *dura mater;* enveloped by the arachnoid membrane, communicating, through the *infundibulum*, with the third, as well as all the other ventricles of the brain, and, by the continuity of surface of the arachnoid membrane, with the entire surface of the cerebral mass. I should also observe, that it appears to be in direct communication with the *Pineal* gland, or central ganglion; that the pedunculi of the gland can be traced down towards the *infundibulum.* (See plate.) It may be said no nerves can be detected in the arachnoid membrane; but the same objection holds good with respect to the *pericardium, pleura,* and peritoneum. However, when these membranes, as well as the arachnoid, are in a state of inflammation, the exquisite pain proves, beyond a doubt, the existence of nerves,; the vascularity shows the presence of blood-vessels, although such could not be previously discovered; and the effusion of lymph, serum, or pus, demonstrates that secretion is vigorously carried on, and the subsequent removal of these substances points out the activity of the absorbents.

It will be perceived the semilunar ganglia perform in the abdomen the same kind of duties the pituitary gland or ganglion does in the cranium. These ganglia further resemble one another in being located in secure positions, being in the proximity of large blood-vessels; in being at some distance from the organs they supply with nerves. The *white* bands constituting the pedunculi of the Pineal gland, as before stated, can be seen proceeding towards the *infundibulum*, which passes down from the third ventricle to the pituitary gland; the internal carotid arteries pass by the sides of the pituitary gland, surrounded by a plexus of nerves derived from the superior cervical ganglia, if any of the branches of the plexus enter the gland, and I am certain they do: so, then, a complete communication would be established between all the ganglia in question.

I will not trespass for some time on the readers of the GAZETTE. I therefore expect whatever blunders I have committed, (and they are not a few,) or presumption I may be deemed guilty of, will be

magnanimously pardoned by all, not excepting those who are inclined
to split hairs, and who regard everything savoring of originality
aduncis nasis.

230 FOURTH STREET, Washington Square, }
    15th *August*, 1859.   }

FIG. 1.—Appearance of Cerebrum and Cerebellum after the removal
of the Calvarium and Dura Mater.

1, 1, Cerebrum.   2, 2, Cerebellum.

FIG. 2.—Similar View as Fig. 1, with rule and needle describing the
method for finding the Pineal Gland or Ganglion.

FIG. 3.—Hemispheres of the Cerebrum removed on a level with the
Corpus Callosum. The posterior lobes of the brain drawn
upward and forward with the Corpus Callosum, so as to bring
into view the Pineal Gland and its peduncles.

1, 1, Cerebrum.   4, Pineal Gland.
2, 2, Corpus Callosum.   5, 5, Nates.
3, 3, Pedunculi Pineal Gland.   6, 6, Testes.

FIG. 4.—Vertical Section of the Brain, showing the anatomical relations of the Pineal Gland.

1, 1, 1, Cerebrum.   6, Nates.
2, Corpus Callosum.   7, Testes.
3, Fornix.   8, Cerebellum.
4, Pineal Gland.   9, Fourth Ventricle.
5, Opticus Thalamus.   10, Medulla Oblongata.

FIG. 5.—View of the Base of the Brain, showing Position of the
Infundibulum.

1, 1, Cerebrum.   7, Medulla Oblongata.
2, 2, Olfactory Nerves.   8, Fifth Pair of Nerves.
3, Optic Commissure.   9, Facial Nerve.
4, Infundibulum.   10, 10, Sixth Pair of Nerves.
5, 5, Third Pair of Nerves.   11, 11, Ninth Pair of Nerves.
6, Pons Varolii.   12, 12, Fourth Pair of Nerves.

FIG. 6.—Horizontal Section of the Brain.

1, 1, Cerebrum.   8, 8, Plexus Coroides.
2, Anterior Commissure.   9, 9, Nates.
3, 3, Corpus Striatum.   10, 10, Testes.
4, Infundibulum.   11, Valvi Lucens.
5, 5, Pedunculi of Pineal Gland.   12, Medulla Oblongata.
6, Pineal Gland.   A, A, A, Lateral Ventricle.
7, 7, Optici Thalamici.   B, Middle Ventricle.

FIG. 7.—View of the Base of the Brain, showing the Connection of
the Infundibulum with the Pituitary Gland, after its removal
from the Sella Turcica.

1, Pituitary Gland.   2, Infundibulum.

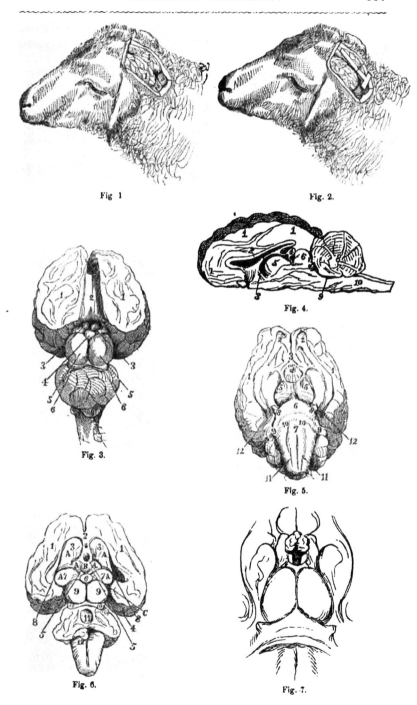

Fig 1

Fig. 2.

Fig. 4.

Fig. 3.

Fig. 5.

Fig. 6.

Fig. 7.

BOOK NOTICES.

A Treatise on Venereal Diseases, by John Hunter, F.R.S., with copious Additions by Dr. Philip Ricord, &c. Translated and edited, with Notes, by Freeman J. Bumstead, M.D. Second edition. Phila.: Blanchard & Lea. 1859.

The genius of John Hunter opened a new path to the investigation of venereal diseases, and to the general principles relating to the therapeutic applications most appropriate to them. But since his day various revolutions have taken place in the minds of medical men, who have devoted their time to the study of this most important and difficult subject. To the labors of Ricord a great debt is due for developing the views of Hunter, settling some points of controversy, and enlightening us on some questions of doubt and obscurity. The edition before us, we are informed, contains a *résumé* of Ricord's recent lectures on chancre. This epitome was gleaned from a volume of notes published by M. Fournier, Interne of the Hôpital du Midi, of Paris. The long-contested question of the unity or the duality of the syphilitic virus receives a considerable share of attention; and the influence of the chlorate of potash in preventing and arresting mercurial ptyalism, is also mentioned. What is offered by the American editor upon the last-named subject adds nothing essential to the knowledge already in possession of very many medical practitioners of this country. Even some who live *in the bush* have for years been familiar with the therapeutic qualities of this salt, not only in mercurial stomatitis, but in other morbid conditions within the mouth.

While it is universally admitted that Ricord has done great service to the cause of modern science, as related to syphilis, his opinions on not a few points are utterly at variance with other writers of the highest distinction. He, himself, has often revoked some of his *immutable laws* appertaining to syphilis, and has fallen back to a state of uncertainty, or has embraced the identical views which he had for years repudiated and ridiculed. With all his brilliancy of genius, his quick powers of perception, his fascinating style as a lecturer and author, he cannot be followed as a safe guide by the inquiring student. His imagination at times seems to transcend his judgment, and he is led away into false and dangerous conclusions. Up to the present moment, Velpeau, Gibert, Dapaul, Sigmund, Wilson, and many others of highest repute in the medical world, have steadfastly opposed his views as wholly untenable, and leading to most demoralizing consequences. And now it seems that Ricord has very lately abandoned the position which he has so long and so doggedly maintained in regard to the contagiousness of secondary syphilis. At a meeting of the Imperial Academy of Medicine of Paris, held in the early part of June, he read a paper which astonished everybody. It was an abandonment of his former notions on the non-transmissibility of the secondary lesions of syphilis. It is reported that this change in his opinions nearly knocked him over.

Wherein Dr. Bumstead confines himself to the business of translator of Ricord, he executes his task in a satisfactory manner. But when he assumes the office of teacher, and steps upon the platform to proclaim his own opinions and to instruct us, while we prefer to lend an ear to a maturer and more deliberate voice, and to a more unbiased and comprehensive experience, we confess our dissatisfaction; and we do not hesitate to say, that, in our estimation, his own "forth-puttings" are calculated to mar the popularity and usefulness of the book.

We must here take occasion to express our disgust at some of the statements made by Dr. Bumstead, in the lectures delivered by him at the College of Physicians and Surgeons, of this city. These lectures abound in too many vulnerable points to be discussed here. We will mention only one. In his second lecture, Dr. B. says: "Strange as it may appear, most women who communicate gonorrhœa to men, do so without having it." Such an announcement may be well suited to lewd prostitutes, and to those who visit and support them, in their abodes and practices of filth and beastly licentiousness. But we can scarcely resist the thought that the lecturer made use of this unwarrantable and insulting language as a sort of advertisement for business among certain classes, who may be induced to consult him, and look to him to shield them in their wickedness. Whatever motive prompted the remark, we consider it in the highest degree censurable, and derogatory to the position occupied by Dr. B. "Let him that thinketh he standeth, take heed lest he fall."

A SYSTEM OF SURGERY: PATHOLOGICAL, DIAGNOSTIC, THERAPEUTIC, and OPERATIVE. By Samuel D. Gross, M.D., Professor of Surgery in the Jefferson Medical College of Philadelphia, &c. Illustrated by 936 engravings. In two volumes. Philadelphia: Blanchard & Lea.

This work has just appeared, too late for thorough examination in time for this number, and we can therefore only announce it as in readiness. We hail it with pleasure as an American work, original, elaborate, thorough, and practical, embodying a complete system of surgery, in all its phases. The author has acquired distinction and eminence as a teacher and practitioner, and by his contributions heretofore made to our literature has earned a high reputation. This great work cannot fail to add to his renown, as, from its completeness, it is likely to be the standard in the schools of our country for a long time to come. We refrain from any criticism at present, for obvious reasons; but we have sufficiently perused it to commend it as possessing great merits, and in some respects it is superior as a text-book to any other work of its class.

It is published in two royal octavo volumes, of nearly 1,200 pages each, on superior paper, with large type, and the illustrations are multitudinous and excellent. Messrs. Blanchard & Lea have evidently spared no pains or expense in bringing out these huge volumes; nor is it necessary to bespeak for them a wide circulation, as they will be everywhere in demand.

LETTER TO ALEXANDER H. STEVENS, M.D., LL.D., by a Retiring Physician. Shot to Dhu Glas.

This is the title of a pamphlet, which, apart from its pithy contents, is calculated to make a sensation, by the elegant taste of its typography and the superior style in which it is issued. It purports to be "some account of a *Secret Society* in New York, entitled the Kappa Lambda," and the author conceals his name, thus giving an air of mystery, which enhances the interest of the publication among the people, who will read it. It will prove the epitaph of the conspiracy.

A MICROSCOPIST'S COMPANION.—Dr. John King, of Cincinnati, is at his old tricks again, plagiarizing by wholesale and retail, which seems to be a trade with him and the "*Eclectics*," a name which appears to mean *pirates* of books, including the text, notes, plates, and all. If there is in this work the ghost of an idea, thought, or expression, which is not stolen bodily, we have not the ken to discover it. We marvel that any publishers can be found capable of putting their imprint to such grand larceny, after the conviction and punishment of the literary thief, in the case of the robbery of Wood & Bache, &c. And we marvel still more that any one of the journalists can have the effrontery to commend this book, which ought to be burned by the common hangman.

We are forcibly reminded of the broom-seller, who, being undersold by a rival in the trade, expressed his wonder how it could be done, seeing that he *stole the stuff* of which the brooms were made, and hence could afford to sell cheap. His competitor unraveled the mystery, by confessing that he *stole the brooms ready made!* This is precisely what Dr. King and his publishers deserve the credit of doing in the book trade; and to buy this book, but for the defect in human laws, would make the purchaser *particeps criminis* in the robbery.

EDITOR'S TABLE.

THE LOUISVILLE DAILY JOURNAL

Is edited by our friend Prentiss, who treated the profession so handsomely in May last, that we were half inclined to forgive him for having allowed his paper to be used as a vehicle for puffing a certain doctor last year for Staphyloraphy and other surgical feats. We hoped that his better knowledge of the ethics of our profession, derived from his recent intercourse with the Convention, would have prevented him from being caught again in the same snare. But as we found the same journal heralding the same surgeon again for the radical cure of hernia, &c., we ventured to hint to the *Louisville Medical News* that they had professional delinquencies nearer home than New York, and indicated the foregoing illustration in their *Daily Journal*.

Whereupon Mr. Prentiss grows wrathy, for he is notoriously a "fighting editor," and in defending himself and Prof. Goldsmith, the party in question, ascribes our hint, given to the *Medical News*, to somebody in Kentucky, than which nothing can be more unjust. And he insinuates that there is some "little doctor" who has solicited similar puffs for himself, and he owes it to himself to say who he is; for we know but one doctor in Louisville below the average size in stature, but his soul is above all quackery, and he would despise a newspaper puff.

We can only reply to the severities intended by Mr. Prentiss, in his article on the GAZETTE, by distinctly making ourselves understood. When surgeons or physicians are puffed in the secular papers, either by personal solicitation, or that of friends, very great injury is inflicted upon the party lauded, and he loses caste among his professional brethren. The true surgeon has the medical press opened to him for the announcement of his claims to science and skill, and our own Journals are always eager to award honor to either novelty or merit. Such publication is legitimate and reputable, and the true physician needs none other. It is only when neither novelty nor merit is possessed, that a resort is had to newspaper puffing. If Mr. P. wishes to serve any medical man, therefore, we respectfully suggest to him, before announcing any of his surgical feats, that he should inquire whether they have been made known through professional channels, and their claims been submitted to medical scrutiny. Without such course, he will be liable, as in this case, to injure a neighbor, by a public notice of an every-day proceeding, as though it were a novelty; or as though the party puffed had any exclusive or superior skill to his brethren, which would be a sad perversion of the truth. And yet on just such puffs, quackery lives, moves, and has its being.

So much for Mr. P., the political editor, and we append the following for his protégé :

The Last Phase of Charlatanism.

In our last issue we alluded, half playfully, to the practice of a Louisville pretender to surgery, of permitting himself to be puffed in the city papers. This was not the first time he had been taken to task for this breach of honor, held sacred among medical gentlemen. The physicians of that city, disgusted by the frequent nauseous allusions to this pretender's achievements in surgery, in a public print, called his attention to the fact in another city paper. This they would not have condescended to do, but for the fact that the pretender was connected with recognized medical gentlemen, which gave him sufficient consequence to entitle him to this public castigation. The pretender only answered this through his newspaper organ, the editorial containing many flings at the " Code."

This pretender is not to force us into any controversy with his organ, a political newspaper. He shall not use that shield to screen his writhing bacon from the lash. We believe he writes these editorials himself, and for the best of reasons.

1st. Every one of them, those even written to repel invited attacks, contain a puff of himself. The one concerning us embodies a prodigious puff of this Goldsmith as a " bussen" curer.

2nd. The editor of his principal organ has a national reputation for wit and vivacity, while Dr. Goldsmith is notoriously leather-headed, with red eyes, a sodden countenance, and the manners rather of a coal boatman than a gentleman. Now these editorials bear internal evidence of the paternity of the latter rather than of the former. For our allusion to him (though we spared his name) he is out in a low-bred, ill-concocted article in his organ, intended to puff himself, defame . us, and some one he calls a rival in his city. He hopes to draw us into a controversy with his political editor. He is mistaken. Whatever appears there in regard to us or himself we shall believe him to be the author of.

We learn that there are gentlemen in the profession of medicine in Louisville, who recognize and consult with this bloated Harlequin. We are very happy that it is their privilege, and not ours.

ACADEMIC DEGREES.

The reckless and indiscriminate manner in which certain "Botany Bay" colleges in our country are conferring honorary degrees of A.M., D.D., and even LL.D. upon *dunces*, is fast tending to bring academic honors into disrepute. This year we have observed, among numerous degrees worthily bestowed upon gentlemen whose scholarship and prominent usefulness entitle them to academic honors, that there have been too many instances in which mediocrity not merely, but imbecility, and even notorious offenders against the learned professions, have had these distinctions awarded to them. The reasons assigned in extenuation are, the wealth or political or ecclesiastical influence of the party or his relatives, whence colleges expect support as a *quid pro quo* for thus prostituting their honors. A letter before us assigns, as the defence for conferring the degree of *Artium Magister* on one of the weakest men in the profession of medicine, that he and his friends had made, or promised, a trifling subscription to the university! and this honorary A.M. has no pretensions to scholarship of any kind, and could not translate his diploma if sent to him, and is not known at all beyond the immediate circle of his family and the congregation of his church; but having married into the family of a clergyman, who is an officer of the college, he must have a degree!

Another is made LL.D. because he has wealth acquired by the most disreputable of all quackery, as in the case of Dr. Jaynes, of Philadelphia, and others of kindred character. Another LL.D., it is said, was made so before his beard was grown, because a large donation was expected from his wealthy father, a contingent recompense not likely to be realized; while the title of D.D. has been squandered in like manner, and under similar influences.

We are glad to see that the title M.D. is conferred honorarily in very rare instances, as it ought to be. The only exception made by any body to the honorary degrees conferred by medical colleges during 1859 is that made by Dr. Butler, of the *Medical and Surgical Reporter*, who growls at the M.D. bestowed upon Dr. Marsh, of this city, by Castleton Medical College; and only for the reason that he does not advertise in his paper, so far as is apparent, for in education and position, in character and usefulness, Dr. M. is every way Dr. B's superior. The "*Reporter*" will not get the "advertisement," notwithstanding this ruse, for Dr. M. has the wit to know that it will not "pay" to patronize that *weakly* sheet of a provincial town like Philadelphia, and hence he will still advertise his trusses "largely in all the New York journals," and ignore Dr. Butler and his squibs.

NEW YORK QUARANTINE

Is still, as aforetime, the same unmitigated humbug and nuisance, and increasing in its odious and superstitious exactions and extortions, by the stupidity and political conspiracies among its officials. The daily reports of the Commissioners of Health are laughed at as a broad farce, and there is *here* more ignorant panic and prating about yellow fever than in New Orleans or Havana.

There are two sets of Commissioners, and a double corps of hungry medical officers, pampered out of the public crib, with nothing to do. The sapient Health Officer makes a great outcry for a steamboat to carry him on board the floating hospital in his occasional visits, for which an extra $5,000 is paid him beyond his $40,000 reported annual income from fees and perquisites.

The chief resident physician of the Marine Hospital still gets his $5,000 a year, and clamors for *assistants*, with similar salaries, notwithstanding his hospital is abandoned, and the patients all provided for elsewhere. The physician of the floating hospital receives $1,000 per month! and is the only man who earns his pay, though his patients

are few, and far between. And if he is the politician we take him
for, he will have perquisites besides. The Health Commissioner and
Resident Physician of the Board of Health manage to get \$7,000 per
annum between them, so that the medical men connected with the
Quarantine are all well provided with fat salaries at the public expense.
How long the Chamber of Commerce, ship-owners, merchants, and
sailors of this port will submit to be thus robbed by a system which
outrages all sanitary science, and is a disgrace to the civilization of the
age, will be learned at Albany next winter. If asses be still sent to
the Legislature, these abuses will be perpetuated.

DR. BUTLER,

Of the *Medical and Surgical Reporter*, has our sympathy in his recent
disappointment, by the abolition of the office he was seeking at
Blockley Hospital; the Board of Guardians having returned to the
oft-repeated experiment of dispensing with the Chief Resident Physician, rather than appoint Dr. B. or any other of the hungry expectants. But he should not lose his temper and rail at his neighbors on
this account, as he may have better luck next time.

Our harmless *jeu d'esprit* on his tilt with the feminine doctors,
which was intended to relieve him from his " bad eminence," seems to
have "touched him on the raw," if we may judge by his "wincing,"
although we meant it playfully. His defence of Dr. Jewell should
have been sent to the Philadelphia papers, so many of which have
identified him with this war upon the "women-doctors," that our
jocose allusion to him was called for. And as to Dr. Griscom, he had
better leave him to our own picking, now that his supply of " Gas for
the Hydro-oxygen Blowpipe" of Dr. Butler has been exhausted, and
" Gotham" is no more.

The editors of the *Reporter* may spare their counsels to us as to
making our Journal "*pay!*" for this has never been a consideration
with us in its publication. When they recover their temper and manners, we may possibly hint to them why it is that their Journal *does
not pay*, as this seems to be paramount with them. The GAZETTE has
no controversy with the *Reporter*, and does not mean to have any, not
regarding it in any sense as a rival, but would say, with Uncle Toby
to the fly, " Go thy way, there is room enough in the world for us
both."

HEROD OUT-HERODED!

The Homœopaths are themselves all quacks, and yet they are out-quacked by the celebrated Dr. Humphreys, formerly one of the officials at the Auburn State Prison. His advertisements in the *Times, Tribune, Herald,* &c., rival those of Hunter, of inhalation memory, whose epitaph we wrote in the GAZETTE long since; and none so poor now as to do Hunter reverence, seeing that he, his journal, and inhalation itself, are defunct—the last of the Consumption-curers!

But this Humphreys, with his column and page advertisements, has now possession of the secular and·*religious* press, even the *Christian Advocate and Journal* having been bought over to this stupendous quackery of quackdom. A "leetle box" may be had for $2, with all the curables for incurable diseases, so that every fool may become his own doctor! and Homœopathy at that.

It is in vain that the sect denounce Humphreys, *Palmer & Co.,* the peddlers of these boxes of their potenzes and specifics, as quacks, for everybody knows that they are themselves quacks, and have no right to condemn their kindred. Indeed, we think Humphreys & Co. are decidedly ahead in the race, and we like their *combinations* of drugs and specifics, and the cheapness at which they sell the "*leetle boxes;*" especially as we find so many of the reverend clergy, who are *of course* authority in these matters, certifying to the virtues of the infinitesimal fraction of nothing. So long as Humphreys & Co. can *pay* for their advertisements, the humbug will flourish.

We cannot marvel that certain fanatics are thus gulled, for it is said by Humphreys, Palmer & Co. that the little pellets are all prepared with *prayers,* and hence all who have faith in the grace of God should confide in the specifics. Thus Hahnemann himself proclaimed long ago that "sugar of milk was the greatest blessing ever bestowed by Divine Providence upon the afflicted of mankind." *Vive la bagatelle!*

SURGERY BY PROFESSOR CARNOCHAN.

New York seems to maintain her position for important and capital operations. Among those recently performed in this city, we may mention the following which have occurred in the practice of Professor Carnochan: ligature of the common femoral for secondary hæmorrhage, on the fourteenth day after amputation, through the middle of the thigh; excision of the upper fifth of the humerus for caries of the bone; restoration of the entire upper lip, after its removal for cancer;

45

ligature of both the common carotids in the same person, allowing an interval of four months between the operations, for elephantiasis of the head and face; the ligature of the external carotid, for aneurism, by anastomosis of the upper jaw; and two cases of exsection of the second branch of the fifth pair of nerves, beyond the ganglion of Meckel, for protracted and severe neuralgia of the face. The operations have all been successful, and promise to be followed by permanent cures.

NEW YORK MEDICAL COLLEGE.

The retirement of Drs. Barker and Childs from the Faculty of this school has necessitated a partial reorganization, as set forth in the announcement on another page. It will be seen that Drs. Green, Davis, Doremus, Carnochan, and Cox, retain their respective chairs; Dr. Peaslee is transferred to the Chair of Obstetrics, &c., Dr. A. Flint, Jr., taking his place as Professor of Physiology, and Dr. James Bryan becoming the Professor of Anatomy; Dr. C. T. Meier holds the Chair of Surgical Anatomy and General Pathology; while J. Sedgwick, Esq., becomes Lecturer on Medical Jurisprudence. The friends of the College everywhere will regard the changes as favorable to the still greater prosperity of the school, and a larger class than usual may be confidently predicted.

UNIVERSITY OF NASHVILLE, TENN.

The catalogue of the literary and medical departments of this institution has just been published for 1859, and shows a state of unparalleled prosperity under the respective Faculties, especially in the medical school, which, though only eight years old, now ranks second in the country in the number of its matriculants.

PENNSYLVANIA MEDICAL COLLEGE.

The announcement in another column of the prompt reorganization of this school, is the enterprise of the late Faculty of the Philadelphia School of Medicine, who have already taken possession of the building and appurtenances of the old Pennsylvania College, and transferred their labors thither for its permanent re-establishment. We are persuaded that this third school in Philadelphia is needed by the brethren there, and will be sustained by a large class of students, who are learning by experience the disadvantages of attending lectures in a crowd. The present Faculty are able and practical teachers, and, it will be seen, possess every facility for demonstrative and clinical teaching which can be offered by either of the overgrown schools of Philadelphia.

UNIVERSITY OF LOUISVILLE, KY.

The new organization of this Faculty we have already had occasion to notice, and now direct attention to the attractive announcement of the present Faculty, which must be regarded as an improvement, and which cannot fail to restore this great school to its former greatness, when it was the leading medical college of the West. Nashville must look out for its laurels.

THE LATEST HUMBUG.

The panic-makers in and out of the profession of our city are busy in clamoring about the fancied dangers to the public health, predicted from the deterioration of the Croton water, so much complained of in the city of New York. The dry weather has diminished the supply of the Croton River from the springs, and a marshy, swampy taste has been the result. Abundant rains are all that is needed, and meanwhile no evil to the public health is to be dreaded.

MR. DELAVAN,

The new City Inspector, is signalizing his reign by a declaration of war against the hog-styes, piggeries, bone-boiling establishments, and other noisome abuses, which have so long disgraced the upper parts of our city; the detail of his operations being duly chronicled by the public press, in contrast with the care-nothing, do-nothing system of his predecessors. No permanent improvement or radical reform in the sanitary condition of the city can be hoped for by these spasmodic demonstrations, so long as the public health is committed to the care of mere politicians, who are in blissful ignorance of the wants of the city, and without any capacity to apply suitable remedies. Prevention is better than cure.

ATLANTA MEDICAL COLLEGE.

The present class of this school numbers 166! which is beyond all precedent, and authorizes the inference that *summer* schools are needed. If in the South, why not in the North?

INEBRIATE ASYLUMS.

We are glad to learn that the encouraging prospects of Dr. Turner and his numerous friends in the projected hospital for drunkards at Binghamton, in our own State, has prompted similar efforts in several of our sister States, and that our profession is everywhere taking the lead in this good work, as it ought to do.

Our old friend, Professor Dunbar, of Baltimore, is at the head of a movement in that city, designed to be the initiative of an Inebriate Asylum for Maryland, and will be grateful for documentary or other assistance from any quarter. The need of such a remedial measure is becoming so apparent of late, that multitudes who have heretofore withheld any response to the appeals put forth in this behalf by the public press, begin to awaken to its importance and necessity.

Intemperance, it is now more than ever obvious, is the prolific parent of a multitude of the deeds of darkness and blood which are cursing our cities everywhere; it is the giant iniquity of our country and age, imperatively demanding the combined wisdom and power of the pulpit and the press for its suppression; nor can any Christian or philanthropist fail to sympathize with a movement which seeks the rescue of its victims, before it is too late. All that has been done in this behalf heretofore is in danger of being lost, unless some new and more efficient agencies are enlisted; for, with our amazing increase of population, there is a corresponding increase of the means, facilities, and opportunities for the manufacture, sale, and use of intoxicating drinks, whereby the physical, social, and moral mischiefs of intemperance are multiplying on every hand, and the victims are augmenting.

What, then, is to be done ? If by no legislative wisdom or device this pestilence can be stayed; if all our cities must continue to be cursed with licensed or unlicensed snares by the thousand, until "Young America" is in danger of being drowned in a deluge of intemperance; and if our political rulers love to have it so; then, in the name of God and humanity we ask, who shall object to the opening of asylums for the victims of this horrid traffic, so that they, or their friends in their behalf, may have a door open for their escape, without awaiting the ordinary results in the lunatic asylum, the prison, the gallows of the murderer, or the grave of the suicide ?

There are hundreds, if not thousands of our young men in the Atlantic cities, who are annually thus victimized, for whom an Inebriate Asylum would prove a city of refuge, if they could be even temporarily committed, for medical and moral restraint and treatment, before their habits of intoxication have wholly put out their eyes, utterly stopped their ears, totally benumbed their moral sense, hopelessly hardened their hearts, and prepared them for any and every crime. Multitudes are annually perishing for lack of some provision of this kind, literally dying the death of fools and having the burial of asses, who might be restored to their families and in their right minds, if they were timely sent to inebriate asylums, until the delirium of their intemperance might be removed, and the dominion of reason recovered.

> "Man's inhumanity to man
> Makes countless thousands mourn!"

And if an irresistible appeal to humanity is ever made, it is in behalf of those who, having fallen by intemperance, discover their error when too late for self-rescue, and cry imploringly for help to their fellow-men, who have been fortunate enough to escape the demon.

☞ THE PRESENT NO. OF THE GAZETTE ☜

Will be found to exceed any former issue in the number and value of original communications, of which there are *seven*, two of which are illustrated by engravings, and one of which is a translation of signal worth from the German. Our subscribers will thus see an indication of the improvements we have projected, and which are in progress to render this Journal still more worthy of their support.

Those who are still delinquent on our books for 1859 will, we hope, be now stirred up to promptly remitting their dues, unless they are willing to relinquish our monthly visits.

EXCHANGES.

We find ourselves under the necessity of curtailing our list of exchanges, to preserve our files; and this, after again enlarging our edition; nor can we supply back numbers, as all are needed for the integrity of a few volumes which must be preserved. Those, therefore, who have failed to receive our successive numbers, will understand the reason, as the demand upon us forbids the continuance of exchanges to the same extent as heretofore, until our edition is still further enlarged, as we propose at the end of the year.

MEDICAL COLLEGES.

The announcement of *nine* of these will be found in this number, and all are schools of established reputation and regular standing.

MISCELLANEOUS ITEMS.

The New York Journal of Medicine.—The July number is an improvement on any of its predecessors in all respects, as we think, and for which much credit is due to Baillière Brothers, of 440 Broadway, into whose hands it has passed, and by whom it is to be henceforth conducted. It is the only medical journal in the country published anonymously, the name of the editors being withheld from the title-page for some reason; although Dr. Stephen Smith is still understood to retain his connection with it, as one of its editors. Dr. Bumstead is a very large contributor to this number. Somebody ought to be responsible for the review department.

Dr. John Bell, of Philadelphia, has been appointed Physician to the City Hospital.

Dr. S. D. Gross has been elected one of the surgeons to the Howard Hospital of Philadelphia.

Dr. Curry has retired from the Shelby Medical College, and from the *Nashville Medical Record.* Dr. H. Erni takes his place in the former, and Drs. Callender and Maddin succeed him in the latter position, they both becoming associated with Dr. Wright. Professor Ford, of the Shelby College, has sailed for Europe.

A new Medical College is announced at St. Joseph, Missouri, where a medical journal has preceded it.

Ranking's Half-yearly Abstract has just reached us from the press of Lindsay & Blakiston, Philadelphia.

British and Foreign Medico-Chirurgical Review, for July, 1859, is out in good season, republished by S. S. & W. Wood, New York.

Dr. David Sands, a graduate of the N. Y. College of Physicians and Surgeons, recently died in this city, of albuminuria. He was a pious and estimable man in all the relations of life.

The National Medical College at Washington, D. C., has been reorganized. All are new professors, except Dr. Miller, who holds only an Emeritus relation, and Dr. Holston. The Faculty has been filled, however, with able men, some of whom have already made their mark. See the announcement on another page.

RECEIPTS FOR 1859.—Continued.

Drs. Dewees, Johnson, Strew, Powell, Caccarini, Selden, W. Stone, Tilden, P. F. Eve, L. A. Smith, Moseley, H. Lindsley, E. Hartshorne, J. A. Allen.

CONTENTS.

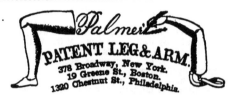

UNIVERSITY OF NEW YORK.
MEDICAL DEPARTMENT.
SESSION, 1859-60.

The Session for 1859–60 will begin on Monday, October 17, and will be continued until the 1st of March.

Faculty of Medicine.

REV. ISAAC FERRIS, D.D., LL.D., Chancellor of the University.

VALENTINE MOTT, M.D., LL.D., Emeritus Professor of Surgery and Surgical Anatomy, and ex-President of the Faculty.

MARTYN PAINE, M.D., LL.D., Professor of Materia Medica and Therapeutics.

GUNNING S. BEDFORD, M.D., Professor of Obstetrics, the Diseases of Women and Children, and Clinical Midwifery.

JOHN W. DRAPER, M.D., LL.D., Professor of Chemistry and Physiology, President of the Faculty.

ALFRED C. POST, M.D., Professor of the Principles and Operations of Surgery, with Surgical and Pathological Anatomy.

WILLIAM H. VAN BUREN, M.D., Professor of General and Descriptive Anatomy.

JOHN T. METCALFE, M.D., Professor of the Institutes and Practice of Medicine.

J. W. S. GOULEY, M.D., Demonstrator of Anatomy.

J. H. HINTON, M.D., Prosector to the Professor of Surgery.

ALEXANDER B. MOTT, M.D., Prosector to the Emeritus Professor of Surgery.

Besides Daily Lectures on the foregoing subjects, there will be five Cliniques weekly, on *Medicine, Surgery, and Obstetrics.*

The Dissecting-room, which is refitted and abundantly lighted with gas, is open from 8 o'clock, A. M., till 10 o'clock, P. M.

Fees for a full course of Lectures, $105. Matriculation fee, $5. Graduation fee, $30. Demonstrator's fee, $5.

NATIONAL MEDICAL COLLEGE,
WASHINGTON, D. C.
(MEDICAL DEPARTMENT OF COLUMBIAN COLLEGE.)

The **Thirty-Eighth Annual Session** will commence on Monday, the 17th of October, and continue until the 1st of March.

FACULTY:

THOMAS MILLER, M.D., Emeritus, Professor of Anatomy and Physiology, and Con. Surgeon.

JAMES J. WARING, M.D., Professor of Obstetrics and Diseases of Women and Children.

JOHN G. F. HOLSTON, M.D., Professor of the Principles and Practice of Surgery.

HENRY WURZ, M.A., Professor of Chemistry and Pharmacy.

JOHN C. RILEY, M.D., Professor of Materia Medica, Therapeutics, and Hygiene.

NATHAN SMITH LINCOLN, M.D., Professor of the Theory and Practice of Medicine.

B. JOHNSON HELLEN, M.D., Professor of Anatomy and Physiology.

WM. E. WATERS, M.D., Demonstrator of Anatomy.

Clinical Lectures will be given regularly during the session by the Professors, (free to all students of medicine,) at the Washington Infirmary.

FEES.

Matriculation, (paid once only,)................................$ 5
For a full course, (single tickets $15,)........................90
Demonstrator's ticket..10
Graduation fee 25

JNO. C. RILEY, M.D., Dean,
453 Fourteenth Street.

ALBANY MEDICAL COLLEGE.

One Course of Lectures will be given at this Institution annually, commencing the *first* Tuesday of *September*, and continuing sixteen weeks. Degrees will be conferred at the close of the term, and also after the Summer Examination in June.

PROFESSORS:

ALDEN MARCH, M.D., Professor of Principles and Practice of Surgery.
JAMES McNAUGHTON, M.D., Prof. of the Theory and Practice of Medicine.
JAMES H. ARMSBY, M.D., Professor of Descriptive and Surgical Anatomy.
HOWARD TOWNSEND, M.D., Prof. of Materia Medica and Physiology.

CHARLES H. PORTER, M.D., Prof. of Chemistry and Pharmacy.
J. V. P. QUACKENBUSH, M.D.,Prof. of Obstetrics and Diseases of Women and Children, and Medical Jurisprudence.
AMOS DEAN, Esq., Prof. of Medical Jurisprudence.

Fees for the full course, $65. Matriculation fee, $5. Graduation fee, $20.

Material for dissection abundant, and furnished to students on the same terms as in New York and Philadelphia. Hospital Tickets free. Opportunities for Clinical instruction are believed to be equal to those afforded by any College in the country. Price of Board from $2,50 to $3,50 per week.

JOHN V. P. QUACKENBUSH, Registrar.

UNIVERSITY OF NASHVILLE.

Medical Department.—Session 1859-60.—The Seventh Annual Course of Lectures in this Institution will commence on Monday, the 2d of November next, and continue till the first of the ensuing March.

THOMAS R. JENNINGS, M. D., Professor of Anatomy.
J. BERRIEN LINDSLEY, M. D., Chemistry and Pharmacy.
C. K. WINSTON, M. D., Materia Medica and Medical Jurisprudence.
A. H. BUCHANAN, M. D., Surgical Anatomy and Physiology.

JOHN M. WATSON, M. D., Obstetrics and the Diseases of Women and Children.
PAUL F. EVE, M.D., Prof. of Prin. and Prac. of Surgery.
W. K. BOWLING, M. D., Institutes and Practice of Medicine.
WILLIAM T. BRIGGS, M. D., Adjunct Professor and Demonstrator of Anatomy.

The Anatomical rooms will be opened for students on the first Monday of October, (the 5th.)
A *Preliminary Course* of Lectures, free to all Students, will be given by the Professors, commencing also on the first Monday of October.
The Tennessee State Hospital, under the direction of the Faculty, is open to the Class free of charge.
A Clinique has been established, in connection with the University, at which operations are performed and cases prescribed for and lectured upon in the presence of the class.
Amount of Fees for Lectures is $105; Matriculation Fee, (paid once only,) $5; Practical Anatomy, $10; Graduation fee, $25.
Good boarding can be procured for $3 to $4 per week. For further information or Catalogue, apply to

W. K. BOWLING, M.D.,

NASHVILLE, TENN., July, 1859.   *Dean of the Faculty.*

CASTLETON MEDICAL COLLEGE.

There are two full Courses of Lectures annually in Castleton Medical College. The SPRING SESSION commencing on the last Thursday in February; the AUTUMNAL SESSION on the first Thursday in August. Each Course will continue four months. Degrees are conferred at the close of each term.

WM. P. SEYMOUR, M.D.,Prof of Materia Medica and Therapeutics.
WILLIAM SWEETSER, M. D., Prof. of Theory and Practice of Medicine.
E. R. SANBORN, M. D., Prof. of Surgery.
WM. C. KITTRIDGE, A. M., Prof. of Med. Jurisp.

CORYDON LA FORD, M. D., Prof. of Anatomy.
P. D. BRADFORD,M.D.,Prof. of Phys. & Pathol
GEORGE HADLEY, M. D., Prof. of Chemistry and Natural History.
ADRIAN T. WOODWARD, M. D., Prof. of Obstetrics.

FEES.—For Lectures, $50; for those who have attended two Courses at other Colleges, $10 Matriculation, $5; Graduation, $16; Board from $2.00 to $2.50 per week.

A. T. WOODWARD, M.D., Registrar.

CASTLETON, VT., Jan., 1859.

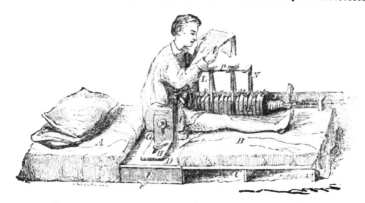

TO PHYSICIANS.

WINCHESTER'S GENUINE PREPARATIONS
OF THE
PURE HYPOPHOSPHITES.

The UNDERSIGNED, having made arrangements for the importation of PHOSPHORUS, directly from the English and French *manufacturers*; and having also completed arrangements for manufacturing the HYPOPHOSPHITES upon a more extended scale than any other Chemist in the United States, offers his preparations to Physicians and the Trade at lower prices than any other manufacturer in the United States.

My preparations now embrace every base suggested by Dr. Churchill, (Lime, Soda, Potassa, Ammonia, Manganese, Iron, and Quinia,) and may be obtained either in the *Crystalline* form or in *Solution*. There can be no doubt that the SOLUTION is the preferable form for exhibiting the Hypophosphites, whether combined, as in my popular "*Preparation of Lime and Soda,*" or separately. I offer to the profession every facility for trying Dr. Churchill's treatment, and guarantee the chemical purity of my preparations.

Experience has instructed the more advanced of the Profession that the chemical changes effected in the Crystalline Salts by exposure, (on account of their eager affinity for oxygen,) impair or destroy their therapeutical efficiency, and that, therefore, these must be *discarded from general practice*, before the world can realize the beneficent revolution to be wrought in medical science by Dr. Churchill's discovery.

As there is much misconception as to all that is *peculiar* to Dr. Churchill's Theory, I beg to set forth a more exact statement than has heretofore been made regarding it, and for this purpose the following extracts from his Treatise are submitted:

EXTRACTS FROM DR. CHURCHILL'S TREATISE:

Page 12, *et sequitur:*—"Occupied, as I have been, since the commencement of my medical career, in researches upon the treatment of *phthisis*, my investigations led me to believe that the tubercular diathesis depended wholly upon some disturbance of the primordial functions of life; that, considering the intimate union which exists between all parts of the body, this disturbance must have, as a proximate cause, some important modification in the *process of sanguification*. The works of various pathologists, especially those of MM. Andral and Gavarret, the correctness of which has since been confirmed by others, indicated *that the variations in the composition of the blood*, in pulmonary *phthisis, had no peculiar and important relation*, as far as its ORGANIC ELEMENTS were concerned. I was, consequently, induced to believe that it was among the INORGANIC ELEMENTS of this fluid that we should look for the *special cause* of this diathesis.

"As the phenomena of this disease, approximating to those of many other morbid states of the body, and especially to chlorosis, appeared to me to be attributable to the loss, or diminution, rather than to the augmentation of some essential constituent, I decided to commence my experiments by increasing, if possible, the quantity of this element; I decided to commence my investigations by the use of phosphorus.

"Admitting that the phosphorized element of the blood, or of organic matter, exists in the body in some other form than that of phosphoric acid, it was evident to me that it performed the double part of an *eminently combustible substance*, and at the same time entered into molecular combination with the other elements of the body, in such a way as to become an integral portion of it. * * * * * * * I think I am justified in drawing the following conclusions, upon which the Academy is requested to pass its judgment:

"THE IMMEDIATE CAUSE, OR AT LEAST ONE ESSENTIAL CONDITION OF THE TUBERCULAR DIATHESIS, IS THE DIMINUTION IN THE SYSTEM OF PHOSPHORUS, WHICH IS FOUND IN IT IN A FORM CAPABLE OF OXYDATION.

"THE SPECIFIC REMEDY FOR THIS DISEASE CONSISTS OF A PREPARATION OF PHOSPHORUS, WHICH PRESENTS THE DOUBLE CHARACTERISTIC OF BEING IMMEDIATELY ABSORBED OR ASSIMILATED, AND WHICH AT THE SAME TIME IS AT THE LOWEST POSSIBLE DEGREE OF OXYDATION."

EXTRACTS FROM DR. CHURCHILL'S LETTERS:

"What I am anxious for is, that the Hypophosphites should be brought, *as speedily as possible*, INTO UNIVERSAL USE, AS I KNOW THAT THEY WILL PROVE NOT ONLY AS SURE A REMEDY IN CONSUMPTION AS QUININE IS IN INTERMITTENT FEVER, BUT ALSO AS EFFECTUAL A PRESERVATIVE AS VACCINATION IN SMALL-POX.

"This assertion no longer rests upon the thirty-four cases with which my discovery was ushered into the world in July, 1857. I can now appeal to the results in upward of one hundred and fifty detailed observations of the disease, collected during the past year at my Public Dispensary, Rue Larrey, Paris.

"To these cases might be added almost an equal number from my private practice. Similar results have, since the publication of my discovery, been announced by Professors Pari-got, of Brussels, and Maestre de San Juan, of Granada, in Spain; as also by Drs. Jacinto Le Riverend and Galvez, of Havana, and Reinvilliers, of Paris.

"If, as I assert, the Hypophosphites be the SPECIFIC REMEDY of PHTHISIS, because at least one of the essential conditions of that disease consists in the *want or undue waste of the oxydizable phosphorus in the animal economy*, it follows that CONSUMPTION WILL BE PREVENTED simply by taking care to keep the system supplied with a due amount of that element. Now, if there existed any certain signs or symptoms by which we might recognize either that Phthisis is impending, or that the phosphorized element is deficient, the prevention of the disease might be effected with *perfect certainty.*"

☞ Prices will be made known by "Trade Circular" to all who address the undersigned, at the sole General Depot for the sale of the pure HYPOPHOSPHITES, manufactured strictly in accordance with Dr. Churchill's method.

J. WINCHESTER, 43 John , N. Y.

AMERICAN
MEDICAL GAZETTE.

Vol. X. **OCTOBER, 1859.** **No. 10.**

ORIGINAL DEPARTMENT.

PROF. OPPOLZER ON ACUTE ATROPHY OF THE LIVER.

Translated from the Report of John Schnitzler, by ALFRED WEILLER.

Acute atrophy of the liver is one of the rarest and most obscure diseases known. The views of the two greatest authorities on pathological anatomy are entirely opposed to each other. Whilst Rokitansky holds that acute atrophy is a peculiar species of disease, with perfect annihilation of the hepatic cells, caused by the blood of the portal vein being overcharged with elements of bile—Virchow contends that the disappearance of the hepatic cells is merely *post-mortem*, and rather a consequence of speedy decomposition; allowing, however, that some diseases are more prone than others to cause this decomposition.

Although the majority of pathologists and clinical writers incline to the theory of Rokitansky, there is little unity of opinion among them as to the causes of this disease.

Henoch supposes that it is owing to an excessive secretion of bile, whereby the biliary ducts are distended, and the latter, pressing upon the blood-vessels, cause a derangement in the nutrition of the hepatic cells, which consequently undergo fatty degeneration.

This view is refuted by both clinical and post-mortem observations. For neither before nor after the atrophy do we find appearances of polycholia; and the idea that the biliary ducts are overcharged, is just as little confirmed by the subject.

According to V. Dusch, the destruction of the hepatic cells depends entirely on the retention of bile, the latter dissolving the former. Prof.

46

Oppolzer has, as yet, not observed this retention; nor does he believe that bile dissolves the hepatic cells. He has instituted several experiments in reference to this subject; and once he placed a piece of liver in bile, taken from a man who had died from acute atrophy, and in this, as in all other experiments, no change could be discovered in the hepatic cells, even after the liver had remained in the bile for a number of days. And this last experiment silences the objection that might be raised, that morbid bile is more destructive than the healthy.

Henle's opinion is not less untenable. He believes that the disappearance of the cells arises from the obstruction of the portal vein; but Prof. Oppolzer has never yet found this, although he has often observed obstruction of the vein where no atrophy existed.

Lebert looks upon the disease as a mere typhoid process. Prof. O. does not concur with this opinion, although he has himself seen a case of exanthematous typhus, with perfect destruction of the hepatic cells; yet, in general, the whole course of the disease, the absence of exanthem, and of all change in the alimentary canal, discountenance this idea.

Prof. Oppolzer is of the opinion that acute atrophy of the liver is merely the termination of a disease, and is most probably an inflammation. That atrophy is merely the termination of a morbid process, is shown by the icterus existing a number of days, sometimes weeks, before the appearance of the more violent symptoms; and the anatomical condition proves it to be an inflammatory process, because the destruction of the cells through fatty degeneration is easily explained, as owing to a previous inflammation, as it is well known that inflammation of the parenchyma often leads to fatty degeneration, and eventually to disintegration. (Virchow's examinations.)

This view, which has been confirmed by the latest experiments of Frerichs, who also proved that, in acute atrophy, exudations form around the hepatic cells, has been accepted by Prof. Skoda.

As we have now explained the character of the disease, we will refer to one particular case.

Anna S., 38 years of age, was, according to her own statement, always healthy, but had suffered some twelve years ago from a slight icterus, which she attributed to her diet. About the middle of May, a. c., she was again troubled with the same, without, however, being able to trace it to any cause. It interfered very little with her general health, her appetite, with all other physical and mental functions, remaining perfectly undisturbed. She therefore stated, that she merely came to our clinic to consult us with reference to the discoloration of her skin. This was on the 17th of May.

We found the patient in a pretty good state of nutrition, the whole surface of the body, as well as the conjunctiva of the eye, somewhat jaundiced. The neck and thorax were well formed, and the physical examination of lungs and heart proved these organs to be in perfectly good condition.

On percussing in the line of the right axilla, we noticed dullness commencing from the lower margin of the seventh rib, and resonance from the lower margin of the eighth rib to the arch of the same in the mammillary and parasternal lines; the resonant sound began between the sixth and seventh ribs, extending to their arches; below this spot, the sound was clear, full, and tympanitic. In the sternal lines, the dullness began at the fifth rib, and extended $1\frac{1}{2}$ inch below the xyphoid process, and about the same distance towards the left side.

The spleen was located in the line of the axilla, between the ninth and eleventh ribs, and was of normal size. The abdomen was not distended, the pulse not accelerated, nor was the temperature increased. Besides the normal qualitative and quantitative elements of the urine, there was a little biliphecin.

It appeared, both from the course and general condition, that we had but a simple icterus to deal with, that was itself unaccompanied by any other symptoms. Almost three weeks elapsed before the slightest change took place in the condition of the patient, when, on the 4th of June, the disease presented quite a different phase.

On the evening of the said date the patient became dizzy and stupefied, and soon afterwards she fell into such a perfect sopor that the most vigorous shaking failed to arouse her.

On the following day we found the patient in the same condition; she lay in the deepest sopor, (coma;) pupils were dilated, light having no effect upon them. All attempts at arousing her proved unsuccessful; even when severely pressed in the region of the liver, she remained perfectly unconcerned. She had passed both urine and fæces involuntarily during the night. Abdomen was somewhat distended. Upon percussing the liver, dullness was found in the line of the axilla, about two plessimeters in extent; in the mammillary lines about one; and in the right parasternal not more than a finger's breadth. In the sternal and left parasternal no dullness was observed.

In this case we could fully prove, by means of percussion, a *sudden decrease* of the liver, although we cannot but ascribe to the meteorism a part of the tympanitic sound noticed in the hepatic region. The yellow discoloration seemed to have increased little, or not at all, since the previous day; the temperature of the skin was rather lessened than heightened; pulse was 64; respiration 20.

The urine taken by means of the catheter possessed very peculiar characteristics; its color was brown, (like beer,) was of ammoniacal odor, and alkaline reaction. Spec. grav., 1:015. Urophæin, uroxanthin, urea and uric acid, in normal quantities; chlorides, plentiful; sulphates lessened; phosphates almost entirely absent.

Abnormal elements were: biliphecin and uroretrin in small quantities; carbonate of ammonia, leucin, and tyrosin, rather abundant.

If we take the symptoms as they present themselves just now, we find: icterus, affection of the brain, sudden diminishment of the liver, and abnormal urine, entirely changed in its chemical composition.

Although these collective symptoms give us the unmistakable description of acute atrophy of the liver, Prof. Oppolzer spoke, as yet, of this diagnosis merely as *probable*, but he endeavored to establish it by excluding all contingent diseases that might lead to error.

1. Icterus is a constant and never-failing attendant, or rather a *precursor*, to acute atrophy; it generally exists in a moderate degree, and does not increase in intensity after the atrophy has commenced. The causes of this strange condition, this disproportion between disease and symptom, Prof. O. attributes to the destruction of the hepatic cells, whereby the formation of bile is stopped. In general, Prof. O. subscribes to the opinion that the bile can only be formed in the hepatic cells, and that the icterus is caused by the retarded discharge of bile and the absorption of the same; which opinion is confirmed by the experiments of the physiologists, Müller, Moleschott, and others. But Prof. Skoda holds to the idea that the bile—or at least certain elements thereof, particularly the pigment—is formed in the blood, and that the icterus is, in many cases, the result of deranged secretion; in others, however, (biliary calculi, cancer, polypus growths or severe catarrh of biliary ducts,) he can but attribute the icterus to the retarded discharge of bile, and consequent absorption.

2. The mental symptoms in this case manifested themselves by depression of the whole nervous system. As before stated, the patient lay in perfect coma, pupils dilated, pulse and respiration lessened in number. The questions, therefore, rise: (1.) Are these symptoms those of acute atrophy, or are they caused by some other disease? and (2.) If they are the symptoms of atrophy, how are they to be explain-

ed, and what has the depression of the action of the brain to do with disease of the liver?

The cases in which we meet with a similar comatose condition are:

a. Apoplexy. This we entirely exclude in this instance, on account of the age and constitution of our patient, and the absence of all muscular paralysis.

b. Convulsive and cataleptic diseases, which are commonly followed by sopor or coma. The history of the patient, and our own clinical observations, preclude this supposition.

c. Typhus as well as all other blood diseases are excluded, because of the absence of all symptoms of fever.

d. Poisoning by narcotics produce the very same symptoms observable in our patient, and the idea of poisoning in this case is not so remote as it might at first appear. For the patient occupies the same ward with about fifty others, each of whom receives different remedies; and it is easy enough, even where the greatest precaution is observed, to confound the medicines; nor is an error on the part of the apothecary out of the question. This morning we could not find the slightest trace of any medicine whatsoever on or near her bed, and consequently the best clue to the discovery of the poisoning is wanting.

Prof. Oppolzer excluded altogether, however, the following poisons:

Opium and its preparations, particularly morphine, usually give rise to sopor, to the same state that we see here, but then the pupils are contracted; and besides, the opiate can, by means of chloride of iron, be detected in the urine as meconic acid.

Belladonna and stramonium cause both sopor and dilatation of the pupils; the pulse is, however, accelerated, and their respective alkaloids (daturine and atropine) can be detected in the urine.

Digitalis causes irregular pulsations of heart and pulse.

Hyoscyamus rather gives rise to hallucinations and delirium than to sopor.

Cannabis indica effects contraction of the pupils, a jovial delirium, and ungovernable laughter.

Alcoholic drinks can easily be detected by the smell of the breath, and they generally cause vomiting, with deep, heavy breathing. The same can be said of chloroform.

The possibility of a poisoning having taken place can be seen by merely referring to these few illustrations, as the discrimination between their effects and the existing state of the patient rests but upon

very trifling points; and when we take into consideration the different
effects these remedies have upon different individuals, in different diseases, we must admit that we could not exclude this idea, had not the
analysis of the urine decided against it, in favor of acute atrophy of
the liver.

The second question, therefore, remains to be answered, viz.: What
has the affection of the brain to do with disease of the liver?

Henle considers it as a consequence of hyperæmia of the brain, but
the experience drawn from post-mortem examinations fails to corroborate this view.   Nor can it be caused by the blood being overcharged
with bile, for we often meet with cases of icterus that have existed for
years, without any sign of disease of the brain accompanying them.
The presence of leusin and tyrosin in the blood cannot be looked upon
as the cause, as neither of these are poisonous, and even when injected
into the blood of animals they do not act as a narcotic.   Prof.
Oppolzer is of the opinion that, as in uræmia, the carbonate of ammonia contained in the blood is the cause of the sopor; and the whole
course of this case, as has been before described, strengthens this view.

3. The third important symptom is the sudden decrease of the liver.
We have already given the different opinions that prevail as to the
cause of this diminution, and therefore there is nothing left to us but
to repeat, that the diagnosis of acute atrophy of the liver should
always be made with the greatest caution, as it is difficult to prevent
error in defining the size of the liver.   Thus, a liver may be *naturally
small*, or it may be pressed or covered with gas-filled intestines.   We
can therefore only be certain of its being acute atrophy, *when the liver
diminishes as it were under our eyes*, and thereby the possibility of error
excluded; and this was the reason why Prof. O., despite so many concurring symptoms, merely spoke at first of the *possibility* of such a
diagnosis.

4. The urine.   This contained, as already stated, the following
abnormal elements: Biliphecin, uroretrin, carbonate of ammonia, leucin,
and tyrosin.

The biliphecin was, in this case, of no more than ordinary consequence, as it is to be found, with few exceptions, in the urine of every
jaundiced patient, and merely proves the existence of biliary pigment
in the blood.

The uroretrin is only met with in disease, and, according to Prof.
Oppolzer, mostly in exudative processes; and this opinion has been
confirmed by every case which we have seen this year.

Carbonate of ammonia is found in typhus, but generally not before the later stages. It is always present in uræmia, diseases of the bladder, and sometimes in the convalescent stage of exudative diseases.

Leucin and tyrosin—crystallized remnants of albuminous bodies—were first discovered by Frerichs in the urine of patients suffering from typhus; yet it seems that these two substances are not always present in this disease, as in the typhus-epidemic of this year, we have not once observed it in the urine; whilst in the previous year, we have repeatedly seen it at our clinic. Leucin and tyrosin are also often found in different infectious diseases, and also in acute atrophy, as has been seen in this case. As the urine was taken by means of the catheter, and immediately afterwards examined, we cannot look upon the carbonate of ammonia, nor the leucin and tyrosin, as products of decomposition.

Those symptoms which generally accompany acute atrophy—such as great pain in the hepatic region, manifesting itself on pressure even in sopor, by groaning of the patient and by the working of the fascial muscles; fever, often accompanied by chills and vomiting of bile and blood—were not noticed in this case.

According to Budd's treatment, we ordered the patient drastic purgatives, consisting of calomel and jalap, and directed the whole body to be washed in vinegar.

The next day, (June 6th,) the patient was in quite a different condition; her consciousness had returned the previous evening, but she was still very apathic, and some of her answers were not quite correct. The temperature of her skin was not heightened; pulse was 72; respiration 24. The liver was not painful, even on severe pressure; and as the abdomen was not distended, we were enabled to give it a careful examination.

On percussion, we noticed a resonant tone in the line of the axilla, commencing from the seventh rib, and in the mammillary and parasternal lines from the sixth to the arch below this; and in the sternal lines, downward and left to the xyphoid process, the tone was clear, full, and tympanitic. Thus, each place where two days previously dullness was found on percussion, we had now a full, clear tone, whereby the diagnosis of acute atrophy of the left lobe of the liver was established beyond doubt.

The urine was of alkaline reaction; spec. grav. 1.021. Chlorides were abundant; phosphates and sulphates scarce, although more than on the previous day. Abnormal elements were biliphecin and uroretrin in small quantities; no leucin and tyrosin, nor was there the slightest trace of albumen. The drastic ordered the previous day was suspended, and the patient received a mild cathartic and a cooling drink; and as her digestion had not been in the least interfered with, due consideration was paid to her appetite, which had been from the commencement in an excellent state.

From the 7th to the 10th, the patient felt tolerably well, although she was still somewhat feeble and apathic. The jaundice disappeared gradually. The urine was, during this time, very changeable. The spec. grav. fluctuated between 1.020 and 1.025. On the 7th the reaction was neutral, or rather somewhat alkaline, and somewhat sour at the same time; on the 8th and 9th, rather more sour; on the 10th, more alkaline. Phosphates and sulphates were augmented; biliphecin and uroretrin still in small quantities; and since the 8th, a small quantity of albumen, but no leucin and tyrosin.

On the afternoon of the 10th, the patient became suddenly deliri-ous; her sight failed, and at last perfect amaurosis set in, which, how-ever, disappeared after the lapse of two or three hours; whereupon the patient relapsed into a state of sopor, from which she awoke the next morning, having had, however, during the night, involuntary evacua-tions of both urine and fæces.

On the morning of the 11th we found the patient rather weak; her sight was feeble, and her speech confused; we also noticed a slight tremor of the left hand; the abdomen was very much distended; pulse 72; temperature of the skin not increased. The same drastic purgatives (calomel and jalap) were again administered.

On the afternoon of the same day amblyopia again set in, (it did not get as far as amaurosis,) which disappeared in about two hours, when she again relapsed into a soporific condition, in which she re-mained till the following morning. During the night she passed both urine and fæces involuntarily.

On the morning of the 12th we found the patient very low; the expression of her face apathic; sight feeble; stammering in her speech; tremor in her left hand more marked than on the preceding day, but not the slightest fever. Abdomen was not distended, liver not pain-ful, and on percussion, the atrophy (this time, also, of the right lobe,) could be established with certainty, as the liver did not anywhere reach the arch of the ribs. The urine taken by means of the cathe-ter was of alkaline reaction, contained leucin and tyrosin, but no albumen, uroretrin, nor biliphecin. The medicine of the foregoing day was repeated.

On the 13th the patient felt much better; her sight was less feeble, her answers were clearer, the tremor in the hand had ceased, the icterus was very slight, the urine reacted somewhat sour, and there was nothing abnormal in its contents. The medicine was therefore again suspended.

On the 15th there was scarcely a trace of the icterus left, and the patient felt perfectly well, with the exception of being a little weak. The urine was of sour reaction, sp. gr. 1.024, and contained the qualitative and quantitative normal elements.

From this day the patient rapidly convalesced; and as, on the 20th, the last trace of icterus had disappeared, she was pronounced perfectly restored. (Whereby we refer, of course, to her general condition, not that her liver had resumed its normal shape, by the formation of new cells.)

Prof. Oppolzer concludes his clinical remarks with the following observations:

As soon as the nervous symptoms have appeared, the course of the disease is very rapid, so that very often no more than two or three days elapse between this period and death; sometimes it takes only as many hours. But we should not look upon the disease as acute atrophy merely on the appearance of the nervous symptoms; but rather the general precursors, such as icterus, derangement of digestion, and fever, should be looked upon as the first stage of the disease.

The prognosis was at first very doubtful, nay, even fatal. Prof. O. had as yet not seen one case of recovery from acute atrophy; and in those cases published by Budd, Graves, and Griffin, the diagnosis is doubtful, as the weightiest symptom of all, viz., diminution of the liver, is not mentioned. They were most probably merely severe forms of icterus typhosus, without destruction of the hepatic cells. Prof. O. has himself seen a case of this description, where recovery ensued upon the use of chinin. Consequently, the case just related · is *the first* in which the atrophy has been established through physical examination; and thus, with the aid of art, the further progress of the disease can be stopped, and recovery brought about.

Knowing so little as we do of the nature of this disease, there can be no idea of specific therapeutics. We have, consequently, only a symptomatic treatment, which can be summed up as follows:

The pain in the region of the liver is best relieved by means of narcotics, as long as there is no delirium; should there be hyperæmia of the liver, leeches should be applied; but as soon as the diminution of the liver commences, all bleeding should be avoided. As regards the vomiting, ice, pulv. æroph., aqua laura, cerasi, magisterum bismuthi, and sometimes mustard applications to the stomach, will be found of service. Hæmorrhage from the stomach and intestines should be treated with tannin, alumen, or acetas plumbi, and with ice applications to the stomach.

Should the nervous symptoms appear with or without fever, (as in our case,) drastic purgatives should be given. Are symptoms of febrile excitement present, cold applications to the head, washes, and particularly an opiate, would be serviceable. If the patient is, however, depressed, cold vinegar washes and bathing the head (even internal administration of vinegar) would not be out of place; ether, musk, and other excitants, are also sometimes appropriate.

A New Method of Operating for Varicose Veins.

By E. S. Cooper, Prof. of Anatomy and Surgery in the Medical Department of the University of the Pacific, San Francisco.

From time immemorial wounds of veins have been regarded by the medical profession as a dangerous class of injuries, and until within the past twenty years operations for the cure of varicose veins of the leg were regarded as unjustifiably hazardous by nearly all of the ablest surgeons. Since that period it has been different, and operations upon the vena saphena major and minor have been comparatively frequent, and much of the dread which was entertained in regard to interference with these veins in a varicose state has been removed by the favorable results of the same. But there are still many of our most skillful surgeons who condemn the practice, as too dangerous. And why is this? Is it because they have found anything peculiar in the formation of the veins showing a predisposition to inflammation when injured, or is it because they have found by experience that wounds of veins are disposed to dangerous inflammation, the burrowing of matter into the adjacent parts, pyæmia, &c.? Every one will answer at once that it is the latter, because there is nothing peculiar in the conformation of the veins tending to inflammation.

Why does experience teach that wounds of veins are dangerous?

Because veins are the channels through which undecarbonized blood is conveyed to the heart from remote parts of the body, and a considerable injury to a vein will necessarily cause a stoppage of the blood at that point, and which, collecting day after day, becomes a foreign substance, and source of great irritation. I am fully convinced by experiments upon dogs that a vein can be ligated with as little danger as an artery, when the artery which supplies the veins with blood is also ligated.

Statistics of results of operations for varicose veins show that, in a majority of instances in which fatal results have occurred, there was an extensive burrowing of matter in the immediate region of the operation, even when the patient ultimately died of pyæmia. Any method, therefore, which tends to lessen these dangers in operations upon varicose veins of the leg must be a desideratum. The following is my method:

An incision is made into the vein one and a half inch long, and a small pledget of lint is placed into it. I carry the incision through the walls of the vein into the cellular tissue beneath, and am careful to introduce the pledget of lint into the bottom of the incision. This operation may be repeated at several points along the vein, if thought necessary. The object of using the lint in this way is to make the entire wound become a granulating and secreting surface, by which the accumulation of fluids at the place where the blood is arrested in the vein will be constantly carried off. The accumulation of blood does not cause any irritation for the first four or five days, and at the end of this time the lint should be removed, and a poultice applied. During the time the lint is retained a roller wetted with an evaporating substance is kept tightly applied.

The two methods which have received great favor among medical men are those of Sir Benj. Brodie and M. Velpeau. In the first method, the vessels are simply divided; in the plan practiced by Velpeau, ligatures are placed upon the veins at different points. Both of these methods sometimes cause death, though frequently the patient recovers in a few days, without an inflammatory symptom occurring. But when death does occur, it is always after a high grade of local inflammation has existed for some time, produced by the accumulation of venous blood in the region of the operation.

In the method I practice there is made a secreting surface sufficiently large to carry off the fluids which are disposed to accumulate at the point of operation. There is no bleeding of consequence attending this

ALBANY MEDICAL COLLEGE.

One Course of Lectures will be given at this Institution annually, commencing the *first* Tuesday of *September*, and continuing sixteen weeks. Degrees will be conferred at the close of the term, and also after the Summer Examination in June.

PROFESSORS:

ALDEN MARCH, M.D., Professor of Principles and Practice of Surgery.

JAMES McNAUGHTON, M.D., Prof. of the Theory and Practice of Medicine.

JAMES H. ARMSBY, M.D., Professor of Descriptive and Surgical Anatomy.

HOWARD TOWNSEND, M.D., Prof. of Materia Medica and Physiology.

CHARLES H. PORTER, M.D., Prof. of Chemistry and Pharmacy.

J. V. P. QUACKENBUSH, M.D.,Prof. of Obstetrics and Diseases of Women and Children, and Medical Jurisprudence.

AMOS DEAN, Esq., Prof. of Medical Jurisprudence.

Fees for the full course, $65. Matriculation fee, $5. Graduation fee, $20.

Material for dissection abundant, and furnished to students on the same terms as in New York and Philadelphia. Hospital Tickets free. Opportunities for Clinical instruction are believed to be equal to those afforded by any College in the country. Price of Board from $2,50 to $3,50 per week.

JOHN V. P. QUACKENBUSH, Registrar.

UNIVERSITY OF NASHVILLE.

Medical Department.—Session 1859-60.—The Seventh Annual Course of Lectures in this Institution will commence on Monday, the 2d of November next, and continue till the first of the ensuing March.

THOMAS R. JENNINGS, M. D., Professor of Anatomy.

J. BERRIEN LINDSLEY, M. D., Chemistry and Pharmacy.

C. K. WINSTON, M. D., Materia Medica and Medical Jurisprudence.

A. H. BUCHANAN, M. D., Surgical Anatomy and Physiology.

JOHN M. WATSON, M. D., Obstetrics and the Diseases of Women and Children.

PAUL F. EVE, M. D., Prof. of Prin. and Prac. of Surgery.

W. K. BOWLING, M. D., Institutes and Practice of Medicine.

WILLIAM T. BRIGGS, M. D., Adjunct Professor and Demonstrator of Anatomy.

The Anatomical rooms will be opened for students on the first Monday of October, (the 5th.)

A *Preliminary Course* of Lectures, free to all Students, will be given by the Professors, commencing also on the first Monday of October.

The Tennessee State Hospital, under the direction of the Faculty, is open to the Class free of charge.

A Clinique has been established, in connection with the University, at which operations are performed and cases prescribed for and lectured upon in the presence of the class.

Amount of Fees for Lectures is $105; Matriculation Fee, (paid once only,) $5; Practical Anatomy, $10; Graduation fee, $25.

Good boarding can be procured for $3 to $4 per week. For further information or Catalogue, apply to

W. K. BOWLING, M.D.,

NASHVILLE, TENN., July, 1859. *Dean of the Faculty.*

CASTLETON MEDICAL COLLEGE.

There are two full Courses of Lectures annually in Castleton Medical College. The SPRING SESSION commencing on the last Thursday in February; the AUTUMNAL SESSION on the first Thursday in August. Each Course will continue four months. Degrees are conferred at the close of each term.

WM. P. SEYMOUR, M.D.,Prof of Materia Medica and Therapeutics.

WILLIAM SWEETSER, M. D., Prof. of Theory and Practice of Medicine.

E. R. SANBORN, M. D., Prof. of Surgery.

WM. C. KITTRIDGE, A. M., Prof. of Med. Jurisp.

CORYDON LA FORD, M. D., Prof. of Anatomy.

P. D. BRADFORD,M.D.,Prof. of Phys. & Pathol

GEORGE HADLEY, M. D., Prof. of Chemistry and Natural History.

ADRIAN T. WOODWARD, M. D., Prof. of Obstetrics.

FEES.—For Lectures, $50; for those who have attended two Courses at other Colleges, $10 Matriculation, $5; Graduation, $16; Board from $2.00 to $2.50 per week.

A. T. WOODWARD, M.D., Registrar.

CASTLETON, VT., Jan., 1859.

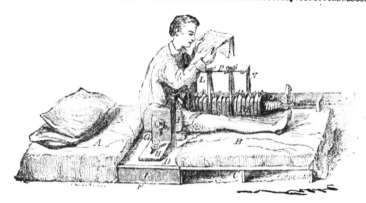

Burge's Apparatus for Fractured Thigh,

INVENTED BY

J. H. HOBART BURGE, M.D., of Brooklyn, N. Y.,

AND

WM. J. BURGE, M.D., of Taunton, Mass.,

has been thoroughly tested in actual practice, and has produced the most gratifying results. It is remarkably simple in its construction, easily applied, comfortable to the patient, adapted to fracture of either limb and to patients of any size. It is free from all the objections to which the ordinary straight splint is liable, and possesses other new features of great practical utility. By it the counter-extending pressure is confined to the nates and tuberosities of the ischia, and does not at all impinge upon the front of the groin, by which means one of the most frequent sources of annoyance and danger is obviated. No part of the body is confined except the injured limb and that to which it is immediately articulated, viz., the pelvis; thus the chest is left entirely unrestrained, and entire freedom of motion granted to the whole upper part of the body, which tends greatly to the comfort and health of the patient.

The pelvis is so secured as not to be liable to lateral motion or to sink in the bed.

Provision is also made for facility of defecation, thus insuring the greatest possible cleanliness, and preventing the necessity of disturbing the patient when his bowels are moved.

☞ Members of the profession may obtain this apparatus, complete in all its parts and nicely packed, by sending FORTY DOLLARS by mail or express to the address of

GEO. TIEMANN & CO.,

63 Chatham St., New York,

C. E. BORDEN,

Taunton, Mass., or

HIGBY & STEARNS,

162 Jefferson St., Detroit, Mich.

For further particulars see Transactions American Medical Association, Vol. X., and New York Journal of Medicine, May, 1857, and September, 1858.

Academy of Sciences, in which he asserts the practice to have been common in Circassia, Georgia, and Greece.

Germany claims vaccination as far back as 1668.

The *Allgemeine Unterhaltungen*, a journal, says that the German, *Goetz*, discovered cow-pox, and that a learned treatise was written on it in Gottingen in 1668.

CHLOROFORM.

In 1681 Papin wrote on surgical operation without pain, and clearly pointed out the anæsthesia, (loss of feeling.) He was afraid to publish it, but gave it to Dr. Bœrner, one of his old friends, and to his heirs. This old manuscript, yellow with age, was fortunately bought by the librarian of the Elector of Hesse for some Louis, and now fills an honorable niche in his library.

HOMŒOPATHY 200 YEARS BEFORE OUR SAVIOUR.

Polybius, the Greek historian, son-in-law of Hippocrates, wrote an Essay on the Nature of Man, in which he gave out the notion of cure by *simili similibi*, like by like, and Hahnemann is supposed to have taken the hint from it. Their recommendations of violent poisons as medicines is borrowed from Avicenna, the Arabian philosopher and physician, who died at 58 years of age, in 1036. He wrote fifty pages a day without fatigue, and on almost every science. He prescribed arsenic in some cases. Paracelsus said, "Mercury to drive out mercury, sulphur sulphur,—not as *water to drive out fire*—by contraries. The celebrated Des Cartes was taken in by this logic of like by like, tried it, and nearly killed himself. He *took brandy to cure a fever!* Heat to heat. Hahnemann was more lucky, for he took *quinquina* to *cure his fever*, and that, he supposed, was the grand secret of Homœopathy.

August 11, 1859.

SELECTIONS.

DR. DURKEE'S TREATISE AND A NEW YORK REVIEWER.

We must express our surprise at the appearance, in the New York *Journal of Medicine*, of an article professing to be a review of the recently published treatise on Gonorrhœa and Syphilis, by Dr. Durkee, of this city. The writer's private griefs, at a manifest eclipse of a certain translation of Ricord on the Venereal, edited by him, might have excused sharp criticisms, but should not have betrayed into un-fairness. To speak of a work which is filled, to an unusual degree, with distinctly announced opinions, the results of thirty years' expe-rience—with admirable and original descriptions of all matters relating to diagnosis—and with the clearest practical directions in regard to treatment, as "chiefly a compilation"—amounts to an interdiction of the use of the English language, every word of which has been again and again used by preceding writers.

A large portion of the review is devoted to fault-finding, because of Dr. Durkee's unwillingness to adopt every specious explanation of pa-tients, and to admit the extreme frequency (though he by no means denies the possibility) of blennorrhagia derived from other sources than impure connection. "We think," says the reviewer, "it is time that every man who has the clap should not therefore be considered a liar, and we maintain that the statements of the majority of venereal pa-tients who come under the care of any physician can be relied upon implicitly." We think, that when any physician has seen this class of patients, (even many of those among them who have no urgent mo-tive for concealment and no delicate sense of shame,) again and again compelled to abandon their subterfuges and *acknowledge* that they have lied, he learns to be somewhat incredulous in regard to specious tales, when they are contradicted by glaring facts, or are opposed to the results of almost universal experience. Are not the works of Ri-cord, and other commentators on syphilis, full of flippant recitals of the devices resorted to for removing the ingenious veil of mystery with which patients had vainly hoped to shroud their disease?

We protest against the attempts of some writers on syphilis to sub-stitute the exception for the rule, and to defend the doctrine, inculcat-ed by the reviewer in another place, "that a man rarely communicates gonorrhœa to a woman unless he has it himself," (*very* rarely,) "while, strange as it may appear, most women, who communicate gonorrhœa to men, do so without having it." We object to such far-fetched ex-planations as that gonorrhœa does not occur more frequently in mar-ried life because of an acquired acclimation between the parties. How is it that men *acclimated* with kept mistresses should be so often vic-tims of this disease? How is it that in married life it should occur so very seldom when the parties are faithful to each other, but should be so readily communicated where one of them has become infected from a third person? We make these protests and objections without re-gard, for the moment, to the bearing of these questions upon public morality; but from a strong aversion, we confess, that we entertain to having the good sense of the members of the profession outraged by attempts to exhibit them as holding opinions which would be considered, by many a shuffling patient, as only worthy to be laughed at as fit for " the marines." We are quite satisfied with the conclusions of Dr. Durkee, " that while the medical man admits that various innocent causes may induce gonorrhœal discharges, he may feel warranted in the opinion that the combined agency of all these causes is quite insignificant, compared with the agency attributable to the one chief cause. Where there is ground for reasonable doubt as to the cause of blennorrhagia, it is right that the suspected party should have the benefit of that doubt."

In the treatment of gonorrhœal ophthalmia, Dr. Durkee is represented as recommending venesection " in a manner not sanctioned by the best modern ophthalmic surgeons." It is true he cites two authorities as placing great reliance on depletion; but he expressly says, " blood-letting is not carried to anything like the extent which was once considered proper," and he goes on to state various reasons *against* heroic use of this means.

The youthful reviewer concludes his task by taking exception to the brevity of the descriptions of some of the symptoms of true syphilis; but we submit that, in a work of but 431 pages, only a limited space can be devoted to details of the features exhibited by well-understood and undisputed phenomena.

To conclude, we must reiterate our formerly expressed judgment in favor of the work of our distinguished fellow-townsman. In our opinion, Dr. Durkee's book is well adapted to the *practical wants* of physicians and students—is both graphic and lucid in style, and is creditable alike to the long experience of the author, and to the medical literature of his country, in which it fills so important a place.—*Boston Med. and Surg. Journal.*

INGENIOUS DEVICE.

We noticed in a New York newspaper an advertisement, half a column long, headed " Health of American Women," setting forth the virtues of the " Graefenberg Medicines." The proprietor of these medicines, or the " Graefenberg Company," represented by Dr. Bridge, a "regular physician, of fine attainments, and of great judgment and discrimination in the treatment of disease," offers testimonials "from the Governors of two States, the Chairman of the Board of Health of New York, one of the surgeons-in-chief of the Bellevue Hospital, many clergymen—including the Rev. N. Bangs, D.D., the Head of the Methodist Church; the State Chemist and Assayer of the State of Massachusetts; the Mayor of New York City; the United States Commissioner to Great Britain; the proprietor of Barnum's Museum, and many other public men," &c. There is nothing surprising in all this, for many of the above names are attached to other quack medicines, and there is a frankness in placing the "proprietor of Barnum's Museum" on the list, which is quite refreshing. We confess, however, we were not a little surprised to see the names of several of the most eminent New York medical men appended to the advertisement. While we were wondering how these names could possibly have been procured, a closer examination showed that though they are printed in a conspicuous manner, so as to appear at first sight as if endorsing the wonderful virtues of the Graefenberg medicines, there is in reality no fraud, since it is only stated that "convincing and unanswerable arguments have been addressed to the leading physicians and surgeons of the day, prominent among whom were Dr. Valentine Mott, President and Professor of Surgery," and half a dozen others. We do not know what reply these gentlemen made to the convincing and unanswerable arguments, but the Graefenberg Company has not seen fit to publish them, perhaps with a view of persuading the public that "silence gives consent."—*Boston Med. and Surg. Journal.*

CORRESPONDENCE FROM THE SEAT OF WAR IN ITALY.

By J. J. CHISOLM,

Professor of Surgery in the Medical College of South Carolina.

MILAN, *July* 21st, 1859.

The hospitals in Milan, which number twenty-four, and all of which are filled with wounded from the bloody battles of Magenta and Solferino, offer a rare opportunity for the study of gun-shot wounds, and also for the comparison of the various modes of treatment instituted by civil and military surgeons. All of these buildings are not equally ventilated; many of them were built for hospitals, and in their time were considered patterns of such institutions. The majority have been pressed into service from the force of circumstances. The facilities for transportation by rail-road are so great, that the wounded, taken from the field, were immediately sent to the neighboring villages and from thence to the large cities, where the conveniences for treatment could be more readily obtained. Milan of course came in for a very large share, and in a few hours all of its hospital accommodations had been disposed of: convents and barracks were soon teeming with sufferers; friend and foe mingling their cries of agony and expressions of sympathy, so suddenly had their condition changed their previous thirst for blood. The medical profession of the city at once volunteered their assistance, and the wounded without delay received surgical aid. At this late day, one month and even more since the wounds were received, much of interest connected with the active treatment has been lost, and the relative importance of the same can no longer be traced; but still, the full wards offer so much material for instruction, that our visit was extremely satisfactory.

We first visited the great Civic Hospital, built in due oblong form, and containing a series of open courts. The building possessed three thousand beds. Many of the wards were very long, and the number of the wounded necessitated two, three, and even four rows of beds, with a very narrow passage between them. Notwithstanding this crowded condition, no offensive odor could be perceived from the suppurating wounds. Cleanliness pervaded the entire establishment. The appearance of the patients was bright, and indicated a progressive convalescence. This hospital was filled with French soldiers, who bore their suffering well, and were chiefly annoyed by their compulsory inactivity. The bright appearance of the wards was partly attributed to the fact that the serious cases had been thinned out, and their places supplied by those of a milder character; still, many very serious ones remained, as the recital of individual cases will show. The wounds were nearly all healthy; a few were cleaning off after an attack of acute gangrene, which at one time had been very rife in the hospital, and to which a great many of the amputated had succumbed. Even now, with rare exceptions, it was in the stumps that the ravages of gangrene were seen. Under this combination, nearly all the amputations of the thigh were fatal. Those of the upper extremity were more successful, although equally attacked by gangrene, as the exposed bones indicated. In one of the hospitals which we visited, formerly a barrack, with rooms accommodating about ten beds, surrounded by long and spacious corridors, hospital gangrene was epidemic. In this institution were now collected one thousand wounded Austrians, whose worn frames and gaunt visages indicated a fearful combat with disease. They had been led to believe that if taken prisoners they would as surely be put to death. Therefore all who had the strength to crawl along after they were wounded · had hid themselves in the ditches or among the thick undergrowth; many remaining on the battle-field two and even three days, living upon ditch water, if they were so fortunate as to be in its neighborhood. When you take into consideration their moral dejection, we may nearly say annihilation; their lymphatic tendencies; their irregularity of living, for scarcity was the common condition of the Austrian camp, and before the battle of Magenta, it was reported that the Austrians had not tasted food for fifty hours; and then their wounds, much more grave than those of the French, as they were made by a much larger ball;* and add to all this the mistaken abstemious diet which was pursued in this hospital, you may understand readily the condition in which we found these unfortunates. The physician with whom we made the visit, believing in the contagiousness of the disease, had isolated these cases in separate wards, and some of them were fearful; thighs transfixed, in the depth of which you could thrust your fist, &c. He stated to us that he had seen patient after patient attacked who were lying in contiguous beds to a case of gangrene, thus clearly proving to him its infectious character, the tendency to attack diminishing with the space of interval. Yet, I saw this physician thrust his dirty, unwashed finger, which one minute before had been bathed in the pus of gangrene from one of the worst cases I ever saw, directly into a healthy wound, to show us the position which the ball had taken. I shuddered at this utter recklessness, and did not wonder at the fearful mortality which had befallen his practice. In the better regulated hospitals, and especially among the victorious troops, many gun-shot wounds healed with surprising facility, and comparatively few were accompanied by much inflammatory reaction. The majority of these now chronic wounds had no induration around them, and a few appeared to have healed by quick union. Most of the wounds were in the extremities, and very few of the trunk; the majority of the latter had been left on the field of battle. Most of the cases which had survived the day had been lost before our visit. Judging from present appearances, the lower extremity was more frequently wounded than the upper. In the greater number, the ball had transfixed the limb and escaped, so that very rarely was it necessary to remove a foreign body.

---

* The rifle of the French Chasseurs carries a conical ball of over two oz. weight.

I saw but two cases in which a ball had been removed by a counter-opening. It appeared to me that the conical ball, which is now coming into universal use, not only moves with much greater velocity, but cuts its way to a greater extent than did the round ball. The wounds made by them have not that mangled appearance, nor are they so tortuous, with eccentric courses. Perhaps we may account in this way for the mild degree of inflammatory reaction and absence of general excitement, which was noted in so many cases. Even where fingers had been amputated by shot, the stumps looked well, the interval of a month no doubt materially assisting. From the same causes secondary hæmorrhage was rare.

It was very interesting to examine the course of balls through the most intricate portions of the body: the neck, the axilla, the groin, in the very midst of the most important blood-vessels and nerves, without leaving any permanent injury. The accounts of the soldiers were that they bled profusely, losing quarts of blood, and were picked up exhausted; yet these injured vessels did not require ligatures, nor did secondary hæmorrhage occur. These wounds of arteries must have healed with great facility. In many instances the entrance and exit of the ball was such, as to warrant the belief that the main arteries could not have escaped; yet, after the first profuse hæmorrhage, the wounds would heal without further trouble. I saw an aneurism of the popliteal vessel, produced by a ball, operated upon very unscientifically by the head surgeon of this great hospital. After the incision through the skin, for which alone he used the knife, he continued and completed the dissection with a scissors, making necessarily a most tedious operation; Scarpa's triangle was selected as the seat of ligature. In the early treatment of all the wounded, cold water had been freely used, and appears to have been the general plan pursued. When suppuration had set in, this treatment gave way to forcing beds of lint, which was the universal practice. This bedding was continued until suppuration, ceased, and the wound cicatrized. Nimia diligentia was everywhere conspicuous. In many of the hospitals two and even three dressings were daily made, the wounds being thoroughly washed, as if excessive cleanliness was the *sine quâ non*. The wound was subjected to this scouring from within as well as without, and I heard one of the surgeons exclaim, with evident satisfaction, when the water injected into a wound came away as clean as when thrown in. I saw some wounds which were so far healed that the new cuticle had .actually formed over it, under a thin scab.

This was torn off, so as to give the favorite charpie something to do. Whilst all this covering up was going on two and three times a day, the surgeons were complaining of the hot summer weather, with its injurious effects upon the wounded. How consolatory is the thought that nature has endowed us with strong constitutions, so that we may have enough and to spare! otherwise, woe to many! Several cases showed very forcibly the pertinacity of human life. They were chiefly chest wounds; not those in which the ball in striking a rib had followed the circumference of the chest, so as to appear serious to a trivial examination. Many examples of such were in the wards. I refer to those in which the chest had been completely transfixed, with its contained lung. In one of these cases, the ball had entered at the posterior edge of the scapula, midway between the lower angle and the spine, and had, after transfixing the chest, escaped behind the anterior border of the axilla, through the outer edge of the great pectoral muscle. The patient had spit up largely of blood, which continued for some days, but had now altogether disappeared. The posterior wound was still discharging—the anterior had healed. By pressure no pus escaped; but during the act of coughing, the diaphragm, assisted by the thoracic muscles, pumped out ounces of frothy pus from the pleural cavity. He was very much reduced by this drain, which had been going on for three weeks, but had strength enough to enjoy his pipe, which we saw him using as we returned by his bed. In another case, the ball had perforated the left side of the chest, on a level with the third rib, and about two and a half inches from the middle of the sternum. Its exit was at the lower portion of the shoulder-blade. This patient had had hæmoptisis for several days, followed by violent inflammation of the lung and coverings. By repeated blood-lettings, the hæmorrhage as well as the inflammation had been controlled, and the patient was ready to be discharged. How the large blood-vessels at the root of the lungs escaped injury, is an enigma. Would not transparency of the tissues develop curious facts in pathological anatomy? Thoracic wounds were comparatively common, whilst very few intestinal wounds existed in the hospital. Most of these had terminated fatally, either upon the reception of the injury, or very soon afterwards. One case of great interest was shown, in which a ball had obliquely entered the abdomen just above the symphisis pubis, escaping near the anterior superior spine of the ilium. The iliac wound had healed quickly. On the second day after the receipt of injury, some coffee which he had taken escaped from the pubic wound; this is his account of himself, and from that time his food has continued to discharge from the opening. In examining the parts, the intestine, which appears to have the lining of the upper portion of ilium, has become intimately adherent to the skin, its mucous surface protruding above the general level. At times it exhibits a lively vermicular motion, an inodorous, colored discharge, consisting of digested food escaping freely at such periods. This case, with others which have occurred, would show either the paralyzing effect of injury upon the motions of the intestine, or the very limited motion which normally exists in the same; otherwise how can we explain the rarity of fæcal extravasation in intestinal wounds? It is proposed to re-establish in this case the continuity of the intestine, by destroying the septum, when the external orifice will close spontaneously. In a case of interest, the entire body of the lower jaw had been crushed by a cannon-shot, which carried away the chin. A large orifice was formed, through which the entire lower jaw, with the exception of the rami, escaped in broken fragments. The tongue hardening, lost its support, and protruded. The wound, two inches in diameter, now looked healthy, and was gradually contracting. The tongue was retained in the mouth by pledgets of lint. With the exception of the frightful deformity, for which there will be no remedy, the patient will do well. In another case the ball had perforated the root of the neck in the posterior triangle, grazing the external border of the sterno-cleido mastoid muscle, having its exit on the back; profuse hæmorrhage followed the injury. Now, after an interval of four weeks, the wounds having perfectly healed, paralysis of the arm exists, with the exception of those fingers supplied by the ulnar nerve, which retain perfectly their sensibility. One soldier was shot in the face, in such a way that the ball entered at one molar, and escaped through the other, passing across the floor of the orbit. The pupils of both eyes were dilated, and vision much impaired; the wounds had perfectly healed.

But a few cases of tetanus had occurred. I saw one convalescent, in which the muscles were still rigid. This person had been shot through the calf, the ball in its passage fracturing the tibia. From a large opening, pus was freely discharging. In this case I saw the head surgeon, who had used the scissors so freely in the morning, further dilate the wound, and for fifteen minutes make continued efforts to remove a piece of dead bone which was not yet detached, and which was imbedded finger deep in the calf. It would be a curious instance, if this excessive additional pain which the tetanic patient was compelled to endure, without the soothing aid of chloroform, quiets the nervous excitement under which he was laboring.

The ladies of Milan are constantly engaged at the hospitals, supplying and manufacturing lint and dressings for the use of the wounded. Not only do they liberally bestow comforts, but give their individual assistance. Many of the wounded were taken to their dwellings, where every attention was lavished upon them. I saw several of these, during convalescence, riding out with their refined hostesses; a striking contrast between the rough soldier of the ranks and the polished courtisane. Their unremitting kindnesses soothed many a pang, and gave that solace which is the peculiar prerogative of women. —*Charleston Med. Journ.*

AUDIBLE KNOCKINGS OF THE MUSCLES.

At a recent meeting of the "Académie des Sciences," M. Jobert de Lamballe read a paper, the subject of which is highly interesting, not only to the surgeon, but also to the non-professional reader. Not very long ago, this distinguished surgeon was called to visit, in consultation, a young girl about 14 years of age, who, for more than six years, had suffered from involuntary movements in some of the muscles on the outer side of the leg. These movements were characterized by pulsations or knocks, having almost the regularity of a pulse, each knock being distinctly heard at some distance, as proceeding from behind the external malleolus. A similar affection manifested itself, not long after the first, at a corresponding point in the left leg, though less intense in degree. There was pain, hesitation, and tendency to fall when walking. When the foot was extended, and on applying pressure to certain points along the course of the muscles, the patient could for a time arrest the throbbing; but this invariably produced a good deal of pain and fatigue in the limb. The parents of the girl had become quite settled in the belief that the peculiar sounds or knocks, which proceeded from the limb, were the result of supernatural agency; and it was not till M. Jobert had made a careful and scientific investigation and fully explained the matter to them, that their minds were disabused of this idea. He found that these sounds were produced solely by the rising and falling of the tendon of the peroneous brevis muscle, while contracting, or in action, and at the very part where the tendon passes along its osseous groove. The involuntary character of these movements he believes to have been owing to some peculiar functional trouble of the muscular fibres, or the nerves supplying them.

M. Jobert believes it possible that, by a little practice, these knocks or pulsations, although in the case in question altogether independent of the volition of the individual, could be produced at will, and that it is to the possession of this peculiar power that the entire secret of mediums and the so-called spirit-rappers is due. These peculiar sounds, he stated, could be produced by the muscles and tendons in ·other parts of the body, and he related the case of a lady who could give rise to them at the hip-joint by assuming a particular position.

M. Velpeau has met with a number of instances of this character, occurring in different localities. The muscles and tendons, both of the shoulder and of the leg, of the upper as well as the lower extremities, were equally capable, in rare instances, of producing these peculiar raps or sounds. Certain conjurers had been known, who could even produce a kind of harmony by a succession of knocks, in this way imitating the tune of a dance or a military march.

M. Jobert brought the history of this interesting case to a close, with a few remarks on the surgical treatment which he adopted. The medical attendant upon the girl had failed to do her any good, although he had employed a great variety of medicines, such as leeching and blistering, continued pressure over the part, etc., together with the internal use of medicines.

M. Jobert treated the case as follows: he cut across and completely divided the body of the peronæus brevis of both legs, by means of a subcutaneous section; then, by means of a suitable splint or apparatus, put up the limbs so as to secure their perfect immobility. When reunion had taken place, the girl recovered the complete use of both members, and no trace of the affection has since appeared. The cure was complete and permanent.

M. Jobert continued his remarks, and observed that a German physiologist, M. Schiff, whose attention had been given largely to this subject, made the discovery, some three or four years ago, as to the seat and origin of these peculiar sounds, which have been so commonly attributed to supernatural agency. Observing that the sounds proceeded from the foot of the bed of the individual who pretended to be influenced by spirits, M. Schiff began to question, and to have serious doubts of their supernatural origin, and was not long in concluding that they were the result of natural causes, to be accounted for and located in the body itself. From his knowledge of anatomy, he was led to think that the seat of these sounds might be the peroneal region, where there exists a bony canal or groove, along which pass the tendons of the peronei muscles. After a little practice, he was enabled, in whatever position he placed himself, to imitate all the tricks and prodigies of spirit-rappers, and he clearly established the fact that these peculiar sounds originate in the tendon of the long peroneous muscle, and moreover that they are dependent on a diminution in thickness of the sheath, or in the total abstinence of the sheath, of this muscle. While agreeing with M.. Schiff as to the seat of these sounds, M. Jobert differs with him, as we have already seen, as regards the particular muscle producing them. The one believes that it is the peroneus brevis; the other is of opinion that it is the peroneus longus, which is mainly·concerned in their production. They differ, again, on another point, viz.: the sounds or knocks observed by Schiff were purely physiological, altogether voluntary, dependent upon the will; in the case of M. Jobert's patient, the movements were of an involuntary nature, painful, consequently morbid. The subject is really one of much interest, and well meriting a further investigation on the part of anatomists and physiologists. When once the purely physical character of these sounds is demonstrated, much may be accomplished in the way of dispelling the absurd superstition connected with spirit-rappings. —*Boston Med. and Surg. Journ.*

CORRESPONDENCE EXTRAORDINARY.

[If anybody needs further light on the subject of the latest failure to crush Dr. Horace Green, let him read what follows. The conspirators might be bought now at half price.]

Letters from Professors J. Hughes Bennett, of Edinburgh, and Carl Rokitansky, of Vienna, on the Post-Mortem Examination of the late S. S. Whitney.

The following opinions relative to the pathological appearances found at the autopsy of the late Mr. Whitney are of great interest, in connection with the history of this remarkable case. Comment is unnecessary. The agreement of both of these celebrated pathologists, whose opinions are here given, upon all the essential points in the case, is conclusive. To both of them was forwarded a copy of the February number of the *Monthly*, containing a full report of the proceedings of the Academy of Medicine when this subject was under its consideration. In addition to this, a copy of the original post-mortem, certified by his Honor the Mayor of New York, was sent to Prof. Rokitansky, by his former pupil and personal friend, Dr. Charles Bernacki, of this city. Dr. Bernacki has kindly placed Prof. Rokitansky's reply at our disposal. The letters are placed in the order of time in which they were received.

PROF. BENNETT'S LETTER.

EDINBURGH, *May* 18, 1859.

My DEAR DOCTOR—I have hesitated for some time as to how I ought to reply to your letter; that is, whether it would be better to enter into a lengthy criticism of Mr. Whitney's case, or simply answer the two queries you have put to me. After carefully studying the case itself, I find so much to comment on in the various branches of diagnosis, pathology, treatment and ethics, that I feel constrained to throw my notes aside, and give up the idea of entering into the matter fully, as it would oblige me to write a treatise rather than a letter.

You request my opinion: 1. As to the tubercular character of the pulmonary abscess; 2. As to whether such effect as Dr. Beales intimates could have been produced by the injection of nitrate of silver, which was employed.

1st. *As to the tubercular character of the pulmonary abscess.*—The description given by Dr. Green of the physical signs on the 25th October, 1858, is remarkably clear, (see *Am. Monthly*, p. 104,) and can leave no doubt as to the existence of condensation of the left lung at the apex, with softening of the tissue. When Dr. Beales was called in, Dec. 14th, he does not seem to have made any physical examination of the chest. At all events, no account of any is given from that time up to the period of the patient's death, (*Monthly*, p. 111 to p. 115.) But he tells us afterwards, that he had previously made such examination (p. 117) towards the end of October; he gives no description of these signs, but only states his opinion, viz., that "he could not discover any tubercles in his lungs, and did not believe any existed." The report of the post-mortem, however, demonstrates that the physical examination of the lung made by Dr. Green was in every respect correct, (*Monthly*, p. 116.) "The whole of the upper part of this lobe (the left) was red, and solid—hepatized." "At the commencement of the bronchial ramifications there was an open cavity, about the size of a small black walnut, of a reddish-brown color, and irregular villous surface, as though a slough had separated." This answers thoroughly for the flat sound, detected two months previously, over the upper portion of the left lung, and the humid râle audible below the left clavicle, on inspiration and expiration.

As to the nature of the disease, Dr. Beales conceives it to have been acute and recent pneumonia, (p. 118.) I cannot think so, when I consider the accurate account of physical signs given two months previously, then indicating the condensation and softening which were subsequently found. It must have been chronic pneumonia passing into gangrene, or a limited tubercular abscess accompanied by chronic pneumonia of the apex. The descriptions given of the lesions do not enable me to say which of these it was. In fact, I consider it a matter of little importance, because a chronic exudation of the apex so readily passes into tubercle, and an old tubercular abscess is so commonly accompanied by chronic pneumonia, that, in truth, it often becomes difficult, if not impossible, to say where tubercle ends and pneumonia begins. It is enough that a chronic *exudation* was there, and that, I consider, Dr. Green fully indicated by his physical signs six or seven weeks before Dr. Beales was called in.

2d. *As to whether the treatment caused the disease.*—Dr. Beales informs us that Dr. Mott told the family, after the post-mortem examination, that they had not seen any disease that might not have been produced within a week, (*Monthly*, p. 118.) According to this idea, it could not have been the injection into the trachea which caused the pulmonary disease, as that operation was performed on the 6th of December, without causing any irritation, and he died on the 21st. Besides, the pulmonary lesion existed on the 25th October, as proved by physical signs. The injection, therefore, could not have caused that lesion. Is it not more probable that, a chronic exudation having existed at the apex, and a cavity formed, this latter perforated the pleura, causing the pleural exudation, followed by the emphysema of the cellular tissue? At what moment did this perforation take place? We are told that Mr. Whitney visited Dr. Green on the 14th of December, after breakfast, (the time is not stated;) the doctor passed an instrument into his throat, and finding some obstruction, he pushed the instrument with some force; he (Mr. W.) felt something give way, immediately experienced *severe* pain about the top of the windpipe, and told the doctor he had " hurt him;" he returned home, informed the family of what had occurred, and was seen by Dr. Beales at 1 P. M., (p. 112.) Dr. Green's account of what happened on the 14th is different.   According to him, (*Monthly*, p. 106,) when the sponge reached the glottic opening, the patient partially closed the throat, so that the instrument did not enter the windpipe at all.   It was at once removed, no more force having been used than that which is constantly employed every day in operations on the air-passages.   The patient, after talking a while with Dr. Foy and myself, and remarking that " the operation hurt him more," or that " he felt it more than usual," he left, with the arrangement that he should return the next day and have the tube employed.   The patient's account to Dr. Beales is, that at the moment the probang was arrested at the glottis, he felt something give way, and experienced *severe* pain about the top of the windpipe, (p. 112.)   But is this consistent with the fact that he talked for a while with Drs. Foy and Green, and went home intending to come next day, &c.?   Again, was the pain, if felt *at the top* of the windpipe, symptomatic of perforation of the pleura in the chest ?   It appears to me difficult to answer these questions, more especially when we read the account of the alarming condition of Mr. W. at 1 o'clock, when first seen by Dr. Beales, (*Monthly*, p. 111.)   I am, therefore, inclined to ask, What occurred in the interval between the patient's leaving Dr. Green and his seeing Dr. Beales ?   This may have been an interval of three or four hours, and of this most important period I can find no account whatever.   It is true, Mr. Whitney seems to have had the impression that his severe symptoms commenced when the sponge was arrested, but this is negatived by the evidence of Drs. Green and Foy, who saw no evidence of severe pain even in the throat.   When, then, did the pulmonary and pleural perforation take place, which induced the emphysema and subsequent symptoms ?   With the facts at present before me, I cannot answer this question, but it is clear to my mind that it may have occurred during the hours not accounted for; that it might have been altogether spontaneous, connected only with the progress of the chronic pulmonary lesion; and that it had no relation whatever to the operation performed by Dr. Green.

In addition to the lesion already referred to, it appeared, on dissection, that there was an abscess behind the larynx, and stretching towards the left of the pharynx, the size of a hen's egg, with an opening at its upper and posterior part, into the pharynx, large enough to admit the end of the forefinger.   This abscess was not discovered before death, by any of his attendants, medical or surgical.   Dr. Mott, a great authority in surgery, asserts that this was an acute abscess.   Dr. Beales distinctly states, (*Monthly*, p. 119,) that in his opinion it was caused on the 14th December, by the accidental laceration of the pharynx by the probang; and his account of the symptoms, as he observed them at 1 P. M. on that day, supports the supposition, especially the intense pain in the region of the larynx, shooting through to the cervical vertebræ, and down the course of the trachea to the chest; he kept grasping the larynx, &c. (p. 111.) Now, as the larynx was shown subsequently to be healthy, it is very probable that these symptoms were connected with the pharyngeal abscess. But how? Is such pain consistent with the first commencement of an abscess, or did it accompany the rupture of an abscess previously formed? By what signs was it pronounced to be acute? Might it not have existed before the operation of the 14th? Might it not have come on subsequently? On all these points I will not venture to speak. But having now used the probang in many hundred cases, and under all circumstances, I am at a loss to understand how its being arrested at the glottis would either lacerate the pharynx, so as to give rise to an abscess, or cause the bursting of an abscess which had already formed—" downward, behind and below the thyroid cartilage." I cannot but think that the application of the sponge had no more to do with this abscess, than it had with the exudation into the apex of the left lung.

Yours, very truly and sincerely,

J. HUGHES BENNETT.

PROF. ROKITANSKY'S LETTER.

MOST ESTEEMED FRIEND—I received your letter on the 8th, along with the documents relating to the sickness and death of Mr. S. S. Whitney, through Mr. Wallner, or rather, as I was not at home, through my wife. First permit me to express my most heartfelt thanks to you, and my tranatlantic friends, for the friendly remembrance which you show in the recognition of my scientific labors, and the honorable confidence reposed in me. And now to my task. I have devoted my entire attention to the documents you sent me, as you will perceive, *absque omni partium studio*.

Certainly the most important point is to determine the nature of the cavity in the left lung, "just at the root, or the commencement of the ramifications of the bronchiæ." This is very difficult, for two reasons: 1. Because the description of the cavity is very imperfect; and 2. Because the whole report (Gesammtbefünd) is very defective, inasmuch as a complete dissection was not made. Neither sufficient local nor sufficient general data are given for a diagnosis.

In the last point of view, particularly, we are not certain whether a tuberculous individual or not is under consideration. It would seem as though no actual tuberculization was present.

If, under these circumstances, I give my opinion in compliance with your request, it can be of value only as a supposition.

1. The abscess in the larynx might be the result of a perichondritis; this abscess broke externally into the contiguous circumjacent areolar tissue. The red point found in the larynx was probably connected with the abscess. The reddening of the mucous membrane of the air-passages is of no importance.

2. I do not consider it as proved that the condition of the upper lobe of the left lung was that of recent hepatization. True, there was noticed a considerable pleuritic exudation on the exterior of the lobe, but I presume that this lobe of the lung had been partially attacked with atelectasis, (obturation,) in consequence of a bronchial catarrh, and was in a state of incipient destruction, (induration.)

3. The cavity in this lung (this lobe of the lung) I would consider as a bronchial sac, or rather as a cavern, (bronchial cavern,) resulting from the ulcerdus destruction of such a sac.

Was this ulcerative process due to a continuous, exacerbating, catarrhal inflammation of the mucous membrane of the sac, or to a tuberculization of the mucous membrane of the same? We are obliged to accept the former solution of the question, inasmuch as the report denies the presence of any tubercles.

This cavernous opening must then be considered, since from it a destruction of both layers of the pleura proceeded, as the source of the extravasation of the inspired atmospheric air into the circumjacent areolar tissues. This, then, is my opinion with reference to the significance of the results of the post-mortem examination. As regards the operative treatment, I have not been requested, in fact, to give an opinion; still, you may perhaps like to hear that also. It is very evident that the two conditions met with, i. e., the abscess in the larynx, and especially the cavity in the left lung, existed before the treatment; and I also believe that the latter (the treatment) was not the cause of the death of the patient.

Your sincere friend,   ROKITANSKY.

VIENNA, *June 14th,* 1859.

[*Amer. Med. Monthly.*

WHO DISCOVERED ANÆSTHESIA?

Nineteen years ago this summer, Dr. L. P. Brockett, a physician now, but then a student in Hartford, Connecticut, having recently had a molar tooth extracted which gave him great pain, was talking with the dentist on various subjects, when the conversation turned on the intoxicating influences of nitrous oxide gas. The dentist remarked, "*that he believed that a man might be made so drunk by this gas, or some similar agent, that dental or other operations might be performed upon him without any sensation of pain on the part of the patient.*" This conversation occurred in August, 1840, and the man who uttered the startling and entirely novel proposition was Horace Wells.

Four years passed by, and in the same city a traveling lecturer (Colton by name) administered to several persons the "laughing gas," amongst others, to a certain dentist. One of the party, while under its influence, received a severe hurt, but did not give any evidences of pain, when the dentist remarked to his neighbor (Mr. David Clark) that he believed "*that a man, by taking that gas, could have a tooth extracted or a limb amputated, and not feel the pain.*" This was on the 10th of September, 1844; and the great idea was again distinctly stated by the same Horace Wells.

On the morning of the 11th of September, (the day after his lecture,) Mr. Colton was requested by a gentleman to go with him to a dentist of Hartford, Dr. J. M. Riggs, and carry some "nitrous oxide." This person sat down in the operating chair, took the bag of gas, and inhaled it until he became insensible, and Dr. Riggs extracted one of his largest teeth. On coming to his senses, he cried out, "*It did not hurt me more than the prick of a pin; it is the greatest discovery ever made.*" On that day the great idea became an embodied fact, and the discoverer proved in his own person the truth of his theory, for the man was Horace Wells.

From that time his restless, excitable spirit knew no peace. Day and night he talked of it, experimented with it, and studied its effects and modes of preparation. In a few months the truth was verified by many successful experiments. Doctors and professors, bishops, members of Congress, and many citizens of Hartford and the vicinity, united with one accord to declare, from personal experience, their perfect faith in the new discovery. Not only in tooth-drawing, but in large surgical operations, was the experiment tested. The thigh was amputated, tumors removed, cancers dissected out of the human body without pain; and for *twenty-two months* no other man opened his mouth, made an experiment, or published a fact with regard to the great discovery about to bestow its priceless blessing on suffering humanity, save the one to whom we owe it—Horace Wells.

This ardent, zealous seeker after truth, often injudicious and extravagant, but ever frank and guileless, had a quondam student, (now friend,) who lived in Boston. His name was W. T. G. Morton. To him he applies for assistance, so that his discovery may be brought before the notice of the great men of the metropolis. Morton gave him the opportunity of using the nitrous oxide in the presence of the medical class of Harvard University. The tooth was extracted, but the patient screamed; and although he afterwards declared that he did not feel the pain, the *students hissed* the trembling adventurer (the unknown dentist) from the hall—and back to his home, heart-broken, friendless, but not despairing, came Horace Wells.

The tale is almost told. Morton sees *his* chance. Wells had proved that *sulphuric ether* has the wonderful power; and fearing to repeat an experiment which had just failed, *he* determines to try the ether. He seeks for an influential friend, and finds him in *Professor* Charles T. Jackson, (God save the mark!) and on the 30th of September, 1846, twenty-two months *after* Dr. Wells proved the fact on himself, Morton pulled out a tooth for Eben Frost without pain. The professor now, however, steps in for his share. The Letheon is patented. The Boston surgeons use it in the hospital. Bigelow sends it to Liston, who telegraphs to Edinburgh—Glory! we have conquered pain. The stolen goods is contended for by the first rogue, who finds himself cheated out of the credit by the second, who is a professor, and has the cards over him. They fight over the glittering prize. Meanwhile, the *world* weeps with joy at the blessed boon, and a thousand thankful hearts throughout the civilized earth send up their grateful prayers to God for the unutterable blessing.

Where is the discoverer—he who thought it first—proved it first— he who ventured all—yea, his life, for the truth—where is Horace Wells?

Defrauded of his honors, betrayed by his friend, deserted by good fortune, his body shattered by the constant use of all sorts of excitants —still experimenting on himself—his mind ill regulated, impulsive, tortured by the cruel fate which seemed to await him; 'twas more than he could bear. Mankind looked here and there eagerly for their benefactor, and found him at last—*in the suicide's grave.*

We bring before you, reader, in a few words, this mournful story, because it is right that *we*, American physicians, who are proud to claim as *ours* this greatest gift to medical science, should not neglect to do honor to its real author. His wife lives yet to pray that this may be done. His son asks that his father's claim shall be closely scrutinized, and, if proved, acknowledged, and published to the world. It is substantiated by evidence* too strong to be overthrown—by facts deposed and sworn to by numerous witnesses above suspicion. Let us, then, individually examine for ourselves, and then unite with one accord to award tardy justice to the memory of Horace Wells.—*Va. Med. Journal.*

DR. HORACE WELLS AND ANÆSTHESIA.

The following preamble and resolutions were unanimously passed at the meeting of the Medical Society of the City of Hartford, on Monday evening, February 7th, 1859:

In view of the former and more recently renewed attempts to deprive the late Dr. Horace Wells, of this city, and his family, of the honor and any reward which might be given them for the discovery and development of the principle of anæsthesia as applied to surgery; and in view also of the efforts made and making to induce unreflecting yet generous individuals to pecuniarily recompense other claimants, *we*, the Medical Society of the City of Hartford, many of whose members were personally acquainted with Dr. Wells, participated in his experiments, and were conversant with the facts from the first, feel it our duty to pass the following resolutions:

Resolved, That having examined the testimony which has been presented in favor of the claim of Dr. Horace Wells, that he originated the idea, and was the first effectually to demonstrate the practicability of inducing a state of insensibility for surgical purposes by the use of substances inhaled, we feel assured that such was indisputably the fact, and that to withhold from Dr. Wells the credit of this discovery, which he generously gave to the world without fee or reward, is unjust and dishonorable.

Resolved, That to bestow pecuniary recompense, or honors of any description, upon those not entitled to such testimonials, to the neglect of the deserving, is a discouragement to virtuous action, and we entreat all who are besought to contribute to other claimants than Dr. Wells,

---

* See Senator Smith's statement of the question, as laid before the committee of Congress, a copy of which, owing to the kindness of a friend, we have before us.

that they candidly examine both sides of the question, believing that if this is done, the cause of truth, which has labored heretofore under many discouragements, will triumphantly vindicate itself.

Resolved, That we consider it unworthy any member of an honorable profession that he should support claims for a patented article, while Horace Wells, nearly two years before, proclaimed the discovery of the principle of anæsthesia, demonstrated its power, gave it freely to the world, and at Boston, in the very amphitheatre of the medical school, urged its use upon the medical faculty.

Resolved, That the pamphlet called " Anæsthesia," or the testimony upon the subject, arranged by the Hon. Truman Smith, collected from a multitude of our fellow-citizens of the highest respectability, is a most satisfactory defence of Dr. Wells' claim, and to it we would refer any who are in doubt as to the rightful discoverer of the aforesaid principle, believing no unprejudiced person can arise from its perusal with other views than those held by this Society.

Resolved, That the thanks of this Society be given to the Hon. Truman Smith for his able, honest, and zealous defence of the truth, and for his aforesaid work on anæsthesia, a work which deserves the thanks of the whole profession, and of every lover of justice.

Resolved, That in approving the foregoing resolutions, we are in no way actuated by any other motive than that desire for truth which should always govern our profession; that the desire of establishing the claim of Dr. Wells for the aforesaid discovery does not arise from the fact that he was a resident of our city, or that this discovery re-flects honor upon it; but we feel that this defence is a solemn duty devolving upon us as a medical body, for on whom should it fall unless upon those personally and best acquainted with all the circumstances of the case, who witnessed the birth of the great idea, and watched its full development ?　　　　　·　　　　　S. E. FULLER, *Clerk*.

By the Proceedings of the Connecticut State Medical Society, just published, we learn that the foregoing report of the County Society was acted on as follows.

[Alas! poor MORTON and his backers !]

Dr. Hooker, Chairman, presented the following report, viz.:

The committee to whom was referred the preamble and resolutions of the Medical Society of the City of Hartford respectfully report: That in their opinion the claim of the late Horace Wells, of Hartford, to the discovery and application of the principle of producing anæsthesia by inhalation for surgical purposes, is supported by incontestible evidence; they therefore recommend to this Convention, for approval and endorsement, the preamble and resolutions referred to them. Report adopted.

CHOLERA.

Cholera in England.—The cholera is again here, and it has arrived by the old route, from Hamburg. One case proved fatal last week on board one of the Hamburg steamers on her passage: another was sent to the *Dreadnought*, and died there, also from a Hamburg vessel; and a third died in a Hamburg vessel on the Thames. Dr. McWilliam, who is doing duty temporarily for Sir Wm. Pym, the Superintendent-General of Quarantine, has done all that he is empowered to do by having vessels from Hamburg boarded at Gravesend, and suspicious cases of disease removed to the *Dreadnought*, or elsewhere, and similar instructions have been sent to our eastern and northeastern ports; but beyond this the Privy Council will not act. The mischief is probably done by this time, and we are not likely to escape an autumn epidemic of cholera; but we have a strong conviction that it would be well to keep all vessels ariving in England from Hamburg, or from any port infected with cholera, under observation for at least three days before admitting their passengers to laud in this country. This would lead to no very great inconvenience or loss, and it would surely be better to err on the side of excessive caution than of culpable neglect.—*Med. Times and Gazette*, Aug. 6th, 1859.

Cholera and Cholerine at Paris.—Considerable alarm has been felt at Paris, under the idea that the cholera has reappeared. It is true that during the great heats a great number of cases have occurred, and several patients have been rapidly carried off. Cholerine, too, prevails on a large scale. Still, the disease has not manifested the character of an epidemic; and there can be little doubt that this sporadic cholera will disappear, as the usually high temperature of the last few weeks has abated.—*Ibid.*

Cholera in Bombay.—Between the 2d and 22d of June 683 persons, of whom six were Europeans, fell victims to cholera in Bombay; and at the departure of the last mail this fatal scourge raged with great violence.—*Ibid.*

A VISIT TO THE LONDON HOSPITALS.

By E. D. Fenner, M.D., of New Orleans.

My Dear B.—I arrived at this great metropolis on the 7th instant, after a very pleasant journey from the time I left home, and have been recently so busy seeing novelties and wonders, that I begin to feel tired of it, and must soon change the scene. Among the many and various interesting objects that have attracted my attention in London, I have not overlooked its great medical institutions, and I beg leave now to offer you the following crude observations upon such of the hospitals and distinguished medical men as I have seen. I must here acknowledge my obligation to our old friend and quondam fellow-citizen, Dr. G. T. Browning, for his very kind courtesy ever since I have been in the city.

ST. THOMAS' HOSPITAL.

June 13th.—Dr. Browning accompanied me to this venerable institution, which dates back to a beginning in the year 1213. It was first an almshouse, but in 1552 was endowed and incorporated by King Edward VI., whose statue now stands in the yard, and was erected in 1737. It looks like the statue of a boy of sixteen years. In the front yard is a statue of Sir Thomas Knight, erected in 1714, one of the earliest and greatest benefactors of this institution. We walked through wards, consisting of very large rooms, with beds on each side. Everything looked very neat and comfortable. The head nurses are very intelligent women, who have very nice apartments, and receive good wages. There is a Magdalen ward for venereal diseases; only seven or eight cases in at present. The general wards were not full. The operating-room is extremely small, plain, and antiquated. We followed some students into the lecture-room, and sat down to hear a clinical lecture by Dr. Barker. There were only four students present when he began, but ten more came in afterwards. He commenced a slow sort of Presbyterian style of reading reports of cases, with minute detail of symptoms, and hardly ever looking up at his audience, which soon produced such a soporific effect on me, that I thought it best to retire, and we did so, I think, without his observing us. I was unable to procure any report of this hospital.

WESTMINSTER HOSPITAL.

Operating Day.—Tuesday, June 14th, 1859.—My friend, Dr. Browning, failing to meet me at two o'clock, I determined to go to the hospital without a conductor. On entering, saw a young man, who told me there was no impropriety, and showed me the way to the operating-room. At the door we met Mr. Holt, one of the surgeons, to whom I introduced myself, and received a polite invitation to accompany him and take a seat near by. There were two other surgeons present, Mr. Brooks and Mr. Morehouse, who belonged to the hospital and had operations to perform.

Operation 1.—*Removal of a small fibrous tumor* from the breast of a young woman. She was put under chloroform, and the tumor soon removed, with a considerable portion of the mammary gland. Two or three small arteries were tied, and the wound sewed up with *silver* sutures.

Operation 2.—*Lithotrity* in a man who had suffered from severe stricture of the urethra, and also stone in the bladder. The stricture had first been relieved, and then the stone was crushed. He had undergone the operation twice before this. He was put under chloroform, and with some difficulty a piece of the remaining stone was found and crushed. Mr. Holt said that he now only performed lithotomy when lithotrity was forbidden by some peculiarity in the case.

Operation 3.—*Stricture in the urethra.*—Man, aged about thirty-five, and rather weak in the lungs. On this account, Mr. Holt would not use chloroform. He used an instrument for *tearing* open the stricture. It was quickly done, and the pain only momentary. Mr. H. has a steady hand, and is a nice operator.

Mr. Brooke now took the stand.

Operation 1.—*Removal of external piles* from a woman. She was put under chloroform, and it was done with scissors.

Operation 2.—*Hydrocele.*—In a man for the third time; a simple puncture with a trochar; no injection afterwards. Mr. B. said it was hardly necessary. Patient's penis had been amputated previously.

Mr. Holthouse, the third surgeon, then took the stand, and had nothing but one operation on the eye of a blind man. He removed a portion of the *lens*, but said it would not do much good.

I walked through the wards of the hospital, and found everything neat and comfortable. The operating-room and lecture-room both very small. There is a school now connected with this hospital, not chartered to confer degrees, but authorized to send applicants to the university as candidates. This hospital has 175 beds, and affords relief to about 2,000 in-patients, and 20,000 out-patients, annually.

MIDDLESEX HOSPITAL.

June 15.—Dr. Browning accompanied me to this hospital at twelve o'clock, being operating day. Found nothing on hand; walked through the wards, and found the usual arrangement of large wards, with about twenty beds in each; low, iron bedsteads, and no curtains, divided into male and female, medical and surgical wards. The amphitheatre, operating or lecture room small, and very plain. Dissecting-room small, and very plain; on the ground-floor of a back building, only one long table, suitable for six or seven subjects. In this building are also the apothecary and chemical rooms. Number of patients about 150. It is a fine hospital. Large number of out-patients, as in the previous.

ST. MARY'S HOSPITAL.

June 15.—This is one of the new hospitals; a fine, large building; large wards, with very high ceiling. I got the last published report, which was for 1857. The number of in-patients for that year was 1,480; out-patients 4,026; average number of in-patients, 143.

Operating Day.—Mr. Coulson, surgeon—a good-looking man, with a smiling countenance, apparently about fifty-five years of age; gray hair.

Operation 1.—*Removal of a small cheloid tumor* from the top of the sternum of a young woman—a simple thing, and soon over. She was put under chloroform.

Operation 2.—*Removal of a large morbid growth,* involving the right labium pudendi. He didn't seem to have any very definite idea about it, but cut out a considerable portion of it. She was under chloroform. In both these operations Mr. Coulson used the silk ligature. These were all the operations he had. The operating-room or amphitheatre is larger and neater than any I·have yet seen.

GUY'S HOSPITAL.

June 17th.—I took breakfast early and got to this celebrated old hospital about nine o'clock, with no other guide than a letter from my friend, Dr. Crawcour, to Dr. Odling, professor of practical chemistry in the medical school. I found a lecture going on by Dr. Oldham, addressing about thirty students in a very fluent and animated style on *deformities of the pelvis.* He is a good-looking man, and is one of the professors of midwifery. The lecture being clinical, he entered fully into the propriety and method of premature delivery. At the close of the lecture we all followed him into one of the wards, and saw him perform the operation.

He did it with a long trochar, and very soon drew off about eight ounces of the liquor amnii. He then examined a new case that had just entered the ward—an intelligent-looking, nervous young woman, with a countenance expressive of much anxiety and suffering. The doctor questioned her minutely relative to the previous history of the case, and then examined by the touch. He almost immediately shook his head, and said aloud to the closely-packed students around, "*Malignant disease to great extent.*" No sooner had he said this, than the poor woman's countenance, which had been lit up with anxious hope, suddenly sunk, and she began to sob most bitterly, as if fully conscious that her doom was sealed. I could not but remember how often the French physicians and surgeons had been condemned for doing this very thing. If he had not pronounced the diagnosis in her hearing, it would have answered just as well, and the poor woman might have enjoyed the *delusion of hope* for some time, which would certainly be preferable to the pang of despair.

I then went into the laboratory, and found Dr. Odling lecturing and demonstrating practical chemistry. Dr. O. is a very handsome and youthful-looking man, a fluent talker, and expert manipulator. He was a classmate of our Prof. Crawcour, and seems to be equally enthusiastic in his branch. At the close of his lecture he greeted me very cordially, and carried me through all the departments of this great hospital. The buildings cover a very large space of ground, and are well arranged into medical, surgical, and maternity wards, laboratory, dispensary, pharmaceutical, dissecting, and lecture rooms, museum and library. The house makes up about 500 beds; the in-patients average 500 constantly, and 5,000 a year. The *out*-patients number about 40,000 a year. All these London hospitals appear to have dispensaries attached to them. The museum at Guy's is very fine, (15,000 specimens,) and the library has eight or ten thousand volumes. The lecture-room would seat about 200. At this hospital is a bronze statue of Thomas Guy, its sole founder, in 1821, and a beautiful marble statue of Sir Astley Cooper.

From this I went to *University College Hospital*, with a note of introduction to Dr. Jenner. I found him busily engaged prescribing for *out*-patients. I sent him my note, and was soon invited to enter. I took a seat, and saw him examine a considerable number of patients, men, women, and children. There was one case of intermittent fever, quite a rarity in these parts. Dr. J. examined the patients with great care before prescribing. All the children had to be stripped naked. He does not attend wards at this time.

Dr. Jenner is a nice, tidy-looking gentleman; hair black, and very thin on the top of his head; of rather low stature, but stout; looks Scotch, but says he is English, and not related to Edward Jenner, of vaccine celebrity. After finishing his service, he kindly took me through the wards of the hospital, and also the university building adjoining. As we went along we passed Dr. Parkes, and on my telling him that he, Dr. Parkes and Dr. Watson, were the men, of all in London, I had most desired to see, he introduced me to Dr. Parkes, whom I found to be a very fine-looking and affable gentleman. I took occasion to mention Dr. H. F. Campbell's report " *On the Nervous System in Febrile Disease,*" and said I would send him a copy if they would review it in one of the London journals, which they promised to do. They gave me their cards, and invited me to call. I found everything about this hospital in nice order. There are generally from 150 to 200 patients in the wards, and a large number of out-patients apply twice a week for advice and medicines.

Having, through the kindness of Dr. Odling, obtained a ticket to the *Royal Institution of Great Britain,* I went at 9 P. M. to hear a lecture by Mr. Faraday, one of the most distinguished philosophers of the day. When I applied, the secretary said he could not refuse me a ticket, but that I might congratulate myself on being an American, as there was hardly any other to whom he would grant the favor, and being the last lecture of the season, the house would be very full. I presume he was influenced somewhat by the fact that this great institution, the first of the kind in London, was founded in 1799 by a few men, among whom was our distinguished countryman, Count Rumford. It was here that Sir Humphrey Davy delivered his celebrated lectures, and announced his great discoveries in chemistry and electricity, which have immortalized his name and conferred honor on the institution. He was followed by Mr. W. T. Brande, and then came Mr. Faraday, who, full of years and honors, still charms and delights the distinguished audiences that always attend his lectures. On this occasion the lecture-room was crowded with the very *élite* of the city, among whom were many noblemen and ladies. The subject was *phosphorescent light*. Mr. Faraday is a very good-looking man, with a profusion of gray hair, fine eyes, and ruddy complexion. He is upward of sixty years of age, but quite active, and one of the most expert and successful experimenters I ever saw. He is very fluent, and speaks rapidly, as if anxious to communicate as much knowledge as possible in the time allowed. His experiments were beautiful, and he was listened to with profound attention. He lectured about an hour and a quarter, and I did indeed congratulate myself on having the happiness to see and hear so great a philosopher. This is a splendid institution, having a fine museum, and a select library of 30,000 volumes.

I here closed my observations for the day; went back to Morley's; jotted down my memoranda, and retired to rest pretty late.

ST. BARTHOLOMEW'S HOSPITAL.

June 18th.—I went to this ancient and celebrated institution about noon. This was the theatre of Mr. Abernethy's great deeds and quaint humor, and is decorated with a fine marble bust and portrait of him. St. Bartholomew's was founded in 1102, and is, I believe, the oldest of all the London hospitals. It receives within its walls nearly 6,000 in-patients annually, and its out-patients and casualties amount to nearly 90,000 annually. It contains 650 beds, of which 420 are allotted to surgical cases, and 230 to medical cases and the diseases of women. The museums of anatomy, materia medica, and botany are extensive, and open daily to students. The library contains upward of 5,000 volumes of standard works, also the chief medical journals. A reading-room is open to students of the school, during the greater part of the day. Among the medical and surgical staff are some names well known in our country, as the venerable Sir Wm. Lawrence, Mr. Stanley, Mr. Skey, Mr. Paget, Dr. Burrows, Dr. West and Dr. Farre. On entering, I was conducted to the room where Mr. Paget was prescribing for surgical out-patients. I sent him my card, and he welcomed me cordially. He dispatched thirty or forty patients in a very short time, and then having a pressing engagement, he asked his assistant to conduct me to the operating-room and wards. It was operating day, and Mr. Stanley now drove up. He saluted me politely, and asked me to walk in and see what was to be done. Mr. S. is rather short and stout, with gray hair and a good face. Having learned from my conductor that there was very little to be done here to-day, I concluded to go at once to King's College Hospital, where there was a prospect of seeing a number of operations.

KING'S COLLEGE HOSPITAL.

When I arrived I found about a hundred spectators in the amphitheatre, and the distinguished surgeon, Mr. Ferguson, commenting on a case upon which he had just operated. Mr. Ferguson looks to be about fifty years of age, robust, well formed, rather bald, and a very cool, self-possessed air. He speaks very deliberately, and not without the disagreeable appearance of affectation. But he is as cool and deliberate in operating as he is in speaking. I witnessed the following:

Operation 1.—*Lithotrity* on a man: third time. The patient was put profoundly under chloroform, and Mr. F. proceeded to extract about a dozen fragments of stone from the bladder. From the manner with which these rugged fragments were dragged through the urethra, I shall certainly not envy this patient the pleasure he will have in emptying his bladder for the next day or two. He was on the table nearly an hour.

Operation 2.—*Amputation of the thigh.*—This was a case of *ununited fracture*, which had resisted all the means resorted to for the purpose of producing bony union. Mr. Ferguson removed the limb with the knife alone, and then sawed off a considerable portion of the bone. After tying the arteries, he closed the stump with silk sutures, and it looked very neat. It was done under chloroform. After the operation was over, he drew from the lower fragment a long ivory peg that had been driven into the bone to cause reunion. Mr. F. did not mention any other means that had been resorted to in this case. I could not but suspect that this poor fellow had lost a leg for the want of skillful surgery.

Mr. Bowman now took the stand, and operated on a young woman for a deformity of the upper lip. It was very tedious, and her beauty was certainly not improved at the close of the operation, though it may be ultimately. Mr. B. is a tall, thin, handsome man, with an intellectual countenance, and apparently about forty. His remarks on the case were very interesting.

Mr. Wood, assistant surgeon, now took the stand, and operated for the permanent cure of reducible hernia on a young man. He took occasion to condemn Wurtzer's operation, and then performed *his own*, which, from the little I saw and heard of it, I am unable to describe so as to make you understand.

Dr. Watson holds the honorary position of consulting physician to this hospital, but does not attend wards. Dr. Budd, his successor, is in service, but I have not had the pleasure of seeing him.

LONDON FEVER HOSPITAL.

June 23d.—This morning my ever kind friend, Dr. Browning, conducted me to this institution. Having seen very few cases of fever in any of the hospitals I have visited, I felt a strong desire to see one specially devoted to this class of disease, which, as you are aware, is the most important of all in our part of the world.

The London fever hospital is rather small, (only about 200 beds,) situated in a high and airy place, and most admirably arranged for ventilation and cleanliness. The visiting physicians are Alexander Tweedie and Southwood Smith; assisting physicians, Wm. Jenner and C. Murchison; resident medical officer, Dr. J. D. Scurrah. The latter received us, and very politely conducted us through the entire establishment. Neither of the visiting physicians was present, which I regretted, as the name of Tweedie and Southwood Smith have long been familiar to us as writers on fever. They are now old men, and rather behind the new lights of the day.

Dr. Scurrah gave me the annual report for 1858, from which it appears there has been a marked decline in the prevalence of fever in the last year or two. Some other diseases besides fever, amounting to more than one-third of the whole, are admitted into this hospital. The admissions for fever last year were 357, viz.: typhus 15, typhoid 180, febricula 44, scarlatina 118. Deaths from fever 59, viz.: typhus 9, typhoid 28, scarlet 22. This shows a mortality from fevers of more than 16 per cent., which certainly does not reflect much credit upon the fever doctors of the great metropolis, especially when we consider that every possible convenience and advantage are here supplied. The only drawback is, that some of the cases are admitted in advanced stages of disease, a thing that occurs at all hospitals. The largest admissions occur in September; the smallest in February. Daily average throughout the year, thirty-eight.

The mortality from typhus fever was upward of 50 per cent., from typhoid 13.72 per cent., and of scarlet fever 19 per cent. Now I would ask whether any respectable practitioner of seven years' experience in any city, town, or neighborhood in our Southern country would ever boast of such success as this in the treatment of fever? Dr. Scurrah says they do not pretend to *cure* fevers at this hospital, but rather to guide them as safely as possible through their natural course. The treatment consists of wine, nourishing broths, sometimes camphor mixture, and astringents when there is diarrhœa.

It is evident that fevers at this day constitute but a small portion of the diseases requiring medical aid in London, so different from the state of things in the days of Sydenham. And this is unquestionably due to the wonderful improvement that has taken place in sanitary measures. In the three weeks I have spent in London I have traversed it in almost every direction, and I must say it is the cleanest city I ever saw. The only place I have seen that could be compared to even Common Street, our great thoroughfare, was around the great fish market of Billingsgate, and even this comparison would be decidedly in favor of the latter. London was once as sickly as New Orleans, but is now one of the healthiest cities in the world; and this is entirely due to her admirable sanitary measures. If our own ill-fated city would only follow her example, there is no telling what great benefit would accrue. I have obtained some valuable reports from the General Board of Health, which I shall bring home with me.

The hospitals named are all I have found time to visit during my sojourn in London, though there are five or six others of high standing. Nearly all of the great hospitals have medical schools attached, and afford fine facilities for instruction. In these schools students are prepared for examination before the royal colleges of surgeons and physicians, which confer the highest degrees upon the successful candidates.

The amount of charity extended to the afflicted poor of London is almost beyond calculation, and reflects great honor upon the liberality of her wealthy citizens. All the great hospitals are free to the poor; but besides these, there are eighty-eight free dispensaries, and other medical institutions of various kinds, devoted entirely to the relief of the poor. From the Medical Directory I learn that in only twenty-one of these institutions the average number of patients for a single year was upward of *one hundred and ninety thousand*. In a single one —the Metropolitan free hospital—the average number of patients was fifty thousand. Many other instances might be given of extraordinary charity and benevolence to the poor. It really appears to me that the poor of this great city are the favorite *pets* of the rich, who bestow on them every imaginable care and comfort.

But I find my letter is getting entirely too long, and lest I should weary the patience of yourself and readers, I will here conclude, with the promise to let you hear from me again, after I shall have visited some of the other seats of medical science in this part of the world.

I start to Edinburgh to-morrow, thence to Dublin, and after that to Paris, where I shall probably write again.

I remain, very truly, yours,

E. D. FENNER.

LONDON, *June* 25, 1859.

[*N. O. Med. News and Hosp. Gaz.*

VALUABLE SURGICAL DISCOVERY.

PARIS, *July* 28, 1859.

A medical discovery of much value, destined to effect a great amelioration in the treatment of ulcers, abscesses, flesh wounds, &c., has lately been made by two former *internes* or house surgeons of the Hospice de la Charité, and by them generously offered to the world without fee or reward. At the last sitting of the Academy of Science, M. Velpeau demanded permission to make an important communication, and announced that the two young practitioners in question, Messrs. Crome and Demeaux, had paid him a visit for the purpose of presenting to his notice their discovery and explaining to him its results. Messrs. Crome and Demeaux have found a process for the complete and instantaneous disinfection of animal matter. The action of the disinfecting agent arrests the progress of decomposition, and effectually prevents the generation of insects. The substance, prepared for use, costs here about one franc for a hundred pounds, and the expense in America would probably be still less. The following is the formula, as given by the inventors themselves:

Plaster of commerce, reduced to a fine powder, 100 parts; coal tar, one to three parts. The mixture of the two substances is effected with ease by the aid of a mortar, or by any other appropriate mechanical means. The application of this composition to the dressing of sores or wounds requires a particular preparation. A certain quantity of the powder, prepared according to the formula, is diluted with olive oil to the consistency of a paste or ointment. This species of paste or salve is of a dark-brown color, has a slightly bituminous odor, and may be kept in a closed jar for an indefinite period. The oil unites the powder without dissolving it, and the composition has the property of absorbing infectious liquids the instant it is applied to the sore which produces them. The application may be mediate or immediate. In the latter case, that is to say, placing the composition directly in contact with the sore, no pain whatever is produced; on the contrary,

49

the salve has a detersive action, cleanses the sore and favors circulation.

In the course of his remarks, M. Velpeau mentioned the case of a
patient at the Charité, to whom the new process had been applied,
with perfect success. This person was afflicted with a frightful abscess
in the thigh, from which exuded a purulent matter of a most infectious
odor, rendering the operation of the surgeon both painful and difficult.
This matter, mixed with a powder held in readiness by the two experi-
mentalists, was disinfected in one minute, touched with impunity by
the spectators, and applied beneath their noses, without leaving a trace
of unpleasant odor.

As has been seen, the elements of this composition are of the simplest character; and though intelligence of the discovery could not have
reached the medical faculty of the United States in advance of this
letter, your own surgeons will doubtless receive, by the same mail
which carries this, every corroborating particular. My desire is to
make known the event throughout our country, and I sincerely hope
this paragraph may be widely copied by your exchanges. As M.
Velpeau himself observed at the close of his observations before the
Academy, too much publicity cannot be given to so valuable a discovery, as well as the disinterestedness of its authors. In their own
report, Messrs. Crome and Demeaux state that the composition may
be applied in the form of a poultice, or on cotton, and laid on the
wound. They demonstrate that their mode of dressing possesses the
double property of disinfecting morbid products and of absorbing their
liquids. This last circumstance entirely obviates the necessity of lint
—which is one of the most important features of the discovery.—*N.
Y. Express.*

Attempted Abortion and Death from Introduction of Air into the Veins.

One of the most painfully familiar topics of our current medical experience arises from the familiarity and indifference with which the
large mass of community have come to regard the production of abortion; so that everywhere we hear the lament of the honorable physician,
of the unconcern with which he is consulted for this purpose by both
the unmarried female, who may be supposed to have the more anxious
solicitude to hide her shame, and alike the respectably wedded mother,
who has no such motive to afford a plausible pretext.

The danger which is associated with these attempts does not appear to be duly estimated even by the members of the profession, in many instances; and popularly a great many expedients, instrumental and medical, are used and regarded as perfectly innocent and harmless. Every now and then, however, we read of and observe sudden and almost inexplicable death to ensue in çases of this kind.

An instance in point fell under our observation within less than a year in this city. We were summoned, about 11½ o'clock, P. M., (near midnight,) to see a lady, and found her already dead. Upon inquiry, and in the subsequent details of the coroner's inquest, it transpired that she, although a happy wife and mother, had determined not to allow any further additions to be made to her nursery cares. Finding herself, therefore, pregnant, she had consulted one of those dames reputed to be skilled in such matters, and had held repeated private interviews with her for a number of days before her decease. The night of her death, her husband was engaged away from home until about 11 o'clock. The servant-girl remained up until after 10 o'clock. The husband arrived at home at 11, and found his wife deceased and the girl and children asleep. Certain instruments were found about the person of the deceased, which indicated that she had made an attempt to throw up a strong stimulating injection into or about the mouth of the uterus. What she actually did is, however, left in some conjecture, but death must have been very suddenly produced, considering the brief time in which she was left alone, and in view of the fact that the girl in the next room was unawakened.

It will be a happy time when this truth shall become impressed upon the popular mind, that whenever a woman places herself in the hands of "abortion procurers," she positively runs the risk of her life in every instance.

The following case, reported by Dr. John Swinburne, of Albany, N. Y., and which we copy in full from the *Medical and Surgical Reporter*, is in point, and affords some especial light upon the character of danger in these cases, and how death may ensue, and very suddenly:

Miss M. A. S., aged twenty-three, unmarried, was admitted to the house No. 40 Franklin Street, for the purpose of having an abortion procured, on or about the thirteenth of March.

It is ascertained that attempts were made from day to day to rupture the membranes with a blunt steel instrument. These efforts only produced slight inflammation, softening, and partial separation of the membranes and placenta.

On the evening of the twenty-sixth of March, Dr. J. H. Case was summoned in haste to the above-mentioned house, where he found that the young woman had just died. An examination before the Coroner's jury the next morning elicited, among other testimony, the following statements:

Dr. J. A. Case sworn: Knows Mrs. Masten; was called to attend a patient at her house about six months ago; her given name is Oscillea; her ostensible business is an astrologist. The patient whom I visited six months ago was a young woman; she had inflammation of the womb. Was called by Miss Curry last night at 9 o'clock; said that Mrs. Masten wanted I should call as soon as possible, that a lady there had fainted and was very sick; went to 40 Franklin Street, and found Mrs. Masten on the walk; she said she was glad I had come, as the woman was very bad, and she was afraid she was dead; she said it was only an india-rubber that she was using, and that the deceased fell right back dead. Found a body lying on the bed very pallid, and dead to all appearances; Mrs. M. did not go in with me; thought it might be a case of suspended animation; gave her some stimulants, but they did her no good—she was dead; told Mrs. M. so, and she said, " Oh, Doctor, what shall I do ?" The girl Curry then said, wringing her hands, " What shall we do ?" I told Curry that they could do nothing with her; Mrs. Masten said to her, " No, I am to blame; I shall have to stand it." She again asked me what she must do; advised her to throw herself upon the mercy of the law; she asked me if I didn't think it best for her to try and escape; told her that it would be impossible if she undertook it; she also said it was a bad time for her, as she had no time to fight it out or money to escape; but that she expected some on Monday, and if she had that she would clear right out in half an hour; she again repeated that she didn't know how deceased came to die, as she could show me the instrument, and that it couldn't hurt her; went into the bed-room again, and another young lady said she thought deceased was reviving; wanted me to try and revive her; Mrs. Masten turned down the bedclothes and produced a gutta-percha catheter. [The article was produced and identified.] She said that was the instrument she used, and that it could not hurt her; also, that it wasn't the one she generally used; that it was milder, and the girl's death surprised her; that while using it the patient, as she thought, fainted away; that she tried to fetch her to, and failing, had sent for me; think it was about nine o'clock when I got to her house; don't think that over fifteen minutes had elapsed until I saw the deceased, after being called. Mrs. Masten indirectly asked me to loan her money to escape with; I found three or four young girls in the house when I first got there; one of them said that she had got through with her troubles, and that she thought it best for her to get away as soon as possible; asked her if she was able, and Mrs. Masten said she was all right; suppose, from what I saw and heard, that all the young ladies were "in trouble;" think I know one of the young ladies I saw there; believe I prescribed for her some time since.

Assisted by Charles H. Porter, Professor of Chemistry, Dr. C. P. Staats, and my students, Messrs. Mosier and Covel, I made a *post-mortem* examination fourteen hours after death. The following detailed description is given for the benefit of medical readers:

External appearances of body natural, but very pallid. On cutting through the integuments into the cellular tissues, air was observed to issue from the divided veins in the form of a frothy fluid. On exposing the heart, its right cavities were found to be greatly distended with a spumous mixture of blood and air, and slight compression of the heart was seen to force out bubbles of air from the divided intercostal veins. A thorough examination showed that the jugulars, and the veins emptying into them, even to the small vessels of the brain, were all distended with air.

The uterus was found to be of a dark livid or maroon color at its lateral portions, and its veins and sinuses were so fully distended with air, as to give it the appearance of a bag of angle-worms. The sensation communicated to the touch was analogous to that of varicocele, with the exception that in the latter the tissues are soft and distended with liquid, whereas in the case of this uterus the presence of air was unmistakably manifested by its characteristic crepitus when the vessels were compressed by the finger.

The membranes of the ovum were entire, and contained a normal amount of amniotic liquor, and an apparently healthy female fœtus of about five months' growth, presenting no appearance of decomposition, nor any change to indicate death of the fœtus at any period long prior to that of the mother.

On the internal surface of the membranes was a slight exudation of lymph, as from inflammatory action. Externally they were separated from the womb on its right latero-posterior surface, as was also the placenta in part. Beneath the lower border of the latter was an effusion of blood in the form of several small coagula. The os and cervix were open to the extent of two lines, and filled with bloody mucus.

On examining the membranes and their contents, the internal surface of the womb exhibited the following appearances: 1. Slight softening of the tissues; 2. Several abrasions, evidently not natural; 3. A perforation communicating directly with the uterine sinuses, about two inches from the cervix, and in the right latero-posterior region. This opening communicated directly with the veins of the broad ligament, and thus with the ascending cava. The direction of the perforation was parallel with the longitudinal axis of the uterus. All the other organs of the body were in a perfectly healthy condition.

These *post-mortem* appearances, conjoined with the description of the young woman's death, cannot be accounted for by any other cause than that of " air in the veins." Death occurred while the instrument was in the uterus, and was *immediate*, for the woman mistook *death* for *syncope*.

The point of interest in this case is as to the *manner* in which the air was introduced. Several deaths have been reported from ingress of air into the large veins of the neck, and even the subclavian is liable to the same thing under favorable circumstances, such as tension upon the vein from the subject's position during surgical operations, or by traction upon a tumor during excision, the vein being temporarily *canalized*, or prevented from collapsing.

Under all circumstances this canalization of a vein, or its conversion into a rigid tube, is the indispensable condition requisite for the intrusion of air. But this condition is inadmissible in the case of the uterine veins and ascending cava, from the nature of physical laws which govern the movements of the fluids in the body, no less than in inorganic matter.

In the twenty-second volume of *Braithwaite's Retrospect*, on page three hundred and nine, will be found an article by Dr. J. R. Cormack, in which is discussed the possibility of introduction of air into the venous system through the medium of the uterine veins immediately after parturition. He instances the experiments of Legallois upon animals, whereby that author became satisfied of the possibility of the intrusion of air in this way, and by analogy conjectured that many cases of death in the human subject might be accounted for in a similar manner.

He also quotes from Dr. Simpson, of Edinburgh, who reports an autopsy of the body of a female who died after delivery, where the entrance of air through the uterine veins was conjectured to be the cause of death. The examination, conducted carefully, so as to exclude all apparent sources of error, resulted in the discovery that the lower cava, hypogastric, and uterine veins were distended with frothy blood and air.

Dr. Simpson also explains the manner in which air might be forced into the veins by the contraction of the uterus after having been filled with air, which is not seldom the case. This organ being distended with air, the os tincæ being closed either by its own sphincter or by a coagulum of blood; the uterine veins being large and patulous, and the forcible contraction of the organ—these furnish, in his opinion, the mechanism capable of accomplishing the fatal accident. (See *Braith-waite's Retrospect*, xix., page 262.) In the present case no such conditions are furnished, and throwing aside the hypothesis of spontaneous ingress, we are compelled to fall back upon the presumption that the abortionist forcibly inflated the entire venous system, by means of the catheter introduced into the uterus, perforating its parietes, and in contact with the lacerated vessels of that organ. And this presumption is strengthened by the fact that the opinion prevailed, at the time of the coroner's inquest, that abortion might be produced by inflating the space between the membranes and the womb.

The fact of forcible inflation is incapable of proof, there being no third person present at the time of death, and hence no witness. Absolute certainty can only be arrived at from the confession of the guilty woman herself.—*Lancet and Observer.*

DR. J. M. SIMS AND HIS SILVER SUTURE.

[The following just and discriminating article on this subject is from the pen of Dr. Warren Stone, the eminent surgeon of New Orleans. It is extracted from a valuable paper by that gentleman, in the last number of the *N. O. Med. and Surg. Journal.*]

In this connection I will take occasion to express my sense of what is due to Dr. J. M. Sims, for introducing the silver ligature, as well as establishing a successful method of operating for vesico-vaginal fistula and analogous lesions, which is mainly due to the silver suture.

Up to the 'time Dr. Sims laid before the profession his mode of operating for vesico-vaginal fistula, it must be admitted that no successful mode of treatment had been established, and hundreds of females laboring under this most loathsome and painful affliction were left in hopeless misery. It is true that an occasional cure was effected under favorable circumstances, but these cases were rare exceptions to the general rule. Since the method of Dr. Sims has been adopted, all the bad cases that were formerly pronounced incurable are cured with great certainty. The attention of the profession was called a few years ago to the button suture of Dr. Bozeman, of Montgomery, Alabama, which, by many, is considered an improvement, and it has been quite generally adopted. It is not my object to discuss the merits of this improvement. Dr. Sims uses the plain interrupted suture, and no one operates with more success, I believe, than he does; but if others realize more favorable results by the button suture, than by the simple, it is their duty to adopt it. I see nothing in this improvement that detracts from the merits of Dr. Sims, however much it may redound to the credit and honor of the inventor. It would seem that Dr. Sims thought otherwise, and setting aside all his well-founded claims to merit, for his indomitable perseverance in inventing instruments, and simplifying the operation, he bases them entirely upon the introduction of the silver suture. This he set forth in a paper he read before the New York Academy of Medicine, in which he may have indulged in some pardonable egotism, and unfortunately brought forward personal matters that belonged to him and Dr. Bozeman alone. This gave the friends of Dr. Bozeman (who seemed to have been sharp critics) an excuse for a severe criticism, and they not only ridiculed his paper, but his claim to the discovery of the silver suture. Although there was in these criticisms an affectation of rendering some undefined merit to Dr. Sims, the effect with strangers was calculated to do him great injustice. It was urged (and with truth, it must be admitted,) that the silver and other metallic sutures were known long since. Dr. Levert, of Mobile, made experiments as long ago as 1828, and published the results (which were highly favorable) in the *American Journal of Medical Sciences* of that year, but no one acted upon the principle thus established.

When a principle is put to practical use, if it is important, many aspirants spring up for the honor of the discovery. Dr. Simpson, of Edinburgh, on reading the discourse of Dr. Sims, was reminded that he had read somewhere the report of a successful case operated upon in which the silver suture was used. He instituted a correspondence on the subject, and finally found that it was reported in a London journal in the year 1835. Dr. Simpson is a very ingenious man, and ready to adopt any improvement that gives promise of value, but this case passed him unnoticed, and would in all probability never have been thought of again if he had not read the discourse of Dr. Sims. The remarks of Sidney Smith, in the defence of Hamilton, who established a system of education, when the critics denied the originality of the system, are very appropriate. He says, "Whether Hamilton is or is not the inventor of the system that bears his name, or what his claims to originality may be, are questions of very second-rate importance; but they merit a few observations. That man is not the first discoverer of any art, who first says the thing; but he who says it so long, so loud, and so clearly that he compels mankind to hear him. The man who is so deeply impressed with the importance of the discovery that he will take no denial, but, at the risk of fortune or fame, pushes through all opposition, and is determined that what he has discovered shall not perish for the want of a fair trial. Other persons had witnessed the effect of coal gas in producing light; but Windsor worried the town with bad English for three winters before he could attract any serious attention to his views. Many persons broke stone before Macadam, but Macadam felt the importance of the discovery more strongly, stated it more clearly, persevered in it with greater tenacity, wielded his hammer, in short, with greater force than other men, and finally succeeded in bringing his plan into general use."

When Civiale brought before the profession of Paris his admirable surgical operation, called lithotrity, the critics attempted to write him down, and denied that the process of breaking down stone in the bladder was a new invention. After having proved that he was not the inventor of his instruments, they attempted to show that the instruments themselves were detestable, and further, that Civiale did not know how to use them. Civiale, however, was happy in his associations. The eminent Chaussier and Percy concluded their report upon the subject of Lithotrity to the Academy of Science, in these words: "Lithotrity is glorious for French surgery, honorable to its inventor, and consoling to humanity;" and a writer, in reply to these critics, who would deprive Civiale of the merit of originality, says: "In effect, the only true proprietor of a surgical improvement is he who applies it successfully, all theoretical reasonings and the cavilings of chronologists to the contrary notwithstanding."

Whether Dr. Sims bases his claims for distinction upon his indomitable perseverance under repeated failures and disappointments, ill health and other impediments, in endeavoring to establish the curability of vesico-vaginal fistula, or merely upon the introduction of the silver suture, as embracing the whole merit, he is clearly entitled to it, and these just acknowledgments no more detract from the merit of those who have made valuable improvements, than those improvements detract from the merits of the original inventor.

I have made these few remarks in justice to the profession, rather than from any partiality for any individual member. Whatever an individual member may do that redounds to his honor, sheds a proportionate lustre upon the whole profession, and nothing detracts from it so much as our own bickerings and injustice to each other.

* * *

[From the Nashville Medical Journal.]

DR. BUTLER AND THE MEDICAL REPORTER.

" UNFAIR."

Under this caption, the *Medical and Surgical Reporter*, of Philadelphia, makes much ado about the republication of a Philadelphia newspaper article on the medical classes of that city last winter, in the New York *Medical Press*, New York MEDICAL GAZETTE, and finally the Nashville *Journal of Medicine and Surgery*. He says it was very unfair to republish that newspaper article, without at the same time republishing his editorial effort at a refutation. Our friend has very singular ideas of "fairness." We did him the justice, as did the AMERICAN MEDICAL GAZETTE, to say that he contradicted it, and this was an extension of courtesy for which any reasonable man would have been grateful. Had not the journals, any of them, a perfect right to reprint what a newspaper editor said about students of medicine in Philadelphia, or anywhere else, without attaching to it what Dr. Butler, or any one else, chose to say about it in his journal? This gentleman certainly attempts the inauguration of a new dogma in the metaphysics of fairness.

The case stands thus: A Philadelphia newspaper, speaking of the medical students there last winter, says:

" Their education, it must be allowed, is (in the majority of cases) neither finished nor respectable. They will pardon us for so severe a statement, but we make it because it is true—we make it because it ought not to be true, and because we wish to do them some good. It is true. A visit to the lecture-rooms of our colleges will prove it to be true. What description of young men are to be seen in these places? The roughest we ever saw in our lives. Most of them have a Texan Ranger look. Nobody in the world would pronounce them to be refined, liberally-endowed young gentlemen. Hair as long as that of a savage, moustaches as fierce as the whiskers of a tiger, a reckless expression of the eye, a long, shuffling, clumsy gait, sword-canes, dirk-knives, revolvers, attire very unfashionably made, hard swearing, hard drinking, coarse language, cigars, tobacco quids, and pools of tobacco spittle, are too prominent barriers for the formation of so flattering a judgment. The picture is not overdrawn. We might make it a great deal less flattering, and then we would be absolutely true."

The *Reporter* copies it, and comments upon it in a manner to suit itself. We copied it, and commented upon it in a manner highly satisfactory to us at the time, and since, as we have reason to know, eminently satisfactory to a host of others. This, the *Reporter* says, is very unfair, for in fairness we ought to have copied his reply. Why, it was public property: a newspaper publication that we had just as much right to as Dr. Butler, and we were under no more obligation to quote his comments upon it than he is to quote ours. So unfair does Dr. B. consider it, that he has to dive down deep in the mud to hunt up a motive for it. It can't be, he thinks, that we are prompted by personal hostility. No, that won't do. He cannot believe that he is personally offensive. It must be something else. It must, he thinks, " BE JEALOUSY OF THE MARKED SUCCESS OF THIS JOURNAL." ! ! !

Now we ask Dr. Butler, in all soberness, if he does believe that we are jealous of the marked success of his journal? Our conscience bears us witness that we were as ignorant of such "marked success" as an unborn child. That could not, therefore, had we been the most jealous of mortals, have been the cause for reprinting a newspaper article concerning medical students, without Dr. Butler's comments. We have shown that we were not unfair to Dr. Butler, or any one else, in republishing a newspaper article that was no more to him than to us, and to which we had as much right as he. Had the publication anything to do with him or his, the matter would have assumed another aspect, and his comments, in justice to him, ought to have gone along with the republication. But it had no reference to him, whatever, and his attaching himself to it no more constituted him a part of it, than the fixedness of a bur in a sheep's tail constitutes it a part of the sheep. We have never even read Dr. Butler's comments.

We have shown that had we been unfair in not copying his comments in a newspaper article—that every one except himself knows he had better never have commented on at all, and which no other Philadelphia editor, *from some cause*, did comment upon—that we could not have been influenced by "*jealousy of the marked success*" of the *Reporter*, because that startling fact was positively unknown to us at that time.

But these absurdities, gross as they are, are only introductory to still greater blunders, in this editorial of the *Reporter*. He speaks of "the meanness which has led them" (the New York journals and ours) "to convey the impression through their pages that *we* circulated a vile slander against the medical students that attended lectures here last winter." But did we, though, Dr. Butler? And if we did not, is it not a pitiful "meanness" in you to say so? And in saying so, if it is untrue, did you not, in its utterance, "circulate a vile slander" against medical gentlemen? The charge is, that we conveyed the impression through our pages, that the editor of the *Reporter* circulated a vile slander in the form of the above newspaper article, against medical students at Philadelphia last winter. Now, the AMERICAN MEDICAL GAZETTE said concerning this newspaper article—and we quoted every word of it—that "The editor of the *Reporter is very indignant at this onslaught on the students*, and insists that they are A VERY WORTHY CLASS OF YOUNG MEN." (The italics and capitals are ours.) Now, with this staring him in the face, what is to be thought of the candor and manliness of the editor of the *Reporter*, to charge upon us the "meanness" of conveying the impression through our pages that *he* had circulated a slander against the students? We are not in the mood just now of bandying epithets, nor shall we; but unless Dr. Butler has sold himself, body and soul, to an interest he supposes we may possibly damage, and has degenerated from a high-toned medical editor into a whining and yelping partisan scavenger, he will take back this charge of "meanness" against us; and if he does not do so, we politely beg him to consider the above from us as standing charges against him.

But this gentleman, in the very blaze and smoke of his blunderbuss, between her "operations"—vulgarly called "*discharges*"—takes time audibly to eulogize her own omnipotence and integrity. "We have the consolation," says he, "of knowing that we occupy the vantage-ground over them all, by reason that OUR EXTENSIVE CIRCULATION in the West, South, and North gives us an opportunity of reaching a large portion of their readers, and exposing their meanness," &c. Well, did you not also occupy the vantage-ground over that newspaper editor, by reason of your extensive circulation in beer-cellars, tap-rooms, and canal-boats, and thus securing you an opportunity of reaching his readers, and exposing his meanness? And if you had not, for what purpose did you follow him?

The vantage-ground of us all by reason of his extensive circulation! That is talking tolerably loud for a two-year-old next spring. We went once, when we were less pious than we are now, to see the farce of the mummy, where an artificial mummy, provided for the occasion, is placed beside a real one.

> "The coffins stand like open presses,
> And show the dead in their last dresses."

The stage being clear, the live mummy pokes his head round the edge of his coffin in the most quizzical manner, and a just-between-you-and-me air, and asks his brother mummy, "How much does yer git fur being uv a mummy?" So, when we remember how gallantly our young friend bore himself on the decks of the *New Jersey Reporter*, which under his guidance won an enviable national reputation, mindful alone of the great interests of the medical profession, beyond and above the dirty waters of medical school politics, and see him now in a fishing smack, befogged in the murky atmosphere of the Schuylkill, doing for others what they consider a condescension to do for themselves, while the whole benefit, if any, inures to them, and uttering great swelling words, as "vantage-ground," "West, South, and North," "extensive circulation," "jealousy of our marked success," etc., etc., being ourself an old medical campaigner, and slightly up to snuff, the temptation becomes irresistible to make the inquiry, "Brother, how much do you get for being a mummy?"

HOW IS IT?

The editor of the Philadelphia *Medical and Surgical Reporter* says he is "the second oldest medical editor in the United States, our senior being Dr. Isaac Hays, the veteran editor of the *American Journal of Medical Sciences*."

In the *New Jersey Medical Reporter* for February, 1854, its editor, Dr. Joseph Parrish, says, "The name of S. W. Butler, M.D., appears for the first time upon the title-page as editor." He says Dr. Butler had "proved himself worthy of the confidence and gratitude of the profession, by his unwearied toil as publisher. As he has succeeded in this department so far beyond the expectations of the friends of the *Reporter*, we hope he may excel in the editorship. We bespeak for the new editor a hearty support from the profession."

In the same number of the *Reporter*, Dr. Butler says, in a very handsome salutatory, " Promises the subscriber has none to make. If, in his hands, the *New Jersey Medical Reporter* shall continue to be worthy the support of the profession, as it has been under the editorial conduct of his predecessor, he will confidently *expect* that support," etc.

How, with these published facts before him, Dr. Butler can say he has been an editor for nine years, we cannot perceive. Dr. Butler has been an editor less than six years, while we were in the editorial harness in January, 1851. If Dr. Butler will insist that he is an older *man* than we, not a word in opposition shall escape us. We will yield that point to any one who claims it. Dr. Reese, of the AMERICAN MEDICAL GAZETTE, we think commenced his journal in 1850.—*Ib.*

[Yes. And this man Butler knew it! but his impudence and mendacity are alike unscrupulous. Nor will he now take back the falsehood, for it serves his purpose.]

RUSH MEDICAL COLLEGE—PROF. ALLEN.

[The following manly tribute to the newly-appointed professor at Chicago is merited, and yet reflects credit on its author, Dr. Gunn, of the *Peninsular Journal*.]

If the balance of the new appointments in Rush Medical College are as judicious as that of Prof. Allen to the Chair of Theory and Practice, the School will offer attractions of a very high order; and large classes will be likely to convene annually under the droppings of an institution which adopts the celebrated Rush as its patron saint. Prof. Allen was identified with the organization of the Medical Department of the University of Michigan, and for four years continued his labors in that institution. As a scientific lecturer, he is, in our judgment, unsurpassed; at least, it has never been our fortune to listen to his superior. His lectures are always strong, clear, and convincing. His style is terse and axiomic. Conceiving in his own mind a clear and definite idea of the subject under consideration, separating truth from error, and reducing facts to general philosophy, he never fails to present truth with a clear and bold outline, and in a highly assimilative form. His acquisition is fortunate for the Rush Medical College; and while we regret that Dr. Allen leaves Michigan, we can but commend the sagacity which secures his services, and express our sincerest wishes for his personal welfare.   G.

COMMUNICATIONS.

Is a Study of the Classics essential to the Physician?

"Si vacat, et placidi rationem admittitis, edam."—Juv.

The indispensable utility of a classical education to the attainment of the end of scientific progression is so manifest as to render almost untimely any comment, and to insure for the author of any remarks relative to this fact the distinction of having overstepped the bounds of legitimate duty. But when we consider the mutability of human affairs, and the obliterative tendency of the human intellect, it will be a pardonable presumption to state, that the few subjoined observations may start out into bold relief a truism, which would seem in the memories of many to be undergoing an oblivious process.

Its consideration not only appertains to every profession having for its avowed object the well-being of the community, but directs itself in a special manner to the members of that confraternity which justly prides itself on the number of successful encounters it has had with the legions of malady and death.

To the liberally educated the reason is obvious. For as Time, and the unerring sage, Experience, unremittingly teach that the development of the intellectual faculties is best promoted by a rigorous study of the Grecian and Roman exemplars, it would be a step from the sublime to suppose that the difficulties peculiar to each profession could be surmounted without a due knowledge of such models.

They invigorate and refine the mind; accustom it to habits of maturely deliberating; impregnate it with those philosophic principles which stamp the foremost celebrities of every age; and lavish upon it those excellences rarely to be met with in the offsprings of commercial instruction.

If these be the sources from which spring, in great measure, true greatness, and a portion of the fruits which complete the sum of human happiness, who than the physician needs more to explore them? The very nature of the functions he has to discharge, essentially requires it. His profession without it, "stat nominis umbra." Without it, how, in the name of reason, will he comprehend those physiological dogmas which are constantly absorbing the attention of the most astute intellects? Will he, without a proper classical training, moralize on subjects that cannot be developed but by those who, so to speak, identify themselves with philosophy? To imagine that a knowledge of them is spontaneously acquired, would be an insult to the understanding. It would be something akin to mental alienation, to expect solutions of the mighty problems interwoven with the physiology of the human fabric, from individuals unschooled in metaphysics, and strangers to that habit of logically reflecting, acquired only by the closest study of Athenian and Roman literature. If it require a philosopher to teach and explain philosophy, it no less requires the recipients of such instruction to be intimately acquainted with the writings of those who "waged the bloodless war of arts." Otherwise he might diligently, but with little avail, endeavor to controvert the moral of the adage, which advises the village master to employ his time more profitably by drilling a millstone with a sponge, towards striving to impart knowledge to a fossilized cerebrum.

So is it in the study of medicine, where nearly every function of the animal economy is a subject of philosophic analysis, and where every prescription *should* be the result of a philosophic examination. According to the tenor of recorded experience, where such is not the case, we perceive nothing but the grossest blundering; nothing but the veriest quackery.

The contemplation of man corporeal is one of the many subjects worthy the noblest efforts of the human intellect; and in proportion to the amount of natural endowments and classical attainments that is directed to the contemplation of the unnumbered phenomena blended in the human body, will be the instruction and pleasure derived therefrom. Hence the necessity of attending to the literature of remote eras, so conducive to the expansion of the mental faculties. It is to an unpardonable negligence in this department that the decadence of the medical profession, and the dearth of qualified physicians in this country, is to be imputed. Individuals endued with a very contracted share of intellectual ability, and yet that little void of anything like educational refinement, are indiscriminately admitted into our temples of medicine to "rack their brains for lucre, not for fame." Owing to this it is, and the oversight for which the instructors in our medical institutions are strictly amenable, that our profession has become a synonym for imposition, downright hypocrisy, and empiricism. Such persons, no matter how prolific of her bounties Nature may have been to them, are utterly incompetent to discharge those duties which absolutely need the joint aid of experience and erudition.

A radical reform is loudly called for—one that will stem the torrent of illiterate incumbents that annually flood our halls of medicine. The prolongation of human existence, so often sacrificed upon the altar of ignorance and injudicious medication, the inevitable and woeful consequences of a defective education, demand this from the medical association. And until such be effected, life will be in perpetual jeopardy, and the public still continue to be the victim of misplaced confidence.

The policy of such a reform needs not the deductions of reason. Inexorable time has long since suggested it, by pointing out the evils, now reaching a fearful magnitude, that accrue from the pernicious system that has heretofore regulated our medical establishments.

In proof of the marked deterioration of the profession in this country, we have but to glance abroad, where the standard of medical tuition is much higher. The system is more substantial, and the requirements of each candidate for Hippocratic honors are in accordance with the principles it embodies. In England, Ireland, and France, an adequate knowledge of the classics is a *sine quâ non*. So far, even, is this principle borne out, that the pharmaceutists are constrained to familiarize themselves with the defunct languages—an obligation to which must be mainly attributed the exceedingly rare occurrences of poisoning in those kingdoms.

No matter from what stand-point we view the subject, the necessity of classical instruction forces itself upon us with an equal momentum. No keen observer of human actions is needed to perceive at a glance the validity of the foregoing assertions. They enshrine living facts. Cast the eye whereon we will, the most imbecile intellect will not fail of discovering the leading men of every community, whether social, political, or religious, to be well grounded on the legitimate principles embodied in the classics; and it is worthy of note, that most of the luminaries of our profession have not only studied the unfading beauties of the ancient models, but have actually devoted a portion of their lifetime to a communication of the same to well-inclined students. Herein lies the secret of the success of such men. The mental superiority imparted to them by studying the classics enlarges their sphere of action, and compels the objects of their philanthropy and skill to

50

repose in them unbounded confidence. Enjoying the advantages of a liberal education, the acquirement of knowledge is facilitated; their sober judgments accumulate it, and their charity and discretion dispense it with a prodigality that elicits wonder and appreciation.

Feeling it, therefore, to be the sacred duty of every physician to secure and promote the welfare of his profession, nothing but a profound veneration for "peace and science" have elicited the preceding observations. That a thorough knowledge of ancient literature, which it should be the mission of every lover of the fine arts to disseminate, is essential to the advancement of every profession, and in particular to that of the healing art, must be evident to every unbiased and discerning mind. And till such be registered among the acquisitions demanded of each aspirant to Esculapian laurels, in vain may we fondle the hope that the ends of science are forwarded by a liberal profusion of medical honors on unqualified applicants.

To regain the wonted prestige of our profession in America, to behold with delight once more its pristine splendor, a rigid adherence to those principles upon which true science is founded and fostered must be observed. To derive benefit from any other policy, we might

——" as soon
Seek roses in December, ice in June."

GALEN.

EDITOR'S TABLE.

THE FREQUENCY OF SUICIDES.

A suicidal epidemic would seem to be widely prevalent all over our country, if we may judge by the recent multiplied instances reported through the public press. We have seen numerous attempts to point out its cause or causes, but none which indicate either the true source, or remedy for the shocking evil.

It is idle to assign *Insanity* as the cause of all suicides, as is often flippantly done by those who assume that no one in his senses ever commits this crime. Very many of the cases lately published detail unmistakable proofs to the contrary of this theory. In some, the reasons are assigned by the criminal which impel to the act, while a full recognition of its guilt is admitted in the plea made in mitigation. And this in terms which prove the party to have been possessed of his reason, and preclude all suspicion of irresponsibility, by its deliberate justification, and the pains taken to excuse the deed of blood in the minds of survivors.

Nor, indeed, will insanity, or any other physical disease, supposed to be increasing in the community, furnish an adequate source for the frequency of suicides, although individual instances have been thus occasioned; and it is important that this view of the evil should be impressed upon the public mind, if a preventive remedy is to be sought. Let it be conceded that excess in drinking ardent spirits, in smoking and chewing tobacco or opium, and other vices which shall be nameless, may produce physical disease, and thus result in suicidal mania; yet very many of the cases reported are exempt from any evidence to this effect, and, moreover, present infallible evidence that the source of the crime is a *moral,* and not a *physical* one, at all. The party was in good health, with *mens sana in sano corpore,* by every reliable test. But the deed is done, and its justification sought on the ground of the ills of life being no longer bearable, by reason of some calamity or bereavement; or the detection and exposure of concealed crime being dreaded; or the disappointment of some cherished hope; or the anticipation of poverty, and the like intolerable evils, whether real or imaginary.

These and the like causes will be found to characterize a very large proportion of suicides; and, as their source is in the *moral,* and not in the physical nature of man, the remedy is to be found in *moral* means, and prevention is the work of the pulpit and the press;—the philanthropist, and not the physician, is to be looked to for arresting this terrible crime against all laws, whether human or divine.

Thus far, we express what we believe to be worthy of all acceptation; but, in entering upon our own theory on the subject of causes and remedy, it becomes us to be more qualified in what we say, though our convictions on the subject have been formed after much observation and reflection. Others will estimate them at their true value.

We never saw, heard, or read of a deliberate suicide, who, at the time of committing the deed, left any evidence that he had any belief in a future state of rewards and punishments. But, on the contrary, in nearly all such cases we have ever known, the party had persuaded himself, on some theory, to believe that there was no accountability in the future world. One such, we knew, who left this record by his lifeless body, viz.:

"*I am nothing! God is nothing! I gò to nothing!*" this being, in fact, his cherished creed. Is it any marvel that he lived and died as he did, ending a life of crime, by his own hand, when exposure overtook him? Many others, and some of those in the avalanche of suicides, whose history has lately been reported, were in this category.

Will it be called cant or fanaticism to say of all such cases, that a settled belief in future accountability would have prevented suicide? If not, then the preventive remedy against this and other heinous crimes is the training up a generation in the full belief of future rewards and punishments in the next world; or, in other words, indoctrinating the whole people into the future accountability which is taught in the Christian revelation. This is the work of religion and philanthropy, and devolves upon the pulpit and the press. If Divine Wisdom and Goodness has revealed a future punishment to deter men from crime, it is because such revelation was necessary.

Happy is he, whose lifelong career has been guarded by an unshaken belief in his own accountability hereafter, for the deeds done in the body. He will never be a suicide, whatever other calamity may overtake him. They who teach the contrary sentiment, under any device, or on any pretext, have reason to fear the responsibility of multiplying suicides. For poverty, disappointment, misfortune, calamity, and calumny are the inheritance of so many of our race, that to escape from life and its burdens by suicide, in multiplied instances, would be the instinctive promptings of despair, if the grand redeeming idea of a future state, "another and a better world," did not assuage the anguish of a broken heart by the reflection that "earth knows no sorrows which heaven cannot heal." And even heathen morality taught that it is "better to bear the ills we suffer than rush to others that we know not of." Alas for the hapless suicide! neither ancient nor modern religion come to his aid, else the vision of a future state had stayed his hand and arrested his sad fate.

DR. S. W. BUTLER,

Senior editor of the *Medical and Surgical Reporter*, a weekly issue from Philadelphia, is so effectually disposed of and extinguished by Dr. Bowling, of the *Nashville Journal*, in the article we copy in this number, that we cannot find it in our heart to add to the infliction. Not even his recent provocation, libelous as it is, can tempt us to do more than to "leave him in the worst of all possible company—in company with himself!" "*Pauvre diable!*" said Uncle Toby to the fly.

OUR THREE MEDICAL COLLEGES

Are preparing for their usual winter session, the preliminary course having commenced, and the students beginning to congregate. The preparation for medical teaching in New York is this year more extensive than usual. The colleges are vying with each other in their arrangements for practical anatomy and clinical instruction, the points in which, especially, they are ambitious to excel. Preparatory schools and private teaching never before were so promising, and there is every indication that the superior advantages afforded in New York will attract a larger share of pupils than usual, and from the class of students who can appreciate the privilege of learning their profession in the largest city in the country, and profiting by the most numerous and extensive hospitals, infirmaries, and dispensaries to be found in America.

PROFESSIONAL QUARRELS.

It is not often that medical controversies result in any other or worse consequences than spilling ink, or defacing pure white paper with the perversion of type, for the purpose of assault or defence. In a recent instance at New Orleans, however, two of the brethren, viz., Dr. Choppin and Dr. Foster, both hospital surgeons so called, have so far forgotten themselves, as to attempt to kill each other with pistols, several shots having been fired on both sides, and this at the very door of the hospital. The former was dangerously wounded, while the latter escaped unhurt. The quarrel arose in relation to a patient upon whom both wished to operate with the scalpel, and in the scramble they concluded to operate on each other with revolvers and Derringers, for which surgery they seem to have prepared themselves. It cannot be that hospital surgeons, when on duty, go armed to the teeth, or that they carry pistols in their pocket-cases of instruments, as well as lancets. Such surgeons should be dismissed from any hospital, whether North or South, as unworthy of so high position, and we hope to hear that this penalty has been inflicted in this case.

DR. MARSH

May, after all, find it necessary to send on a small *advertisement* to Dr. Butler, of the *Medical and Surgical Reporter* of Philadelphia, by way of black mail. "Give that dog a bone," or he will never cease his barking.

QUARANTINE AFFAIRS.

These appear to be coming to a head. Since our last issue, the Physician to the Marine Hospital, Dr. Jerome, has provoked the Commissioners of Emigration, who have prayed the Governor to remove him—not from his *office*, but from his salary; the former having been abolished long since. Dr. Gunn, the Health Officer, has been hunting for the yellow fever all the summer, among persons and *fomites!* but with his deputies and Dr. Harris to help him, we have only heard of one death by yellow fever in 'the Marine Hospital; all the rest, which came up to the city and died here, being reported "typhoid and bilious remittent." *Vive la bagatelle!*

NEW YORK MEDICAL COLLEGE.

The preliminary course at this school was opened by Professor Carnochan with a lecture on Surgery, after which an operation of some magnitude was performed in the clinique. About 70 students are said to have been present, and as a month is to elapse before the opening of the regular course, this augurs well for the prospective class.

MR. ALEXANDER CUSHMAN

Announces, in this number of the GAZETTE, several of the Chemicals, and Pharmaceutical preparations, to the manufacture of which he is devoting very special attention. He is known to us as well skilled in every department of his profession, and, as a practical chemist, he has few superiors.

We have extensively used many of his preparations, especially his Syrup of the Superphosphate of Iron, which we have heretofore taken occasion to commend, and which we have proved to be a remedy of great efficiency. All his preparations will be found reliable, being made under his own supervision. Our medical brethren will find his establishment in Broadway and 22d Street, at the St. Germain Hotel, supplied with an ample stock in his line, and himself worthy of all confidence.

COLLEGE OF PHYSICIANS AND SURGEONS.

A course of lectures, by Dr. Cooper, on Medical Botany, has been in progress here, which is highly spoken of.

HYPOPHOSPHITES.

Whatever may be the estimate placed on Dr. Churchill's theory of the adaptation of this class of remedies to the cure of phthisis, yet all will be impressed with the importance of giving them a fair trial. The announcement of Mr. Winchester, in our advertising columns, will enable physicians to procure them, prepared strictly by Dr. Churchill's method, and thus test their value. Mr. Winchester is worthy of all confidence as a Chemist, and devotes himself enthusiastically to these preparations in all their variety of combinations,

DR. TAYLOR,

Whose advertisement is on the 4th page of our cover, is cultivating mechanical surgery, with special reference to the treatment of spinal curvatures. He claims to have had great success, and his instrument appears to us to promise more than any we have seen, in the relief of these intractable cases.

OPHTHALMIC HOSPITAL.

Dr. Stephenson, one of the surgeons of this institution, announces in this number his eighth course of lectures, improving the clinical opportunities for the benefit of students, as heretofore. The annual classes in attendance at these lectures continue to increase.

CONTENTS.

UNIVERSITY OF NEW YORK.
MEDICAL DEPARTMENT.
SESSION, 1859-60.

The Session for 1859–60 will begin on Monday, October 17, and will be continued until the 1st of March.

Faculty of Medicine.

Rev. Isaac Ferris, D.D., LL.D., Chancellor of the University.

Valentine Mott, M.D., LL.D., Emeritus Professor of Surgery and Surgical Anatomy, and ex-President of the Faculty.

Martyn Paine, M.D., LL.D., Professor of Materia Medica and Therapeutics.

Gunning S. Bedford, M.D., Professor of Obstetrics, the Diseases of Women and Children, and Clinical Midwifery.

John W. Draper, M.D., LL.D., Professor of Chemistry and Physiology, President of the Faculty.

Alfred C. Post, M.D., Professor of the Principles and Operations of Surgery, with Surgical and Pathological Anatomy.

William H. Van Buren, M.D., Professor of General and Descriptive Anatomy.

John T. Metcalfe, M.D., Professor of the Institutes and Practice of Medicine.

J. W. S. Gouley, M.D., Demonstrator of Anatomy.

J. H. Hinton, M.D., Prosector to the Professor of Surgery.

Alexander B. Mott, M.D., Prosector to the Emeritus Professor of Surgery.

Besides Daily Lectures on the foregoing subjects, there will be five Cliniques weekly, on *Medicine, Surgery, and Obstetrics.*

The Dissecting-room, which is refitted and abundantly lighted with gas, is open from 8 o'clock, A. M., till 10 o'clock, P. M.

Fees for a full course of Lectures, $105. Matriculation fee, $5. Graduation fee, $30. Demonstrator's fee, $5.

NEW YORK MEDICAL COLLEGE,
East 13th Street, near 4th Avenue.

The Tenth Annual Course of Lectures in this Institution will commence October 18th, 1859, and continue till the first week of March, 1860.

The Preliminary Course will begin September 19th, and continue till the opening of the Regular Course; during these four weeks *practical* instruction will be offered in important departments, to which the attention of students is particularly called.

FACULTY:

Horace Green, M.D., LL.D., President of the Faculty, and Emeritus Professor of Theory and Practice of Medicine, and Professor of Diseases of the Respiratory Organs.

Edwin Hamilton Davis, M.D., Professor of Materia Medica and Therapeutics.

R. Ogden Doremus, M.D., Professor of Chemistry and Toxicology.

J. M. Carnochan, M.D., Professor of the Principles and Operations of Surgery, with Surgical Pathology.

Edmund R. Peaslee, M.D., Professor of Obstetrics and the Diseases of Women and Children.

Henry G. Cox, M.D., Professor of Theory and Practice of Medicine and of Clinical Medicine.

Austin Flint, Jr., M.D., Professor of Physiology and Microscopic Anatomy.

James Bryan, M.D., Professor of Anatomy.

Carl T. Meier, M.D., Professor of Surgical Anatomy and General Pathology.

John Sedgwick, Esq., Counsellor at Law, Lecturer on Medical Jurisprudence.

M. Bradley, M.D., Demonstrator of Anatomy.

B. L. Budd, M.D., Assistant Lecturer on Chemistry.

S. Carey Selden, M.D., and S. Abrahams, M.D., Prosectors to the Professor of Surgery.

C. F. O. LANDIN, Janitor.

ALBANY MEDICAL COLLEGE.

One Course of Lectures will be given at this Institution annually, commencing the *first* Tuesday of *September*, and continuing sixteen weeks. Degrees will be conferred at the close of the term, and also after the Summer Examination in June.

PROFESSORS:

ALDEN MARCH, M.D., Professor of Principles and Practice of Surgery.
JAMES McNAUGHTON, M.D., Prof. of the Theory and Practice of Medicine.
JAMES H. ARMSBY, M.D., Professor of Descriptive and Surgical Anatomy.

HOWARD TOWNSEND, M.D., Prof. of Materia Medica and Physiology.
CHARLES H. PORTER, M.D., Prof. of Chemistry and Medical Jurisprudence.
J. V. P. QUACKENBUSH, M.D.,Prof. of Obstetrics and Diseases of Women and Children.

Fees for the full course, $65. Matriculation fee, $5. Graduation fee, $20.

Material for dissection abundant, and furnished to students on the same terms as in New York and Philadelphia. Hospital Tickets free. Opportunities for Clinical instruction are believed to be equal to those afforded by any College in the country. Price of Board from $2,50 to $3,50 per week.

JOHN V. P. QUACKENBUSH, Registrar.

UNIVERSITY OF NASHVILLE.

Medical Department.—Session 1859-60.—The Seventh Annual Course of Lectures in this Institution will commence on Monday, the 2d of November next, and continue till the first of the ensuing March.

THOMAS R. JENNINGS, M. D., Professor of Anatomy.
J. BERRIEN LINDSLEY, M. D., Chemistry and Pharmacy.
C. K. WINSTON, M. D., Materia Medica and Medical Jurisprudence.
A. H. BUCHANAN, M. D., Surgical Anatomy and Physiology.

JOHN M. WATSON, M. D., Obstetrics and the Diseases of Women and Children.
PAUL F. EVE, M. D., Prof. of Prin. and Prac. of Surgery.
W. K. BOWLING, M. D., Institutes and Practice of Medicine.
WILLIAM T. BRIGGS, M. D., Adjunct Professor and Demonstrator of Anatomy.

The Anatomical rooms will be opened for students on the first Monday of October, (the 5th.)
A *Preliminary Course* of Lectures, free to all Students, will be given by the Professors, commencing also on the first Monday of October.
The Tennessee State Hospital, under the direction of the Faculty, is open to the Class free of charge.
A Clinique has been established, in connection with the University, at which operations are performed and cases prescribed for and lectured upon in the presence of the class.
Amount of Fees for Lectures is $105; Matriculation Fee, (paid once only,) $5; Practical Anatomy, $10; Graduation fee, $25.
Good boarding can be procured for $3 to $4 per week. For further information or Catalogue, apply to

W. K. BOWLING, M.D.,

NASHVILLE, TENN., July, 1859. *Dean of the Faculty.*

CASTLETON MEDICAL COLLEGE.

There are two full Courses of Lectures annually in Castleton Medical College. The SPRING SESSION commencing on the last Thursday in February; the AUTUMNAL SESSION on the first Thursday in August. Each Course will continue four months. Degrees are conferred at the close of each term.

WM. P. SEYMOUR, M.D.,Prof. of Materia Medica and Therapeutics.
WILLIAM SWEETSER, M. D., Prof. of Theory and Practice of Medicine.
E. R. SANBORN, M. D., Prof. of Surgery.
WM. C. KITTRIDGE, A. M., Prof. of Med. Jurisp.

CORYDON LA FORD, M. D., Prof. of Anatomy.
P. D. BRADFORD,M.D.,Prof. of Phys. & Pathol.
GEORGE HADLEY, M. D., Prof. of Chemistry and Natural History.
ADRIAN T. WOODWARD, M. D., Prof. of Obstetrics.

FEES.—For Lectures, $50; for those who have attended two Courses at other Colleges, $10; Matriculation, $5; Graduation, $16; Board from $2.00 to $2.50 per week.

A. T. WOODWARD, M.D., Registrar.

CASTLETON, VT., *Jan.*, 1859.

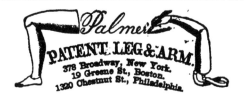

Palmer
PATENT LEG & ARM.
378 Broadway, New York.
19 Greene St., Boston.
1320 Chestnut St., Philadelphia.

"In the *mechanical compensation of lost parts, this admirable mechanism deserves particular notice,* combining lightness and A SUCCESSFUL IMITATION OF THE MOTIONS OF THE NATURAL LEG."— *World's Fair, London,* 1851. Award, PRIZE MEDAL.

WM. LAWRENCE, ESQ., } London.
JOSEPH H. GREEN, ESQ., } London.
M. ROUX, } Paris.
M. LALLEMAND, } Paris.
Surgeons and Judges.

"By a peculiar arrangement of the joint, it is rendered little liable to wear, *and all lateral or rotary motion is prevented.* . It is hardly necessary to remark, that *any such motion is undesirable in an artificial leg, as it renders its support unstable.*"—*Committee on Science and Art, Franklin Institute, Philadelphia.* DR. RAND, Chairman.

Palmer's Artificial Arm

is a new, beautiful, light and useful substitute for a lost arm, imitating closely the natural hand and arm, and performing every office which an artificial appliance can.

MESSRS. PALMER & CO. have a new, light and useful appliance, made to imitate the natural limb, for elongating limbs shortened by diseased hip, &c., (Pott's disease,) instead of the cumbrous shoes and stirrups commonly used.

Pamphlets containing valuable information, reports, testimonials, references, etc., sent gratis to all who apply to

PALMER & CO., 378 Broadway, N. Y.

Since the last number of the "*Bane and Antidote*" was issued, we have received two American Patents—one for the Arm, the other for the Forearm or Hand. We have also been honored with several valuable letters from eminent surgeons and men of scientific attainments, and numerous flattering reports from ladies and gentlemen wearing these Patent limbs.

The reception these inventions have met is most encouraging, while their utility, as voluntarily set forth by the wearers, exceeds their fondest anticipations and *our own.*

We have already received several hundreds of applications, and persons desiring limbs should have their names registered at the studio immediately, if they would be supplied within six months. We deem it important to mention these facts, as applicants will be required to exercise a little patience till we can enlarge our means of supplying, so as to meet the requirements of such an unexampled demand.

The letters from persons wearing the arm and hand are very flattering; some of them being written in terms of praise so extravagant that we have to make some allowance for the fact that they were written in those first days of joy and gratitude, when the writers felt the liveliest appreciation of the benefits conferred upon them. We never ventured to hope for such utility in a false arm as these letters indicate. One gentleman, O—— V——, Esq., of Illinois, whose arm is applied below the elbow, informs us that, although his *left* hand is the artificial one, he has with it "written some letters" to his relatives (in New Hampshire,) "to show them what he can do," and states that he "would not part with it for the best farm in Illinois." Another, P—— B—— S——, Esq., (son of a distinguished Ex-Governor of Virginia,) whose arm was amputated *very near the body,* makes an equally gratifying report, though he cannot, of course, use the arm with the same facility. Several ladies have given similar pleasing accounts of their success in using the inventions.

The Patent Arm and Hand are therefore no longer *experiments,* but useful substitutes for the fairest mechanism of nature, giving, in every articulation and shape, as well as in delicacy of appearance, a very perfect imitation of the original member, both in form and motion.

Full particulars given by letter. Address,

B. FRANK. PALMER,

Surgeon-Artist, Inventor, &c.
Philadelphia.

DR. McMUNN'S ELIXIR OF OPIUM.

THIS IS THE PURE AND ESSENTIAL EXTRACT FROM THE NATIVE DRUG.

It contains all the valuable medicinal properties of Opium in natural combination, to the exclusion of all its noxious, deleterious, and useless principles, upon which its bad effects depend. It possesses all the sedative, anodyne, and antispasmodic powers of Opium.

To produce sleep and composure. To allay convulsions and spasmodic action.
To relieve pain and irritation, nervous excitement and morbid irritability of body and mind, &c.

And being purified from all the noxious and deleterious elements, its operation is attended by

No sickness of the stomach, no vomiting, no costiveness, no headache,
Nor any derangement of the constitution or general health.

Hence its high superiority over Laudanum, Paregoric, Black Drop, Denarcotized Laudanum, and every other opiate preparation.

In consequence of the exclusion of those deleterious principles from the Elixir of Opium, it is not liable to derange the functions of the system, and will be found invaluable for all cases in which the long-continued and liberal use of opiates is indicated and necessary to allay pain or spasmodic action, and induce sleep and composure, as in cases of fractures, burns, scalds, cancerous ulcers, and other painful affections.

The Elixir of Opium is greatly superior to Morphine,

1. In its containing all the active medicinal virtues of Opium in native combination, and in being its full representative; while Morphine, being only one of its principles, cannot alone, and that in an artificial state of combination, too, produce all the characteristic effects of so triumphant a remedy, when several of its other valuable principles are excluded.

2. In its effects, the Elixir is more characteristic, permanent, and uniform, than any of the *artificial compounds* of Morphine.

3. And as a *Preparation*, it is not liable to decompose or deteriorate like the *Solutions* of Morphine; and thus is obviated a serious objection, which has prevented the latter from being used with precision and effect.

To speak summarily, the Elixir of Opium, as a remedy, may be adopted in all cases in which either Opium or its preparations are administered, with the certainty of obtaining all their salutary and happy effects, without being followed by their distressing and pernicious consequences.

The following letter from Dr. Reese fully confirms the above, and commends itself to the attention of the profession and the public:

NEW YORK, *January* 11, 1859.

Messrs. A. B. & D. SANDS: *Gentlemen*—I have been familiar with the history of the "Elixir of Opium" from the time it was first introduced to the profession by Dr. McMunn, and have continued to prescribe the same in public and private practice since he disposed of his interest in it to you in 1841. Of its value, and the purity of the drug from which it is prepared, the best evidence is found in its wide-spread popularity and use among the profession in our own and other countries, and in all our civil and military hospitals, in which it has become a standard article. It is now prescribed by physicians and surgeons everywhere, when the positive medication of Opium is indicated, without the drawbacks in certain pathological conditions involving the nervous system, by idiosyncrasy or otherwise, which are inseparable from the ordinary spirituous or vinous Tinctures, or the salts of Morphia. Its extended use has led to the introduction of spurious imitations, against which you have done well to guard the profession and the public. The fact that the pharmaceutical journals have so frequently proposed and announced "substitutes" for McMunn's Elixir of Opium, and published so many formulæ for its officinal imitation, is the very highest attestation to the merits of the article as prepared by you. Knowing as I do its merits, I most cordially express my desire that its remedial virtues may be more extensively known.   Yours, respectfully,

D. MEREDITH REESE, M.D., LL.D.,

Late Vice-President of the American Medical Association; Resident Member of the New York Academy of Medicine; Editor of the American Medical Gazette, &c.

☞ NOTICE.—A. B. & D. SANDS having purchased of Dr. McMunn all his right, title and interest in this article, and having been the sole Proprietors since 1841, and by whom it has been prepared during that period, respectfully inform dealers and consumers that no Elixir of Opium will hereafter be genuine, unless having their signature on the outside wrapper; and all orders from the "Trade" must be addressed, as heretofore, to A. B. & D. SANDS, Wholesale Druggists, 141 William Street, corner of Fulton, New York.

SOLD ALSO BY DRUGGISTS GENERALLY.

AMERICAN
MEDICAL GAZETTE.

| Vol. X. | DECEMBER, 1859. | No. 12. |

ORIGINAL DEPARTMENT.

A Philosophical Argument against the Contagiousness of Yellow Fever.

DR. REESE—Among the various proofs which have been alleged against the contagiousness of yellow fever, during the recent discussion of that question, there is one which is worth all the rest, and that one forms the subject, particularly, of Dr. Griscom's paper which was read at the last meeting of the New York Academy of Medicine, and published in the AMERICAN MEDICAL GAZETTE for November. I quite agree with Dr. Griscom that the argument is *conclusive*, but do not agree with him as to its *origin*, or that what he himself has said has not been published before. The idea was originally suggested by Dr. Miller, who is quoted to that effect by Professor Paine, in his *Medical and Physiological Commentaries*, (1840,) where it is developed by the latter, and reproduced in his *Institutes of Medicine*, (1847.) The conclusiveness of the argument is such, that I shall substantiate my statement as to the matter of priority by submitting to your readers the following parallel columns, and leave to them such other conclusions as the parallels may suggest:

DR. PAINE's *Institutes*, 1847.	DR. GRISCOM's *Paper*, 1859.
After inculcating (as throughout the work) the great axiom that *like effects require like causes*, Prof. Paine goes on to say, that	Dr. Griscom remarks in his paper:
"Animal or vegetable poisons, if natural or healthy, are the product of natural organic actions; if morbid, they	" In the next place, I would present a single argument against the *possibility* of yellow fever being a contagious disease. This argument I have seen *alluded to only in two works*—that of Prof. Smith on Epidemics, and

56

are generated by diseased actions; if altered from the foregoing conditions, they are more or less the product of chemical decomposition. Since, also, every *specific* disease requires its *exact cause*, and as every cause of disease which is elaborated by the living organism requires a certain precise state of the organic properties and functions for its production; or if more or less of a chemical nature, it has lost its natural peculiarities—it follows that the disease which is produced by a healthy animal or vegetable poison cannot be generated by a morbid one, and *vice versâ;* nor can a chemical product become the cause of a disease which is induced by poisons that are exclusively the product of organic action, as in *small-pox, measles,* yellow and typhus fevers, &c. And since *small-pox* is produced by a morbid organic product, and can never, therefore, arise from another cause, and can be alone propagated by contagion; so, also, as the foregoing fevers depend, in certain known instances, upon the products of *vegetable decay,* they can never be of a communicable nature. Nevertheless, other causes may predispose the body to the operation of the more specific predisposing agents, so that small-pox, measles, &c., may be unusually epidemic and malignant. Healthy animal poisons, therefore, are never generated by the diseased processes which they excite; but the morbid ones are *reproduced* by such processes, and by no other, and mostly by individuals of the same species; while the same law of individuality is universal as to healthy animal poisons.

"For the foregoing reasons, no contagious disease can ever be propagated by any other cause than such as is generated by that precise modification

that of Dr. La Roche on Yellow Fever, (1855,)—and yet, in neither, in my judgment, is the argument pushed so completely to its conclusion as it appears capable of being; and it seems, *to my mind, that had it been presented in its full effect, the mooted question might have* LONG AGO BEEN SETTLED. To understand fully the nature of the argument, we must first know the real meaning and application of the word *contagion,* as now generally received." —"Nowhere, probably, shall we find a more distinct and comprehensive definition of it than in the first four lines of the body of the work entitled 'Elements of the Etiology and Philosophy of Epidemics,' by J. M. Smith, M.D. This definition is in the following words:

"'Contagion is a poison generated by morbid animal secretion, possessing the power of inducing a like morbid action in healthy bodies, whereby it is *reproduced* and indefinitely multiplied.'"

"Applying this definition to certain well-known diseases—*small-pox,* for instance, or *measles,* or *scarlatina*— and we have a full and distinct comprehension of its different points. The virus of *variola,* whencever it came originally, responds completely to them all. It is a poison *reproduced* in and secreted by a *living,* not dead, or decomposed tissue. It is an animal, and not a vegetable production. Infused into a healthy body, it reproduces *small-pox et præterea nihil.*"

"Admitting the broad distinction thus drawn between these two sources of disease, contagion and infection— the one the product of living animal action, the other the result of the decomposition of dead animal or vegetable matter, or of both combined— can these two classes of poisons, so dis-

of the vital states which constitutes the essence of the disease. By the same inductive process, all those affections which have for their causes the products of laws which govern inorganic matter, can neither be regarded as contagious by the philosopher, nor shown to be so by the man who doubts everything but his senses. The laws of life and the laws of chemistry are as wide as the poles from each other. No organic action can form the chemical combinations of dead matter, nor can the forces of chemistry imitate the morbid any more than the healthy products of life.

"Since, therefore, miasmata produce yellow fever, plague, typhus, &c., it clearly follows that the *living* system, when affected by those diseases, cannot generate a poison capable of producing the same affection in others, since the poison depended ORIGINALLY upon *vegetable decomposition*."—PAINE'S *Institutes of Medicine*.

tinct in their chemical and physiological characteristics, produce the same results, when absorbed into the healthy body? Are they convertible influences?"

"It may be stated as a medico-etiological axiom, that two different and distinct causes cannot produce the same effect.

"Now, what is the original source of yellow fever? I say the original source—is it a secreted animal poison, generated by morbid animal action? On the contrary, it is universally accredited, even by the advocates of its contagious power, to a poison derived from vegetable 'putrefaction,' terrene exhalations, or both combined, aided and controlled by certain meteorological circumstances. If, then, it has no other origin than *vegetable putrefaction* or terrene exhalations, it cannot, according to the axiom before announced, have any other source; and, furthermore, admitting, for the sake of the argument, that a body laboring under yellow fever produces any secretion, or aura, or poison in any shape, (though this has never been proved,) that poison has a living animal, and not a dead vegetable origin, and it cannot produce the same disease as the *original* poison produced, and it must, therefore, if anything, produce something different from yellow fever, which is a *specific* disease, the result of one specific cause. *Quod erat demonstrandum*." — GRISCOM'S *Paper*, &c.

By publishing the foregoing in your December number, it will much oblige

Very truly yours,

"QUOD ERAT DEMONSTRANDUM."

[The article to which Dr. Cooper alludes having been published before the receipt of the following letter, we need only now insert the latter, which has been delayed on the route.]

SAN FRANCISCO, CAL., 30th Sept., 1859.

D. M. REESE, M.D., LL.D.:

Dear Sir—A short time since I sent you a communication headed (I think) "A New Mode of Curing Varicose Veins by Incisions, &c." Since that time, on examining more carefully the history of the operation, I find that Richerand and others have practiced the incisions on a still bolder score than is done by myself. I would have my communication headed thus: " On Incisions in the Treatment of Varicose Veins, &c."

The paper contains more extended views in regard to the after-treatment in operations for varicose veins than is found in the books, and may not, therefore, prove practically unimportant.

The practice of the method of Richerand was often attended with serious symptoms, and occasionally with fatal results, which I think was attributable to defective after-treatment.

I shall be much pleased if this reaches you in time for the correction named to be made, though the distance is so great I fear it may not.

We feel very much isolated here from the medical world, but would fain use our feeble efforts to the utmost extent to join our brothers abroad in their efforts to advance the cause of our noble profession.

Very respectfully yours,   E. S. COOPER.

A Case of Uterine Tumor weighing Twenty-one Ounces Removed by means of a Modification of the Ecraseur.

By E. S. COOPER, Prof. of Anatomy and Surgery in the Medical Department of the University of the Pacific, San Francisco.

The removing of large tumors attached to the uterus by means of the ligature is always exceedingly troublesome, and occasionally impracticable, when the tumor is not pedunculated; and in several instances I have known surgeons of some experience to abandon such cases as hopeless, because of the impossibility of removing them by ligature on the one hand, and the dangers of hæmorrhage from using the knife on the other.

Such would appear to have been the condition of the patient whose case I am about to relate, as four of our most prominent medical men in this city tried to remove a uterine tumor by the ligature, which was kept applied for seven weeks, until the patient became too much exhausted to permit further attempts at strangulation, without affecting either the size or hardness of the tumor to any great extent. Two years subsequently, the patient consulted me. She was very much debilitated in both mind and body, and desirous of having the tumor cut out at whatever hazard to her own life, but refused positively to submit again to a trial of the ligature.

Cutting it away I considered unjustifiably hazardous. In this dilemma, I concluded to try the *écraseur*. I could not succeed in throwing a metallic ligature around the tumor, and found great difficulty in doing so with a silken one in connection with the *écraseur* of Chassaignac, which, however, being finally accomplished, I attempted to detach it, but had not made the cord very tight before it was divided by the sharp edges at the eyelet-hole of the instrument.

Finding it impossible to succeed in this way, I ordered an instrument made according to the following plan: A straight shaft of about twelve inches long, connected with a curved extremity six inches long, curved to suit the shape of the inside of the pelvic bones.

The end of this, through which the eyelet-hole was made, instead of being flattened as in Chassaignac's instrument, was almost globular, with a corresponding hole through it, care being taken to have no sharp edges by which the ligatures could be cut in twain.

In all other respects, the instrument was made like that of Chassaignac's.

The instrument, being armed with a silken ligature about two lines in diameter, was introduced with ease by the side of the tumor.

It was, however, with much difficulty that I succeeded in throwing the ligature around the tumor, which, however, I finally succeeded in doing by the aid of a small whalebone rod perforated in the end, to which a small loop of twine was fastened, and through this the cord was carried entirely around the uppermost part of the tumor, which was then slowly separated from its place of attachment, after which I removed it by means of obstetrical forceps.

The patient was very comfortable immediately after the operation, and able to walk in three or four days. She recovered completely in less than two weeks. In fact, the rapidity of her recovery astonished every one.

No hæmorrhage occurred from first to last during the treatment, and not one untoward symptom of any kind.

There were present at the operation Drs. Atkinson, Hertell, Pitt, and McGrath, together with some medical students.

The tumor was fibrous and exceedingly solid, even for one of that class.

OUR PHILADELPHIA CORRESPONDENT.

No. 15.

"The profoundly wise do not declaim against superficial knowledge in others so much as the profoundly ignorant; on the contrary, they would rather assist it with their advice than overwhelm it with their contempt; for they know that there was a period when even a Bacon or a Newton were superficial, and that he who has a little knowledge is far more anxious to get more than he who has none."—COLTON.

DEAR GAZETTE—Having a little leisure, on account of the general healthy condition of the people in this beautiful month of October, I am occupying a few hours in perambulating the medical colleges of our city, to pick up a few notes for the GAZETTE. The first introductory of the season was delivered by the Professor of Institutes to a very respectable crowd of beardless and bearded boys, in the lower room of the mammoth Jefferson College. The usual amount of literary excellence, didactic ingenuity, and pleasing anecdote characterized this production of the eloquent professor and voluminous author.

The popular and eloquent Professor of Chemistry in the University dilated on the qualities and properties, real and fanciful, of the atmospheric air. "It was the cradle and the grave of all human beings." The Professor of Anatomy in the same school "was there to teach, the students were there to learn; and if they loved to learn as well as he liked to teach," they would mutually have a jolly old time. From this characteristic beginning the learned professor plunged immediately *in medias res,* or rather *in medias cellulas, monades, corpuscules, vibriones, fibrillas, et id genus omne corpusculorum minimorum.* In other words, a comparison was sketched between organic and inorganic molecules; the manner of classifying animals was given—man, of course, being placed at the head of creation, and at the tail. A running disquisition and a non-committal discussion was carried on on the old and vexed question (old as Lucretius!) of the spontaneous and genetic origin of living beings. The experiments of Cross, in England, and others in France and Germany, were balanced against each other, together with "my experiments," which seemed pretty decidedly to throw the balance of the argument in favor of the genetic theory.

The assertion of Lucretius, " *Omnia animala ex ovo,*" was thus extended to every living thing; and a large puff-ball was exploded, and the dust blown into the eyes of the audience, in order to prove the invisible and innumerable character of the *semina vegetarum*, referring at the same time to the indestructible character of these minute receptacles of sleeping life, until the proper circumstances of heat, moisture, and light set their dynamic forces in action, adjusted the polarities of their ultimate molecules, and started them on the race of metamorphoses called life. These primary movements, whether in seeds, eggs, or living animals, originated in a liquor or plasma, in which the cytoblasts began their existence, and to assume the forms of organizing life-bodies. Your nucleus, nucleolus, fibril, cell, granule, &c., there first begin to exist, and the king of these, the organic cell, with its caudate appendage. The latter little embryo is endowed with some wonderful faculties, such as absorption, nutrition, elimination, and reproduction. Some seven functions distinguish every and all living beings, and these belong to the above-named cell, as well as to the mighty Leviathan of the deep, &c., &c.

We could not help reflecting on the unfortunate necessity that exists in human nature, in the pursuit of science, to confine itself almost exclusively to one course of thought; thus building the mind up in one direction, like a great fungus, to the dwarfing of it in every other.

In the evening, a friend from your State, who is desirous of visiting our lions, and hearing them roar, desired us to accompany him to the Homœopathic College, to listen to an Introductory Lecture on the Practice (Homœopathic) of Medicine, by J. Redman Cox, Jr., son of the venerable Professor of the University, author of " Cox's Dispensatory," editor of the " American Museum," &c. The fame of the father led us to listen to the son. He defended the theory of Homœopathy, character of Hahnemann; indignantly repelled the idea of his disciples being quacks; advocated progressive medicine; deplored the blind butcheries of the Allopaths; said their medicine cured on Homœopathic principles; attempted to prove this by reference to Allopathic authorities—in which medicines were said to produce certain diseases, for which these medicines were themselves specifics; referred to an insulting remark made by the Professor of Surgery in the University in *his* Introductory; and after showing that the assertion proved both impudence and ignorance in the learned surgeon, added, in the language of Sancho-Panza, that it was " impossible to make a silk purse out of a sow's ear."

To-day we listened to what is supposed to be the last Introductory Lecture of the learned Professor of Practice in the University. We listened to his *first* lecture in that chair, and remember his desire that his audience would turn away their eyes from the blaze of glory which surrounded the setting sun of Nathaniel Chapman, that they might thus the more easily appreciate his own small but growing light. From that time to this, now nine years, the annual tirades of some of the faculty of that school against the practitioners of Homœopathic medicine have been repeated in its halls, re-echoed at the firesides of our citizens, and excited feelings of indignation and opposition sufficient to charter and build up a school to teach its peculiar doctrines, and also to assist in extending his practice until now, it is said, that not less than 200,000 of our citizens, many of them wealthy and intelligent, employ Homœopathic practitioners and advocate their theories.

The lecture to-day was characterized by the usual bitterness—"pity" and "scorn" of these "charlatans," "mountebanks," and "impostors." The severest terms of condemnation, the most bitter denunciations against their characters as men, were freely used by the lecturer.

We could not help asking ourselves whether this bitter denunciation and unmerciful contempt, poured without stint upon the devoted heads of these men, were the true weapons to use in a warfare which the world considers an intellectual rather than a moral one. The charging of moral obliquity and every kind of iniquity on men who have a different medical faith from ourselves, appears to me to be illogical, irrational, and unwise. To make a man a martyr or a scoundrel for his opinions will neither convince him of his error, nor prevent his friends from sympathizing in his persecution; yet we believe this has been the policy of this school since its foundation. The moral and social standing of its real or supposed foes have always been of the worst character, and its history is signalized by aggravated aggressions on the very existence of individuals and institutions. So much for our Alma Mater, several of whose chairs will soon be vacant through resignations, death, and old age.

This evening we have listened to a lecture, by the Professor of Practice in the Jefferson College, which was in striking contrast in every respect with that delivered from the same chair in the University. The eloquent diction, the graceful rhetoric, the learned and literary allusions, with the liberality of sentiment and general research, distinguished the author and his production in the highest degree. His subject was Death: its nature, its causes, and prevention. Diseases, War, Intemperance, Poverty—such a picture of the latter as could be drawn only by a master hand—were described and illustrated in a way to command the breathless attention of some 600 young men, for more than an hour.

Lastly, we listened to the Professors of Surgery and Anatomy in the same college. The former delivered a learned lecture on the life and times of Parè, the father of French surgery; and the latter presented a sketch of the life of his friend and late colleague, Dr. Thos. Dent Mütter. The former was a running description of Parè, Vesalius, and others; and the latter presented the family connections and professional history of Dr. Mütter.

It is reported that the number of students here is larger than usual; it has not appeared so to me. The rooms are not as full as formerly at the Introductions. SENECA.

MEDICAL EDUCATION.

[The approaching session of the American Medical Association, at New Haven, Ct., to be held on the 4th of June, 1860, promises to be by far the most important in its history. Very great interest in the expected action of that body is manifested all over the country, in view of the fact that three several committees are charged with the duty of considering the subject of *Medical Education*, and from each of these Reports are expected, viz.:

1. Standing Committee on Medical Education.
2. Committee of the Convention of Professors.
3. Committee of Conference with the latter, appointed by the Association.

The latter committee would seem to be at work already, and an informal meeting has lately been held in Boston, at which both the *special* committees were represented, and some fifty members of the profession were present, and a free interchange of opinion was had.

We insert the following article from the *Boston Med. and Surg. Journal*, which will serve to show the *status* of the parties; and that a *joint* meeting of the two special committees is called at New York on the 1st day of June, 1860. An excellent *volunteer* article on the subject will be found in the present No. of the GAZETTE, which will repay perusal.—ED. GAZETTE.]

Among the subjects which have held a prominent place in the transactions of the American Medical Association is that of *medical education*, and if no definite results have as yet been obtained from the efforts which have been made in its behalf, it is gratifying to see that its great importance is fully recognized by the Association, and that the failure to recommend some uniform standard of medical instruction is more owing to the inherent difficulties of the subject, than to any want of interest or zeal on the part of members. To show this, it is only necessary to refer to the printed volumes of the Transactions of the Association; and, as many of our readers may not be aware of the efforts which have been made in this direction, we propose to give a condensed statement of what has been done, both by the Association and by the two medical conventions which took place before its organization in 1847.

In the first volume of the Transactions are the Report and Resolutions of the first Committee on Medical Education, consisting of Drs. Haxall, Cullen, Patterson, A. Flint, Perkins, Wing, and Norris. The report embraces 13 pages, and concludes with thirteen resolutions, recommending, among other things, six months courses of lectures, three years' study, seven professors to each college; dissections, cliniques, and hospital attendance to be required, and colleges refusing to comply with these requirements not to be admitted to fellowship. These resolutions were adopted. In the same volume is the Report of a Committee on Preliminary Education, occupying four pages, and containing three resolutions. Preceptors are to require certificates of good moral character, of a good English education, and of a proper knowledge of natural philosophy, of the elements of mathematics, of Latin and Greek.

In Vol. II., page 257, we find a report of 123 pages, of another committee on medical education, of which Dr. C. F. Stewart was chairman. It consists of five sections, and two addendas. Medical education in this country is compared with that abroad. The requirements of the U. S. Army and Navy are stated. The legal requirements in the several States are mentioned, and also sundry other matters. The committee approve of boards of examiners, and of the conferring of two degrees. Appended to the report are eleven resolutions, recommending, among other things, that college cliniques should not be allowed as a substitute for hospital instruction; that examinations for degrees be public; that pharmacy should be a required study; and that boards of examiners should be appointed for each State. The report and resolutions were referred to a committee, who reported seven resolutions, together with an eighth, moved by Dr. E. T. Bond, Jun., recommending private medical institutions, and dispensary practice. In these resolutions the Association reiterates its approval of the resolutions in reference to medical education adopted in 1847; college cliniques are not to be substituted for hospital instruction; six months' hospital attendance to be required for graduation; a meeting of teachers to be held before the next annual meeting, to present a plan for elevating the standard of medical education. Appended to the report are two papers: the first, from the medical faculty of Harvard University, in favor of a four months' course of lectures, and signed by John Ware, Jacob Bigelow, and O. W. Holmes; the other, consisting of facts and arguments in favor of a six months' course, and signed by Samuel Jackson, John S. Atlee, and Alfred Stillé, a committee appointed to answer the above.

In Vol. III., page 145, we find another report on this subject, chiefly confined to the discussion of three points—preliminary education, the character of professional instruction, and the question whether the Association shall prescribe terms of admission into the colleges. Schools of pharmacy are recommended. The report says it is doubtful whether any uniform plan of education or admission to the profession can be established. This report gave great dissatisfaction, and led to a long-continued debate. Resolutions were passed, reaffirming the former action of the Association, and opposing the sentiments of the report. The next volume of the Transactions contains a report of 32 pages on the same subject, by a committee of which Dr. W. Hooker was chairman. Appended to it were seven resolutions, which may be briefly stated as follows: abuses demand consideration; good results from discussion; reform necessary in public sentiment, both professional and lay; our own organizations the proper channel for the profession; the Association has confidence in judicious efforts; former action reaffirmed; a steady onward progress recommended. The report was accepted, the resolutions concurred in, and all State Societies were recommended to republish it for general distribution.

Vol. V. contains no report on medical education. In Vol. VI. is a report by Dr. Pitcher and others, in which a knowledge of the elements of medical science are recommended to be acquired before attendance at hospital; and the advantages of hospital and private teaching are urged. The President (Dr. Wellford) recommends State boards of examination, and legislative action is invoked, to pass a general law of uniformity.

Vol. VII. contains a report of 28 pages, with six resolutions, the principal points of which are, daily *office examinations*, clinical instruction, an enlarged curriculum, and a uniform system of examining candidates for degrees.

Vol. VIII. contains no report. In Vol. IX. is a short report, recommending the preparation of an elementary work on anatomy, physiology, and pathology, for the use of students before attending lectures.

In Volume X. is the report of a discussion on the subject of medical education, which was followed by the appointment of a committee of five, unconnected with any school, to devise a system of medical education, and to report at the next annual meeting. The report of this committee is to be found on page 249, Vol. XI. It recommends primary schools, with daily office instruction, seven professorships, a lecture term of six months, liberal primary education, &c., and proposes that a delegation from colleges should meet in convention at Louisville, at the annual meeting in 1859.

The above nine reports occupy 239 octavo pages of the Transactions; and over fifty members have been appointed on educational committees. Where so strong an interest is manifested, we cannot believe that the difficulties in the way of adopting some uniform system for recommendation are too great to be overcome. It is true, the Association cannot, perhaps, enforce any such system, but its influence is yearly becoming greater, and its recommendation may be almost equivalent to a law. We do not mean that the exact course of study is to be prescribed, but certain conditions should be, and probably will be insisted upon, such as a uniform standard of preliminary education, a three years' course of study, with attendance on two full courses of lectures in separate years, sufficient clinical attendance, regular examinations or recitations, &c., &c.; and such schools as do not conform to these recommendations will be regarded in the same light as an individual practitioner who violates the code of ethics adopted by the Association.

At an informal meeting of medical gentlemen, held in this city last week, the subject of medical education was discussed, and a free interchange of opinion took place. About fifty members of the profession were present, including Dr. Crosby, of Dartmouth College, Hanover, the President of the Teachers' Convention; Dr. Hooker, the Dean of the Medical Faculty of Yale College; and Dr. Blatchford, Chairman of the Committee of Conference, appointed by the Association to meet the Committee of the Teachers' Convention, before the next annual meeting.* A large number of letters which have been received by the Chairman of the Convention Committee, from various gentlemen, on the subject of medical education, were read, expressing various opinions, and offering different plans, which were freely discussed by those present. On one point, the necessity for a full three years' course of study, under the direction of a regular practitioner, as a prerequisite to graduation, all were agreed, and the value of a uniform system of registration to secure proof of this. There was some difference of opinion at this meeting upon matters of detail. The chief topic of discussion was the appointment by State Societies of delegates to attend the examinations made by professors, and also the impracticability of taking from medical schools the duties of examining and recommending candidates for degrees. One obvious reason for this is to be found in the fact that the State Governments are the sources of the power of conferring the degrees, and have intrusted it to boards appointed by themselves, to whom the professors recommend candidates. Harvard University has had, for more than two hundred years, the power of conferring the degree of Doctor in Medicine. The corporation, composed of seven persons, of whom only one member at the present time is a physician, nominate the professors. The board of overseers, composed of thirty-seven, the Governor and Lieutenant-Governor of the State, the President of the Senate and Speaker of the House of Representatives, being ex officio members of this board, confirm the nomination, and these two boards confer degrees, voting on those recommended by the Medical Faculty. A committee of this board, composed of physicians, visits the medical school every year, and receives from every professor a report of the instruction given in his department. The professors of Yale and of Dartmouth Colleges explained to the meeting the modes of influence and supervision exercised by the profession and laity in their respective schools. The advantages of the plan were urged by gentlemen connected with schools where it had long been in successful operation. At Hanover (Dartmouth College) two examinations are appointed by the New Hampshire State Society, who are paid by the faculty, at the rate of one dollar for each student. The delegates may examine, if they please, and they are always consulted when there is any difference of opinion as to the merits of a candidate, but they have no vote;

---

* These Committees will meet at New York, on the Friday (June 1st) preceding the next annual meeting of the Association.

they are present by courtesy, extended by the College to the State
Society. A similar system is adopted successfully at Yale College.

The difficulties in the way of carrying out this system in colleges
which graduate a large number of students are obvious. In some of
the schools in Philadelphia, for example, two or three hundred are
graduated at a time, and it is customary for each candidate to call on
the professors separately, the examination sometimes lasting for weeks.
Here it would be impossible to establish a supervision by a board of
delegates. It is true the method of examination might be altered; a
much larger number of students is examined at Harvard College, at
the close of each term, under the supervision of boards of examiners,
but these boards are composed of some two hundred persons, arranged in sixteen committees. There can be no doubt that the thing is
practicable, if the wants of the community demand it, although it may
be for the interest of certain schools to resist such an innovation. We
are inclined to think that the system of examiners appointed by State
Societies, while it may answer well in certain schools, is ill adapted
for others. The standard of education is regulated, to a considerable
degree, by the requirements of the community. Those whose field of
labor is to be among a sparse population, with limited notions about
medical attainments, and moderate ability for remuneration, will seek
a school where they can be graduated on the easiest terms. On the
contrary, a physician who is to practice in a thickly settled community,
where the standard of education is high, and the competition great,
will find it an advantage to have graduated at a school in which the
examinations are thorough, and whose degrees are evidence of high
qualifications for practice.

We regret that our limits will not allow us to report in detail the
remarks, both on this subject and on others connected with medical
education, which were made by various gentlemen present at the meeting referred to. We can only say, that the fullest appreciation of the
importance of the subject of medical education was manifested. We
have no doubt that the Teachers' Convention will be able to recommend, at least, some general plan, which shall obtain the endorsement
of the American Medical Association, and of the profession generally,
and which public sentiment will compel all schools to adopt. There
certainly can be no doubt that the number of imperfectly educated
and incompetent doctors of medicine has been largely on the increase
within a few years. The records of examinations made by the navy
and army medical boards fully sustain such an assertion.

Two circulars sent to the members of the two committees are appended, that our readers may know the precise points which will be before these committees at their meeting on Friday, June 1st.

BOSTON, *October*, 1859.

DEAR SIR—A Committee was appointed at the meeting of the Convention of the Medical Schools of the United States, held in Louisville, Ky., on Monday, the second day of May, 1859, to consider the matters brought before the Convention, so as to propose a definite course of action at the adjourned meeting of the Convention to be held in New Haven, Ct., on Monday, the fourth day of June, Anno Domini 1860.

At a meeting of this Committee, held in Louisville, soon after their appointment, it was unanimously agreed upon to propose the adoption, by the Convention of Medical Schools, of a rule, requiring from every candidate for the degree of Doctor in Medicine, certificates of the study of medicine during a period of at least three full years, under the direction of a regular practitioner of medicine, who shall certify to the same, under his own hand, and of attendance on two full courses of lectures at a medical school recognized as regularly organized by this Convention, with an interval of at least seven months between the termination of one course and the commencement of the second.

It was proposed, also, that a resolution be passed, that any school which does not adopt and enforce this rule shall not be allowed to send delegates to the Convention of Medical Schools, nor to the American Medical Association, and that its graduates shall not be recognized as regular practitioners of medicine.

It was thought advisable to recognize the deficiency in preparatory education on the part of many who offer themselves as students of medicine, and that all practitioners of medicine, as well as all professors, should be exhorted to do all in their power to impress upon those wishing to study medicine the importance and great advantage of intellectual and moral discipline and culture, as well as of a good knowledge of their own mother tongue and of some acquaintance with the Latin language, and with the elementary truths of mathematics and physics.

It has been also suggested to the Committee to propose a mode or plan for the enrolment and registration of students to be recommended for general adoption. Will you be good enough to furnish the Committee with an account of what is done in your school in this respect, and generally to make any suggestions to them of matters which you think it well to bring before the Convention? .

TROY, 26th September, 1859.

MY DEAR DOCTOR—You doubtless know of your appointment at the Louisville meeting of the American Medical Association, as one of " a Committee of five to confer with the Committee of Medical Teachers, and report at the next annual meeting."

As Chairman of that Committee, I should be pleased to learn your views upon the subjects referred to us.   They are, I believe—

1st. The Resolutions of the New Jersey State Medical Society, recommending Boards of Censors for each Judicial District.

2d. The Resolutions appended to the last year's report on Education, by Dr. James R. Wood.   ˙

3d. Dr. Davis's Resolution concerning Preliminary Education; and

4th. Dr. Sayer's Resolution, recommending the appointment by each State Medical Society, of Examination Delegates, &c.

It has occurred to me that an *early conference* of the joint Committee is essential to any satisfactory result.   Let us meet at some central point and talk over the whole subject in a friendly way, viewing it in all its bearings, and it is possible we might reach a conclusion satisfactory to both Colleges and the Profession at large.   A hasty meeting the day before the annual meeting is too contracted to accomplish much.   I remain yours truly,

THOS. W. BLATCHFORD.

The Life and Character of Humboldt.

Professor Alfred Stillé, M.D., has recently delivered an address before the Linnæan Association of Pennsylvania College, which has been published. It portrays the traits of character which marked the history of the venerable devotee of Nature, so recently departed from a world which he had blessed by his researches, and adorned by a long life of scientific exploration and usefulness.   Humboldt's name was not born to die. _ He was an honor to the two centuries in which he lived and labored; and as a veritable cosmopolite, he belonged to the whole world, though Berlin, of Prussia, claims the honor of his birth, and is honored by his tomb.   Nowhere will his memory be cherished more affectionately than in America, and no fitter eulogist could be found than our friend Dr. Stillé, of Philadelphia, has proved himself to be, by this touching and eloquent oration.

The Relative Value of the Different Methods of Amputation of the Leg, as regards Mortality and the subsequent Utility of the Limb.

Translated from the German, by ALFRED WEILLER.

Dr. Boeckel, of Strasbourgh, has taken this question into consideration, having published a pamphlet entitled "Les Avantages et les Inconvénients de l'Amputation de la Jambe au lieu d'élection comparée aux Amputation sus Malléolaire et partielles du Pied."

He states that all the statistics lately collected by different authors go to prove the superiority of the supra-malleolar amputation (from the commencement of the lower third to the malleoli) over that immediately, or three or four inches, below the knee-joint; showing that the mortality of the latter is double that of the former. (Fenwick says the relative proportions are 1 in 4.5 and 1 in 2.5.) This decided difference in favor of the first method Dr. B. attributes—

(1.) To the wound being further away from the body.

(2.) To the surface of the wound being smaller; and

(3.) To the comparatively rare occurrence of pyæmia and phlebitis.

As regards the utility attainable subsequent to these operations, Dr. B. thinks the advantages are decidedly on the side of the supra-malleolar amputation, as there is a far better support for artificial contrivances. It is true that some patients, after the latter operation, have to leave off their artificial foot and resort to a wooden leg, in consequence of ulceration of the stump; but, in the majority of cases, Dr. B. attributes this to the badly-constructed apparatus, in some of which, for instance, the *end of the stump* is made the point of support. And even in those cases where, on account of the tenderness of the stump, and inclination of the same to ulceration, no other apparatus can be used than the wooden leg, the disadvantages and inconveniences arising from the supra-abundant length of the stump are not so great, but that they are compensated by the difference of mortality, which gives this operation so great an advantage over the higher one.

As regards the operation in the middle third, Dr. B. thinks, without, however, being able to bring any facts to bear upon his opinion, that the large surface of the wound is just as dangerous as in the higher amputation. And, as the stump is not more adapted to an artificial foot, and less so to a wooden leg, he prefers the operation in the upper third to this.

In tibio-tarsal exarticulations, according to good statistical authorities, the average mortality is 1 in 7.2 operations. Out of thirty-two cases cited by Dr. B., four died consequent upon the operation, gangrene of the flaps ensued in three, and in four the caries returned. Out of the two last categories, five cases went through secondary amputation of the leg in loco electionis; ten patients could, after cicatrization of the flaps, use their stumps to more or less advantage; ten could, after some time, walk on the stump without any inconvenience. Dr. B., consequently, comes to the conclusion that this operation is far preferable to the amputation of the leg, provided there is no particular danger of the return of the caries; although, in the former operation, cicatrization goes on slower, and necrosis and suppuration of the sheaths of the tendons take place oftener than in the latter. He also prefers the planta-flap, of Syme, to the dorsal, of Bouden.

The exarticulation below the astragalus, and Pirogoff's operation, are not sufficiently numerous as to allow of a definite conclusion. Dr. B. speaks of seven cases of the first, all of which terminated favorably; and of nine of the latter, one of which was fatal.

In Schopart's operation, the average fatality is one in nine. As regards the usefulness of the limb after this operation, out of thirty-three cases, seven could walk tolerably well immediately after the healing of the wound; in seven, the same result was attained at a later period. In most of the remaining nineteen cases, organic disease of the joint set in about the period of cicatrization, (in some later;) in all, retroversion of the heel took place, which interfered more or less with locomotion; in five, secondary amputation was performed, in consequence of returned caries. From further observation of these nineteen and other similar cases, Dr. B. infers that the retroversion of the heel depends least upon the contraction of the gastrocnemius, as in most cases the division of that muscle failed to remove the difficulty; and only in part does it arise from inflammation of the tibio-tarsal joint and the deep-seated muscles of the leg at the period of cicatrization. The chief cause, however, is, in his opinion, the action of the weight of the body upon the astragalus, which is no longer supported by the anterior part of the foot, and consequently, in walking, it is dislocated forward. The highest degree of retroversion he attributes to the relaxation of the articular ligaments. This opinion has been confirmed by experiments upon the subject. His advice is, therefore, not to choose this method in cases of organic articular disease; when, however, this mode is used, the astragalus should be kept, during the period of cicatrization, in a strongly-flexed position; the patient should not be allowed to walk for some time, and then only with a boot the sole of which is considerably heightened in front.

The amputation at the metatarsal bones, and Lisfranc's tarso-metatarsal exarticulation, produce better results than all other partial amputations of the foot.

The exarticulation between the os naviculare and os cuneiformis cannot now be passed upon.

SELECTIONS.

A FAIR HIT AT FIGHTING DOCTORS.

A fight between two ferocious surgeons in New Orleans has furnished a fine opportunity to editors, few of whom are doctors, to display at once their abhorrence of dueling and abilities of derision. As Christians we cannot but be gratified at the unexpected change of sentiment on the subject of unlawful combat, manifested by the conductors of our partisan newspapers, who heretofore have been rather conspicuous for mediæval notions of chivalry; and as lovers of fun and fine writing, we could not but enjoy the comic descriptions and sarcastic comments of our brilliant and unsparing cotemporaries. Nevertheless, we feel for the fraternity of which, for many years, we were an unworthy brother. We know them well; far better than lawyers or unprofessional editors can know them. They seldom transact business with the gentlemen of the bar except when the latter need aid and counsel, and with political editors physicians have the least possible acquaintance. Of all professional men we know them to be the most provoked and least quarrelsome; the worst treated and least resentful. They are known only to one another; as the angels are; to whom good doctors, and a large proportion are good, bear a close moral resemblance. They are the most liberal and self-denying of mankind; men of sound mind and wide information; the best of counselors and the truest of friends; a class of whom the world declares itself altogether unworthy by patronizing quacks and denouncing science. If all the lawyers any secular editors were to be removed from us in a night, we would feel some inconvenience, but enjoy much relief. Let the doctors be removed, and we would gladly compound for their return by surrendering all the blessings conferred on us by the complicated machinery of court-house justice and the political sagacity and partisan industry of the newspaper press.   It is the glory and the peculiarity of the medical man that he is always seeking truth or acting upon it when found.   The clergyman has a system; the advocate a cause; the statesman a party; the doctor has nothing to divert him from the truth or prejudice him against it.   Having once been a physician, we feel at liberty to pay this just tribute to a profession which we abandoned, not because we did not believe in Medical Science and esteem those who practice it, but because the public did not understand the value of the one nor properly respect the services of the other.   We endured for twenty years a great fight of afflictions, and then gracefully succumbed to the exhausting demands upon our patient, and truthful and righteous spirit.   Whatever the ill-natured may say, we did not retreat because our provisions were consumed, and a lean and hungry multitude of homœopaths, water-curers, and pill venders, were caterpillaring on the fair lands before us.   We could have held out on rye bread and dumplings, and scorned to yield to carnal considerations, had our moral nature been sustained by the intelligent co-operation of the people for whom we were working as only doctors work.   But we retired, and however great was the loss to the community, it is irreparable now, and they must blame themselves for it all. · But we will always love and respect doctors, (of medicine,) and we will not let them be ridiculed and tormented without lifting a voice in their behalf.

But the lawyers have the inside track on the present occasion, and are disposed to make the most of it.   Our witty neighbors of the *Exchange* often furnish us with editorials of great strength and high flavor.   Without committing ourselves to an opinion upon their politics and policy, for we learned when a doctor to be prudent in doubtful matters, we cannot refrain from acknowledging the excellence of their writing and giving our readers a specimen of it.   Happily, our medical friends afford few opportunities for reasonable satire, and it is rather complimentary to them that so much effort is made to improve this one.   We seriously hope that our sprightly friends of the *Exchange* will never give the surgeons an opportunity to retaliate upon their "jugulars" or "subclavians."   Dueling and pistoling are not more reasonable and efficient when perpetrated by gentlemen of the bar and editors of newspapers, than when ventured upon by excited sons of Esculapius.   Men may as well do mayhem and murder about an aneurism as about an epithet. The selfishness that seeks glory from the scalpel is not less worthy of a man than that which dreads infamy from a pen. When thwarted purpose, or wounded vanity, or fear of opinion moves a man to attempt the life of his ene-my, the wickedness and absurdity cleave to the thing and not to the cir-cumstances; to the act, not to the actor. To invade the strictly reserved prerogatives of the Almighty and take vengeance into our own hands, is a daring act of impiety; a hideous ostentation of infi-delity which no cause can justify. We gladly assume, from the spirit of the subjoined article and of a similar one copied into the *Patriot*, that the opinions of the lawyers who conduct these influential papers is so positively against dueling, that no inducement, not even "an aneurism," will tempt them to imitate the bellicose doctors whose deeds they so properly chronicle. Gentlemen do not need the threat of a pistol to make them courteous, and bullies should not be permit-ted to use it to protect their impudence. We are glad to find our editors laughing at the " code of honor," a code never needed for hon-orable men, for it is a code of *threats;* a system of compulsion under which it is presumed that men will be made to act like gentlemen, though they should not feel like them. As to ourselves, we renounce it. We have a more excellent way. With gentlemen we will show ourselves gentle ; with the " froward" we know how to deal in another fashion, "but thereby hangs a tail." We have a regularly appointed fighting editor in our office. We selected him because he has none of the instincts of a gentleman; has no manners; is gruff and short of speech; obtrusive in his habits; constitutionally pugnacious, but not morally brave; and has no more sense than to fight all comers. Withal he is an inveterate office-seeker, and is not more generous in his feelings than others whose lives are devoted to struggles for place. Any communications that may come to us from similar parties will be referred to him, and anybody seeking corporeal "satisfaction" from us can be accommodated by our deputy. Though he is a dog, he will descend to the level of any biped who may exhibit suitable canine tem-pers and propensities. We advise our friends of the secular press to get rid of the duello, and procure a dog, and let him do all the snarl-ing and throttling incident to the office. Should he get killed it would be but a dog less in the world; but good writers, good lawyers, and good fellows like our friends of the *Exchange* and *Patriot*, cannot be spared. We wish them to live to be good Christians, if they are not such already—good citizens and good editors, and ever, through abounding grace, good Methodists. If any lawyers here should ever fight a duel, we give fair notice, that as they have not spared our brethren the doctors, we will feel at liberty to ridicule, roast, and raddle them to the utmost of our poor ability—and now we will indemnify our readers for reading this homily, by giving them the enjoyment of the following editorial from the *Exchange*:

" That doctors disagree sometimes, we all perfectly well know; but how and why they fall out, they generally abstain from mentioning. Neither are we informed of the methods adopted by them to settle their little disputes. They have, for the most part, too keen a sense of the pain inflicted by a half-ounce ball, and too shrewd a perception of its effects upon the system, foolishly to ask or accept of what is so queerly called ' satisfaction.' Their quarrels are usually hushed up among themselves, and the world is none the wiser. It is with uncommon interest, therefore, that we have perused the history wherein are duly related the causes which led lately to a direful combat between two ' great medicines' in New Orleans. Drs. Foster and Choppin, says the *Delta*, are both connected with the Charity Hospital, and it then proceeds to account for the ' strong animosity' which, for ' upward of two years,' has existed between them. The beginning of the quarrel was in this wise. One of Dr. Choppin's students was fatally wounded in an affray and carried to the hospital, where, under the regulations, Dr. Foster ' had the right' to attend him. The former, however, took him in hand, and when the latter came in and heard of this unwarrantable interference with his subject, his wrath waxed warm. The youth was Choppin's pupil, but he was Foster's patient. The one might sympathize with and soothe him, but it was the privilege of the other to salve over his bodily hurts. Neither would waive his pretensions, and so they immediately sought to adjust matters by having ' a severe fist encounter in one of the rooms of the hospital.' Extraordinary as it may seem, we are told this did not prove ' satisfactory to either party.' With men so very hard to please it was difficult to deal, and their friends, seeing that they could never beat each other into more amicable relations, arranged for them to go out and shoot at one another the next morning. This process was gone through in due form, and strange to relate, these impracticable doctors were no more affectionate afterwards than before. Time only served to strengthen their mutual enmity, which, however, did not display itself in any further violence until a few weeks ago. A circumstance then occurred which aggravated them beyond endurance.

The cause of quarrel was, in truth, a grave one, and well calculated
to have set even saints by the ears. It was an aneurism, which rendered necessary the taking up of the subclavian artery. No senti-
mental difference about a pair of bright eyes, nor any stupid misun-
derstanding over their claret, would probably have roused to frenzy
the hate which lay hidden in the hearts of these rivals. It was an
aneurism supplied from the subclavian artery that brought about the
trouble, and what more than the knowledge of this fact is required
from the justification of the combatants? But let us proceed with our
narration. The unhappy man, with the aforesaid aneurism, was
brought to the hospital, where an operation was determined on. He
was not under the charge of either of our bellicose practitioners. The
operation being a serious and most dangerous one, and the chief surgeon of the institution being absent, it had been delayed from day to
day until a week elapsed. Now, Dr. Choppin, of course, desired to
keep his hand in, and was very anxious to have a cut at this particular aneurism. The patient's wife heard of the doctor's willingness to
make the experiment on her afflicted spouse, and called to see him
about the matter. To her great delight, doubtless, this good Samari-
tan not only agreed to take the husband to his own infirmary, and
keep him free of charge until the result of the operation was known,
which would, in all likelihood, have been about two minutes and a
half, but he, moreover, offered to pay $50 for the privilege of exer-
cising his skill upon the abnormal artery. Here was a temptation
irresistible to man or woman, and accordingly the twain posted down
to the hospital gate, intending to direct their steps to the infirmary
in question. But they had calculated without their host, for Dr.
Foster, upon an intimation of the contemplated removal, had given
orders to detain the interesting aneurism. Nor did he in this abuse
his authority, for it is claimed, says the *Delta*, that all who enter the
Charity Hospital, without paying, place themselves under the control
of the institution, and 'the doctors can retain them until cured or
dead.' Paupers, it appears, are not to be discharged when convalescent. Perhaps the prescriptions in their cases are so potent as to kill
or cure at once. However this may be, the poor patient was still
sitting in the gateway, unable to depart, when his benevolent patron
drove up. He was furious at the detention of his subject, and, as an
officer of the hospital, he immediately wrote his discharge himself, and
then waited to answer any one who might question him. He was not
left long to enjoy his triumph, for out came the indomitable Foster,

armed, as it afterwards appeared, with a five-barreled revolver. Choppin, as became his name and his profession, carried a bowie-knife, in addition to two small pistols. 'Are you looking at me, sir?' says Choppin. 'Yes, sir, I am looking at you,' replied Foster. 'And what do you think of me?' rejoins the former. This polite interrogatory the latter answered by expressing an opinion so unfavorable to Choppin, and couched in such ferocious and wicked language, that we cannot quote it, any more than the reviled doctor could bear it. Simultaneously 'both gentlemen drew their pistols,' and in the interchange of shots that followed, Dr. Foster, being a little quicker or cooler than his adversary, inflicted two ugly wounds upon him, which may yet prove fatal. Instead of taking up arteries, and giving $50 and board gratis for the desirable privilege, Dr. Choppin had to submit that day to have his own 'exterior jugular vein tied up,' and a ball hunted up somewhere in the 'iliac region.' It is pleasant to know that the 'man afflicted with the aneurism retreated down the street' when the affray began, and as far as we can discover, did not find his way again into the Charity Hospital, nor did he pursue his journey towards the private infirmary. Such is the story of this difficulty which professional etiquette originated, and professional rivalry precipitated to a bloody ending. The battle may almost be said to have been fought in the cause of science. For no such pitiful prizes as gain or glory did the combatants contend, but they were animated solely by the noble desire to attain through the subclavian artery a higher rank and reputation in the medical fraternity."—*Baltimore Christian Advocate.*

MEDICAL EDUCATION.

By T. J. COGLEY, M.D., Madison, Ind.

I have selected the above short caption for a text, and, without laying the subject off into "heads," I shall take the widest latitude which suits me. Judging from its frequent discussion, in all sections of our country, during the past ten years, it must be a very important subject, in reference to which, between the profession at large and that portion of it who devote more or less exclusive attention to teaching, there has been a great deal of crimination and recrimination. It is much to be regretted that it is not unusual to meet with such language as the following in published "Reports" from committees, appointed by State Societies to report upon the subject in question, and especially as it *seems* to have received the sanction of the Society, whilst it has not:

"*Our Medical Schools, looking only to pecuniary considerations, have become the nurseries of quackery. Many able men are educated in them, but by far the greater number are wholly unfit to practice the profession.*" Again: "*It is notorious that every year students are rejected from physicians' offices, as unfit to aspire to a place in the profession, and are placed upon an equal footing with the brightest ornaments of the profession, by our medical schools, from one end of the land to the other, almost, if not entirely, without exception;*" and the reason assigned is because the "*income of these professional teachers is proportioned to the number of pupils and of graduates. In this way, the love of money is made to operate to the reduction, instead of the elevation, of the standard of preliminary, as well as professional, education.*" Still further: "*The student, driven from the physician's or private teacher's office, for want of essential requisites, goes at once to one of our medical schools—and it matters not to which of them—and, by paying for two courses of lectures and the graduation fee, although he may not hear a dozen of the lectures, he may in eight months obtain a diploma, certifying his full qualification to practice every department of the profession.*" "Or he may, after four years' *pretended* practice, obtain a diploma, by paying for a single course of lectures, and *claim* an equal standing with any." The foregoing, it will not be denied, are tolerably unambiguous charges.

On the other side of the question, the friends of the schools—the teachers—are reported to have said: "We are doing well enough, we desire no change; our halls are full." And some of them are said to have "intimated to the profession at large, that it is none of their business to be meddling with medical education; that they—the teachers—know better than all others the wants of the profession; that all practitioners have to do is to be careful in the selection of their pupils, and very diligent in their instruction; if none but students of good preliminary education and professional training seek diplomas, it will follow, as a natural consequence, that the undeserving will cease to receive them."

The foregoing is selected, not from any desire to give notoriety to any particular person or committee, but because it is recent and at hand; such expressions are readily attainable, in great abundance, emanating from various sections of our country. I refer to all, under the above selections. What we have selected, from both parties, might with propriety be said to be a good illustration of the adage,

that "doctors will differ." And who shall untie this Gordian knot?
Methinks the very best way to dispose of it is to do as Alexander did
with the knot in the harness of Gordius, King of Phrygia—cut it
asunder. Alexander, being a warrior, used his sword; we hope to
lay open this knot with a much more peaceful weapon; but it is much
to be feared that, though one should be successful in unraveling the
inextricable difficulty in question, his reward would be incomparably
less than it was in the case to which allusion has been made.

As those who have preceded me all claim to have "no desire, no
aim, save *to find the truth*," I beg leave to say that I can have no
other object than the development of the truth, for I utterly disregard, further than civility, the opinion either of the profession in general,
or of professors; that is, as regards my opinion as to which of them is
right, having never asked, and never expecting to ask, any special
favor of either. And now having, as I will not deny, made a rather
lengthy exordium, I shall proceed to remark upon the quotations I
have made, for they have a direct bearing upon my "text."

And in the first place, is it true that "*our medical schools, looking
only to pecuniary considerations, have become the nurseries of quackery?*"
It is a very grave charge, and, if true, can doubtless be substantiated,
and it ought to be; but enlightened communities always demand evidence before they convict, for we all know that there are defamers
and detractors in the world; nor do we consider it impossible that such
might happen to be put upon a committee on Medical Education; nor
would we respect a slanderer any more in the capacity of a committee-
man, than as a most loathsome member of society. However this
may be, I can but say, that so far as I am capable of judging, I have
never seen anything in print that was a greater perversion of the
truth; that it cannot be substantiated, and that the converse is susceptible of demonstration.

Twenty-five years ago, when I first became a resident of Indiana,
there were, according to my best recollection, but two medical schools
west of the mountains—the Ohio Medical College, at Cincinnati, and
the medical department of Transylvania University, at Lexington,
Ky. The profession was at that time legalized in Indiana, and by
law the State was divided into districts, in each of which there was
a legally organized medical society, in which, besides the usual officers, there was a Board of Censors, whose duty it was to examine all
applicants, and license them to practice medicine, if deemed worthy.
In this way, at their annual meeting, I had an opportunity of seeing

nearly all of the physicians in one of the districts, which consisted of probably more than half a dozen counties; and although they were highly respectable, and as well acquainted with medicine as physicians generally throughout the Western States, yet I am sure they would unite with me in saying, that their knowledge of the science of medicine was very much inferior to what it would be found to be in a corresponding number of physicians, occupying the same district, at the present day. There was not a member of the Board of Censors who had ever heard a lecture on medicine, and but a very small number in the district who were graduates. About that time medical schools began to multiply; those which existed were better attended, and graduates became much more numerous, so that for many years past they have greatly outnumbered those who have not graduated; and although some may have obtained diplomas who were not prepared for the practice, yet I must say that I never met one who did not make the impression on my mind that he had acquired a familiarity with the science which is seldom if ever attained outside of a medical school. I am not more confident of anything, than that nineteen-twentieths of the physicians who, at the period above named, composed the said medical district, would coincide with me in the opinion that the general intelligence and fitness of physicians for the practice has been enhanced in the above period more than fifty per cent.; and they will also agree with me that the difference has been brought about by the medical schools. If this has not been the agent by which this great change has been wrought, I confess myself entirely ignorant of the cause. "Nurseries of quackery!" I am astonished at the audacity of the assertion. It really seems to me to imply a contempt of moral restraint. And although the circumstances would seem to preclude the possibility of such a supposition, it is difficult to suppress a suspicion of disappointed ambition; but it is fair to say that these sentiments are tinged with the effect of having been previously laid on the table by an almost unanimous vote; and now, although referred to the publishing committee, the "general principles" alone are concurred in, so that it is but the expression of an individual or two, and not of a society.

That some undeserving persons have obtained diplomas from medical schools, I do not doubt; but that the effect of the multiplication of medical schools and graduates has been other than the more general diffusion of sound medical knowledge, and not to fill the country with quacks, is not to be believed for a moment; neither is it, nor can it ever be believed by the great mass of the profession, committees on medical education to the contrary notwithstanding. I have abundant reason to know that, in the cheapest and poorest of the medical schools, as correct principles as are known have been taught, and their students rendered far more fit for general practice—or rather, more fit to learn how to practice—than they could possibly have been without having any connection with these so-called "nurseries of quackery."

Is it true that "by far the greater number of graduates turned out by the medical schools are wholly unfit to practice the profession?" In an extensive acquaintance with practitioners in Pennsylvania, Ohio, Indiana, and Kentucky, during twenty years, I have always been struck with the superior accomplishments and qualifications of those who had graduated in the meanest of the medical schools, when contrasted with the great majority of those who had never attended lectures at all, and I have often heard the same opinion expressed by highly respectable and disinterested persons, perfectly capable of judging correctly; nay, I have often heard it admitted by respectable physicians, who have never had it in their power to attend lectures, or witness anatomical or surgical demonstrations. Doubtless there are, in all graduating classes, various degrees of fitness for practice, and if it were possible, I believe it would be wise to have first, second, and third degrees specified in diplomas, as is the case in some of the smaller German schools or hospitals, for it would be a most powerful incentive to close application. Yet after all, as a general remark, when a young man has graduated with as much honor to himself as possible, he is only fit to *begin to practice;* hence the great importance of hospitals in connection with lectures, of observing and taking part in much hospital practice before taking upon one's self the responsibility of private practice; but to say that "by far the greater number of graduates turned out by the medical schools are wholly unfit to practice the profession," is an exaggeration of the truth which is wholly inexcusable and highly reprehensible.

And there is another thing, which others as well as myself have observed: that some of those who barely passed the green-room, will be found in after years to have almost distanced "brighter ornaments" of the same class, as skillful and successful practitioners, which is owing to their fondness for the study of the science, added to untiring industry and perseverance. I know physicians who, although much engaged in practice, have read profitably on an average four or five hours in every twenty-four, for twenty years, and others who have not during the same time averaged half an hour in each day. Supposing the former to have been barely fit to commence the practice, and the latter as fully prepared as he could be by hearing lectures, where would their relative positions be now as practitioners, especially if the former took delight in the profession, and the latter delighted more in the pleasures and enjoyments of life than in its duties? "Wholly unfit to practice the profession!" I am not an advocate of short preparations, or of hastily entering the profession—the farthest from it possible; but take two young men of equal talents and education, equal ambition to obtain a knowledge of science, and one may "read medicine" in some physician's office for two or three years if he chooses, and let the other attend carefully but one course of lectures in any respectable medical school, and at the end of that time, short as it is, and of course altogether too short, I will forfeit all claims to the possession of common sense if the latter does not know more of the science, and is not better prepared to commence practice, than the former can possibly be.

Is it true that "it is notorious that every year, students, who are rejected from physicians' offices as unfit to aspire to a place in the profession, are placed on an equal footing with the brightest ornaments of the profession, by our medical schools?" Within the scope of my observation during twenty-five years, "the rejection of students from physicians' offices, as unfit to aspire to a place in the profession," has not been by any means so common as to be "notorious;" it is, however, *notorious* that too many have been, by physicians, allowed to aspire to a place in the profession, who were *notoriously* unfit to learn the very alphabet of the same; and it is very clear that, so long as physicians continue to admit unsuitable persons to commence the study, all systems of Medical Education will fail to supply the people with skillful and reliable physicians; besides, the literal truth of the allegation is impossible. All students, on entering a medical school, are required to give the name of their preceptor, if they have not been a practitioner for four years. I have looked over hundreds of catalogues of medical students, and find this to be true; besides, I know the fact; and although I admit it might be possible for a young man occasionally thus to impose upon a faculty, yet to say that it is of such frequent occurrence as to be notorious, is simply ridiculous. I have known young men graduated who did not merit a diploma, but never have I known one to enter a medical school who had been refused entrance upon the study by a physician. It would be well-nigh impossible for a young man to enter a medical college who had neither a preceptor nor any previous preparation, and profess he had either; if he did, he would soon be detected. It would be well for "reporters" of committees to make statements which would at least bear the semblance of truth; this, in our opinion, does not; it is too absurd to dwell on. And if it were true that students rejected by physicians are allowed to enter medical colleges, is it true that they are thereby "placed upon an equal footing with the brightest ornaments of the profession?" Certainly not. If not endowed with the same talents and acquirements, no earthly power can place them on an equal footing. Go where they may, they cannot sustain themselves in practice so well as the really "brighter ornaments," where success is desirable; for it is just as true of physicians as it is of books, they will ultimately find their proper level. In an enlightened community, each will, as a general remark, be appreciated according to his merits, although they may hold diplomas from the same school.

That "students, driven from the physician's office, just go to any of our medical schools, and, by paying for two courses of lectures, obtain, although they may not have heard a dozen of the lectures," a diploma, simply for money, is a monstrous charge, which I hope and believe is not true. If it be true of any, or all the medical schools, it should be proven, and should operate greatly to their disadvantage. But no proof has been offered. The schools, so far as I know, have treated the charge with silent contempt; and, indeed, if untrue, it is too contemptible to notice.

"Or he may, after four years' *pretended* practice, obtain a diploma by paying for a single course of lectures." My present impression is, that the custom of allowing persons who had been engaged in a reputable practice for four years, to become candidates for graduation, originated with Dr. Drake and his compeers; of course supposing that such persons had previously spent a reasonable time in reading medical books, in the office of some reputable physician, all of which seem indispensable in order to be possessed of a *reputable* practice. But wherever it may have had its origin, it has been practiced in at least all the Western colleges for nearly a quarter of a century, and to my certain knowledge has been considered fully equal, in all important respects, to one course of lectures. I have heard several of the most distinguished professors west of the mountains express their decided approbation of this course, under certain circumstances, and give it as their opinion that such physicians *might* be, if observant, studious and in earnest, better fitted for practice, after attending one full course, than any man could be by attending two full courses in succession, without any practice; and I fully endorse all I have heard in favor of the possibility in the case in question. I have known intimately quite a number of physicians who, after having read well, had practiced over four years reputably, and then, after attending one course of lectures, graduated with distinguished honor. Some of them I have known all the time I have been in the profession, and do not hesitate to assert that they are the most skillful and successful physicians I have ever known. Of one of this class I heard the most celebrated surgeon west of the Alleghanies say, " I believe him better qualified to practice than any physician I have known to graduate in twenty-four years," during which period he had been a professor in a first-class school. I believed the opinion was correct—time has served to confirm it. I know many of the same kind who are in the front rank of physicians, and deservedly so. Doubtless this privilege afforded by the colleges has been abused. And pray, what privilege has not been abused? I admit that I, many years ago, knew an individual who had, to my knowledge, been engaged in farming, milling, and speculating all his life, to impose upon a respectable medical faculty by representing himself to be a practitioner of more than four years' duration, and who, after attending one full course, obtained a diploma. Nor will I say that even he was " wholly unfit" to practice, for he was intelligent, by no means devoid of talent, studied closely, and must have learned a great deal in one course. But that he, by obtaining a diploma, was " placed on an equal footing with the brightest ornaments," was far from being true, for with all the influences he could bring to his aid—and they were numerous—he proved to be incapable of sustaining himself " on a level with " his competitors. He remained but a brief period in any one place, and wherever he located somehow the manner in which he hurried into the profession soon followed him, and he lacked very much of being of " an equal standing with any." So that even though medical schools may occasionally err in conferring degrees, the recipients are not so formidable as some seem to suppose, for medical schools, whatever else they can do, cannot give men brains, and this is, after all, the great distinguishing characteristic of the better class of physicians; and, whether I have been mistaken or not, I have sometimes thought that some of those great reporters on Medical Education had not a great deal more of the article than was necessary.

If the schools have said that the profession in general have no right to be "meddling with medical education," I am not prepared to gainsay. I say, let physicians do their duty in selecting and preparing their students for the colleges, and the latter will seldom have it in their power to graduate those who are unfit. There is undoubtedly the starting-point; that being wrong, the whole superstructure is wrong; hence it appears to me self-evident that if preceptors cease receiving into their offices uneducated, brainless students, the profession must cease to be supplied with such materials. If this be not the fountain and origin of all defects in Medical Education, then have I failed to untie or cut the knot.

Among the most offensive as well as most mischievous characters I have met with in the profession, are those physicians who manufacture doctors in their offices. I have happened to know some of these great men—great in their own estimation because they were so reputable as to have students—endowed with a much larger proportion of omentum than brains, who, on account of having acquired a *township-wide* reputation as surgeons, had frequent applications from ambitious young loafers, wholly devoid, it is true, of all kinds of education save that which enabled them to appear to an advantage in a restaurant, yet conscious that they possessed as much as the class of physicians to whom I refer—to become students of medicine; and I have known scores of young men, wholly unprepared to commence the study, after spending a few months in the offices of these great surgeons, to "locate," and become practitioners. Many of the villages, cross-roads, and other public places in the West, are infested by just such "practitioners," who have never seen a medical school nor a dead subject, unless they may have assisted in laying out one of their preceptor's defunct patients. The physician who will countenance—especially who will *entice* illiterate young men to commence the study of medicine, is guilty of all the evil results which inevitably follow the attempts of such to practice medicine, and they should in some way be accountable. I have often seen these young candidates riding around with their teachers, "learning the practice;" they just sit in the buggy, while the surgeon runs in a moment and orders "some more calomel and ipecac." These distinguished surgeons, while in their offices, study the latest novel with intense interest, or perhaps indulge in that very important and useful game called backgammon, about the propriety of removing the ovaries in a desperate case of nymphomania.

Dr. Warren mentioned, in connection, the case of a young man who performed castration on himself by first making an opening in the scrotum with a penknife, and then squeezing out the testicles. Immediately after the operation, the patient repaired to a restaurant and ate heartily of beefsteak, and subsequently attended a public meeting, and was in the act of making a, speech, when he fainted. A surgeon was called, who, on examining the scrotum, found it greatly enlarged, and distended with blood. The coagula being removed, a vessel was tied, and he was removed to the hospital.

Dr. Warren saw him on the following day. There was no further hæmorrhage, and he recovered rapidly, without any bad symptom.

He quoted Scripture in defence of his course, and did not regret it. —*Boston Med. and Surg. Journal.*

Extracts from the Records of the Boston Society for Medical Improvement.

By F. E. Oliver, M.D., Secretary.

June 13th.—*Castration as a Means of Cure for Satyriasis.*—Dr. H. J. Bigelow read the following letters, one from a physician in a neighboring State, requesting his opinion as to the propriety of castration in a case of erotic mania; and the other from Dr. Bell, containing his opinion as to the operation in this affection.

"*Sept. 27th,* 1856.

"Dr. H. J. Bigelow—You will confer a favor on me and my neighborhood if you will give me some information on the following case:

"There is a young man living near me who has been, I suppose it might be called, partially deranged for nearly a year past; his mind runs altogether upon having sexual intercourse with females, and he . grows worse. His conversation and thoughts are on that subject. He will attack any female he sees, and keeps himself indecently exposed when females are present. He is now worse than he was three months ago. He was at the Insane Hospital at —— about four months, but came home worse than he was when he went. Application has been made to me with regard to castration. What do you think of it? I shall wait anxiously for an answer from you, and hope to get one by return of mail. I am, &c."

"P. S.—This young man is sane on other subjects, and will work on the farm some days; but most of the time he is wandering about,

reporters on Medical Education had not a great deal more of the article than was necessary.

If the schools have said that the profession in general have no right to be "meddling with medical education," I am not prepared to gainsay. I say, let physicians do their duty in selecting and prepar-ing their students for the colleges, and the latter will seldom have it in their power to graduate those who are unfit. There is undoubtedly the starting-point; that being wrong, the whole superstructure is wrong; hence it appears to me self-evident that if preceptors cease receiving into their offices uneducated, brainless students, the profession must cease to be supplied with such materials. If this be not the fountain and origin of all defects in Medical Education, then have I failed to untie or cut the knot.

Among the most offensive as well as most mischievous characters I have met with in the profession, are those physicians who manufacture

to peace of mind and energy was produced.

"On the other hand, in all the lunatic hospital cases where I have known it done, no valuable results followed. At the Ohio Hospital, some years ago, it was tried on quite an extensive scale. No case of improvement followed. Indeed, Dr. Awl told me that in one patient, who previously was quiet and contented, a permanent and dangerous condition of irritability followed. He averred that 'they had done some d——d thing or other to him, so that things didn't work as they used to.'

"I knew the young woman you allude to, as Dr. ———'s patient. She eventually came to the McLean, and finished her wretchedness by suicide. I am satisfied that her disease was more cerebral than ova-rial, and that nothing would have been gained by an operation of re-moving the ovaria.

"I confess that I should recoil from the kind of remedy suggested. I have found that heavy doses of opium, long continued, do control that nymphomaniacal disposition, dependent on no local irritation. And I should certainly desire to see this tried to its fullest extent be-fore the other was decided on. A man so afflicted ought, by every consideration of public safety, to be shut up in a lunatic hospital, and the laws are adequate to this end.

"I am, dear sir, very faithfully yours,   L. V. Bell.
"Dr. Bigelow."

In the case of the young woman referred to in the above letter, Dr. Bigelow had been consulted, by a distinguished physician of Boston, about the propriety of removing the ovaries in a desperate case of nymphomania.

Dr. Warren mentioned, in connection, the case of a young man who performed castration on himself by first making an opening in the scrotum with a penknife, and then squeezing out the testicles. Immediately after the operation, the patient repaired to a restaurant and ate heartily of beefsteak, and subsequently attended a public meeting, and was in the act of making a speech, when he fainted. A surgeon was called, who, on examining the scrotum, found it greatly enlarged, and distended with blood. The coagula being removed, a vessel was tied, and he was removed to the hospital.

Dr. Warren saw him on the following day. There was no further hæmorrhage, and he recovered rapidly, without any bad symptom.

He quoted Scripture in defence of his course, and did not regret it. —*Boston Med. and Surg. Journal.*

FAILURE OF HOMŒOPATHIC VACCINATION.

(Letter from Dr. R. DRUITT to the London Medical Times and Gazette.)

SIR—Last week I vaccinated two children, aged respectively three and one years, who were born in New Zealand, and have just arrived in this country. The point of interest is, that these children were vaccinated homœopathically at their place of birth; which operation consisted in making them swallow some globules which were alleged to contain vaccine matter. They were afterwards inoculated with some matter said to be taken from a cow, without any effect; and the failure of this operation was assumed to be a proof that the previous swallowing of the globules had rendered them proof against any further dose of the vaccine poison.

This theory was set at naught, however, by the fact that my vaccination produced the most perfect vesicles; thus showing that the children were utterly unprotected from that poison, and from small-pox.

I have thought it worth while to make this the subject of a short communication to you, to show, as a matter of fact, the worthlessness of this homœopathic practice. On what experimental evidence such a proceeding has been adopted, I know not; but unless there is such evidence in existence, (which I do not believe,) the persons who resort to it ought to be punished for fraud.

It is worth noticing, too, that every eruption in the cow is not cow-pox; and that, as a general rule, it is safest to get the vaccine matter from a healthy child, than to resort to the dairy.

AMPUTATION AT THE HIP-JOINT.

By A. H. BUCHANAN, M.D., Prof. of Surgical and Pathological Anatomy and Physiology in the Medical Department of the University of Nashville.

"Ad extremos morbos extrema remedia."—HIPPOCRATES.

A youth, 14 years of age, of a lively, nervous temperament, who was chiefly occupied in driving a cart, was seized with a severe pain in the thigh, in the early part of last June, and in a day or two was confined to his bed, and called in medical advice. He was attended by several physicians of the city, as his thigh was in a very short time much inflamed, swollen, and exceedingly painful. In the course of a few weeks it was evident to Prof. Winston, who now attended him, that suppuration had taken place, and that the abscess needed opening. He was in this situation when I was called on to open the abscess. My son, Dr. T. B. Buchanan, accompanied me, and opened the abscess about four inches above the outer condyle, and nearly a quart of most offensive pus was discharged. Upon a further examination of the thigh at this time, it was evident that a large osseous tumor existed at the middle and upper third of the femur, and it was also diagnosed that it was either of a malignant character, or a result of severe inflammation and suppuration, originating in the medullary cavity of the bone, and followed by a softening and expansion of its external compact structure; and further, that amputation at the hip was the only hope for him. We heard no more of him during the summer, except that a tent was kept in the opening, and occasionally withdrawn for the discharge of pus. Early in September it was discovered that a spontaneous fracture or suppuration of the femur had occurred near its middle, and he was brought to the State Hospital for further advice. I was requested to see him, and found him reduced almost to a skeleton, with a pulse over 120 beats per minute, with hectic, and still suffering severe pain, especially when the diseased parts were touched, and also discharging a most offensive, thin, yellowish-green, ichorous fluid from the abscess, through the original opening, amounting daily to half a pint or more. Upon a further examination, it was ascertained that the tumor, which was so large in July, had now nearly disappeared, and that only a portion of the fluid contained in the abscess was daily discharged, as the affected limb was four times as large as the sound one, and œdematous up to the groin. Being in this hopeless condition, I did not hesitate to explain to him and his mother that death was inevitable without an operation at the hip-joint, and that it was the *only hope* for him. Impressed, however, with the high responsibility of performing so formidable an operation, I did not urge it upon him until my opinion was fully concurred in by a very large proportion of the most enlightened physicians and surgeons of Nashville. Indeed, there could be but one opinion. The greatest fear we all had was that he would die on the operating-table, for it was evident to all that in his extreme emaciated condition he could not lose a pint of blood and live.

All the dangers of the operation being fully explained both to the mother and the boy, the little fellow said he had taken his resolution to have it removed. We now desired him to take about an ounce of whiskey and water, with thirty drops of laudanum in it. He was brought into the operating-room of the hospital on the mattress upon which he slept, and placed upon the operating-table. Dr. Conwell and Prof. Bowling administered to him chloroform and ether, mixed in about equal proportions. From some cause, at least an hour was occupied in the inhalation before he became anæsthetized, notwithstanding he breathed freely of it. Being now completely under its influence, his nates were brought down to the end of the table, and the diseased leg held by Mr. Krœschell, the intelligent janitor of our college, who understood precisely what I wished him to do, as he had assisted me the day before in performing the operation several times, at the college, on the dead subject. Prof. Briggs was requested to arrest the hæmorrhage from the posterior flap, and my son from the anterior flap; it being understood by all present that I designed to perform what is generally called Liston's operation, that is, by the anterior and posterior flap. All being ready, a sharp-pointed knife, with a blunt back and narrow blade, of suitable length, was entered about half way between the anterior superior spine of the ileum and trochanter major, and carried directly across the joint, beneath the great vessels, in an oblique direction, and its point brought out on the inner part of the thigh, above the tuberosity of the ischium. The anterior flap was then formed by cutting downward, forward, and outward, about four inches. My son, whose thumbs were compressing the external iliac, during this time, upon the os pubis, followed with his fin-

gers the back of the knife, and as I cut out the flap, had already
secured the vessels, by compression with his hands. In cutting this
anterior flap the tremendous gush of most offensive matter and venous
blood—not less than a quart—was horrible, and more than some of
the lookers-on could withstand. The head of the bone was now
readily disarticulated by a few strokes of a strong scalpel, and by carrying the knife on the posterior part of the neck of the bone, and severing the capsular ligament, we, with a few more incisions, separated all
the muscles attached to the trochanter. The long knife was now
passed behind the trochanter, and carried downward, and close to the
bone, a suitable distance, so as to form the posterior flap, which was
made, not by cutting outward, but by withdrawing the knife, and
cutting from the periphery towards the bone. Prof. Briggs followed
the back of the knife while forming this flap, and very effectually prevented hæmorrhage. The limb being removed, the arteries were
ligated as rapidly as possible. Those on the anterior flap were for
the most part secured first; indeed, there were only a few arteries on
the posterior flap that required the ligature. In this part of the operation we received valuable assistance from Drs. Mayfield and Hatcher.
Eleven arteries were ligated, and the amount of hæmorrhage was
quite small; it is supposed not to have been more than six or eight
ounces. The time occupied in removing the limb is said by those
present to have been something more than a minute. The whole
operation was performed, and the boy placed up upon his mattress
without being the least conscious of the operation, the anæsthetic
having in this case the happiest effect. His pulse, neither during nor
after the operation, was perceptibly diminished, but nevertheless we
gave every now and then a sup of whiskey and water, with laudanum
in it. In about half an hour after the operation he threw up the contents of his stomach—half-digested food, whiskey and all. About
half a grain of morphine was now administered, and a sup or two of
whiskey and water. At the end of an hour he complained of severe
pain in his groin; more laudanum was administered. In another hour
the wound was examined by separating the flaps, which, up to this
time, were simply laid together, and covered with cloths dipped in cold
water. On the under surface of the anterior flap an oozing of blood
was discovered from quite a large artery, which was at once, and
easily, re-ligated, and the hæmorrhage entirely ceased. The internal
surfaces of both flaps were now gently sponged over with cold water,
and no further hæmorrhage could be discovered. The cotyloid cavity

at this time was half filled with a sero-sanguineous fluid, which was removed by a small soft sponge. The flaps were now laid together again, and dressed as before with cold cloths.

At the end of two more hours (during which time he was quite comfortable) the wound was again examined as before stated, and not one drop of blood had escaped. The surfaces of the flaps were exuding in a slight degree a sero-sanguineous fluid, and appeared glazed over. The cotyloid cavity, as before, was half-filled with fluid, which was removed. The larger arteries could be seen pulsating with force against the ligatures, and even the smaller arteries, not larger than a hair, could be seen pulsating in great numbers, their extremities appearing to be permanently closed by black specks of coagulated blood, as if by ligatures. Feeling assured that we had nothing to fear from hæmorrhage, as there was now full reaction, (unless some ill-condition of the wound should hereafter arise,) we dressed the wound by binding together the flaps with sutures and adhesive strips, previously placing a tent of lint cloth, as recommended by Baron Larrey, between them, about the size of a common pencil, and extending from the cotyloid cavity an inch or two beyond the lips of the wound. The ligatures were all brought out at one point, which served as another drain. No bandages or other dressings were now used. The boy was made comfortable upon the mattress without removing him from the operating-room, in which he remained all night and slept well; passed urine quite freely at daylight, soon after which he vomited freely. He now drank half a glass of London porter, and soon threw it up; also fresh milk, which he also threw up. At the suggestion of Dr. Winston, he used occasionally a spoonful of milk and lime-water, which remained with him. Removed him at 10 o'clock to his room. Drank occasionally a few spoonfuls of brandy and milk, which he retained. And suffice it to say, that from this time on he gradually improved, taking good, wholesome food, and daily, for the first few days, a little brandy and milk, or porter. The wound continued gradually to heal, and discharged a thick, laudable pus, by no means excessive in quantity, or, indeed, as much as I expected. The tent was removed on the fifth day, and pus discharged through the opening for several days, as well as along the ligatures, and at the upper end nearest to the cavity of the joint. One of the ligatures came away on the ninth day, another on the tenth, and all came off by gently pulling at them with the forceps on the 11th day. From this time he has daily improved, and is now considered entirely out of danger. The wound is nearly cicatrized, and he has returned home in fine spirits and quite hearty. The operation was performed on the 14th of last month, and twenty-nine days have elapsed up to writing. It is remarkable that up to this time he has not taken any kind of medicine since he was removed from the operating-room on the day after the operation. His appetite has continued good, and all his secretions appear to be as natural as those of one in perfect health.

This is the first operation of the kind, so far as we know, that has ever been performed in the State of Tennessee. It was first performed successfully in 1773, by M. Perrault, of Sainte Maure, France, in a case of traumatic gangrene, (Cooper's Surg. Dic.,) since which time, and until the introduction of chloroform, it has been regarded with much more horror, and proved much more fatal, than at the present day, not more than six in twenty formerly surviving it. Sir Charles Bell thought it was an operation that ought never to be performed. The celebrated Percival Pott said, "I have seen it done, and I am now very sure I shall never do it, unless it be on a dead body." Callisen and Richerand held like opinions. Henning, in his military surgery, says, "Obliged as we are coolly to form our calculations in human blood, there is still something in the idea of removing the quarter of a man at which the boldest mind naturally recoils; and yet there are cases in which we have it only left to balance between certain death and this tremendous alternative." The first operation at the hip-joint in the United States was performed by Walter Brashear, of Bardstown, Ky., in 1806. The operation was successful, as well as that of Dr. Mott, of N. Y., who next performed it, in 1824. But it has failed in the hands of such men as Mr. Guthrie, Dr. Emery, Mr. Brownrigg, Baron Larrey, Baron Græfe, Sir Benjamin Brodie, Mr. Carmichael, Drs. Blick and Cole, Baron Dupuytren, MM. Gensoulclat, Roux, Delpech, Pelletau, Dieffenbach, Syme, Velpeau and Walther. (Cooper's Surgical Dic.) Some of the above surgeons have, however, been successful.

Since the introduction of chloroform this operation has been performed with greater success, both in America and Europe, although it is yet one of the most unsuccessful operations in surgery, as the following statistics, taken from Erichsen's last edition of Surgery, (1859,) will show. He says, "Amputation at the hip-joint has been performed, so far as I can ascertain, in 126 cases; of these 76 died. In 47 cases it was for injury; of these 35 proved fatal. In 42 cases in which it was done for chronic disease, 24 recovered and 18 died. According to Dr. S. Smith, the mortality from this operation has been much less of late yerrs than was formerly the case, and this is doubtless the case so far as amputation at the hip-joint for *disease* is concerned; but in cases of *injury* the procedure is still a highly unsatisfactory one. In all the 12 cases, in which it was done in the Crimea, it proved fatal." More than half the cases, therefore, so far as the statistics are known, have died; there being 76 deaths and 50 recoveries of the 126 cases.

In publishing our case, we do so with no feeling of vainglory, or desire for notoriety, or laudation; on the contrary, we sincerely hope we may never be driven to the necessity of performing, or of even witnessing, this dreadful operation again. But we publish it as a great achievement of our noble profession, and as especially creditable to the science and art of surgery, to thus preserve from *certain death* the life of a sprightly and intelligent boy, who may yet live to become a worthy and useful citizen.

[The *Nashville Journal*, from which we copy, contains a plate and description of the diseased bone, which we are obliged to omit.]

MEDICAL REGISTRATION.

We are happy to find that a preliminary meeting has been held, and proceedings commenced, towards the formation of a Medical Registration Society for Birmingham and the Midland Counties. All the speakers united in admitting the great advantage of being furnished with a list of the impostors who impose upon the public by assuming titles to which they have no legal right, and inflict upon the deluded sufferers incalculable loss. This object should be steadily kept in view by these Societies. They must not degenerate into prosecuting Societies for the mere protection of professional interests. The nonsense talked lately by the magistrates about the interested motives of medical men in prosecuting quacks cannot be corrected too soon. It is the public we protect, not ourselves. We do not sell alum and urine at fabulous prices as a certain cure for incurable deafness. The public is not cheated by respectable members of our body; and it is for the national good, not for individual benefit, that the public should know who are legal practitioners, and who are illegal pretenders.—*London Med. Times and Gaz.*

From the Proceedings of the Eighth Annual Meeting of the American
Pharmaceutical Association.

The Committee on Home Adulterations, by Chas. J. C. Carney, of
Boston, reported. Adulteration was defined, in the language of Dr.
Hassell, of London—substitutions, impurities, and accidental contam-
inations being excluded—as "the intentional addition of an article,
for purposes of gain or deception, of any substance or substances, the
presence of which is not acknowledged in the name under which the
article is sold." Great scientific skill is shown in many of the adulterations; in other cases the most pernicious articles are substituted
for the genuine. A list of articles of food habitually adulterated was
given as follows :

Colored Confectionery—Adulterated with emerald or scheeles green,
arsenite of copper.

Beer—with coculus indica and nux vomica.

Pickles and Bottled Fruits—with verdigris and sulphate copper.

Custard Powder—with chromate of lead.

Tea and Snuff—with the same.

Cayenne and Curry Powder—with red oxide of lead.

Sugar Confectionery—with gamboge, orpiment, or sulphuret of
arsenic, and chloride of copper.

Flour and Bread—with hydrated sulphate of lime, plaster of Paris
and alum.

Vinegar—with sulphuric acid.

Sugar—with sand and plaster of Paris.

Milk—with chalk, sheep's brains, ground turmeric.

Arrowroot—with ground rice.

Chocolate—with rice flour, potato starch, gum tragacanth, cinabar,
bals. Peru, red ox. mercury, red lead, carbt. of lime, and the red
ochres to bring up the colors.

Mustard—with ground turmeric, to give it a brilliant color.

Butter—with potato starch, mutton tallow, carbt. lead, and sugar
of lead.

While the committee hesitated to give the names of the parties
guilty of this practice, it was recommended that the Association
should take some action in reference to the subject.

Some curious instances of adulteration had come to the knowledge
of the committee during the year.

During the past year, in a wood-turner's shop, in Boston, was seen more than a barrel of East India rhubarb, which was being turned down into " true Turkey."

This rhubarb was sold for genuine and real Turkey rhubarb.

A druggist was applied to by a man for a situation as a porter in his store.

" What can you do? What have you been doing at your last place ?" were the questions asked.

" O," replied the man, " I have done everything about the store that was needed, until the past year, I have worked up stairs in *the room* making Turkey rhubarb."

" Making Turkey rhubarb, what do you mean by that ?"

" Why," replied the man, " we used to take the East India and *file* and *bore* it into true Turkey."

The man was not engaged.

The following list of drugs adulterated was presented:

Acetate of morphia is adulterated with acetate and phosphate of lime.

Benzoic acid, with asbestos, carbonate and sulphate of lime, hipponic acid and sugar.

Citric acid, with oxalic and tartaric acid and sulphate of lime. It often contains sulphuric acid and salts of lead or copper. In 1850 M. Pennes discovered the presence of lead in this acid, obtained of three highly respectable dealers. The acid was very white, and was intended to prepare the purgative lemonade.

Tartaric acid, with cream of tartar, and sulphate of potassa and with lime.

Aloes, with colophony, ochre, extract of licorice, gum-arabic, and calcined bones.

Starch, with carbonate and sulphate of lime or alabaster; the more common fraud is, however, to saturate it with moisture.

Arrowroot, with potato starch and rice flour.

Asafœtida, with gum resins of poorer quality of sand, and other inert substances.

Balsam Copaiva, with the resinous extract by decoction of the bark of branches of copaisera, turpentine, colophony, and fat oils.

Balsam Peru, with colophony, turpentine, benzoin resin, alcohol, and fixed oils.

Balsam Tolu, with turpentine, colophony, and other resins.

Chloroform, with chlorhydric ether, hyphochlorous acid, hydrocarbonated oils, compounds of methyle and aldhyde, and fixed substances.

Beeswax, with resin, Burgundy pitch, earthy pitch, flowers and sulphur, starch and amylaceous substances, tallow, stearic acid, yellow ochre, calcined bones and sawdust.

Tart. emetic, with cream tartar, oxide antimony, tartrate of iron, chlor. calcium and potassium, and sometimes is contaminated with salts of copper and tin.

Essential oils, with alcohol and fixed oils.

Iodide potassium, with chloride of potassium and sodium, and calcium, carbonate of potassa and bromide of potassium. The latter salt being sometimes in so large a proportion, owing to its lesser price, as to *replace* almost entirely the iodide.

Manna, with glucose or starch sugar, and starch. The large flake manna is sometimes made from a mixture, consisting of a little manna, flour, honey, and a purgative powder; these are boiled together to a syrupy consistence, and then moulded in form of "flakes;" common "sorts manna" has been converted into "flake" by being boiled in water, clarified with charcoal, and moulded into proper form.—*Med. News.*

POOR BUTLER AGAIN!

OLD AGE IS HONORABLE.—Our friend of the *Medical and Surgical Reporter* says, concerning his being the oldest editor but one in the United States, that "Our first statement was correct." Well, his "*first* statement" was made in 1854, in his "salutatory." But we suppose when he says his "first statement," he means his *last* statement; for, in proof of its correctness, he now says that "The burden of editorial labor on the *Reporter* rested on our shoulders almost from our first connection with the enterprise," etc. "This labor first began in July, 1850. The first day of the month was publication day. The first number of the MEDICAL GAZETTE is dated July 6, 1850. * * * But the same number of the *Reporter* contains a notice of the MEDICAL GAZETTE." This is beyond our arithmetic. Dr. Butler commenced his labors on the *Reporter* in July, 1850. "The first day of the month was publication day." "The first number of the GAZETTE is dated July 6th." "But the same number of the *Reporter* contains a notice of the GAZETTE." That is, a publication made on the 1st of July, 1850, contains a notice of a publication made six days afterwards! "This," says Dr. Butler, "shows that either the GAZETTE was a case of premature labor, or that the *Reporter* was one of prolonged gestation." Assuming that Dr. B. was editor of the *Reporter* in July, 1850, he cannot pretend that that publication was a case of prolonged gestation. The gestation that terminated in his birth as editor he says occurred in 1850. But the child did not cry, or give other signs of life, until 1854. This quiet sleep of the child for four years after its birth would go to prove that it came into the world prematurely. Why its existence at all was kept a secret for four years "in the family," we leave to Dr. B. to explain. A birth of that kind is not usually a matter of boast in after years.—*Nashville Med. and Surg. Journal.*

EDITOR'S TABLE.

☞ RED INK.

We repeat, in this number, the new device of using RED INK, on the wrappers of the GAZETTE, as the most polite and delicate intimation to those who are thus designated, that they are *delinquent* subscribers, and in *arrears* on our books.

All who have paid for 1859, receive their Journals *free of postage;* while our *non*-paying subscribers are still *taxed* for postage; a hint which has not proved successful, so that we now try the *Red Ink.*

The year has nearly closed, and unless remittances are now mailed, all who do not pay in advance will be stricken from our mail book for 1860.

The present number, issued December 1st, is the last of the present year, and closes our 10th volume.

☞ The advance subscriptions of all are now due, and prepayment for 1860 will secure the prepayment of postage for the year. Only *two dollars* per annum, in advance.

NEW YORK ACADEMY OF MEDICINE.

The Anniversary Oration before this body was delivered in the 9th Street Dutch Reformed Church, on the 3d ult., by Wm. C. Roberts, M.D. It was an "Eulogium on the Medical Profession," and is spoken of as an able production by all who heard it. It will doubtless be printed.

THE ANNIVERSARY DINNER

Of the New York Society for the relief of the widows and orphans of deceased physicians, was celebrated Nov. 16th, at the Metropolitan Hotel. It was attended by a large body of the profession, including many who are not members, but thus annually manifest their interest in the benevolent objects of the organization, which is to establish a vested fund, the revenue of which is to be available to the families of deceased members who are not otherwise provided for, or who may need to become beneficiaries. Only two such are now receiving its benefits, and the fund already accumulated amounts to $27,000, which is secured by bond and mortgage at seven per cent. The annual dues of members are $10, life members $100, and $150 or upwards constitutes a patron, of which honor many have availed themselves.

At this annual dinner, Dr. Isaac Wood, President, was in the chair, supported on the right and left by representatives of each of the liberal professions—of the Army and Navy of the United States—of the colleges and hospitals, and other dignitaries as invited guests. Over 130 medical men were present at the dinner, which was served in the best style characteristic of the Messrs. Leland, and conducted throughout in a manner reflecting the highest credit on the stewards.

A band of music enlivened the entertainment, cheering the sentiments and speeches, which many thought rendered this one of the most successful anniversaries in the history of the Society.

Rev. Mr. Weston responded for the Clergy, the Hon. Mr. Evarts for the Bar, Dr. Stevens and Dr. Francia for the Medical Profession, Dr. Latimer for the Army, Lieutenant Mayo for the Navy, Dr. J. R. Wood for the Hospitals, and Dr. Bedford replied to the closing sentiment, Woman. All the speeches were excellent in matter and manner, and all were received with cheers.

In the course of the evening there was an agreeable surprise by the announcement that Professor Palmer, of the University of Michigan, was present, having just landed on his return from a professional tour in Europe. He was forthwith pressed into the service, and though not in the programme, he made a most happy and effective speech on the subject of Medical Education as he had observed it abroad, indicating the advantages of the foreign system of teaching over our own, and advocating the propriety of our improving by their example. The points dwelt upon were, 1. Better preliminary instruction before admission as students. 2. A longer term of study, four years instead of three. 3. A more extended course of lectures, nine months of each year instead of four, with fewer lectures in the day; and lastly, that the school should be the hospital, and the hospital should be the school, and that true clinical and demonstrative teaching should, to a great extent, take the place of didactic lectures.

These improvements being engrafted on our system, and the crowning improvement of requiring repeated examinations of students by their teachers, and as an indispensable prerequisite to *a degree or license*, a final examination by a Board *other than their teachers*, who should have the exclusive power of deciding upon qualifications to practice, Prof. Palmer thought we should then have a system here every way superior to anything he saw abroad. And, in conclusion, he deprecated the idea of young men being sent to Paris to finish their education, which he judged detrimental to their physical, intellectual and moral health, and dangerous to the last degree, although there are many honorable exceptions, who have escaped these dangers.

His remarks were received with acclamation, and our veteran, Dr. Stevens, promptly endorsed these views of medical education, which he had favored, and would continue to advocate, until these Reforms should be carried out in this city and country, and all of which he believed would sooner or later receive universal adoption.

The readers of the GAZETTE are no strangers to any of these suggestions, and yet their presentation on this festive occasion, by Prof. Palmer, was most opportune, and met a hearty response.

At the close of the exercises, it was announced that a number of new members had offered, and that Dr. Alexander N. Gunn, the present Health Officer, had done himself the honor of becoming a patron of the Society by the payment of $150.

MEDICAL STUDENTS.

We hear from all quarters that the classes in our medical colleges throughout the country are as large, or larger, than last year, although it is too early in the session for figures.

Professor Paine, of the New York University.

An article which opens this number of the GAZETTE is from a correspondent, who lets the gas out of Dr. Griscom's balloon, by exposing his plagiarism, and characteristic mendacity, in his late speech before the Academy on yellow fever, contagion, and fomites. The writer proves that Professor Paine's works contain all that Dr. Griscom says with such a flourish of trumpets, thus stripping the jackdaw of his plumes; and by parallel columns he then demonstrates that, in the facts and arguments in proof of non-contagion, neither Dr. Griscom nor his friends can have any possible pretence to originality, since Professor Paine had anticipated and published long ago the whole of what they know on the subject, although he purposely ignores the source whence he derived his wondrous discovery. We trust this brief article will be read, that the profession may profit by the information it gives, and that this reclamation for Dr. Paine of the merit of originality may brand the infamy of literary theft into the forehead of the guilty poacher, and reform his habit of stealing other men's thunder.

SANITARY ASSOCIATION.

This anomalous body has now betrayed the animus ascribed to its leaders in the beginning, and the *selfishness* of which was so palpable last year, that his Honor the Mayor was constrained to defeat the bills which they were laboring to lobby through the Legislature at Albany. At the late meeting the Association went over bodily into the political market. Dr. McNulty was the mover of a committee to catechise the candidates of the several factions in politics, and learn their whereabouts in relation to the Sanitary Bill. He was, of course, backed by Dr. Griscom and Prosper M. Wetmore, Esq., both of whom have been office-holders or office-seekers for a time beyond the memory of our oldest inhabitant. That bill, or any other they will prepare, will create fat offices for themselves, and if they can pledge the candidates in advance for their bill, their selfish designs will be thus promoted. As a *quid pro quo*, the idea is held out that ballots containing the names of the pledged men are to be sent to all our physicians; and the papers have already announced that the Academy of Medicine can command 5,000 votes at the coming election! a price sufficient to secure half the candidates for Senate and Assembly from any party, or in any district. Whether the fish will all bite at this bait will soon be known; but how many of the 5,000 votes promised from the Academy of Medicine, as a "power in the State," will be given to either of them, is a problem unsolved. But all is fair in politics, and this trading is only a fair business transaction.

If any improvement is made in the Sanitary or Health Laws of this city, it must be gained by withdrawing the whole subject from party politics. And this unworthy course taken by the Sanitary Association has proven that they are not the men, nor theirs the means, to effect any salutary reform. Nevertheless, they may thus keep themselves before the people as standing candidates for public office, but self-aggrandizement is the animus of the leaders, and its detection will again defeat them at Albany, as heretofore. " A good cause has fallen into bad hands," as was said last winter in Albany by high authority. 'Tis true, a pity, and pity 'tis, 'tis true.

LONG ISLAND COLLEGE HOSPITAL.

The following letter, which comes from " One of the Committee of Organization," may be regarded as exhibiting their side of a question upon which there are two sides. We regret to learn that both Hospital and College are abandoned as the result of the controversy, each party blaming the other for the failure.

" DEAR DOCTOR—It is almost impossible to conceive how facts could be so misrepresented as to justify, in any degree, your remarks on the Long Island College Hospital, published in the November number of the GAZETTE. But that such misrepresentations have been made, is proved, by your feeling justified in making such statements, and that, too, in a manner which evinces confidence in the sources of your information.

" It is unnecessary to inform one of your experience in such matters, that to establish a charitable institution of any kind upon a *permanent basis*, is always a difficult undertaking; and of all these, that of a hospital is perhaps the most difficult, in consequence of being burdened at every step with large outlays.

" You are also well aware, that to establish *satisfactorily* a medical college, which, by your own showing, is an expensive luxury to the professors, is perhaps a no less difficult enterprise. ALL institutions of charity, or of learning, must necessarily struggle during their early history against many adverse circumstances, unless abundantly endowed from their beginning.

"It is not a matter of surprise, therefore, that an undertaking which contemplates the formation of both a hospital and a medical school in one organization, should meet not only the difficulties peculiar to each, but others also, growing out of their combination. And in the case of the Long Island College Hospital, it is not necessary to suspect the agency of ' squabbles,' or ' émeutes,' or ' coups-de-main,' to explain its ill success. Had all the efforts of the Regents and medical officers been directed to the complete founding of either the Hospital or the College, there is no question but an honorable result would have been attained; for, so long as their attention was confined to the Hospital alone, everything progressed favorably. It was not until an attempt was prematurely made to engraft a school upon an imperfectly established hospital that any trouble was experienced.

"The difficulties which arose in the efforts to organize the College were such as could not have been foreseen; and when met, they could not be obviated without sacrificing something of the high character which it was intended the College should possess. They sprung entirely from a *pre-existing state of things in the profession*, of which the officers of the institution were, for the most part, ignorant. This 'state of things' was not created by those officers, but was found already existing, and was felt at every step taken to organize a college in dependence upon the hospital faculty. By making the faculties in a great degree independent of each other, all difficulties seemed to disappear, and the *medical officers, with perfect unanimity*, agreed upon such a plan of organization.

"This course, however, was disapproved by a minority of the Board of Regents, and their disapproval, in connection with a coexisting want of funds, led to the closure of the Hospital. Had there been no difference of opinion among the Regents, the lack of funds could have been undoubtedly remedied; or, if the Hospital had been permanently established, the majority could have decided all questions.

"There is, therefore, no occasion for imputing bad motives to those who have acted to the best of their judgment for the good of the institution, although, to the deep regret of all concerned, the result has been unexpected, and the high anticipations of many disappointed.
                                        "VERITAS."

Our article in the last No. of the GAZETTE, to which the foregoing letter is a reply, was founded on communications from the other side; and though we hesitated to publish those articles, it was not because they were not authenticated, but because they contained the names of numerous gentlemen, with personalities which we could not consider relevant. Hence we substituted a paragraph of our own, which indicated the views of the writers and our own estimate of the unfortunate controversy, with the light we then had; but we refrained from naming the parties, whose real or nominal relations to the College were criticised by our correspondents.

The facts as we now understand them are, that both the Hospital and College were projected by *two* physicians of Brooklyn, who, with the help of a *third, selected* the Council and Regents, obtained the charter, founded the Hospital, were appointed Professors to the Hospital, and became its Surgeons and Physicians. They have been looking for and urging the organization of a Medical College in connection with the Hospital, in accordance with the charter. Of course they expected to be included in the Faculty of said College, but when the Council attempted the organization these founders of the institution were not included in the proposed Faculty, it being found impracticable to obtain Professors for the College, unless the Medical Staff of the Hospital were left out. The objections to these gentlemen seem to have been prompted solely by personal hostility; but they were found to be insuperable, and hence the Council had no alternative but to make the College an independent organization, distinct from the Hospital, or utterly fail in securing, either in New York or Brooklyn, such a Faculty as they judged essential to the success of the new College. The Council reported to the Regents their nominations for Professors, and they might have been elected, and both the College and Hospital have been in full operation under separate organizations; but the disaffections which were apparent, and the pecuniary liabilities already incurred for the Hospital, led to a resolution to abandon the whole enterprise, sell the property, and go into liquidation.

While disposed to place the most favorable construction on the motives of all concerned, we think it singularly unfortunate that the Hospital, so much needed and capable of such extended usefulness, must be overthrown, for no better reason than the "pre-existing state of the profession" in Brooklyn and New York. The new Professors, who were nominated, but not elected, and whose prospective lectures are not to be forthcoming, merit sympathy in their disappointment; which they must feel almost as keenly as do Drs. Ayres, Bauer, and Byrne, whose cherished hopes have so ingloriously perished with the extinction of the Hospital. But until a better "*state of the profession*" can be inaugurated hereabouts, all hopes of establishing a great medical school in Brooklyn, or even a Hospital, may be abandoned. We earnestly recommend the Regents, Council, and embryo Faculty to turn their attention to the much needed reform in the "state of the profession" among us, which it is here shown has defeated their well-meant efforts. Our profession in this region is so sadly cut up into cliques, who claim either to rule or ruin, that it has been said of us, with more candor than politeness, that we "*live like crabs in a basket, by* PINCHING *one another*."

PHYSIOGNOMY ANNIHILATED BY BEARDS.

Lavater might have spared himself the labors of a lifetime, and the preparation of his huge volumes on Physiognomy, which cost him prodigious toil, if he could have anticipated that men of this age would conceal and disfigure the " human face divine" by hirsute appendages, such as characterize no animal but the goat, unless it be certain species of the baboon.

In his day, and long after, the razor was justly deemed an element of civilization, and the science of Physiognomy discovers and describes the *features* as they appear in a face cleanly shaven; and among these the most expressive are those of the *lips, mouth,* and *chin,* whence are derived indications of the mental and moral proclivities of the individual, which awaken in the beholder admiration or distrust, respect or suspicion; and the experience of the discerning among mankind has proved that the science is never at fault when applied by an expert. Women are generally physiognomists by nature, and their instinct in reading character by the face, when this is visible, is proverbially reliable; so that wise men everywhere refuse to confide in anybody, whom their wives pronounce from the face alone to be unworthy of trust.

But for physiognomical observations, the razor must first have removed both beard and moustache, since these, if allowed to grow, conceal the most expressive features. He whose chin, mouth, and lips are rendered invisible by neglecting the daily use of the razor, wears a mask, which conceals his character from the observer, and destroys his identity as effectually as though he perpetually wore a domino. All men, who are similar in size and dress, look alike if their beard and moustache be of the same color, and cannot be distinguished from each other, especially in the dark; much less can a physiognomist detect their characteristics, for the features on which he relies are concealed.

The different colors of the beard and moustache, often light, yellow, brown, red, or gray, when the hair of the head is dark or black, or as in some cases contrasted with baldness, constitute a repulsive deformity. The use of dye for securing uniformity of color is readily detected, and is as much a subject of ridicule as the coloring matters which antiquated and faded beauties apply to the skin; while the rough, grizzly hair or bristles which some men allow their faces to be covered with are a positive nuisance to the eye of taste or refinement. They who are hideously deformed, or the lower features of whose face designate an animal and sensual nature by unmistakable signs, and such alone, have any excuse for wearing either beard or moustache. But to see a man of intellectual and even classical face with his lips covered with hair, and a beard concealing his mouth and chin, which would else give expression to his emotions, is an absolute monstrosity.

Professional men, of all others, should be most scrupulous of personal appearance, and cleanliness. Physicians, lawyers, and even clergymen, in a few instances, have of late abolished the razor from their toilette, and in this country the younger and weaker brethren are falling into the snare. For lawyers and other public speakers, the impediment to speech and hindrance to articulation render the moustache intolerable; while a clergyman thus disfigured is a coxcomb or a dotard in the pulpit, which he should not be permitted to enter until he is shorn of the deformity.

But it is with medical men we have to do, among whom a beard and moustache are the chosen insignia of quackery. Even in France, where barbers, dancing-masters, and *soi disant* counts are unshaven, no physician or surgeon of the Parisian hospitals has thus degraded himself, for we have the portraits of them all in our library, and neither beard nor moustache is in sight.

The *reasons* for abandoning the razor by the few who have thus dishonored their profession are wholly unreasonable and discreditable. They are too indolent to shave—cannot consume so much time—want to look like foreigners—to have a *distingué* appearance—unlike the common herd—and dislike old fogyism. These are the true reasons, whatever they may assign. But while any of our fraternity persist in thus masking themselves, we shall not cease to denounce them as unprofessional and quackish. And we point them to the notorious quack, who first defied public opinion in New York, by beard and moustache, and long hair, when he had no imitator for years, except a few of his brother Homœopaths. Let that tribe follow their file-leader in this as in other tomfooleries. But the physician or surgeon who adopts this fashion will find sooner or later that he has lost caste among his brethren; that his presence in the sick-room is repulsive to the women, terrifying to the babies, and insufferable in a consultation. The habit of stroking his beard and twisting his moustache, with people of sense, is regarded with disgust and loathing; and physicians should never be in this category, as ridiculous as the ancient folly of looking wise under a powdered wig, and with a golden-headed cane poised beneath the nose or chin; or the more modern folly of placing a huge oyster-lamp before the door, instead of having the *light* within.

Let all men cease from Physiognomy, and henceforth study Beards.

The Medical and Surgical Reporter—Kappa Lambda Societies—Moral Insanity, &c.

Our readers are aware that on the appearance of the new weekly at Philadelphia, "*The Medical and Surgical Reporter*," we extended to it and the editors a cordial greeting, and wished it success, a wish we have frequently repeated since. Our courtesies have never been appreciated, but repaid by a repetition of assaults in every conceivable form, both by the editor and his correspondents. Our forbearance was censured by many, and at length more than one of the Journals expressed the surprise which was so generally felt at our silence, until the *Nashville Journal*, having been assailed conjointly with the GAZETTE, by a most unfounded and malicious attack, the veteran editor of that Journal volunteered in our defence while making his own, and read the *Reporter* a homily he can never forget, justly rebuking his arrogance and injustice, his inflated conceit and impudent falsehoods, of all of which he convicted him by his own columns. This article we *copied*, only appending our opinion that the castigation had ample provocation, and was well merited. Whereupon, leaving his bones to Dr. Bowling's own picking, we pursued the even tenor of our way, until, followed up ever since by offensive and disgusting personalities from week to week, we have at length condescended to show how much we defied and despised the *Reporter* and its impotent editor, by hurling back some of his Parthian arrows into his own camp.

As he and his correspondents have now renewed their assaults upon the AMERICAN MEDICAL GAZETTE and its editor, we propose here to dispose of Dr. Butler and his Journal, and thus dismiss both from our columns hereafter.

And first as to the Kappa Lambdas. We have for many years heard nothing on this subject until during the last year, when the old pamphlet of the New York County Medical Society was resurrected, after a sleep of twenty years, and sent to us. Our readers are familiar with all we said about it, and know how we summarily disposed of a subsequent pamphlet and the whole subject, after merely reciting the history and recording its epitaph, as we supposed, for we never could be made to feel the least interest in the subject, and we could only laugh at those who did, or were weak enough to fear it. Hence our duty as a journalist being performed, we heard no more of it until a letter, similar to that inserted in the *Reporter* of the 29th of October, was sent to us, in relation to the overthrow of the Long Island College Hospital, and which we *rejected*, partly because it charged the conspiracy against the Kappa Lambdas, when we *knew* that they had nothing to do with it, and moreover that only one physician of Brooklyn ever belonged to this secret society. Dr. Butler, however, eagerly published the article sent to him, after we had *declined* it, and probably he inserted it for *this reason*.

What will our readers think, with these facts before them, when they learn that in his last number this same Dr. Butler, finding himself under the necessity of apologizing for inserting the Brooklyn article, and also of publishing an elaborate defence of the ancient fraternity in Philadelphia, has the temerity and mendacity to assert, that "the first he ever heard of Kappa Lambdas was through the MEDICAL GAZETTE," and attributing to us "the origin of the raid against them," and commiserating his Brooklyn correspondent for being misled by the GAZETTE, and this when he knew all the facts? This he does for the purpose of basing his personal calumnies against us, as having had private griefs to resent, which are wholly in his morbid surmisings. Happily, our record for thirty years in New York is clear; and as to "position," social and professional, it is quite equal to our ambition, and ever has been to our deserts. And while hostile to secret organizations in a liberal profession, yet we number among our dearest friends many past and present members of the Kappa Lambda associations, nor have our professional intimacies ever been disturbed thereby. The other insinuations of the *Reporter* merit only our contempt.

But it now only remains to demonstrate still more clearly, that the editor of the *Reporter* has entered upon a crusade against the GAZETTE and its editor with so venomous a spirit that there is no possibility of pleasing him.

In our November number we copied from the *Reporter* a full report of the late discussions on yellow fever, &c., in Philadelphia and New York, substituting their report for our own. Of course we gave that journal due credit, and very highly praised the promptness with which it appeared, and added that it was a "very creditable feat in journalism." Now this is *a way we have*, of always doing justice, even to an enemy; and the ten years' history of this journal will prove that we never in a single instance withheld the meed of praise to merit, no matter what relations the party sustained to us. And so in the present instance, had we ignored Dr. Butler and his journal, by giving him no credit for this long extract, he could not even then have railed at us more bitterly than he does in his last number. And because, forsooth, the same number contains a reply to one of his latest assaults upon us—a palpable hit, by the way—he judges us to be insane as Ossowatomie Brown, or "morally" insane like Gerrit Smith. Luckily for us that a hundred miles separates us from that mad-house at Blockley, of which he is *chief!* He is so implacable about our playful reiteration of his "oxy-hydrogen blowpipe," that if we were once in his hands, even his tender mercies would be cruelty. "So much for Butler," and our readers will not again hear from us on a subject which has been too personal for our taste. Our new volume will "seek peace and pursue it."

Marshall Infirmary in the City of Troy, N. Y.

The Charter and By-Laws of this excellent charity have been published. The institution is located on Mount Ida, within the city of Troy, and occupies large buildings erected for the purpose, at an expense of $77,000, more than half of which, together with the nine acres of ground, were the gift of the late Benjamin Marshall, Esq., a benevolent citizen, whose name it bears.

It includes four departments, viz.: one for lying-in women; one for ordinary diseases; one for pestilential and contagious diseases; and the fourth for lunatics.

It is in the care of a Board of Governors, and has the following medical officers at present, viz.:

Attending Physicians—Alfred Wotkyns, M.D.; Thos. W. Blatchford, M.D.; James Thorn, M.D.; Thomas C. Brinsmade, M.D.

Resident Medical Superintendent—Le Roy McLean, M.D.

Medical Assistant—John R. Gregory, M.D.

AMERICAN MEDICAL ASSOCIATION.

Dr. Stephen G. Hubbard, of New Haven, has been appointed by the President of the Association to the office of Junior Secretary, in the place of Dr. Eli Ives, who declined the office. The Senior Secretary is Dr. Bemis, of Louisville, Ky.

THE MEDICAL SCHOOLS,

So far as heard from, have opened with increased classes, although we are only able as yet to approximate the numbers on the authority of rumor, and the full report will doubtless exceed the figures. Soon after the opening we hear that already the matriculations were, at

Jefferson Medical College.........................500
University of Pennsylvania.......................400
University of Nashville...... 400
University of New York....... 300
College of Physicians and Surgeons, N. Y...........150
N. Y. Medical College............................ 75
University of Buffalo............................. 70

From these indications we infer general prosperity in all the schools. We have not heard from either of the other colleges.

AMERICAN MEDICAL MONTHLY.

Our neighbors very flippantly insert the following dogmatic averment in their editorial last month, which they gravely intend as a summary disposal of the questions recently discussed in Philadelphia and New. York:

"THE FACT IS, *that yellow fever is sometimes, in the latitude of New York, communicated from the sick to the attendants, or to persons in the vicinity.*"

The above "fact" we pronounce one of the "false facts" by which superficial thinkers blunder on in antiquated error. It is *not true* in any sense, in which the following is not also true, viz.:

"The fact is, that FEVER AND AGUE is sometimes, in the latitude of New York, communicated from the sick to the attendants, or to persons in the vicinity."

Now, if our neighbors mean no more than this, the statement is wholly irrelevant as regards contagion. If they do mean what they say to imply more, then we pronounce their "fact" to be a fiction, and challenge the proof.

NEW YORK COUNTY MEDICAL SOCIETY.

The following officers were elected November 15th, 1859, viz.:

OLIVER WHITE, M.D., *President.*
H. D. BULKLEY, M.D., *Vice-President.*
HENRY S. DOWNES, M.D., *Recording Secretary.*
SAMUEL A. PURDY, M.D., *Corresponding Secretary.*
B. R. ROBSON, M.D., *Treasurer.*

College of Physicians and Surgeons, in New York.

The Catalogue of the Alumni, Officers, and Fellows of this College has been published, including all from 1807 to 1859. Of the 2,303 names in the catalogue, 1,702 are supposed to be living; while of the alumni, numbering 1,733, 276 are known to be deceased, leaving 1,473.

The largest class of alumni was in 1819, numbering 75. Ten years after, in 1829, it had fallen to 23. In 1839 it was still 23. In 1849 it had reached 45; while in 1859 the alumni only number 39 for the year! This class is the smallest in the history of the college, since 1842-3, when it numbered only 19.

The first Commencement was in 1811, so that the College has been in operation nearly half a century.

A PRIZE MEDAL

Is offered by Dr. George T. Elliott, one of the physicians of the Bellevue Hospital, for the best preparation showing the *Fascia of the Pelvis*, and the competition is open to the students of either of our New York colleges. See announcement in this number, for particulars.

PRIVATE MEDICAL TEACHING.

In addition to the Preparatory Medical School, there are private classes, more or less connected with each of our colleges, in which all the various departments are taught by examinations, cliniques, &c.; so that the students who avail themselves of these helps, have very little leisure time during the college course.

The Boston Medical and Surgical Journal

Seems to be in a fog, in relation to a case of death from a bayonet wound which they reported from "an authentic source," and when their article was replied to and its errors exposed, the editors decline an opinion until they have the case in an "authentic" shape. This is as clear as mud. A correspondent, calling our attention to the subject, inquires whether expulsion from the County and State Medical Society is necessary to constitute a man an "authentic source" for a medical report, imputing malpractice to one or more of its members who remain in good fellowship with their brethren. Perhaps our confreres will condescend to explain.

ALCOHOL: ITS PLACE AND POWER. By James Miller, Professor of Surgery in the University of Edinburgh, &c. From the *nineteenth* Glasgow edition. Philadelphia: Lindsay & Blakiston. 1859.

THE USE AND ABUSE OF TOBACCO. By John Lizars, late Professor of Surgery in the Royal College of Surgeons. From the eighth Edinburgh edition. Philadelphia: Lindsay & Blakiston. 1859.

The worthy publishers merit the thanks of the American public for simultaneously sending out these two kindred publications, written as they are by two of the most eminent men in the surgical world, and upon subjects of vital importance to the present and future generations. They are but little volumes, issued in a neat and portable form, and exactly adapted to general circulation. They are the best "Tracts" which have ever appeared on Alcohol and Tobacco, without any semblance of fanaticism or cant, thoroughly scientific, rigidly accurate and logical, and yet overwhelming in their arguments and proofs for the rejection of these destroyers of the human race, these enemies of health and life, from the position they have acquired by habitual, excessive, and vicious indulgence. If they could be read and heeded by the rising generation, so forcible and demonstrative are their appeals to the young, that a revolution might be hoped for in the habits of millions, which would arrest premature mortality, and furnish examples of longevity such as neither we nor our ancestors have ever known.

AN INTRODUCTION TO PRACTICAL PHARMACY, designed as a text-book for the Student and as a guide for the Physician and Pharmaceutist, with many Formulas and Prescriptions. By Edward Parish, Principal of the School of Practical Pharmacy, &c. Philadelphia: Blanchard & Lea. 1859.

This well-known book now appears in a second edition, greatly enlarged and improved, and having 246 illustrations. The author has evidently bestowed great pains in the preparation for the reissue of this work, which is now an octavo of over 700 pages. The former edition was popular and useful, so that increasing patronage will doubtless reward the publishers for bringing it out in so handsome style. It should be forthwith placed in every apothecary-shop in the land, and it will be a valuable addition to every medical library.

THE PHYSICIAN'S VISITING LIST AND DIARY, AND BOOK OF ENGAGEMENTS, FOR 1860. Philadelphia: Lindsay & Blakiston.

We are indebted to the publishers for our copy of this perennial Annual, which has so long been our daily companion, that its loss would be indeed a privation. Various imitations and substitutes have been contrived, issued, and puffed, but we have never seen one which in all respects was equal to that of Lindsay & Blakiston; nor have any of them contained any real improvement, but only additional matter, which has neither novelty nor merit, and yet makes the book too cumbersome for the pocket. We have never known any of the brethren who had tried this little Annual once, who could be induced to exchange it for any other; and many of them, we know, make it serve the purposes of day-book, cash-book, expense-book, journal, and ledger, besides being a diary of business and engagements. Ours provides for fifty patients daily, which, we are fain to confess, is more than we have ever found to *pay*, and more than we can find time to visit, when they are scattered over so large a space as New York and its surroundings. The smaller size, with blanks for twenty-five patients, can be had of the publishers, and it is worth double its cost to any physician. Each copy contains an Almanac, Marshall Hall's Ready Method, Poisons and their antidotes described, and a Table to calculate the periods of utero-gestation, prefixed to the blank leaves for Diary, Memoranda, and Engagements.

LECTURES ON SURGICAL PATHOLOGY, delivered at the Royal College of Surgeons of England. By James Paget, F.R.S., &c. Philadelphia: Lindsay & Blakiston. 1860.

This is the second American edition of what will long be regarded as a standard work, and must be invaluable to students who aim to excel in pathological science. It is more minute and complete than any other book ever written in this department, and its form of Lectures enables the author to condense much information on each topic in small compass. Hypertrophy, Atrophy, Repair, Inflammation, Mortification, Specific diseases, and Tumors, are all treated of here, by an expert worthy the name. We cordially recommend the book to the profession.

THE ACTION OF MEDICINES IN THE SYSTEM. By Frederick William Headland, M.D., &c., of London. Philadelphia: Lindsay & Blakiston. 1859.

This work is well known to the profession, as the Prize Essay which received the Fothergillian gold medal, in 1852, from the Medical Society of London. We have here an American reprint of the third edition, revised and improved by the author, availing himself of the criticisms and acquisitions in this department during the seven years past. Without adopting all its theoretic teachings, we commend the book for its ability and utility, furnishing as it does a complete antidote to the various medical heresies so rife during the last half century, and vindicating as it does both the science and art of rational medication from the fashionable frivolities of the know-nothing, do-nothing systems of those who deify Nature, and depreciate the resources and capabilities of Art when guided by the lights of scientific truth and the inductions of enlightened experience. Every medical student should be indoctrinated into the medical faith, by reading this work and kindred productions, to establish his confidence in true therapeutics, and fortify him against popular and professional skepticism in therapeutics and the art of healing. It is issued in the publishers' best style.

TREATISE ON MICROSCOPIC DIAGNOSIS. By Gustaf von Dueben. With 71 engravings. Translated, with Annotations, by Prof. Louis Bauer, M.D., &c. New York: John Wiley. 1859.

This handsomely-gotten-up manual has just been placed on our table. We have had but barely time to give it a cursory perusal, yet even this has convinced us of its eminent practical value for incipient pathologists. Indeed, we rarely meet with a book that conveys so much useful instruction with the same brevity and clearness, and we may well imagine its having rapidly acquired great popularity with the profession in Europe. Dr. Gustaf von Dueben is a Swede, of promising talent; his investigations are characterized by great care and circumspection; his conclusions are cautious, and respectful to the labors of others; and his ultimate aim is to render the microscope a serviceable instrument in diagnosis, which, in our opinion, he has realized as nearly as our present status of knowledge would permit. The engravings are well executed and demonstrative, and the enterprise highly creditable to the publisher.

In comparing this recent product of medical literature with the plagiaristical microscopical companion of Dr. John King, of Cincinnati scholastic notoriety, we can, of course, not hesitate in pronouncing the former a most meritorious and useful addition to a medical library; the latter an imposition, not worthy the notice of the profession.

For access to this useful treatise we are indebted to Dr. Louis Bauer's indefatigable diligence, already favorably known to the profession; and we confess that the style of diction is as pure and perfect as could have been produced by any man not educated in the English language.

TO CORRESPONDENTS.

"BROOKLYN" will find his queries answered in this number, except as to the medical men concerned in the late explosion of the Long Island College Hospital. The Council are Drs. Mitchell, Dudley, Mason, and Henry, all of Brooklyn. The first Faculty chosen by the Council are said to have been Drs. Gilman, Dalton, St. John, Draper, and Sands, all attachés of the College of Physicians and Surgeons of New York. These being unacceptable to the Regents, who desired that Brooklyn might not be ignored, the second Faculty nominated were Drs. Hamilton, Flint, Trask, Hutchinson, Enos, and Chapman, the other chairs being left vacant. The three last named were all of Brooklyn, the others being taken from Buffalo, New York, and White Plains, respectively. We are not informed whether either of the gentlemen named was pledged to accept the appointment. As, however, the whole project, including both College and Hospital, has fallen through for the present, it is unimportant.

"Fordham," "Dutch Doctor," and "Mordecai the Jew," are declined, and will be returned to their authors. The GAZETTE has now said enough on the subject, both sides having an airing in this number.

CONTENTS.

AMERICAN MEDICAL GAZETTE ADVERTISER.

MEDICAL COLLEGE OF OHIO.

SESSION OF 1859-'60.

FACULTY.

L. M. LAWSON, M.D., Professor of the Theory and Practice of Medicine.
JESSE P. JUDKINS, M.D., Professor of Anatomy.
GEO. C. BLACKMAN, M.D., Professor of the Principles and Practice of Surgery and Clinical Surgery.
GEORGE MENDENHALL, M.D., Professor of Obstetrics.
C. G. COMEGYS, M D., Professor of Institutes of Medicine.

JOHN A. MURPHY, M.D., Professor of Materia Medica and Therapeutics.
H. E. FOOTE, M.D., Professor of Chemistry and Toxicology.
B. F. RICHARDSON, M D., Professor of Diseases of Women and Children.
JAMES GRAHAM, M.D., Professor of Clinical Medicine.
WILLIAM CLENDENIN, M.D., Demonstrator of Anatomy.

L. M. LAWSON, M.D., *Dean*, Northwest corner Sixth and Walnut Streets.
GEORGE MENDENHALL, M.D., *Registrar*, 197 Fourth Street.

OPENING OF THE COURSE.

The Fortieth Regular Course will open on the 18th October, and terminate on the last of February. Students are earnestly advised to be in attendance, especially those who expect to be candidates for Graduation, as credit for a full course cannot be allowed unless the pupil matriculates at an early period, and observes regular attendance on the Lectures   Clinical Lectures will be delivered at the Commercial Hospital and City Dispensary, during September and October, previous to the commencement of the Regular Course.

The public Commencement will take place early in March, with as little delay after the close of Lectures as practicable.

RESIDENT PHYSICIANS AND SURGEONS.

At the close of each Session, two or three graduates will be elected to act as Resident Physicians and Surgeons in the Commercial Hospital for the ensuing year.

Two Resident Physicians will be appointed to St. John's Hotel for Invalids, and the graduates of this College can compete for the places.

Two advanced Students will be elected at the close of each Session to act as Resident Pupils at the Dispensary, for one year, who will have rooms supplied them in the College building.

FEES.—For the whole Course, $90: Dissecting Ticket, $6; Graduation Fee, $25.
The Student can take one or more Tickets, as may suit his purposes.
The Dissecting Ticket is optional, except that the candidates are required to take it once.

Students. on arriving in the city, by calling at the College, (on Sixth Street, between Vine and Race,) will be conducted to good boarding-houses, where they can be accommodated with board, at from $2.50 to $4 00 per week.
Further information may be obtained by addressing

L. M. LAWSON, M.D., Dean.

CINCINNATI, OHIO, 1859.

ATLANTA MEDICAL COLLEGE.

PREPARATORY COURSE.

In addition to the regular Course of Lectures, which opens on the first Monday in May, a Preparatory Course of Instruction has been established. the second Session of which will commence on the first Monday in November next, and continue until the last of the following February.

Lectures will be given daily by the regular Professors of the College, with examinations and Dissections and Clinical Lectures, conducted as in the Regular Summer Course of Lectures.

This Preparatory or Winter Course will not count as a full Course in the requisites for graduation; neither is it obligatory, in order to be admitted to examination at the end of the Summer Term.

The fee for the Course is *Fifty Dollars*, which amount will be deducted from the fees demanded of those who may take the regular Summer Course.
For further information, address

J. G. WESTMORELAND, Dean.

ATLANTA, GA., Sept. 15, 1859.

UNIVERSITY OF NEW YORK.
MEDICAL DEPARTMENT.
SESSION, 1859-60.

The Session for 1859–60 will begin on Monday, October 17, and will be continued until the 1st of March.

Faculty of Medicine.

REV. ISAAC FERRIS, D.D., LL.D., Chancellor of the University.

VALENTINE MOTT, M.D., LL.D., Emeritus Professor of Surgery and Surgical Anatomy, and ex-President of the Faculty.

MARTYN PAINE, M.D., LL.D., Professor of Materia Medica and Therapeutics.

GUNNING S. BEDFORD, M.D., Professor of Obstetrics, the Diseases of Women and Children, and Clinical Midwifery.

JOHN W. DRAPER, M.D., LL.D., Professor of Chemistry and Physiology, President of the Faculty.

ALFRED C. POST, M.D., Professor of the Principles and Operations of Surgery, with Surgical and Pathological Anatomy.

WILLIAM H. VAN BUREN, M.D., Professor of General and Descriptive Anatomy.

JOHN T. METCALFE, M.D., Professor of the Institutes and Practice of Medicine.

J. W. S. GOULEY, M.D., Demonstrator of Anatomy.

J. H. HINTON, M.D., Prosector to the Professor of Surgery.

ALEXANDER B. MOTT, M.D., Prosector to the Emeritus Professor of Surgery.

Besides Daily Lectures on the foregoing subjects, there will be five Cliniques weekly, on *Medicine, Surgery, and Obstetrics.*

The Dissecting-room, which is refitted and abundantly lighted with gas, is open from 8 o'clock, A. M., till 10 o'clock, P. M.

Fees for a full course of Lectures, $105. Matriculation fee, $5. Graduation fee, $30. Demonstrator's fee, $5.

NEW YORK MEDICAL COLLEGE,
East 13th Street, near 4th Avenue.

The Tenth Annual Course of Lectures in this Institution will commence October 18th, 1859, and continue till the first week of March, 1860.

The Preliminary Course will begin September 19th, and continue till the opening of the Regular Course; during these four weeks *practical* instruction will be offered in important departments, to which the attention of students is particularly called.

FACULTY:

HORACE GREEN, M.D., LL.D., President of the Faculty, and Emeritus Professor of Theory and Practice of Medicine, and Professor of Diseases of the Respiratory Organs.

EDWIN HAMILTON DAVIS, M.D., Professor of Materia Medica and Therapeutics.

R. OGDEN DOREMUS, M.D., Professor of Chemistry and Toxicology.

J. M. CARNOCHAN, M.D., Professor of the Principles and Operations of Surgery, with Surgical Pathology.

EDMUND R. PEASLEE, M.D., Professor of Obstetrics and the Diseases of Women and Children.

HENRY G. COX, M.D., Professor of Theory and Practice of Medicine and of Clinical Medicine.

AUSTIN FLINT, JR., M.D., Professor of Physiology and Microscopic Anatomy.

JAMES BRYAN, M.D., Professor of Anatomy.

CARL T. MEYER, M.D., Professor of Surgical Anatomy and General Pathology.

JOHN SEDGWICK, Esq., Counsellor at Law, Lecturer on Medical Jurisprudence.

M. BRADLEY, M.D., Demonstrator of Anatomy.

B. L. BUDD, M.D., Assistant Lecturer on Chemistry.

S. CAREY SELDEN, M.D., and S. ABRAHAMS, M.D., Prosectors to the Professor of Surgery.

C. F. O. LANDIN, Janitor.

UNIVERSITY OF LOUISVILLE.
MEDICAL DEPARTMENT.
TWENTY-THIRD SESSION.

BOARD OF TRUSTEES:

Hon. JAMES GUTHRIE, President.
WM. S. VERNON, Esq., Secretary.

MEDICAL FACULTY:

The Medical Department of the University of Louisville will enter upon its twenty-third Session on the first Monday in November. Lectures preliminary to the regular course will be delivered at the University and Marine Hospital, free of charge, and will be commenced on the 1st of October. The Dissecting Room will also be opened at that time. The session will close, as heretofore, on the last of February. Extensive opportunities will be afforded for the study of Clinical Medicine and Surgery.

Lecture Fees, $105; Matriculation, $5.00; Graduation, $25.00; Hospital, free.

For further particulars, address

J. W. BENSON, M.D., Dean of the Faculty.

PENNSYLVANIA COLLEGE—MEDICAL DEPARTMENT.

Ninth Street, below Locust, Philadelphia.
SESSION OF 1859-60.

FACULTY:

The Session of 1859-60 will commence on Monday, 10th of October, and continue, without intermission, until the first of March. The Commencement for conferring Degrees will take place early in March, causing as little detention of the Graduating Class, after the close of the Lectures, as possible.

There will also be an examination of candidates for graduation on the 1st of July; the Degree, in such cases, being conferred at the ensuing Commencement in March.

The rooms for Practical Anatomy will be open early in September.

The College Clinic will be conducted on every Wednesday and Saturday throughout the Session.

The Register of Matriculants will be open in the College Building early in September. The Janitor will always be present at the College, to give every necessary assistance and information (as regards board, &c.) to students, on their arrival in the city.

FEES.—Matriculation, (paid once only,) $5.00; for each Professor's Ticket, $15.00; Graduation, $30.00.

LEWIS D. HARLOW, M.D., Dean,

No. 1023 Vine, below 11th Street.

UNIVERSITY OF BUFFALO.

Medical Department.—The Annual Course of Lectures in this Institution commences on the FIRST WEDNESDAY IN NOVEMBER, and continues sixteen weeks. The Dissecting-rooms will be opened on the first Wednesday in October.

Clinical Lectures at the Buffalo Hospital throughout the entire term, by Professors HAMILTON and ROCHESTER.

FACULTY.

JAMES P. WHITE, M.D., Professor of Obstetrics and Diseases of Women and Children.

FRANK H. HAMILTON, M.D., Professor of the Principles and Practice of Surgery and Clinical Surgery.

GEORGE HADLEY, M.D., Professor of Chemistry and Pharmacy.

THOMAS F. ROCHESTER, M.D., Professor of Principles and Practice of Medicine.

EDWARD M. MOORE, M.D., Professor of Surgical Anatomy and Surgical Pathology.

THEOPHILUS MACK, M.D., Lecturer on Materia Medica.

SANDFORD EASTMAN, M.D., Professor of Anatomy.

AUSTIN FLINT, JR., M.D., Professor of Physiology and Microscopy.

BENJ. H. LEMON, M.D., Demonstrator of Anatomy.

Fees—including Matriculation and Hospital Tickets, $75. Demonstrator's Ticket, $5. Graduation Fee, $20.

The Dean is authorised to issue a perpetual ticket, on payment of one hundred dollars.

Students who have attended a full course of Lectures in this or any other Institution, will be received on payment of $50. The fee from those who have attended two courses elsewhere is $25.

For further information or circulars, address

THOMAS F. ROCHESTER,

BUFFALO, 1859.   Dean of the Faculty.

THE ELLIOT PRIZE,
BELLEVUE HOSPITAL.

THE PRIZE OFFERED BY

DR. GEORGE T. ELLIOT

to the Matriculated Students for the Terms 1858-9 and 1859-60, in the College of Physicians and Surgeons, 23d Street, University College, 14th Street, and the New York Medical College, 13th Street, for the best

Preparation of the Fasciæ of the Female Pelvis,

to be placed in the MUSEUM of BELLEVUE HOSPITAL, will be awarded by the Professors of Surgery and Anatomy in the above Colleges, on

MONDAY, MARCH 5th, 1860.

TIMOTHY DALY,
Warden of Bellevue Hospital.

NEW YORK, *Sept.* 26, 1859.

DR. GEO. T. ELLIOT
HAS REMOVED TO
No. 19 West Twenty-ninth Street.

MEDICAL INSTRUCTION

AT

BELLEVUE HOSPITAL.

The Winter Course of Medical and Surgical Instruction, illustrated by Clinical Practice, will commence on Monday, the 17th of October, at 1½ P.M., precisely, at the new Anatomical Theatre of Bellevue Hospital, when the opening address will be delivered by John W. Francis, M.D., President of the Medical Board. Drs. Chandler L. Gilman and John T. Metcalfe will also address the students. The Medical Profession, Students of Medicine, and others interested, are invited to attend.

TIMOTHY DALY,

Warden of Bellevue Hospital.

NEW YORK, *Oct. 15th,* 1859.

THE WOOD PRIZES,

BELLEVUE HOSPITAL.

THE PRIZES OFFERED BY

DR. JAMES R. WOOD

to the Matriculated Students for the Terms 1858-9 and 1859-60, in the College of Physicians and Surgeons, 23d Street, University College, 14th Street, and the New York Medical College, 13th Street, for the best

ANATOMICAL OR SURGICAL OPERATION,

to be placed in the MUSEUM of BELLEVUE HOSPITAL, will be awarded by the Professors of Surgery and Anatomy in the above Colleges, on

MONDAY, MARCH 5th, 1860.

TIMOTHY DALY,

Warden of Bellevue Hospital.

NEW YORK, *Sept.* 26, 1859.

J. O. BRONSON, M.D.,

HAS REMOVED TO

No. 79 East Eighteenth Street,

Second Door from the Clarendon Hotel.

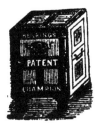

NEW YORK OPHTHALMIC SCHOOL.

THE DRUG STORES,

510 Grand Street and 32 Catharine Street.

EDWARD C. PASSMORE

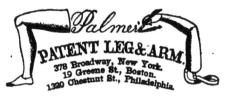

Palmer
PATENT LEG & ARM.
378 Broadway, New York.
19 Greene St., Boston.
1320 Chestnut St., Philadelphia.

"In the *mechanical compensation of lost parts, this admirable mechanism deserves particular notice,* combining lightness and A SUCCESSFUL IMITATION OF THE MOTIONS OF THE NATURAL LEG.' — *World's Fair, London,* 1851. Award, PRIZE MEDAL.

WM. LAWRENCE, ESQ., } London.
JOSEPH H. GREEN, ESQ., }
M. ROUX, } Paris.
M. LALLEMAND, }
Surgeons and Judges.

"By a peculiar arrangement of the joint, it is rendered little liable to wear, *and all lateral or rotary motion is prevented.* It is hardly necessary to remark, that *any such motion is undesirable in an artificial leg, as it renders its support unstable*"—*Committee on Science and Art, Franklin Institute, Philadelphia.* DR. RAND, Chairman.

Palmer's Artificial Arm

is a new, beautiful, light and useful substitute for a lost arm, imitating closely the natural hand and arm, and performing every office which an artificial appliance can.

MESSRS. PALMER & CO. have a new, light and useful appliance, made to imitate the natural limb, for elongating limbs shortened by diseased hip, &c., (Pott's disease,) instead of the cumbrous shoes and stirrups commonly used.

Pamphlets containing valuable information, reports, testimonials, references, etc., sent gratis to all who apply to

PALMER & CO., 378 Broadway, N. Y.

Since the last number of the " *Bane and Antidote* " was issued, we have received two American Patents—one for the Arm, the other for the Forearm or Hand. We have also been honored with several valuable letters from eminent surgeons and men of scientific attainments, and numerous flattering reports from ladies and gentlemen wearing these Patent limbs.

The reception these inventions have met is most encouraging, while their utility, as voluntarily set forth by the wearers, exceeds their fondest anticipations and *our own.*

We have already received several hundreds of applications, and persons desiring limbs should have their names registered at the studio immediately, if they would be supplied within six months. We deem it important to mention these facts, as applicants will be required to exercise a little patience till we can enlarge our means of supplying, so as to meet the requirements of such an unexampled demand.

The letters from persons wearing the arm and hand are very flattering; some of them being written in terms of praise so extravagant that we have to make some allowance for the fact that they were written in those first days of joy and gratitude, when the writers felt the liveliest appreciation of the benefits conferred upon them. We never ventured to hope for such utility in a false arm as these letters indicate. One gentleman, O—— V——, Esq., of Illinois, whose arm is applied below the elbow, informs us that, although his *left* hand is the artificial one, he has with it "written some letters" to his relatives (in New Hampshire,) "to show them what he can do," and states that he "would not part with it for the best farm in Illinois." Another, P—— B—— S——, Esq., (son of a distinguished Ex-Governor of Virginia,) whose arm was amputated *very near the body,* makes an equally gratifying report, though he cannot, of course, use the arm with the same facility. Several ladies have given similar pleasing accounts of their success in using the inventions.

The Patent Arm and Hand are therefore no longer *experiments,* but useful substitutes for the fairest mechanism of nature, giving, in every articulation and shape, as well as in delicacy of appearance, a very perfect imitation of the original member, both in form and motion.

Full particulars given by letter. Address,

B. FRANK. PALMER,

Surgeon-Artist, Inventor, &c.

Philadelphia.

DR. McMUNN'S ELIXIR OF OPIUM.

THIS IS THE PURE AND ESSENTIAL EXTRACT FROM THE NATIVE DRUG.

It contains all the valuable medicinal properties of Opium in natural combination, to the exclusion of all its noxious, deleterious, and useless principles, upon which its bad effects depend. It possesses all the sedative, anodyne, and antispasmodic powers of Opium.

To produce sleep and composure. To allay convulsions and spasmodic action.
To relieve pain and irritation, nervous excitement and morbid irritability of body and mind, &c.

And being purified from all the noxious and deleterious elements, its operation is attended by

No sickness of the stomach, no vomiting, no costiveness, no headache,
Nor any derangement of the constitution or general health.

Hence its high superiority over Laudanum, Paregoric, Black Drop, Denarcotized Laudanum, and every other opiate preparation.

In consequence of the exclusion of those deleterious principles from the Elixir of Opium, it is not liable to derange the functions of the system, and will be found invaluable for all cases in which the long-continued and liberal use of opiates is indicated and necessary to allay pain or spasmodic action, and induce sleep and composure, as in cases of fractures, burns, scalds, cancerous ulcers, and other painful affections.

The Elixir of Opium is greatly superior to Morphine,

1. In its containing all the active medicinal virtues of Opium in native combination, and in being its full representative; while Morphine, being only one of its principles, cannot alone, and that in an artificial state of combination, too, produce all the characteristic effects of so triumphant a remedy, when several of its other valuable principles are excluded.

2. In its effects, the Elixir is more characteristic, permanent, and uniform, than any of the *artificial compounds* of Morphine.

3. And as a *Preparation*, it is not liable to decompose or deteriorate like the *Solutions* of Morphine; and thus is obviated a serious objection, which has prevented the latter from being used with precision and effect.

To speak summarily, the Elixir of Opium, as a remedy, may be adopted in all cases in which either Opium or its preparations are administered, with the certainty of obtaining all their salutary and happy effects, without being followed by their distressing and pernicious consequences.

The following letter from Dr. Reese fully confirms the above, and commends itself to the attention of the profession and the public:

NEW YORK, *January 11*, 1859.

Messrs. A. B. & D. SANDS: *Gentlemen*—I have been familiar with the history of the "Elixir of Opium" from the time it was first introduced to the profession by Dr. McMunn, and have continued to prescribe the same in public and private practice since he disposed of his interest in it to you in 1841. Of its value, and the purity of the drug from which it is prepared, the best evidence is found in its wide-spread popularity and use among the profession in our own and other countries, and in all our civil and military hospitals, in which it has become a standard article. It is now prescribed by physicians and surgeons everywhere, when the positive medication of Opium is indicated, without the drawbacks in certain pathological conditions involving the nervous system, by idiosyncrasy or otherwise, which are inseparable from the ordinary spirituous or vinous Tinctures, or the salts of Morphia. Its extended use has led to the introduction of spurious imitations, against which you have done well to guard the profession and the public. The fact that the pharmaceutical journals have so frequently proposed and announced "substitutes" for McMunn's Elixir of Opium, and published so many formulæ for its officinal imitation, is the very highest attestation to the merits of the article as prepared by you. Knowing as I do its merits, I most cordially express my desire that its remedial virtues may be more extensively known. Yours, respectfully,

D. MEREDITH REESE, M.D., LL.D.,

Late Vice-President of the American Medical Association; Resident Member of the New York Academy of Medicine; Editor of the American Medical Gazette, &c.

☞ NOTICE.—A. B. & D. SANDS having purchased of Dr. McMunn all his right, title and interest in this article, and having been the sole Proprietors since 1841, and by whom it has been prepared during that period, respectfully inform dealers and consumers that no Elixir of Opium will hereafter be genuine, unless having their signature on the outside wrapper; and all orders from the "Trade" must be addressed, as heretofore, to A. B. & D. SANDS, Wholesale Druggists, 141 William Street, corner of Fulton, New York.

SOLD ALSO BY DRUGGISTS GENERALLY.

Lightning Source UK Ltd.
Milton Keynes UK
UKHW021514121118
332200UK00013B/845/P